The Therapeutics of Mineral Springs and Climates

Isaac Burney Yeo

THE THERAPEUTICS OF

MINERAL SPRINGS

AND

CLIMATES

THE THERAPEUTICS

OF

MINERAL SPRINGS AND CLIMATES

BY

I. BURNEY YEO, M.D., F.R.C.P.

Emeritus Professor of Medicine in King's College, London
Consulting Physician to King's College Hospital
Hon. Fellow of King's College; formerly
Professor of the Principles and Practice of Medicine
and of Clinical Therapeutics in King's College, and
Examiner in Medicine at the Royal College of Physicians

Author of "A Manual of Medical Treatment"
"Food in Health and Disease" etc. etc.

CASSELL AND COMPANY, LIMITED
LONDON, PARIS, NEW YORK
AND MELBOURNE. MCMIV

PREFACE.

THE author in his "Manual of Medical Treatment" has dealt *generally* with the subject of Clinical or Practical Therapeutics; in his work on "Food in Health and Disease" he has treated *specially* of the Therapeutics of Food; in the present volume he has taken for his subject "The Therapeutics of Mineral Springs and Climates." These three works therefore cover a large portion of the wide field of practical Therapeutics.

The use and selection of baths and climates in the treatment of Disease are topics which have long engaged the attention of the author; indeed, the present work is founded on an earlier treatise of his on "Climate and Health Resorts," which has been many years out of print. A long self-imposed winter holiday has afforded the author the leisure needed to revise, re-model, and, to a great extent, re-write the former work so as to render it more systematic, complete, and helpful as a guide to the selection, for invalids, of suitable resorts for climatic or mineral-water treatment.

This work is divided into two parts. The first is devoted to the study of mineral springs; and as the introductory chapters are concerned with certain general considerations, including the *classification* of mineral waters, it has been possible to adopt the obviously convenient plan of describing the vast number of mineral-water resorts in alphabetical order, and those resorts that have appeared, for various reasons, to be of minor importance to English invalids have been printed, in smaller type, at the end of each alphabetical group, and described as briefly as possible.

The second part is concerned with the subject of Climates. It has no pretension to be a systematic or exhaustive treatise on climatology. (The reader who desires to consult such a work must be referred to Professor Hann's "Handbook of Climatology," an

English translation of which, by Ward, has been published by Macmillan, New York, 1903.) But this part follows more closely the method adopted by the author in his former work, and its chief object is to serve as a practical guide to the characters and applicability of such climatic resorts as are fairly accessible to and likely to be visited by English invalids.

With regard to the mode of action of natural mineral waters, there is a manifest tendency in the present day to look upon this subject from a wider point of view than that which has hitherto been furnished by available chemical analyses. In a recent article in the *Lancet* (January 30th, 1904) it is pointed out, with truth, "that the effects of the salts in natural mineral waters are such as cannot be obtained from any artificial imitation of them," and it is aptly suggested that the "newly-discovered property of radio-activity which is in all probability possessed by all natural waters" may account for much that has hitherto seemed unaccountable, especially in the action of the so-called "indifferent" springs. Professor Oscar Liebreich has also expressed his belief "that minimal quantities of substances in mineral waters may be of importance," and speaks of the "fallacy of the old-fashioned notion that springs, the chief ingredients of which are the same, have the same therapeutic effect even though differing in some minor ingredients;" and he also refers to the fact that two mineral waters, otherwise identical, will be found to differ as regards electrical conductibility. More remarkable still is the conclusion, arrived at by experimental physiologists, that *absolutely pure* water—that is, water without traces of mineral substances—is poisonous!

But the time is not yet ripe for any positive, practical pronouncement on this subject. We must be content to wait until further scientific research, combined with wider experience, shall afford us more reliable data.

HERTFORD STREET, MAYFAIR
March, 1904.

CONTENTS.

Part I.

MINERAL SPRINGS.

SECTION A.

INTRODUCTORY.

CHAPTER I.

PAGE

THE NATURE, COMPOSITION, AND CLASSIFICATION OF MINERAL SPRINGS 1

CHAPTER II.

MODES OF APPLICATION AND ACTION OF MINERAL WATERS 22

CHAPTER III.

ACCESSORY MEASURES EMPLOYED IN CONNECTION WITH MINERAL-WATER CURES 43

SECTION B.

DESCRIPTION OF THE PRINCIPAL MINERAL SPRINGS (IN ALPHABETICAL ORDER) 52

SECTION C.

THE APPLICATION OF MINERAL WATERS AND BATHS TO THE ALLEVIATION AND CURE OF DISEASE . . 382

Part II.

CLIMATE AND CLIMATIC RESORTS.

CHAPTER I.

CLIMATE AND CLIMATES 457

CHAPTER II.

SEA OR MOUNTAIN? 478

CHAPTER III.

PAGE

SEASIDE RESORTS IN THE UNITED KINGDOM 492

CHAPTER IV.

CONTINENTAL SEASIDE RESORTS 538

CHAPTER V.

MOUNTAIN CLIMATIC RESORTS: ST. MORITZ AND THE ENGADINE—DAVOS PLATZ, AND THE MOUNTAIN-AIR CURE FOR CONSUMPTION 555

CHAPTER VI.

OTHER MOUNTAIN HEALTH RESORTS: FOR WINTER AND SUMMER CURES 581

CHAPTER VII.

WINTER QUARTERS: A REVIEW OF SOME WINTER HEALTH RESORTS 609

CHAPTER VIII.

THE WESTERN RIVIERA: A STUDY OF ITS CLIMATE AND A SURVEY OF ITS PRINCIPAL RESORTS 665

CHAPTER IX.

SEA VOYAGES, AND SOME DISTANT CLIMATIC RESORTS . 697

CHAPTER X.

THE APPLICATION AND SELECTION OF CLIMATES—TREATMENT IN AND LIST OF SANATORIA 715

INDEX TO PART I. 747

" " II. 755

Part I.

MINERAL SPRINGS.

SECTION A.

INTRODUCTORY.

CHAPTER I.

THE NATURE, COMPOSITION, AND CLASSIFICATION OF MINERAL SPRINGS.

DEALING first with the **nature** of mineral springs, we may point out that, strictly speaking, all waters found in nature are *mineral* waters, for as water is a universal solvent, even rain water, which is the purest natural water known, contains minute amounts of mineral substances and gases in solution, which it meets with in the atmosphere.

All springs are dependent on rain. A portion of the rain which falls on the surface of the earth sinks into the soil, and thus there exists, in a greater or less proportion, in different districts, masses or accumulations of subterranean water. *Springs* are the outflow of this subterranean water from openings, natural or artificial, made on the surface of the ground.

All springs, then, are more or less mineral springs, and contain mineral substances which the rain water has dissolved in its passage from the surface, through the porous or soluble substances it has encountered in its subterranean course.

Here and there the surface water finds its way down to great depths in the earth, into those intensely hot regions from which lava streams proceed, and we may conclude that hot (thermal) springs have a deeper origin in the earth than cold springs, and that the hotter the spring is, the greater is the depth from which it flows. It is also highly probable that at those great depths a part of the water may be decomposed by the intense heat, and forced to enter into chemical combination with parts of the melted rocks, etc., and thus many of the gaseous and solid substances found in mineral waters may originate.

It is obvious that the nature and amount of the mineral substances found in solution in natural springs will depend on the nature of the soil, or the structure and composition of the subterranean rocks through which the water of these springs has percolated.

In ordinary *spring* water the mineral substances most commonly found are salts of *lime*, chiefly the bicarbonate and sulphate, and, in smaller proportions, often some salts of soda and magnesia, and especially sodium chloride. In limestone districts the amount of lime salts in the "spring" water is occasionally considerable, imparting to the water what is known as "hardness." In some instances the amount of lime salts in such springs will reach to two parts in 1,000! Now, when one considers that the celebrated Pavillon spring at Contrexéville contains only 2·4 per 1,000 of mineral constituents, and that 2 of these consist of sulphate and bicarbonate of lime—the very same constituents which we find in our hard "spring" waters—it will be seen how difficult it sometimes is to define and distinguish a so-called "mineral" water from ordinary spring water by its chemical composition. This is even more strikingly manifest in connection with "mineral" springs of very feeble mineralisation, such, for example, as the Evian water, the total mineralisation of which is represented by 0·5 per 1,000, and this consists chiefly of carbonate of lime.

It has always been recognised that "thermality," the possession simply of a high temperature, brings a spring into the category of mineral waters, but the Evian waters are cold.

"Mineral" springs have been defined as those which contain a sufficient amount of mineral substances to make them *taste* of them, or to deposit them as they evaporate on objects around; but many popular mineral springs do neither.

For our present purpose we may define a mineral water, or as it is sometimes termed, a "medicinal" water, as a water which either from its chemical composition or its thermality, or some other quality which experience has proved it to possess, is found useful in the treatment of disease. We must remember that even the absence of mineral constituents, in the most feebly mineralised springs, may be of importance, in some instances, on account of the greater purity of the water and its increased solvent power.

Next, as to the **composition** of mineral springs. In the first place salts of lime are especially common, more particularly the carbonate and sulphate; there is scarcely a spring into the composition of which these compounds do not enter in greater or less proportion. Salts of sodium also are very common—common salt (sodium chloride) is a predominating ingredient in a vast number of mineral springs. Sodium sulphate and sodium carbonate are also frequently met with. Magnesium salts, especially the sulphate (Epsom salts), are also common.

Potassium salts are less frequently met with, but potassium sulphate is often found in combination with sodium and magnesium sulphates. Iron compounds, in small amounts, are very common ingredients in mineral springs, and in some they are present in sufficient quantity to give them distinctive therapeutic properties. The carbonates of iron are the most widely diffused ferruginous compounds, but the sulphates, the chloride, and the crenate are also found.

Silica in small amount occurs in many springs. In waters containing sodium chloride in notable amount other chlorides are often found associated with it, some only in small proportions, such as the chlorides of calcium, magnesium, potassium, lithium, ammonium, manganese, strontium and barium.

Iodine and bromine in small amount are sometimes found in the same class of waters, usually in combination with sodium, potassium, and magnesium.

Sulphur in "sulphur" waters usually occurs as sulphuretted hydrogen or some other binary compound, as sulphide of sodium or calcium.

Arsenic is an important element in a limited number of springs, and is most frequently found combined with sodium, calcium, magnesium, or iron.

Compounds of copper, cobalt, and nickel are occasionally found, and traces, but very rarely, of cæsium and rubidium.

Nitrates, phosphates and borates are occasionally, but not frequently, met with.

Bituminous substances are found in certain springs; in the Salso Maggiore springs there is a considerable amount of petroleum.

Organic substances conferring an unctuous property upon the water are found in many of the French springs, chiefly the thermal sulphur springs, as at Barèges in the Pyrenees, and hence such substances are termed *barégine*, but sometimes *glairine*.

Of the *gases* found in mineral waters, carbonic acid and sulphuretted hydrogen are of chief importance. Free oxygen and nitrogen are also of common occurrence, and the new element argon is often found in those waters that are rich in nitrogen; traces of helium have been found under the same circumstances.

Inflammable gases are occasionally found in some mineral springs, as at Salso Maggiore (*methane* and *ethane*) and a few other less well-known waters.

The *temperature* of mineral waters varies greatly, and a certain degree of thermality is usually a valuable quality in a mineral spring. Some springs issue from the earth at the temperature of boiling water—this is the case with the Great Geyser of Iceland; but there are springs in France which reach a temperature of 180° F. (Chaudes Aigues), and in Germany of 167° (Aix la Chapelle), and in this country of 120° (Bath). The Carlsbad Sprudel has a temperature of 162·5° F. Some very hot springs are found in Russia.

With regard to the **classification** of mineral waters, any attempt at a strictly scientific or precise classification of mineral springs is out of the question, owing to the complexity of their constitution and the great variety of their constituents, both qualitative and quantitative.

The well-known French spa Royat affords a striking example. By some authors it is classed amongst the "muriated alkaline waters," but this gives no indication of the fact that the water contains arsenic, iron and lithium. The French, in order to be more precise, class it under the long and awkward denomination of "*thermale alcaline, gaseuse, chlorurée-sodique, ferro-arsenical, et lithinée*"!

Some grouping, however, of those mineral springs which are related in composition, as well as in physiological or remedial action, is needful, and we shall adopt that mode of classifying them in this work which we consider the most simple and practically useful. But in any classification the grouping will be to a great extent artificial, and the several groups will be found to overlap and to be somewhat ill-defined. It is in the nature of the case that it should be so. Attempts have been made at much more elaborate classification and sub-division, but we think they will be found in practice only confusing and embarrassing.

There are two terms commonly used in the classification of mineral waters which we propose to discard, the one as obsolete and the other as misleading. The first of these is the term "muriated," applied to waters containing common salt or common salt with other chlorides. As this term is no longer used in chemistry or pharmacy, we do not think it should be retained in modern works dealing with the description or classification of mineral waters, and we propose to use the terms "common salt" or "chloride" or "mixed chlorides," as may seem most appropriate, in its place. The other term, "acidulous," is applied in Germany to all mineral waters containing much free carbonic acid gas—and many of these waters are highly alkaline; we therefore prefer to use the term "gaseous," which conveys no impression of acidity as the word acidulous certainly does.

The following is the classification, we believe, that will be found the most simple and convenient:—

1. **Simple or "indifferent" thermal** waters, the "acrato-thermal"* waters of the Germans. These are characterised by their high temperature, varying from about 80° to 150° F., by their very feeble mineralisation, and by their great softness. They are sometimes termed "*indifferent* springs," on account of the absence of any special mineralisation; and sometimes, as they are often found in wild, romantic, wooded districts, they have been termed "*wildbäder*," "wild-baths." They are rarely used internally, and if so employed they are simply intended to exert a solvent purifying influence.

As baths they are very largely employed, and some of the most frequented spas of Europe come into this group.

The following belong to this class:—

GREAT BRITAIN.

Bath.
Buxton.
Bakewell.
Mallow (co. Cork).
Matlock Bath.

* ἄκρατος (κεράννυμι), unmixed—a poor term.

FRANCE.

Aix en Provence.
Alet.
Avène.
Bagnères-de-Bigorre.
Bagnoles de l'Orne.
Bains les Bains.
Campagne sur Aude.
Chaudes Aigues.
Dax.
Evaux les Bains.
Luxeuil.
Néris.
Plombières.
Rennes les Bains.
Sail les Bains.
St. Amand.
St. Laurent les Bains.
Ussat.

GERMANY AND AUSTRIA.

Badenweiler.
Brennerbad.
Buda-Pest.
Gastein.
Johannisbad.
Krapina-Töplitz.
Landeck.
Liebenzell.[1]
Neuhaus.
Römerbad.
Schlangenbad.
Salzbach.
Teplitz.
Topelbad.
Veldes.
Villach.
Voeslau.
Warmbrunn.
Wiesenbad.
Wildbad.

ITALY.

Battaglia.
Bormio.
Ischia.
Monsumanno.
Pozzuoli.
Pré Saint-Didier.
Valdieri.
Vicarello.

SWITZERLAND.

Loeche les Bains.
Ragatz.

SPAIN AND PORTUGAL.

Caldas de Gerez.
Caldas de Oviedo.
Fitero.
Panticosa.
Sacedon.

BELGIUM.

Chaude-fontaine.

Owing to the difficulty in referring many of the foregoing to any particular group, some of the French authors describe these, as well as certain others, as "eaux indéterminées."

2. **Common salt** waters—the "muriated" waters of some authors—the "chlorurée-sodique" of French writers. The term "Salins" is often applied in France to the places in which these springs occur, as "Salins Moutiers," "Salins de Jura," etc.

This is a very large and somewhat artificial class. Owing to the great diffusion of common salt in nature, it is found in varying quantities in a vast number of mineral springs, many of which contain other and more important constituents.

This class includes hot springs like Wiesbaden and cold springs like Homburg. It comprises springs or wells varying in strength from 2 parts of common salt in 1,000 (Baden-Baden) to over 300 parts in 1,000 (Droitwich). The stronger waters are termed "brines," or "soolen," and they are used to prepare brine baths, or "soolbäder." Some of these springs are highly *gaseous* as well as hot (Nauheim), and are given as gaseous (effervescent) "thermal soolbäder."

In many of these springs other chlorides are present as well as sodium chloride, such as chlorides of magnesium, calcium, lithium, etc.; hence the term "muriated" has been applied to this class to indicate that its chief characteristic is the possession of chlorides, or muriates, as they used to be called. But instead of this term we propose, as we have said, to use the modern term "chlorides," and sometimes for greater precision "mixed chlorides."

We shall, therefore, term the springs of this class either "common salt" waters, or "sodium chloride" waters, or "chloride" or "mixed chloride" waters.

Some of the springs of this group contain bromides and iodides in small amount, and are therefore spoken of as bromo-iodide waters, as Woodhall Spa in this country, Bad-Hall in Upper Austria, Wildegg in Switzerland, Kreuznach in Germany, and La Mouillère (near Besançon) in France.

A notable amount of bicarbonate of iron is found

in some of these waters; this is the case with some of the springs at Homburg.

It also sometimes occurs that a so-called sulphur spring is rich in common salt, or that common salt springs are found in company with sulphur springs, as at Harrogate. It is usual in such cases to regard the sulphur as the characteristic constituent, and to classify them amongst sulphur spas.

It will be seen, in the following list of common salt springs and wells, that Germany is especially rich in such waters.

GREAT BRITAIN.

Ashby-de-la-Zouch.
Bridge of Allan.
Droitwich.
Llangammarch.
Nantwich.
Woodhall Spa.

FRANCE.

Balaruc (warm).
Bourbonne les Bains (hot).
Bourbon Lancy (hot).
Bourbon l'Archambault.
Br scous (at Biarritz).
Châtelguyon (warm, gaseous).
La Motte les Bains (hot).
La Mouillère (Besançon).
Lons le Saunier.
Roncas Blanc.
Salies de Béarn.
Salies du Salut.
Salins du Jura.
Salins Moutiers (warm).
Santenay.

GERMANY AND AUSTRIA.

Arnstadt.
Aussee.
Baden-Baden.
Berchtesgaden.
Cannstatt.
Csiz.
Dürkheim.
Durrheim.
Elmen.
Frankenhausen.
Hall (Tyrol).
Hall (Upper Austria).
Hall (Würtemberg).
Hallein.
Heilbrunn.
Homburg.
Inowrazlaw.
Ischl.
Ivonicz.
Jagstfeld.
Juliushall.
Kiedrich.
Kissingen.
Koesen.
Kolberg.
Kreuth.
Kreuznach.
Munster-am-Stein.
Nauheim (warm, gaseous).
Neu-Ragoczi.

GERMANY AND AUSTRIA (*continued*) :—

Niederbronn.
Oeynhausen, or Rehme-Oeynhausen (warm, gaseous).
Reichenhall.
Rosenheim.
Rothenfelde.
Salzburg.
Salzhausen.
Salzschlirf.
Salzuflen.
Salzungen.
Schmalkalden.
Soden (warm).
Sulza.
Thale.
Traunstein.
Wiesbaden.
Wittekind.

SWITZERLAND.

Bex.
Rheinfelden.
Schweizerhalle.
Wildegg.

LUXEMBURG.

Mondorf (warm).

ITALY.

Abano (hot).
Castro-caro.
Monte Catini (warm).
Salso Maggiore.

SPAIN.

Caldas de Montbuy (hot).
Caldas de Malavella (hot).
Cestona-Guesalaga (warm).

3. **Alkaline** waters.—This is perhaps the most natural of the groups of mineral waters, the characteristic constituent being *bicarbonate of sodium*, together, usually, with a considerable amount of free carbonic acid gas.

It is divided into three sub-classes, which also form fairly natural groups :

(*a*) *Simple alkaline waters*, in which sodium bicarbonate is altogether the predominating ingredient.

(*b*) *Alkaline and common salt* (chloride) waters, which contain an appreciable amount of sodium chloride as well as sodium bicarbonate.

(*c*) *Alkaline and sodium sulphate* waters (sometimes termed alkaline-saline waters), which contain besides sodium bicarbonate a notable amount of the aperient sodium sulphate.

Examples of this class of mineral waters are by no means so common as of the preceding. We do not know of a single example of either of these sub-classes in Great Britain.

Of the *simple alkaline* group, France possesses in Vichy and Vals the two most notable examples.

Ems, in Germany, is a well-known example of the second, or *alkaline and common salt* sub-division; and to this class belong most of the so-called German natural table waters, as Apollinaris, etc.

Examples of the third group, the *alkaline and sodium sulphate* waters, are found chiefly in Austria, and Carlsbad may be named as the type of this class.

(*a*) *Simple alkaline waters* ("*bicarbonatées sodiques*" of French waters).

FRANCE.

Le Boulou.
Marcols.
Montrond.
Vals.
Vichy (warm).

GERMANY AND AUSTRIA.

Bilin.
Birresborn.
Fachingen.
Fellathal-quellen.
Neuenahr (warm).
Obersalzbrunn.
Preblau.
Radein.

SWITZERLAND.

Passugg.

RUSSIA.

Borjom.

ITALY

San Marco.

PORTUGAL.

Vidago.

(*b*) *Alkaline and common salt springs.*

FRANCE.

Royat (warm).
St. Nectaire.
Vic-le-Comte.

GERMANY AND AUSTRIA.

Assmannshausen.
Ems.
Gleichenberg.
Lipik.
Luhatschowitz.
Offenbach.
Sanct Lorenz.
Szeawinca.
Toennisten.

ITALY.

Casamiccola.
Pozzuoli.

RUSSIA.

Essentuke.

(*c*) *Alkaline and sodium sulphate waters.* No examples of this sub-class are found either in Great Britain or France.

GERMANY AND AUSTRIA.

Bertrich.
Carlsbad (hot).
Elster.
Franzensbad.
Marienbad.
Rohitsch.

SWITZERLAND.

Tarasp.

4. The next class also is a rather small one; it consists of the waters known in Germany as **bitter** waters on account of the bitter taste given them by the magnesium sulphate (Epsom salts) they contain. They are also known as sulphated waters, as their chief constituents are the aperient sulphates of magnesium and sodium. They often contain, too, some aperient chlorides, and these are sometimes termed "muriated sulphated." The chief examples of these waters come from Austro-Hungary, but there are one or two representatives of the class in Great Britain and France. Some of the following are only used for export, and do not represent drinking spas:—

ENGLAND.

Cheltenham (chlorides also).
Leamington (chlorides also).
Melksham.
Purton Spa.

FRANCE.

Montmirail.
Brides (chlorides also).
St. Gervais (chlorides also).

GERMANY AND AUSTRIA.

Æsculap.
Apenta.
Franz-Josef.
Friedrichshall (chlorides also).
Grenzach (chlorides also).
Pullna (chlorides also).
Salzerbad (chlorides also).
Saidschitz.
Sedlitz.

SWITZERLAND.

Birminstorf.
Mulligen.

SPAIN.

Carabana.
Condal.
La Margarita.
Rubinat.
Villacabras.

5. The class of **iron** or **chalybeate** waters is a large one, as iron is very widely diffused in nature, and minute amounts of iron occur in nearly all mineral waters ; but the springs rightly admitted to this class should contain iron in such amount and in such combinations as render them therapeutically useful as blood restorers. In the most serviceable and popular of the chalybeate springs this iron exists as bicarbonate, and is kept in solution by an excess of free carbonic acid. The presence of an abundance of free carbonic acid greatly increases the value of an iron spring, as it renders the water more palatable and digestible.

Iron occurs in some springs, but not often, in the form of sulphate or chloride or crenate.

Many spas, classed amongst other groups, possess springs containing iron, which is often associated with aperient or other salts, as at Harrogate, Elster, Marienbad, Franzensbad, and elsewhere.

It would be useless to attempt an exhaustive enumeration of the immense number of springs which contain iron, in some form or other, and enjoy limited local reputation as chalybeate springs, but those of chief use and resort will be found amongst the following. England and France are remarkably poor in *typical* chalybeate springs.

ENGLAND.

Flitwick.
Shanklin.
Tunbridge Wells.

FRANCE.

Forges-les-Eaux.
La Malou (warm).
Orezza (in Corsica).
Renlaigne.

BELGIUM.

Spa.

GERMANY AND AUSTRIA.

Alexandersbad.
Antogast.
Augustusbad.
Bartfeld.
Berka.
Bocklet.
Borszek.
Bruckenau.
Cudowa.
Driburgbad.
Elopatak.
Elster (aperient sulphates also).
Freyersbach.
Frienwalde.
Flinsberg.
Godesberg.
Griesbach.
Imnau.
Koenigswart.
Kohlgrub.
Langenau.
Liebenstein
Liebwerda.
Petersthal.
Pyrmont.
Reinerz.
Rippoldsau.
Schandau
Schwalbach.
Steben.
Teinach, and many others.

ITALY.

Recoaro.
Santa Catarina.

SWITZERLAND.

Acqua Rossa.
Ander-Pignieu.
Farnbuhl.
Fideris.
Morgins.
San Bernardino.
St. Moritz.

Iron occurs in some springs, as we have seen, in the form of sulphate. These are not esteemed of the same value as the preceding, as they are more difficult of digestion. Those in Great Britain have only a restricted local reputation. Of these may be mentioned: Flitwick, in Bedfordshire; Sandrock, Isle of Wight; Gilsland Spa, Cumberland; Horley Green, Yorkshire; St. Anne's Well, Brighton; Dorton, Bucks; Lady Ida Well, Knockin, Salop. In Scotland there are Hartfell Spa, Moffat and Vicar's Bridge, near Dollar. In North Wales, Trefrew, in the Vale of Conway.

Sulphate of iron is also found in the springs of Katzes and Mitterbad in the Tyrol, Parad in Hungary, Alexisbad and Muskau (Hermannsbad) in Germany, and in a few others.

6. The next class—the **earthy** or **calcareous group**—is a somewhat artificial one, as the lime compounds they contain are found also, though in smaller amount, in most of the *simple thermal springs* as well as in those of other groups. Indeed, it is not always easy to determine whether a mineral spring shall be described in this or in the simple thermal group. If it is a hot spring and used chiefly for baths, it is likely to be included in the latter; if cold, and used mainly for drinking, then in the former.

The characteristic constituents of this group of natural waters are calcium carbonate and sulphate and magnesium carbonate. When sulphate of lime is the chief ingredient they are sometimes termed "gypsum" waters, and when carbonates of lime and magnesia are in notable excess, they are often described as "*alkaline* earthy springs."

When, as is not unfrequently the case in France, springs contain sodium bicarbonate as well as carbonate of lime and magnesia, it is usual to describe them as "*eaux bicarbonatées mixtes.*" France is particularly rich in these earthy or calcareous springs.

ENGLAND.

Bath (hot). Also in Class I.

FRANCE.

Audinac (warm).
Aulus.
Bagnères-de-Bigorre (warm).
Capvern.
Cransac.
Contrexéville.
Martigny les Bains.
Pougues les Eaux.
Siradan.
Vittel, and others.

ALGIERS.

Hammam-R'Irha (hot).

GERMANY AND AUSTRIA.

Auerbach.
Grau.
Inselbad.
Krynica.
Lippspringe.
Szkleno.
Wildungen

ITALY.

Chianciano (warm).
Lucca (hot).

SWITZERLAND.

Bergun.
Faulen-see Bad.
Loeche les Bains.
Peiden.
Saxon.
Weissenberg.
Vals (Grisons).

7. The class of **sulphur** waters is a very large and artificial one. It comprises waters differing very greatly from one another in chemical constitution and in physiological action. It includes springs like Aix les Bains, which are extremely feebly mineralised, containing only 0·49 of solids per 1,000, and having close affinities with the "simple thermal" group, its mineral constituents consisting chiefly of carbonate and sulphate of lime—and springs like the "old sulphur spring" at Harrogate, which contains, besides other constituents, 12·7 per 1,000 of sodium chloride. The only common character which serves to bring these springs into the same group is that they contain either sulphuretted hydrogen, or some other binary compound of sulphur, such as sodium or calcium sulphide, and possess the characteristic odour of sulphuretted hydrogen.

Many of the sulphur waters, like those of Harrogate, contain varying proportions of sodium chloride, and to some of these springs, such as Uriage, the French authorities apply the term "*chlorurées sodiques sulfureuses.*"

There are a vast number of *warm* sulphur springs in France, especially in the Pyrenees, their characteristic constituent being, for the most part, sodium sulphide. These waters are very prone to *degenerate,* as the French say, on exposure to the air. The sodium tends to combine with the carbonic acid in the water and the air and form sodium carbonate, and part of the sulphur thus set free is precipitated and gives a milky or flocculent aspect to the water, while another part of the sulphur combines with hydrogen from the water and escapes in the form of sulphuretted hydrogen. Some of the sodium sulphide also becomes oxidised into hyposulphite, sulphite, and finally sulphate of sodium, so that after a little time the water contains only sodium carbonate and sulphate in solution, and becomes distinctly alkaline. Such waters are then said to have *degenerated.*

It is especially in the French warm sulphur springs that those low forms of vegetable life occur which give rise to the substances we have already referred to under the names of *glairine* or *barégine.*

There are no *warm* sulphur springs in England.

GREAT BRITAIN AND IRELAND.

Askern Spa.
Ballynahinch.
Builth.
Harrogate.
Lisdoonvarna.
Llandrindod Wells.
Lucan.
Llanwrtyd Wells.
Moffat.
Strathpeffer.

FRANCE.

Aix les Bains (warm).
Allevard.
Amélie les Bains (hot).
Argelès-Gazost (warm).
Ax les Thermes (hot).
Bagnols (warm).
Barbotan (warm).
Barèges (hot).
Barzun (warm).
Cadéac.

FRANCE (*continued*) :—

Cambo (warm).
Cauterets (warm).
Challes.
Digue (warm).
Eaux Bonnes (warm).
Eaux Chaudes (warm).
Enghien.
Euzet.
Gréoulx (warm).
Guagno (warm), Corsica.
Labassère (warm).
La Preste (warm).
Luchon (warm).
Molitg (warm).
Olette (hot).
Pierrefonds.
Pietrapola (Corsica).
Prechacq les Bains (hot).
Puzzichello (Corsica).
St. Boes.
St. Honoré les Bains (warm).
St. Sauveur (warm).
Uriage (warm).
Vernet les Bains (hot). And many others.

GERMANY AND AUSTRIA.

Abbach.
Aix la Chapelle (hot).
Altenberg.
Baden, near Vienna (warm).
Bad Boll.
Bentheim.
Buda-Pest (warm).
Eilsen.
Hercules-Bad (warm).
Innichen.
Kainzenbad.
Ladis.
Langenbrucken.
Langenfeld.
Langensalza.
Meinberg.
Nenndorf.
Parad.
Pystjau (warm).
Reutlingen.
Warasdin-Teplitz (warm).
Weilbach.
Wipfield. And others.

SWITZERLAND.

Alveneu.
Baden.
Gurnigel.
Heustrich.
Lavey.
Lenk
Lostorf.
Le Prese.
Schimberg.
Schinznach.
Sernens.
Stachelberg.
Yverdun. And others.

ITALY.

Acireale.
Acqui (hot).
Cività Vecchia.
Porreta (warm).
Sciacca (hot), Sicily
Tabiano.
Vinadio (hot).
Viterbo (warm).

SPAIN.

Caratraca.
Ledesma.
Montemayor.
Panticosa
Santa Agueda.
Trillo. And many others.

PORTUGAL.

Caldas de Rainha (warm).
Caldas de Vizella.
San Pedro do Sul (hot).

RUSSIA.

Bousk.
Bragoun.
Piatigorsk (hot).

GREECE.

Thermopylæ (hot).

NORWAY.

Laurvik.
Sandefjord.

BOSNIA.

Illidze.

EGYPT.

Helouan.

The following subdivision of sulphur waters is sometimes adopted :—

(*a*) Those in which *sodium sulphide* is the binary sulphur compound present, giving to the springs their special character. This condition prevails in most of the sulphur baths of the Pyrenees, as Barèges, Cauterets, Luchon, etc.

(*b*) *Sulphuretted hydrogen* springs, in which H_2S is the characteristic constituent, as represented by Aix les Bains, Schinznach, Strathpeffer, etc.

(*c*) *Sulphur and sodium chloride* waters, which contain a certain amount of sodium chloride as well as H_2S. Such springs are found at Aix la Chapelle, Harrogate, Uriage, and elsewhere.

8. There is a small group of mineral waters which are termed **arsenical**, as they contain arsenic, generally in small, but in varying proportions. The arsenic usually occurs in alkaline waters, commonly in the form of sodium arsenate, as in La Bourboule ; sometimes in association with iron, as in Levico and Roncegno water. In some springs arsenic occurs in quantities so minute as to be practically of no

importance, but certain of these are, notwithstanding, occasionally termed "arsenical."

In the following list the arsenical waters are arranged as nearly as can be in the order of their strength :—

(*a*) Containing *arsenious acid* :—

Roncegno, Austria ..	0·1150 grammes per litre arsenious acid + (0·1090 *sodium arsenate*).
Levico, Austria ...	0·0086 grammes per litre „ „
Srebernik, Bosnia ...	0·0060 „ „ „ „
Linda Pausa, Germany	0·0030 „ „ „ „

(*b*) Containing *arsenates* :—

La Bourboule, France	0·0282 grammes per litre sod. arsenate.
Sylvanés	0·0160 „ „ arsenate of iron and magnesia.
Court St Etienne, Belgium	0·0097 „ „ sodium arsenate.
Vic sur Cère, France	0·0080 „ „ „ „
Civilina, Italy ...	0·0080 „ „ arsenate of iron.
Ceresole Reale, Italy	0·0057 „ „ sodium arsenate.
Royat (St. Victor) ...	0·0045 „ „ „ „
Vals (Dominique), France	0·0030 „ „ „ „
Cudowa, Germany...	0·0025 „ „ arsenate of iron.
Val Sinistra, Switzerland	0·0019 „ „ sodium arsenate.
Bussang, France ...	0·0012 „ „ arsenate of iron.
Mt. Dore, France ...	0·0010 „ „ sodium arsenate.

Traces of arsenic are found in many others.

There is another small group of waters containing *iodides* and *bromides*, most of which will be found enumerated under the *common salt* class. It may be convenient to mention them here.

Woodhall Spa in England.

Challes, La Mouillère, Salies de Béarn, Salins du Jura, in France.

Heilbrunn, Krankenheit-Tolz, Kreuznach, Salzbrunn, Salzschlirf, in Germany.

Hall, in Upper Austria.

Lipik, in Hungary.
Ivonitch, in Galicia.
Castro-caro, Salso Maggiore, in Italy.
Wildegg, in Switzerland.

Having, in the foregoing groups or classes, enumerated most of the mineral water resorts treated of in this work, we shall be enabled, for purposes of description and reference, to adopt in Section B, which begins on page 52, the system of *alphabetical* arrangement, which has a great and obvious advantage.

CHAPTER II.

MODES OF APPLICATION AND ACTION OF MINERAL WATERS.

Modes of Application: Bathing Cures—Douches—Gas and Vapour Baths—Inhalations—Drinking Cures—Action of the Different Classes of Mineral Waters Externally and Internally.

BEFORE proceeding to the description of individual springs, it will be desirable to consider the modes of application and action of mineral waters in a general sense. And first as to the modes of **application.**

Although, in the great majority of instances, the waters of a spa are applied both externally and internally, in a certain number the *external* method and in a few others the *internal* method is especially relied upon. Indeed, in most cases, one or other method predominates.

For example, at Salso Maggiore there is no *drinking* of the waters, whereas at Eaux Bonnes and at La Bourboule there is very little bathing, these being essentially drinking cures. At Gastein, at Aix les Bains, at Nauheim, the treatment relied upon is almost wholly *external;* at Neuenahr, at Contrexéville, at Cauterets, it is almost wholly *internal,* baths being only regarded as accessory measures. It is true, however, that where the patients are made to inhale the dense vapour and finely divided spray of the water, in special apartments devised for the purpose, some of the constituents of the water may be absorbed *internally* through the respiratory mucous membrane, and this, at such spas, is claimed to be so.

In the preparation of baths, if the spring is naturally of too high a temperature, its temperature is reduced to a suitable degree either by the addition of ordinary water, or water from a cooler spring, or by allowing the water to remain in the bath until it has cooled sufficiently; and if the spring is naturally cool or cold, its temperature is raised to the needful point either by the addition of ordinary hot water or by heating the water of the mineral spring by means of special contrivances.

In the case of cold springs rich in free carbonic acid gas, when it is important to retain as much of the gas as possible in the water of the bath, the heating of the water is usually effected either by what is known as the Schwarz method, in which hot steam is introduced between the double bottom of the metal bath, as at Schwalbach, or by Pfriem's method, in which steam under high pressure is directly introduced into the water of the bath; or a third method may be used, which consists in passing the hot steam through pipes situated in the angle between the floor and the sides of the bath.

Baths are also given either in the form of full baths, or half baths, or local baths, *i.e.* limited to one limb or a definite part of the surface of the body.

Full baths are given either in what the French term a *baignoire, i.e.* a bath adapted to the form of the body like the ordinary domestic bath, or in a *piscine, i.e.* a well-shaped bath, usually lined with tiles, into which one descends by steps, and in which the patient can either stand or sit or move about. Such baths may be large enough to receive several persons at the same time, and when very large may be used as *swimming* baths.

As we shall see in the next chapter, mineral water baths may be modified or fortified by the addition of various substances either of the same nature, as the concentrated *Mutter-lauge*, or salts extracted from the spring itself; or by adding quite different substances to the water, as mud, or *Moor*, or pine extracts.

Mineral waters are also applied externally in various forms of *douches* of varying temperature and pressure. There are *jet*, *fan*, and *spray* douches; *vertical*, *horizontal*, and *ascending* douches, a modification of the ascending douche may be used for internal "irrigations." What is known as the "Scotch douche" (*douche écossaise*) is one by means of which hot and cold streams are applied *alternately* to the same part of the body. What is termed by the French a *submarine* douche is a douche applied beneath the surface of the bath, and which may be either hotter or colder than the water of the bath.

Gas baths and douches are also given in some spas, the gas, usually carbonic acid, being obtained from the springs.

In many spas, where diseases of the respiratory organs are treated, the mineral water is administered by *inhalation*, as well as by drinking, and various forms of apparatus are employed to reduce the water to a fine spray or dust (*poussière*), which is inhaled, mixed often with the vapour of the water, or with such gases as it may contain.

The hot vapours given off by some of the springs of naturally high temperature are, by means of convenient appliances, sometimes inhaled as they come directly from the source, and such vapour is also in other instances used for the preparation of hot vapour baths and douches, general or local.

As we have already said, in most but not in all spas, a certain amount of the water of the mineral spring is taken daily internally, and the treatment is therefore both *internal* and *external*.

We shall, in the next place, consider in a *general* sense, the **action** of mineral waters, first, when applied externally, and secondly, when taken internally.

As to their **external action**, the idea which formerly prevailed that a portion of the substances, dissolved in the mineral water of the bath, was absorbed by the skin into the blood, has been negatived by repeated experimental observations. It is therefore incorrect to suppose that the action of mineral water baths can be, in any way, dependent on absorption of their constituents through the skin, for it has been proved that the sound and healthy human skin is not permeable to water, or the fixed substances dissolved in it, even after prolonged immersion. It must, however, be borne in mind that volatile or gaseous constituents of mineral baths may be absorbed through the respiratory organs, and indeed it seems probable, from experimental observation that the skin itself is permeable to certain volatile and gaseous constituents of baths, as for example carbonic acid gas and sulphuretted hydrogen.

It has been asserted by some that the skin has been found permeable to water and watery solutions in *fine spray* at an elevated temperature, and it has been suggested that the force with which the spray has been thrown upon the skin has influenced the absorption.

Doubtless absorption in the bath may be promoted by removing from the skin the fatty layer derived from the secretion of the hair follicles and sweat glands, together with the superficial epidermal scales which hinder absorption, and this may be done by friction with soap and water; and much the same result would probably follow friction of the skin in a hot bath consisting of an *alkaline* mineral water. A high temperature of the bath by causing dilation and fulness of the cutaneous capillaries would also favour absorption. But it must be repeated that in an ordinary mineral water bath no absorption of the water, or the fixed substances dissolved in it, takes place through the healthy and unbroken skin.

The action of a hot mineral water bath, especially of the "simple thermal" class, must be much the same as, if not altogether identical with, that of a bath of ordinary water of the same temperature. It tends to cause dilation of the capillaries of the skin, and so promotes the circulation of blood in the cutaneous vessels, and may thus indirectly contribute to relieve congestion of deep-seated organs. It macerates the epidermis, and promotes the shedding of its superficial scales, while it stimulates the excretion of the cutaneous glands, and causes diaphoresis in proportion to the temperature of the bath, or of the atmosphere into which the patient passes after the bath. It is therefore a powerful agent of cutaneous elimination.

If the water of the bath is tepid only, it has a soothing effect on the endings of the peripheral nerves, and tends to equalise the distribution of blood.

But when the mineral water of the bath contains constituents capable of exercising *chemical* stimulation or irritation of the skin, then we have additional effects to consider besides those dependent on its thermality, and we must, in the next place, pass on to the consideration of the action of the different classes of baths.

1. The "**indifferent**" **thermal** springs act like ordinary warm baths, their effects being mainly due to their temperature; but it is quite possible that the small amount of solids they contain, especially when these render the water faintly alkaline, exercise some influence; and some influence may also be attributed to the maintenance of a *constant* temperature during the bath, which is provided for in suitably arranged baths. As to the suggestion so often put forward that some of these springs exert a specific electrical effect, this view has never been established, and is not accepted by the most competent authorities. The contributory influence of climate and altitude must, however, never be overlooked in estimating the suitableness of such baths.

The baths of this class may be divided into two sub-groups, according to their temperature—

(*a*) Those of "indifferent" temperature, *i.e.* below the body temperature of 98·6° F., and (*b*) those which tend to raise the body temperature, and are therefore above 98·6° F.

(*a*) Baths belonging to the first group (Buxton,

Ragatz, Schlangenbad) do not disturb the body temperature, they therefore stimulate mildly the cutaneous nerves, and tend, reflexly, to soothe the central nervous system. They exert a limited and mildly stimulating action on metabolism. Such baths, if long protracted, serve also to macerate the epidermis in certain chronic skin affections (psoriasis, eczema), and by soothing the nerve endings, improve the capillary circulation. They also prove of use in slow convalescence from acute disease, in the debility attending some chronic constitutional affections, in premature senility, and in irritable neurotic or hysterical conditions associated with neuralgia, dysmenorrhœa, insomnia, etc. In this respect their action is analogous to that of ordinary hydrotherapeutic treatment. They are often also prescribed in certain forms of chronic spinal disease, as in the early stage of tabes and in cases of pseudotabes, as well as in cases of peripheral neuritis.

(*b*) The second group of hotter springs (Gastein, Teplitz, Bath) tend to raise the temperature of the body, quicken the circulation in the skin, increase cutaneous excretion, and produce a stimulating effect on the circulatory and nervous systems. In this way they promote the absorption of chronic exudations, either of rheumatic and gouty or traumatic and inflammatory origin. They are often employed to relieve chronic joint affections in connection with gout, rheumatism and rheumatoid arthritis, chronic peritoneal exudations, and chronic uterine and peri-uterine and other pelvic inflammations. They are constantly used in the treatment of sciatica and other forms of neuralgia, and in these and other cases their action is usually reinforced by certain accessory measures such as local hot douches, friction, and massage; the warmth of bed after the bath is also beneficial when it is desired to maintain and promote its diaphoretic action. The temperature of the water should be kept constant during the continuance of the bath, and it is usually thought undesirable that the water of the bath should reach much higher than the waist; indeed, some bath physicians think it advisable to apply cold compresses to the head and precordium during the bath.

Therapeutically allied to this class are the natural hot vapour baths, such as are found at Lucca, Monsumano, and Battaglia, in Italy.

2. We must, in the next place, consider the action of **common salt** or **brine** baths, the second of our groups of mineral springs. These *brine* baths (Germ. *Soolbäder*) are prepared from mineral waters containing sodium chloride, usually associated with other chlorides in smaller quantity. Some of these springs are hot, and those that are cold are heated artificially. A few are gaseous, being charged with free carbonic acid. Salt springs vary much in strength. A brine or salt bath should contain at least 1·5 per cent. of saline constituents. If it does not contain more than 2 per cent. it is a *weak* brine bath; if it contains from 3 to 6 per cent. it is a moderately strong one. Springs stronger than this require dilution before using as baths. From the stronger springs of this class *brine salts* are extracted, and also what is known as "*mother lye,*" or *Mutter-lauge* (Germ.), or *eaux mères* (French), or *aqua madre* (Ital.). These can be used for fortifying the weaker salt baths. *Mother lye* is obtained by concentration of the salt water by boiling and evaporation. Much of the sodium chloride crystallises out, and is used in commerce; and the residue contains, besides sodium chloride, the other more soluble salts in higher proportions. These are usually calcium and magnesium chlorides, together with whatever iodides or bromides may be contained in the spring. Brine salts are obtained by further concentration of the *mother lye.* Strong brines are also sometimes prepared by graduation, containing from 16 to 20 per cent. of salts.

The action of these salt baths depends in part upon their temperature, but mainly on the *chemical irritation* or *stimulating* action of the dissolved salts on the skin and the peripheral cutaneous nerves. The salt of the water soaks through the epidermal layers, and acts as a chemical stimulant to the nerve endings in the skin. The cutaneous sensibility and blood pressure are usually raised, and the production of carbonic acid is said to be increased. Differences of opinion exist, amongst observers, as to whether these baths do or do not increase nitrogenous metabolism.

In certain hypersensitive persons the stronger salt baths may cause urticarial or eczematous eruptions; they should then be diluted or interrupted. Similar eruptions sometimes occur after sea baths; indeed, warm sea baths are closely related in their action to the class of baths we are considering. Their therapeutic action has been found favourable to the removal of chronic exudations, of scrofulous glandular enlargements and chronic inflammatory thickenings and indurations. They are useful in rickets and other maladies associated with lymphatism and tuberculosis in children. They are found beneficial in chronic inflammatory disorders of the female pelvic organs. They are used for the removal of gouty and rheumatic exudations about joints and elsewhere, and in some forms of neuralgia and paralysis of rheumatic origin. They are considered to have a strengthening effect on the skin, and to render it less sensitive to chill. The strength of the bath must be graduated to the individual; delicate, sensitive persons require the weaker ones, and lymphatic scrofulous patients often need those of greater strength.

The *gaseous thermal salt baths*, which do not need artificial heating, are especially valuable when our object is to rouse the nervous force as well as improve the general nutrition; they are therefore frequently prescribed in neurotic cases, in some cases of paralysis, in spinal irritation, in tabes, and recently they have been largely recommended in the treatment of cardiac affections. The presence of free carbonic acid in these baths enables them to be borne of a lower temperature than other brine baths owing to the stimulating effect of this gas on the skin. The inhalation of the spray of these waters, produced by suitable mechanical contrivances, is found of much value in chronic catarrhal conditions of the air passages.

3. The waters of the next group, the **alkaline** waters, are almost exclusively relied upon for their *internal* use, and when employed for baths it is only as an accessory measure. As baths they exert a more cleansing action on the skin than ordinary warm water, and the free carbonic acid gas which is present in many of them produces no doubt a mildly stimulating effect on the skin. Like other warm baths they exert a soothing effect on the nervous system. Those of the alkaline chloride group (Ems) are often used in catarrhal conditions of the female pelvic organs. The same may be said of the alkaline sodium sulphate group, and these latter are also prescribed and thought useful in the treatment of obesity.

4. The class of "**bitter**" waters have no special action as baths. They are, however, often prescribed as auxiliary to the drinking cure.

5. In estimating the action of **iron** or **chalybeate** baths, the idea that any absorption of iron takes place by the skin must be set aside.

The action of the iron waters that are especially used as baths, as well as for drinking, is mainly due to the free carbonic acid contained in them and which exerts a stimulating or irritating effect on the skin as its bubbles accumulate upon and are discharged from the surface of the body. Owing to the effect of the free carbonic acid on the skin these baths can be given of a lower temperature (77° to 90° F.) than would otherwise be practicable; they are then believed to promote metabolism and to be made capable of remedial application in debilitated and anæmic conditions. A reflex action extending from the periphery to the central nervous system renders these baths valuable in irritable neurasthenic states. They are found to increase the appetite and promote nitrogenous assimilation, as less urea is eliminated; they therefore favour the "nutritive retention of organic matters in form of albumen" (Kisch).

They are prescribed with advantage in cases of debility, associated with anæmia and chlorosis, in neurasthenic states, and in the disorders of menstruation connected with anæmia. Care is taken, as we have already pointed out, in heating these baths, to adopt methods which shall prevent the loss of carbonic acid, and for the same reason the bather is recommended to remain still in the bath, so that this gas may have a better effect on the skin.

In the few chalybeate baths in which the iron occurs in the form of sulphate, the astringent properties of these waters may be utilised in the treatment of vaginal leucorrhœa, and in strengthening and bracing up the skin in persons with a tendency to excessive perspiration. In these instances where weak iron waters, containing no free carbonic acid, are administered as baths, the effect can only be the same as that of the indifferent thermal baths.

6. The class of **earthy** or **calcareous** springs exercise no specific effect when used as baths. The action of most of the springs of this class when administered as baths is identical with that of the *indifferent thermal* springs, to which class, indeed, some of these spas might be referred. They are employed in the same class of cases.

In those instances in which they are prescribed as very protracted baths (Leukerbad) for the cure of chronic skin diseases, such as psoriasis and eczema, they must act simply by imbibition and maceration of the epidermal scales and cleansing of the skin. They may also exercise a sedative effect on the irritated cutaneous nerves.

7. Next, as to the action of the large class of

sulphur baths, in which we must include those springs which contain a certain amount of sodium chloride, as well as sulphur compounds.

There seems some difference of opinion amongst authorities as to the precise action of sulphur baths, and it is certain that this action must differ considerably according to their strength, their composition, their thermality, and the manner in which they are applied.

The action of the very weak sulphur waters probably scarcely differs at all from that of the simple thermal springs; but when they contain much sulphuretted hydrogen and are applied at a high temperature, they exercise a powerful stimulating or even irritating effect on the skin, causing cutaneous hyperæmia, increased transpiration, and desquamation of the epidermis; they therefore excite and increase the function of the skin and promote absorption. If the patient is kept in a warm bed after the bath, marked diaphoresis often occurs, with diminished diuresis, and a considerable amount of urea has been found in the perspiration.

Those sulphur baths that are alkaline also cleanse the skin of fatty and pigmentary substances, and inspissated excretions adhering to it. This would favour absorption from the bath—if it were possible.

The *germicidal* action of some of the sulphur waters is likely to be of importance in certain cases—especially in parasitic skin affections—and may account for the ancient reputation which many of them possess for promoting the healing of wounds received in battle. It is more especially in connection with these baths (but not exclusively) that what is termed "a crisis" occurs after a week or so of treatment. This is simply a form of artificial dermatitis, induced by the action of the hot sulphur water on the skin.

At one time sulphur baths were believed to be useful in the diagnosis of latent constitutional syphilis, and of specific value in its treatment; they are now no longer credited either with the power of making latent syphilis apparent or with exerting any specific influence over the disease. We shall have to return to this subject in a later section (Section C).

In the treatment of gout by sulphur baths and the internal use of sulphur waters, the elimination of uric acid has been stated to be markedly increased.

Besides gout and constitutional syphilis, sulphur baths are recommended in the treatment of chronic rheumatic affections, rheumatoid arthritis, chronic metallic poisonings, some scrofulous disorders, the sequelæ of traumatic lesions, and in some chronic affections of the nervous system, as tabes and certain motor and sensory neuroses.

Very vigorous and various methods of treatment are carried out in connection with sulphur baths; they are often applied at a high temperature up to 107° F. They are used in all forms of douches. The natural vapours and gases given off by the thermal springs are collected or allowed to pass into suitable cabinets for the purpose of giving vapour or gas baths, and the vapours as well as the fine spray to which the water is reduced by mechanism devised for this end, are used for *inhalations*.

We must now, in the second place, pass on to consider the action of these mineral springs when taken **internally**. It must, however, always be kept in mind that the remedial or beneficial action of mineral waters is largely dependent on the associated conditions, such as alterations in diet, climate, exercise, social surroundings, etc. These are by no means unimportant factors in the results obtained in the treatment of chronic diseases. They are probably more worthy of consideration in many instances than small differences in the chemical composition of the mineral springs. There can be no doubt that many mineral waters, whose curative effects are in themselves wholly insignificant, have been raised into importance by the intelligent and skilful accessory methods attending their use. Even in mineral waters containing active and energetic constituents, much of this efficacy depends on the watchful regularity and continuity of their application, and the absolute and faithful devotion of the patient, for the time being, to the system of cure. Apparently inert and very feebly mineralised springs, when thus systematically and regularly applied, may be attended with unexpectedly good results.

In all *drinking* cures we must not overlook the value and curative action of the amount of *water* itself which is consumed.

To persons unaccustomed to the use of pure water as an ordinary beverage, the daily drinking of a large quantity of this highly important solvent, apart from the mineral substances it holds in solution, must have most influential physiological and therapeutic effects. It must, for one thing, stimulate healthy metabolism by assisting in the removal of waste products accumulated in the organism, and by flushing and cleansing the excretory channels. In this way the blood itself must be washed and cleansed. Considerations such as these enable us to explain the good results obtained from drinking these mineral springs, which contain less mineral constituents than ordinary spring water, their solvent action being on that account greater than that of more strongly mineralised springs.

There is, then, one consideration common to all drinking cures, and that is the *quantity of water* that is consumed.

It has been stated, in connection with the effect of "indifferent" springs, that "sipping" has a remarkable effect in abolishing the inhibitory action of the vagus, and so quickening the heart beat. This statement has been too hastily and unquestioningly received. We have ourselves made repeated test observations with wholly negative results, except in highly nervous subjects prone to the influence of *suggestion*.

1. The **"indifferent" thermal** springs are mainly

prescribed, as we have seen, for baths and bathing cures; they are sometimes ordered also for drinking, in cases needing only mild treatment. Their effect is mainly that of the ingestion of a certain amount of warm water; they help to remove waste products, they flush the excretory organs, they tend to keep the intestinal contents more fluid, and so assist in remedying constipation. They are sometimes found to exert a soothing action on the gastro-intestinal mucous membrane, and to relieve certain forms of gastralgia and enteralgia. They are also found useful in some forms of atonic gout and rheumatism.

2. Of the **sodium chloride** waters, only the weaker ones, or those of medium strength, are employed undiluted internally. The stronger ones are too irritating to the gastric mucous membrane. The presence of a considerable amount of free carbonic acid in many of them favours their internal use, makes them more pleasant to take, and augments their stimulating effect on stomach digestion. Some of these springs (*e.g.* Homburg) contain a fair amount of iron, which commends their use in the anæmic.

These waters, taken fasting, increase gastric tone and function, and increase the renal secretion, and the stronger and rather more concentrated ones (Kissingen) augment intestinal secretion and act as aperients. They improve nutrition, and do not, like other aperient waters, cause emaciation. They should therefore be preferred for emaciated dyspeptics. They are used in forms of atonic dyspepsia and chronic gastro-duodenal and intestinal catarrh, in abdominal stasis and hæmorrhoids, in chronic catarrhal affections of the respiratory organs (in these it is often advisable to add a little hot milk or whey to cold springs), in scrofula and rachitis (especially those springs containing iodine and bromine), and in some gouty arthritic conditions.

3. The whole of the **alkaline** class of waters are of great importance for *internal* use, whether we

consider (*a*) the simple alkaline waters, (*b*) the alkaline common salt waters, or (*c*) the alkaline sodium sulphate waters.

These all owe their alkalinity to the presence of sodium bicarbonate. The *simple alkaline* group contain also a considerable amount of free carbonic acid. Vichy and Vals are types of this group.

These waters act as antacids in gastric hyperacidity; they allay gastric irritability, and stimulate and regulate the gastric functions. They also, especially when warm, exert a cleansing action on the gastric mucosa in catarrhal conditions, dissolving stringy mucus adhering to the gastric walls and washing it away. They also tend to counteract abnormal fermentative processes; they are therefore used largely as remedial agents in dyspepsia and gastric and gastro-intestinal catarrhs. They dilute the bile and promote its secretion and its free flow by flushing the bile ducts, and are thus found of great service in the treatment of gall stones and catarrh of the bile ducts.

The colder springs are more diuretic. These waters are useful in neutralising hyperacidity of the urine and in liquefying accumulations of mucus in the bladder, and are therefore of value in the treatment of cases of vesical catarrh dependent on hyper-acid urine—they act as solvents of uric acid (Pfeiffer), and are of great value in cases of uric and oxalic acid renal calculi.

They increase temporarily the alkalinity of the blood, promote nutritive metabolism, cleanse the blood and the tissues, and are therefore useful in some forms of gout and of the uric acid diathesis, and are especially serviceable in cases of gouty glycosuria and diabetes.

The warm springs are recommended in the treatment of chronic catarrhs of the air passages, pharyngeal, laryngeal, and bronchial, because of their solvent and liquefying effect on thick and inspissated mucus, so that they prove effective expectorants.

The second group of alkaline waters—the *alkaline and common salt* waters—are employed in much the same class of cases as the first, but the presence of a notable but not a large amount of *sodium chloride* modifies the action of the alkaline water, and determines to a certain extent its applicability.

It has been pointed out that the weaker waters of this class approximate in composition to that of a physiological saline solution. They are regarded as less likely than the preceding group to cause loss of flesh, as sodium chloride promotes the absorption and assimilation of nutritive substances; also as less depressing, and better adapted therefore to atonic conditions; and as less likely to render the urine too alkaline.

The presence of sodium chloride is believed to increase their solvent action on uric acid, and to inhibit its precipitation. They are found to be more applicable to the treatment of atonic gout (Royat), and to be more particularly indicated in the treatment of chronic and subacute catarrhs of the respiratory passages (Ems), as they exercise a greater fluidifying effect on the secretion of the respiratory mucous membrane. They are frequently prescribed for gargling and inhalation (sprays).

The springs of the third group—the *alkaline and sodium sulphate* waters—are of great therapeutic importance. They are amongst the most effective and reliable of mineral waters.

In full doses they have a purgative action, the cold ones being more active in this respect than the warm. They stimulate intestinal peristalsis and liquefy the intestinal contents. This effect is believed to be due to the small amount of the salts absorbed in the stomach and upper part of the alimentary tract, so that considerable portions pass on into the large intestine. The cold springs also have a marked diuretic effect. The *warm* ones are less aperient and less diuretic.

The metamorphosis of fat is increased by these springs. Like other alkaline waters, they exert a stimulating effect on the flow of bile and a solvent action on uric acid. These springs are found of great service in cases of abdominal plethora with constipation and hæmorrhoids, especially in "high feeders." The *cold* and more purgative waters are best suited to such cases. They also have a more powerful effect in the reduction of fat, and are largely frequented by obese patients (Marienbad).

The warm springs (Carlsbad) are more suitable to the treatment of gastric and intestinal catarrh, cases of catarrhal jaundice, of gall stones, of hepatic congestion and hypertrophy, as well as splenic hypertrophy, the sequel of malarial fever; of cases also of uric acid gravel and gout and gouty or fat diabetics.

The close attention to diet which is usually observed at these spas contributes largely to the good results obtained.

4. The next class of mineral waters distinguished by the considerable amounts they contain of the **aperient sulphates** of magnesium and sodium, and often named "bitter waters" because of the bitter taste of the magnesium sulphate, are largely employed for their purgative effect in the treatment of habitual constipation. Many of the best known and most active of this class are not drunk at their sources, but are imported in bottles and taken in comparatively small doses (three to six ounces) at home. Some of these springs contain also considerable quantities of sodium chloride (Friedrichshall) and smaller amounts of other less active salts. The few springs of this class that are drunk at their source (Brides, Leamington) are much weaker than those that are imported for home use.

Their action is mainly purgative; they exert a stimulating effect on the secretions of the intestines, and tend to liquefy the fæces as well as to excite peristaltic action. They are employed for the same purpose as other aperients. They have been found useful in the treatment of obesity (Apenta, Brides les Bains). Courses of the milder springs (Brides, Leamington) are sometimes prescribed as alternatives to the alkaline sodium sulphate waters in gastric and hepatic affections.

5. The internal use of **chalybeate** waters is very efficacious in the treatment of many forms of anæmia and chlorosis. The most useful of the iron springs are those which contain bicarbonate of iron together with a large amount of free carbonic acid. The combination is an important one, and promotes the digestion of the water and therefore the assimilation of the iron. It is certain that the use of such waters for some weeks is followed by an increase in the number of red blood corpuscles and in the amount of hæmoglobin. An increase in the elimination of urea and in the body weight has also been noted, and the frequency of the pulse has been observed to increase, as well as the body temperature by one or two degrees Fahrenheit. There is generally some improvement in appetite, but a tendency to constipation has often to be guarded against by the simultaneous administration of some gentle aperient, or in some obstinate cases it may be better to select a spring which contains some aperient constituents as well as iron (Franzensbad, Rippoldsau).

With regard to the selection of an iron spring, the important conclusion has been arrived at by several observers, that in springs which contain relatively small amounts, the iron is absorbed more readily than in those which contain large quantities.

Authorities are not agreed as to the manner in which chalybeate waters exert their remedial influence—whether they act directly in increasing the formation of hæmoglobin, or by protecting the iron taken in the food from decomposition, or simply by stimulating the blood-making organs.

Iron waters are especially indicated in cases of

anæmia and chlorosis following loss of blood, or accompanying retarded convalescence, after acute disease, or when the sequel of malarial attacks, or associated with general exhaustion from overwork, or neurasthenic states; also in amenorrhœa and other disorders of the sexual system accompanied with debility. The choice, where possible, of suitable climatic conditions, adapted to these various morbid states, will exercise an undoubted influence in the results obtained.

6. It is somewhat difficult to realise what is the precise mode of action, when taken internally, of the class of **earthy** or **calcareous** springs, as some of the cold members of this group differ but little in composition and physical characters from ordinary springs of "hard" water, the "hardness" of which is due to the presence, in considerable amount, of calcium carbonate and sulphate—the same salts as form the characteristic constituents of these springs.

It should not be lost sight of, moreover, that it is especially in the application of waters of this class that very large quantities are prescribed, as we mention in our notice of Contrexéville, and it can scarcely be doubted that the large quantity of water thus introduced into the alimentary canal exercises *per se* an important influence in the results obtained.

It is generally thought that the presence of calcium and magnesium carbonate in mineral waters corrects or inhibits the production of acid in the stomach, and that these waters are therefore of use in the treatment of some forms of dyspepsia and intestinal catarrh (chronic diarrhœa). Owing to the astringent effects of the calcium salts these springs tend to lessen excessive secretion from the respiratory and urinary as well as the alimentary tracts, and they are therefore prescribed in cases of chronic bronchial catarrh with profuse secretion, and in cases of catarrh of the bladder and urinary passages. It is doubtful whether they possess the power claimed for them of inducing the breaking up and expulsion of urinary calculi, or of inducing changes in the urine leading to the solution of uric acid. They are, however, largely prescribed in cases of urinary concretions and in cases of gout and the uric acid diathesis.

7. Authorities are by no means agreed as to the mode of action of **sulphur** waters when taken internally. We do not propose to occupy space in discussing the various unsustained hypotheses put forward by many—chiefly German—writers.

It seems to have been established, however, that even such small amounts of sulphur as are present in sulphur waters are capable of producing stimulating effects on healthy organs, and it has been inferred that even smaller amounts may excite reaction in diseased organs which may be attended with remedial effects (H. Schulz). The beneficial effects that have been observed to follow the use of these waters in syphilis and in cases of chronic metallic poisoning have been referred to an augmented eliminatory action by the kidneys, intestines, and skin.

The advantages to be obtained from them in cases of abdominal plethora, with constipation, hæmorrhoids, and enlarged liver, have been stated to be due to their stimulating effect on intestinal activity and to their causing an increased secretion of bile; this aperient effect, however, differs much in different persons, and this may account for the fact that, while they agree with some patients, they utterly disagree with others. It has also been suggested that they exert an internal antiseptic action.

It is certain that the internal use of the warm sulphur waters, combined with inhalations of the warm spray, especially those springs which contain also some sodium chloride, proves of much service in the treatment of chronic catarrh of the respiratory passages—pharynx, larynx, and bronchi. No doubt the solvent action of the hot water and the sodium salt goes for much, but the belief that the sulphur exerts a specific effect on the respiratory mucous membrane is widely entertained by the physicians practising at some of these spas.

Little need be said, in this place, as to the action of the so-called *lithium*, the *iodine* and *bromine*, and the *arsenical* springs. These mineral substances may be taken to have the same physiological and therapeutic effects as when given in the ordinary pharmaceutical preparations.

The fashion of claiming important remedial effects, in gouty states and in tendencies to uric acid depositions, for waters containing minimal amounts of *lithium* salts is rapidly passing away, having been pushed to the verge of absurdity.

The *iodo-bromine* waters are applicable to the treatment of precisely the same cases as those treated by the ordinary preparations of those drugs. The same may be said of the waters containing arsenic; they certainly often present the means of giving very mild and prolonged courses of this remedy in connection with climatic conditions calculated to enhance its remedial effects. Those containing arsenic in association with sulphate of iron (Levico) are regarded as very efficient blood restorers in anæmic and chlorotic states, and in associated enlargement of the lymphatic glands and the torpid forms of scrofula, in malarial cachexia, and in neuralgias.

CHAPTER III.

ACCESSORY MEASURES EMPLOYED IN CONNECTION WITH MINERAL WATER CURES.

Medicated Baths—"Moor" or Peat and Mud Baths—Sand Baths—Gas Baths—Sun and Light Baths—Electric Methods—Massage and Mechanical Exercises—The "Terrain-Kur" Diet—Climatic Conditions—Hydrotherapy—After-Cures.

In this chapter we propose to pass in review the many accessory measures that are applied in numerous spas to supplement, strengthen, enhance, or modify the effects of the mineral waters. And first, with regard to the preparation of *aromatic* and *medicated* baths. In these baths, substances are added to the mineral water, for the purpose of exercising some remedial influence on the skin and peripheral nerves, over and above that which may be expected from the mineral water itself. The *pine-needle* bath is one of the most familiar of these. It is made by adding to the bath a decoction of the needles and young shoots of firs or pines, or the addition of the ethereal oil (fir-wood oil), or the tincture or spirituous extract acts as well. It is believed that the volatile ethereal constituents penetrate the epidermis, stimulate the cutaneous circulation and the peripheral nerves, and are eliminated through the renal, pulmonary, and cutaneous channels. Similar effects follow the addition of aromatic herbs to the bath water—as camomile, wild thyme, elder-flower, sweetflag, peppermint, spearmint, lavender, sweet marjoram, balm, sage, etc. For a full bath about 1½ to 2 lb. of the herbs are tied up in a bag and infused in a gallon of boiling water, the juices expressed, and the infusion added to the bath. The addition of the *equivalent* quantity of the spirituous extract or tincture of those herbs answers as well. *Alkaline* or "*lye*" baths are sometimes prepared by adding common washing soda to the bath in the proportion of about forty to sixty grains to three gallons of water. This mixture is often used for local *foot* baths as a derivative measure in cases of cerebral congestion or congestion of the thoracic viscera. Decoctions of *bran, starch,* or *malt* are also sometimes added to baths to allay irritation.

Astringent baths are likewise prepared by the addition to the water of the bath of decoctions of oak bark, elm-willow bark, or walnut leaves.

In many Continental spas baths are prepared of "peat" or *Moor* (the term used in Germany) or "mud," with which the mineral water is mixed.

Mineral peat consists of decomposing vegetable soil that has been for a very long period in contact with mineral water, so that it has undergone peculiar chemical changes, and is found to contain certain acids and salts, such as sulphuric and formic acid, iron sulphate and phosphate, sodium chloride, aluminium, silica, resin, and other substances. The peat, after exposure to the air and weather, becomes disintegrated, and is in this state mixed with hot mineral water until it acquires the consistency needed. The composition of these peat baths must necessarily vary considerably, according to the salts in the mineral spring mixed with them, the character of the decomposing vegetable substances which form the principal portion of the peat, etc. Peat has been described as *saline* peat when the earth is especially rich in alkaline sulphates and earthy salts, *ferruginous* peat when it contains much iron sulphate, and *sulphurous* peat when sulphur or sulphuretted hydrogen is present in it.

"Mud" baths are prepared with the deposits which are precipitated from many mineral waters, as the "fango" at Battaglia, or from muddy deposits in the neighbourhood of mineral springs, as at

St. Amand, Dax, etc. These muds are mixed in suitable proportions with the thermal water.

It has been suggested that these baths act like large poultices to the surface of the body, and that, besides the influence of their temperature, the weight of the peat exerts a considerable mechanical effect on the skin through compression and friction, while the saline and acid substances in the peat may have a stimulating effect on the cutaneous nerves. Kisch noted as a result of his observations on the effect of the peat baths at Marienbad, that the *pulse* was *accelerated* eight to twelve beats a minute, the *blood pressure* increased in proportion to the density of the peat, the *respirations* increased in frequency, the temperature of the body elevated, the perspiration increased, the secretion of urine lessened, its solids increased except the phosphates; and in women there was augmentation of the menstrual flow.

These baths are appropriate to cases in which it is desired to raise the body heat and to produce powerful stimulation of the skin. They prove useful, therefore, in gout and rheumatism, and in neuralgias of gouty or rheumatic origin; in some forms of peripheral paralysis, in rheumatic, gouty, and other exudations. They have been found useful in some chronic affections of the *female sexual organs*, as metritis, parametritis, and disorders of menstruation.

The *sulphurous* peat baths, in addition to their suitability to cases of chronic gout and rheumatism, are also useful in traumatic cases, and the *sulphurous* mud baths in diseases of the joints, neuralgias, and paralysis.

In some of the Continental seaside resorts thermal baths are prepared from *sea-mud*. Hot sand baths are also applied in some resorts, as in Ischia. They have been introduced, too, at Lavey in Switzerland.

In some spas dry *gas baths* are given with the gases proceeding from the springs, chiefly either carbonic acid or sulphuretted hydrogen. It is doubtful if these are of any great utility, but some bath physicians think them of service. These gases are also applied as local douches.

The cabinets used for gas baths are made of wood, and are furnished with a lid in which there is an opening for the neck or chest, and the patient is seated in the bath so that only the lower portion of the body below the waist is enclosed, the head or the whole of the upper part of the body remaining free. The patient, except that he removes his shoes, does not undress, for the gas readily penetrates the clothing and reaches the skin. The bath usually lasts about ten to twenty minutes, care being taken that the gas is not inhaled.

Such baths of carbonic acid are said to cause capillary congestion and stimulation of the activity of the skin and of the cutaneous nerves, with an increase of general sensibility; but if too prolonged, a depressing effect on the circulatory and respiratory functions becomes manifest, probably from absorption of the gas through the skin.

They are prescribed (at Franzensbad, Marienbad, and elsewhere) in cases of neuralgia and peripheral paralysis, in nervous impotence in the male, in vesical atony, in some torpid skin affections, and in menstrual derangements, as amenorrhœa, dysmenorrhœa; and vaginal douches of the gas are given in some forms of vaginismus. When used as local douches to the surface the skin should be kept moist over the painful parts.

Sulphuretted hydrogen gas is applied in the same way, but it is generally mixed with carbonic acid or nitrogen. Its action is sedative to the cutaneous nerves, and therefore reduces general nervous irritability. At the same time circulatory and respiratory activity is lessened.

It must be remembered that the gas may be absorbed by the skin and by inhalation, and may cause toxic effects if absorbed in too large quantity.

These baths are used (at Aix la Chapelle and

elsewhere) in cases of general hyperæsthesia, hysteria, neuralgia, and certain chronic exanthemata.

Steam baths, hot-air baths, spray baths are well known and familiar therapeutic agents which form an essential part of the treatment in many spas, and can hardly be regarded as accessories.

Sun and light baths.—We are not aware that "sun" baths have been generally utilised in connection with mineral waters, but at Veldes, Ober-Krain, Austria (station Lees-Veldes, an hour from Lerbach), a "sun and air" cure is established, and there the patients, very lightly clothed, or practically naked, are, in fine weather, in the open air, exposed, in an enclosure, to the direct sun heat. Being much in the open air in a sunny locality no doubt proves a valuable auxiliary to many mineral water cures, without going to the extent of such exposure as is practised at Veldes.

In many spas, such as Harrogate, for example, *radiat heat and light* are largely used as accessories to the mineral water cure, by means of the incandescent *electric light bath* or cabinet. It is said to have "no equal as a sudorific measure" (Kellogg), it promotes the absorption of exudations, and acts, in some cases, as a tonic and stimulant to nutrition. It increases oxidation and improves metabolism, and is on that account of service in the treatment of gout, rheumatism, and hepatic inadequacy ; also in obesity and fat diabetics. It is of great value in sciatica and many other forms of neuralgia, as well as in cases of autointoxication and metallic poisonings. "In chlorosis and anæmia the most excellent results are obtained" (Kellogg), and it is of use in some forms of nephritis by its derivative effect on the skin.

It is certain that the *electric incandescent light* bath is a most important and valuable accessory to mineral water treatment.

Much difference of opinion exists as to the value of the application of the older *electric bath* as applied in many spas ; but there can be little doubt that the use of the various electric methods, as employed by skilled operators, at such baths as Gastein, Bath, Buxton, and Aix, has been found of eminent service.

Nowadays there are few, if any, mineral water cures that do not rely upon *massage* or some form of *mechanical exercise* as indispensable auxiliaries to the course.

Massage may be either general or local. The former enters largely into our ordinary daily practice, and it is the latter that is practised most commonly in connection with mineral water cures. It is applied in a great variety of morbid states—neuralgias and myalgias, passive effusions, exudations, stiff joints, chronic rheumatism and gout, constipation, muscular wasting, and loss of power, etc., etc.

At Aix les Bains was instituted a combination of massage with the hot douche—a method which has been introduced into many other spas. At Bourbonne les Bains the thermal douche is applied with such force that it is said to have the same effect as massage.

At many spas (Baden-Baden, Nauheim, Ragatz, etc., etc.) " Zander institutes " have been established for Swedish gymnastics and with mechanical appliances for graduated exercises in great variety. At other spas (Homburg, etc.) Ling's system of Swedish gymnastics is applied ; and at Nauheim the now well-known " resistance exercises " * are carried out in the treatment of cardiac affections. Oertel's " Terrain-Kur " has been organised at certain spas situated in suitable hilly countries (Aussee, Baden-Baden, etc.) for graduated uphill walks especially intended for the treatment of cases of cardiac debility associated with obesity. The extent and nature of the exercises undertaken by such patients are determined by the bath physician, and should by no means be left to the discretion of the patient. Unfortunately, serious consequences have occasionally followed the adoption

* Described in the author's " Manual of Medical Treatment," vol. i., p. 396 *et seq.*

of this method, and we hardly think it can be claimed to have yielded many brilliant results. A certain amount of regular muscular exercise is a valuable accessory to mineral water treatment in cases of glycosuria in the robust. It helps to use up the sugar circulating in the blood; but feeble and thin diabetics often bear muscular exertion very badly.

The importance of establishing and carrying out a suitable *diet*, or of initiating desirable changes in dietetic habits, in connection with courses of mineral waters, cannot be over-estimated. And although the indiscriminate application of a rigid system, to all patients alike, cannot be commended, the experienced guidance and direction of the spa physicians should never be disregarded. The acquirement of more wholesome and rational dietetic habits during a course of mineral waters, and their maintenance afterwards, is one of the great advantages attending this method of treatment.

At spas where the gouty, the dyspeptic, and the obese are sent in large numbers (Carlsbad, Vichy, Marienbad, etc.), a more or less rigorous diet is essential to the success of the cure, and is usually accepted and followed; but it would certainly be an advantage, at most other mineral water resorts, if the physicians were enabled to exercise some control or direction over the food supplied to, or taken by, the patients.

Altered *climatic conditions*, the "change of air" and surroundings, often prove of the greatest service as auxiliaries to mineral water treatment. Many popular mineral springs are situated in mountainous districts, at considerable elevations. St. Moritz, in Switzerland, is at an elevation of nearly 6,000 feet; Tarasp, 4,000; Bormio, in Italy, about 4,500; Gastein, in Austria, 3,300; Mt. Dore, in France, 3,400; Buxton, in Derbyshire, 1,000; and Llandrindod, in Mid-Wales, about 700 feet. In these situations the tonic, bracing influence of mountain air undoubtedly enhances the good effect of the mineral treatment, or counteracts, in other instances, any exhausting tendency it may have. In many other instances we find that the most frequented spas are situated in the midst of romantic and picturesque forest, or mountain, or lake scenery, which has a soothing, restful, and advantageous moral effect on the visitors. We have only to mention such resorts as Baden-Baden, Wildbad, and others in the Black Forest, Luchon and Eaux Bonnes in the Pyrenees, Royat in Auvergne, Spa in Belgium, Strathpeffer in the Scottish Highlands.

Then we find in, or adjacent to, many home and Continental spas institutions for the application of the methods of hydrotherapy, as a substitute for, or as supplementary or complementary to, the mineral water courses. There are well-known "hydros" at Harrogate and Buxton, and the same is the case in many French and German mineral water stations.

Finally, we may here refer to the subject of "*after-cures*" as an essential part of most courses of mineral waters. It is certainly most undesirable, after a course of mineral waters and baths, to return at once to the cares and anxieties of business, or household management, or to fulfil social engagements. A period of calm and repose, in cheerful surroundings, is most useful in consolidating and confirming the good effects of bath treatment.

In selecting a suitable place for an "after-cure," regard must be had to the nature of the patient's malady, to the locality and its neighbourhood in which the "cure" has been carried out, and to the local knowledge, experience, and counsel of the bath physician. In many cases it will be desirable, in returning from the Continent, to select a resort conveniently placed on the homeward route, so as to divide the journey and lessen the fatigue of travelling. Often suitable mountain resorts exist close to the spa, and therefore very accessible, as the stations on Mt. Revard, close to Aix les Bains. On returning from French baths, there is Fontainebleau and St.

Germain, inland resorts, or Dieppe on the Channel, or our own south coast resorts, including the Isle of Wight. On the way back from Germany there is Spa, with beautiful surroundings for drives and walks; or, on the sea coast, Ostend, Blankenberghe, Neukirke, Scheveningen; or Ramsgate, Folkestone and Hythe on our own coast.

Except for some anæmic and neurasthenic cases, we do not consider places situated at great elevations (5,000 to 7,000 feet) well adapted for "after-cures." The air often proves exciting and irritating, the rapid changes of temperature are keenly felt, and in cold seasons and in persons with feeble circulations, chilliness and depression are apt to be complained of. Medium elevations of 3,000 to 4000 feet, such as Mt. de Caux or Les Avants, above Montreux, or Beatenberg, above Thun, or Engelberg, near Lucerne, or the Dolden, near Zürich, and the numerous Black Forest resorts, such as St. Blasien, Triberg, etc., are safer and more generally suitable. But in the choice of an "after-cure" many considerations personal to each individual have to be weighed and discriminated.

SECTION B.

DESCRIPTION OF THE PRINCIPAL MINERAL SPRINGS.

WE now proceed to give some account of the chief mineral springs, arranged in alphabetical order. The less important ones will be found in smaller type at the end of each alphabetical group.

Aix la Chapelle (Aachen), now united with Borcette (Burtscheid) into one community (Aachen-Burtscheid), is a well-known *thermal sulphur* bath, situated on the railway between Brussels and Cologne, and conveniently accessible from London in eleven or twelve hours. Aachen is now a large town with about 140,000 inhabitants; it is pleasantly situated, at an elevation of 530 feet, on the slopes of the Lousberg, and is surrounded by wooded hills ranging from 750 to 1,120 feet high. It lies on the western frontier of Germany, on the borders of Holland and Belgium. The soil on which it is built is of porous sand, which readily absorbs heavy downfalls of rain, leaving the streets and paths quickly dry again. It has a medium temperate climate, not very hot in summer, and the cold of winter is said to be mitigated by the heat given into the atmosphere by the hot springs.

Its history as a bath stretches back into a remote antiquity. Charlemagne, whose remains repose in its cathedral, has been regarded not only as the founder of the town but as the discoverer of the springs, but there exist evidences (relics of the stone age) near the hot springs that they were used by the primitive inhabitants of the country; there are also ruins of Roman baths, showing that they were utilised in later times by the Romans.

The characteristic components of the numerous springs are *sodium chloride* and *sodium sulphide*, together with sulphuretted hydrogen; they differ only in temperature and the relative amounts of the sulphur compounds they contain.

If we take the strongest of the springs, the Kaiserquelle, we find it contains 4·1215 grammes of salts per litre, *sodium chloride* 2·639, sodium bicarbonate 0·918, sodium sulphate 0·152, *sodium sulphide* 0·011, calcium bicarbonate 0·227, magnesium bicarbonate 0·077, bicarbonate of protoxide of iron 0·013, minute amounts of lithium chloride, strontium sulphate, and sodium bromide and iodide, silicic acid, and organic matter. Its temperature is 131° F. A temperature of 172° F. has been found in connection with one of the springs—the Schwertbad—which is said to be the hottest spring in Central Europe. In the great bath establishments, of which there are several, we find both hotel accommodation and baths combined — an arrangement obviously of great convenience to the patients. The Kaiserbad, the chief of these, is supplied by the Kaiser-spring, so also is the Neubad and the Königin von Ungarn. The drinking fountain, Elisenbrunnen, in the Elisen Gardens, is also supplied by pipes from the Kaiser-spring.

The Quirinusbad possesses three springs.

The Rosenbad spring supplies also the Comphausbad and in part the new and very complete Corneliusbad. These bath-houses belong to the city of Aix la Chapelle.

There are several bath-houses at Burtscheid where the hottest springs are found; twenty-eight are in use!

It is as well to be aware that there are a "Kaiserbad" Hotel, a "Rosenbad" Hotel, and a "Neubad" Hotel at both Aachen and Burtscheid, and visitors must give explicit directions as to which they wish to be taken to.

The thermal waters are administered here, as

elsewhere, as ordinary baths, varying in temperature according to the doctor's prescription; and as douche baths, in which systematic friction and gentle massage are combined with the douche—the massage is applied while the bath is filling and the patient remains in the bath for a time afterwards. This is found to be a most efficacious and agreeable form of bath when applied by a skilful attendant. The Scotch douche (alternately warm and cold) is given, as well as other forms. Vapour baths also are used. Those who drink the waters take them about an hour before breakfast. It is usual to take some exercise between each glass.

Inhalation and pulverisation rooms and apparatus for the local application of the water to the nose, larynx and other parts are also provided.

There is at Aix a "Zander" institute for the application of Swedish gymnastics. Mud baths are given in the Schlossbad.

As to the maladies suitable for treatment here:—Chronic catarrhal affections of the respiratory and gastro-intestinal mucous membranes are benefited by the inhalations, the baths, and the internal administration of the alkaline chloride of sodium and sulphuretted waters. Chronic arthritis, rheumatic or gouty, stiff joints, and muscular pains are greatly advantaged by the hot baths, together with the douche-massage as applied there.

Chronic skin diseases are sent there, as to other sulphur baths; eczema, acne, and psoriasis especially; and it must be borne in mind that the doctors at Aix do not hesitate to use, at the same time, the ordinary medicinal remedies for such affections. Certain forms of neuralgia, paralysis, and tabes are treated there.

Finally, Aachen has a very *special* reputation in the treatment of syphilis. Weber says that "70 per cent. of the patients visiting the Spa are syphilitics"! By regular, free mercurial inunction a vigorous anti-syphilitic treatment is systematically carried out, and the hot sulphur baths, by promoting absorption and favouring change of tissue, aiding nutrition and stimulating elimination through the skin and other excretory organs, influence powerfully the curative action of specific remedies.

A table water is manufactured from some of these springs by the removal of sulphur and the addition of carbonic acid gas.

The season at Aix la Chapelle is practically all the year round.

The charges at the private bath-houses at Aachen-Burtscheid are less than at the municipal bath-houses at Aachen. For details apply to the "Kur Director," Aachen, Germany.

Aix les Bains, or Aix in Savoy, is one of the most important bathing resorts in France. Its reputation is universal; and situated as it is on one of the great European highways between the north and the south, between Italy and France, it is most easy of access to that great stream of travellers who annually migrate, in search of health or of pleasure, from the north to the south of Europe, or even to Africa and the Far East. Thus it is that Aix is far more cosmopolitan than any other bath in France, and with our own people it is especially popular, partly, no doubt, from its great repute in the treatment of those very English maladies, rheumatism and gout. Its attractive site and picturesque neighbourhood, its excellent hotels, its large and gay casino, and the brilliant society which may frequently be found there, combine to render it a town of pleasure, as well as a resort for health.

The train service between Paris and Aix is exceedingly good, as the express trains to Turin, Brindisi, and Rome stop there. The journey takes only between eight and nine hours.

The town itself is about a mile from the small but very picturesque Lac du Bourget, and is 850 feet above the level of the sea and 90 feet above the lake. It lies in a wide open valley surrounded to some extent, but by no means shut in, by the adjacent Alps of Savoy. The town is well built, with wide streets and shady avenues of trees, and gardens surround many of the hotels and private houses. Hotels and boarding-houses and furnished apartments abound, the accommodation being, as usual, proportionate to the price paid for it.

Steamers and rowing-boats take visitors to the different objects of interest on the lake.

Numerous Roman remains are exhibited at Aix, of which local guide-books afford full information. There are many walks and drives, short and long, all full of interest and attractiveness, and many excursions by railway into charming scenery which will delight those who can spare the time to take them.

Aix is said to enjoy a mild and equable climate, an entire freedom from fogs, and to be protected from winds by the surrounding mountains. Nervous subjects find the climate soothing and conducive to sleep, and those who find it too warm and relaxing in the town can resort to the cooler and more bracing atmosphere of the surrounding hills.

The *sources* of Aix (two in number, *Source de souffre* and *Source d'alun*) are *sulphurous*, and their characteristic ingredient is sulphuretted hydrogen, of which there are 2 cubic centimetres per litre. Their temperature ranges from 113° to 115°, and the quantity yielded in twenty-four hours is enormous—as much as four million litres. Their mineralisation is very feeble, only 0·49 grammes of solids per litre, chiefly carbonate of lime. They are rich, however, in organic matter (*barégine*), to which they owe their unctuous feeling, a valuable quality for massage under water.

The so-called "alum" source is badly named, as it contains no alum; indeed the two *sources* are probably branches of a single subterranean canal.

These hot mineral springs are utilised in a variety of ways in an *Établissement Thermal*, which is furnished with every appliance needed for the treatment of the cases that are sent there, and provided with 120 skilled masseurs and masseuses!

The waters are administered internally as well as applied externally, but it is not usual to give them in large quantities, or to enforce them on persons with delicate digestions, who may find difficulty in tolerating them. Two to four glasses a day form the average quantity, and when stronger sulphur waters are indicated it is usual to prescribe the strong sulphur water of Challes. To promote elimination by the kidneys a water resembling the Evian water, "l'eau de Saint Simon," derived from a spring a little distance from Aix, is often ordered to be drunk by gouty patients before or after the baths and douches, or as a table water.

But it is to the mode of application, *externally*, of the hot sulphur springs, especially to the combination of douching and massage, that Aix chiefly owes its reputation—what is known as the Aix *douche-massage*.* The patient sits on a wooden *stool* (or reclines on a *plank*), and one or two *doucheurs* (or *doucheuses*), most of whom are extremely skilful, shampoo and apply *massage* to different parts of the body, over which jets of hot water, varying in temperature, are at the same time propelled.

"It is astonishing," says the late Sir Grainger Stewart, who was himself submitted to the process, "with what skill, what patience, tenderness, and firmness the shampooing and passive movements are performed. When every joint has been moved to the utmost extent possible, the patient is made to stand, while from a distance a powerful stream of water is propelled upon the different limbs, especially about the

* The practice of *massage* is stated to have been introduced at Aix about the beginning of the last century by persons returning from Bonaparte's expedition into Egypt.

articulations chiefly affected. When the bath is over, the patient is rapidly dried, wrapped in flannel sheets and blankets, and is carried back to his hotel in the curious sedan-chair. Having reached his apartment he is lifted into bed, still swathed like a mummy, is covered up with additional blankets and a quilt, and left to perspire for a longer or shorter period. After twenty minutes or half an hour, he is carefully rubbed down by an attendant who had accompanied him to the bath." Other patients are allowed to walk back to their hotel, where they should rest for an hour.

Sometimes a *vapour* bath is applied. The patient "enters an apartment which contains a curious wooden box, with a round hole in its movable lid. After undressing, he steps into the wooden box and finds that he is shut in all except the head, the round hole being occupied by his neck. Immediately a valve on the level of the floor is opened, the hot vapour rises about him, and he soon begins to perspire freely. The perspiration running from his brow, trickles down his face. Presently he feels the stream flowing down his sides and his legs, and presently a feeling of oppression and debility comes on, and after ten or twenty minutes the bath is opened up, the patient is carefully dried and removed to his hotel." There are also chambers, or *étuves*, in which, from the hot mineral water, general vapour baths are produced. These are known as *bouillons*.

Then there is the *local vapour* bath (*Berthollet*). "By ingenious contrivances the bath-man is enabled to steam one arm or one leg. Speedily the limb begins to perspire and the parts become soft and comparatively flexible. Perspiration occurs all over the body, especially in those who have been undergoing other forms of treatment, and so great care requires to be taken to prevent a chill. When the parts have been thoroughly softened, manipulation, shampooing, and passive movement of joints are carefully carried out, just as after the douche, but only confined to one limb.

"On certain days the patient is sent to the spacious and comfortable *swimming baths*, and there he is allowed to disport himself for a longer or shorter time, practising, amid the somewhat warm water, active movements of the limbs. When his swim is ended he may have a cold douche or not, according to the direction of the doctor. He is rapidly dried, and, if well enough, is directed to walk about smartly in the gardens, which are close to the establishment."

Ordinary cold water is used when necessary to lower the temperature of the mineral springs; or Challes water is added if a very strong sulphur bath is required.

Rooms are specially devoted to inhaling the sulphurous vapour of the water (*humage*), and also to the inhalation of the atomised thermal water (spray), which can be directed upon any part of the body, and is especially applied in affections of the nose, throat, face, and eyes, but this form of treatment is more usually carried out at Marlioz. A "Zander" institute for Swedish gymnastics has recently been established at Aix, and adjacent to this is an establishment for the application of "Nauheim" baths and the various forms of electrical treatment now in use.

It is necessary, in the next place, to consider the action of these waters and the kind of diseases to the treatment and cure of which they are applicable, remembering that it has been authoritatively said that "massage plays the principal *rôle* in the medications at Aix."

It is easy to see that the object of such a method of treatment as has been just described must be to promote the removal of waste material and stimulate powerfully the action of the skin, as an agent of elimination. It is as it were a purgation through the skin! Whatever excrementitious matters are retained in the blood, or too slowly eliminated, that can be got rid of through the skin, must be discharged from the system by such active stimulation of the cutaneous surface.

We see also how, by the attraction of the blood to the surface of the body and its retention there in the dilated vessels, congestions of deeper parts must be relieved and a general stimulus given to the circulation of the nutritive fluids of the body; so that indirectly a great stimulus is given to healthy nutrition and normal tissue change. It is necessary, however, to bear in mind that usually the existence of a certain latent vigour and power of reaction are assumed in the application of such stimulating measures.

Indeed, it is this point that most frequently exercises and tests the judgment and discrimination of the physician. If from age, or general exhaustion, or a naturally feeble constitution, this power of reaction is absent, then these modes of treatment only excite and exhaust, and a state of feverish debility is produced, and the patient is left worse, instead of better, for the treatment. So that it is occasionally necessary to resist the not unnatural desire of such patients for active treatment of this kind.

It is not uncommon for the temperature of the body to be raised two or three degrees during the douches, and the pulse thirty or forty beats in the minute; moreover, a slight degree of feverishness is often induced (thermal fever) which needs careful management, especially with respect to diet and exercise.

The period of treatment ordinarily lasts about twenty-five days, with a few days' intermission for rest; but it may be, and often is, necessary to suspend the treatment for a time, so that invalids should allow themselves five or six weeks, and, if everything goes well, the last week may be advantageously spent at one or other of the more accessible mountain resorts in the neighbourhood. Exercise in the open air is insisted upon, a moderate, careful diet, free from any excess, is enjoined, as are also early hours, especially in the damp evenings of the spring and autumn, and aperients are often required by gouty and rheumatic patients, especially when the condition of the urine shows that much waste material is being discharged from the body.

Among the cases best suited to treatment at Aix, chronic rheumatic and gouty affections take the foremost place. The personal observations of the late Sir Grainger Stewart on this head deserve to be quoted:

"The treatment of Aix is of extraordinary value in various rheumatic conditions. *First*, it is of great service in the way of removing the thickness and stiffness which so often remain after attacks of acute rheumatism—a stiffness due partly to changes within the joint, but mainly to thickening of the fibrous tissues round the articulation. *Second*, in case of chronic rheumatism, where a slow inflammatory action is going on in and around the joints, it suffices both to remove inflammatory products and to diminish the tendency to rheumatic inflammation. *Third*, in rheumatic affections of the muscles, fascia, and nerve sheaths, it affords in many cases the most decided and speedy relief. *Fourth*, in the wasting of muscles, which so often occurs in connection with rheumatic processes, the manipulation and shampooing, along with the electrical stimulation which the doctors superadd, generally prove distinctly serviceable; and *fifth*, on the occurrence of slight rheumatic threatenings, it appears that the use of the Berthollet or vapour bath often suffices to prevent the further development of the disease."

Treatment at Aix is, however, of doubtful value in cases of osteo-arthritis, "Rheumatoid arthritis" as it is often termed.

As to the treatment of *gout* at Aix it is admitted that, at the beginning of the course, an acute attack is sometimes induced, necessitating a suspension of the treatment until the severe pain has passed away; but it is maintained that the ultimate result is to diminish the frequency and intensity of the attacks and to eliminate the gouty poison from the system. It is usual, in many of these gouty affections of the joints, to combine with the thermal treatment the application of the continuous electric current to the wasted muscles. Skin diseases of gouty origin, psoriasis and eczema, are especially adapted to the treatment at Aix. It should be remembered that it is especially the *atonic* form of gout that is best suited to treatment at Aix, and that *after* a course of *external* treatment by these hot sulphur waters it is often thought advisable to prescribe an *internal* treatment, at Vichy, Evian, Contrexéville, or Vittel.

Rheumatic forms of neuralgia, and especially *sciatica*, whether of rheumatic, gouty or syphilitic origin, are benefited by the combination of bathing, douching, and shampooing as practised there. Alcoholic and other forms of *peripheral neuritis* are said to be greatly benefited by a combination of douche-massage with electrical treatment.

The presence of cardiac complications in the gouty and rheumatic are not regarded, by some of the physicians at Aix, as contra-indicating the application of *douche-massage*, in certain cases, as it has been observed, experimentally, that douche-massage causes a diminution of arterial tension.

Chronic affections of the nose and throat are also sent to Aix, or rather Marlioz, for amelioration or cure. Chronic atrophic rhinitis is treated by nasal douches, the inhalation of the natural vapour of the hot sulphur springs, and by local application of the aqueous spray; swimming baths also are enjoined, as well as the internal use of Challes water.

Precisely the same method of treatment is applied, with advantage, to cases of chronic inflammation of the pharynx, granular pharyngitis, etc., often associated with a gouty and rheumatic as well as a scrofulous diathesis.

Chronic laryngeal catarrh, with hoarseness and loss of voice, and often some irritative cough, induced by over-fatigue of the larynx in public speaking and singing, or by excessive smoking, or by alcoholic drinks, is benefited by the inhalations of the atomised sulphur water as applied in the *salles d'inhalation* at Marlioz. The climate of Aix and Marlioz is also believed to aid the treatment of these cases greatly.

Some forms of chronic bronchial catarrh are reputed to have been relieved by treatment by the inhalations, etc., at Marlioz, and the same is said with respect to hay-fever and certain types of phthisis.

As an aid to the effect of specific remedies in the treatment of constitutional syphilis, Aix les Bains has always enjoyed a considerable reputation, though Aix la Chapelle surpasses it in this repect; as to the power and influence of this treatment in *revealing latent* syphilis the greatest divergence of opinion exists, and the latest tendency is to a denial of this property. Scrofulous affections of the bones, joints, and glandular system, scrofulous ophthalmia, and even lupus are reported to be greatly benefited and even cured by the course at Aix.

Cases of chronic skin disease which travel all over Europe, from bath to bath, seeking relief, and, it must be added, often finding none or but very little, naturally visit Aix les Bains in considerable numbers. One of the most troublesome and inveterate of these diseases is *psoriasis*, which often affects gouty persons; this disease is rarely completely cured, but they claim at Aix that under the influence of treatment there, the patches become paler, the scales are shed, and the absorption and action of internal remedies are promoted.

In cases of eczema the first effect of the treatment is often to exaggerate somewhat the symptoms, but if the course is prolonged sufficiently the manifestations disappear.

In the relief of acne the swimming-baths, together with the local application of the sulphur water, prove very efficacious.

In hysteria, and in certain chronic uterine affections, in anæmia, and chlorosis, treatment at Aix proves beneficial. In some of these cases removal from home influences, which are not unfrequently injurious, change of air, scene, and food, the regular occupation of bathing and shampooing, and the enforced exercise in the open air, combined with judicious medical supervision, have probably more remedial influence than the *sulphur* in the water.

In certain cases of paralysis, the combined stimulating influence of bathing, shampooing, and the application of the electric current produces a beneficial effect.

Certain cases of traumatic disease of the bones and joints are usefully submitted to the treatment at Aix.

Marlioz is but a quarter of an hour's walk from Aix, and may practically be regarded as belonging to it. Its springs, three in number, are *cold sulphur* springs, and they are used chiefly in the form of inhalation and pulverisation—*i.e.* in vapour and spray. At Marlioz there are special arrangements in the shape of well-arranged *salles d'inhalation* for the application of the vapour and spray of these sulphur springs to the treatment of chronic affections of the respiratory passages, such as chronic coryza, chronic laryngitis and pharyngitis, and chronic bronchial catarrh. Patients following this treatment can either reside at Aix, or, if they prefer a quieter life, they can find comfortable apartments in the *château* and *villa* attached to the *Établissement* at Marlioz, which is situated in pleasant and extensive park-like grounds.

In the bath establishment at Marlioz the usual baths and douches are provided, and every appliance for hydrotherapeutic treatment, either with the sulphur springs or with ordinary water. The Marlioz water appears to contain sulphur in combination with sodium as sulphide of sodium, just like the Pyrenean springs, according to some authorities, while others have found sulphuretted hydrogen in it. Besides carbonate and chloride of sodium it is said to contain iodide and bromide of sodium.

Mountain-air stations suitable for an after-cure are now brought, as it were, to the doors of the patients at Aix. By means of a mountain railway the high plateau on the summit of Mont Revard is reached in an hour, and an excellent hotel is found there at an elevation of 4,900 feet. For those who do not need so bracing a resort, there is Pugny-Corbières, about half an hour from Aix, at an elevation of 2,000 feet, on the border of shady woods, and another climatic station has been established on the *Col du Chat*. The well-known resorts at the eastern end of the Lake of Geneva, Glion, Caux, Les Avants, etc., are also easy of access.

The season is from April 15th to the end of October; the months of July and August are often very hot.

Allevard is an important French *cold sulphur* spring containing much free sulphuretted hydrogen, and employed chiefly in the treatment of diseases of the throat and respiratory organs.

The baths at Allevard in the department of Isère lie about midway between Chambéry and Grenoble, being twenty-three miles from the former and twenty-five from the latter town. A branch line connects it with Pontcharra-sur-Bréda, a station on the line of rail between these towns. It is reached in eleven hours from Paris.

The village of Allevard is built on both banks of the river Bréda, at an elevation of 1,350 feet above the sea. It is in the midst of beautiful scenery, and has many admirable excursions and points of view in its neighbourhood. It has a southern aspect and a mild and rather moist climate. It is not shut in, as many such places are, between high mountains; but the valley is open, and the mountains on each side rise by gentle wooded slopes, behind which stand steep and bare peaks of great height.

The hotels and pensions, most of them situated in a shady park, are good and comfortable; and the simple and quiet life there, and the calm and peaceful surroundings, must be especially grateful and suitable to the more serious class of invalids for whom the cure at Allevard is prescribed. The special application of the mineral springs of Allevard is in the treatment of diseases of the throat and respiratory organs, especially when associated with the rheumatic or gouty constitution: Chronic throat and nose catarrhs, chronic bronchitis, asthma, and even certain forms of consumption are treated there (apyretic forms with general health good) with favourable results.

One of the special modes of treatment in vogue at Allevard is the inhalation of the gases given off by the water of the springs, cold and unheated. This takes place in the *salles d'inhalation froide*.

In these rooms, which are large enough to contain fifty patients at a time, the water, under pressure, is by means of suitable mechanism driven into spray so fine and so diffused that the gases in it become set free into the surrounding air: ninety-five per cent. of the sulphuretted hydrogen contained in the water (there are 24 c.c. of this gas per litre), together with much of the nitrogen and carbonic acid it also contains, is diffused into the atmospheres of these *salles d'inhalation froide*. The respiration of this medicated air has been found of special service in the treatment of tuberculous and other affections of the throat and lungs. The patients are allowed to remain from three to fifteen minutes in this air; and they return to these rooms five or six times in the day, and in the intervals the jets of water are turned off, and the rooms thoroughly ventilated by opening all the windows and doors.

There are also at Allevard, as at Royat and elsewhere, rooms devoted to inhalation of the warm vapours of the water. In these the patients remain, suitably clothed, for half an hour or more; and this method is found particularly serviceable in the treatment of chronic bronchial catarrh and catarrhal asthma. There are also two large chambers for the inhalation of *warm pulverised* water.

Douches for the throat, the nose, the eyes, the face, etc.; a room for gargling; hot foot and leg baths—used here very hot, and prescribed for their revulsive effect to most of the patients; and all the appliances necessary for general bathing, douching, and massage are to be found in this *very* complete bath establishment. Internally the water is drunk in small doses at first—a quarter to half a glass daily, gradually increasing to two or three glasses, either cold or mixed with a little warm syrup or milk.

The Allevard water is, as we have said, a *cold sulphur* spring, its temperature being about 60° F. It contains a considerable amount of free sulphuretted hydrogen, as well as nitrogen and carbonic acid gases; its chief solid constituents are sodium chloride, calcium carbonate, calcium and magnesium sulphate, silica, and traces of arsenic. But it is by no means strongly mineralised.

This water is said to be easily digested, to increase appetite, and to promote nutritive changes. It is maintained that the sulphuretted hydrogen when coming in contact with the bronchial mucous membrane abstracts oxygen and deposits its sulphur, having at first a stimulating and afterwards a sedative effect, the latter being also contributed to by the carbonic acid and nitrogen contained in the water.

A long list of maladies are treated at Allevard —in addition to those already named: chronic pharyngitis and tonsillitis, adenoids, laryngitis, hay-asthma, enlarged bronchial glands following whooping cough or measles; amongst skin affections, eczema and impetigo.

The season is from June 1st to Sept. 30th—the best time being from June 15th to Aug. 20th. There is a casino with theatre and the amusements usually found at a French spa.

Amélie les Bains.—A *thermal sulphur* bath in the Pyrénées Orientales, at an elevation of about 900 feet, in a valley enclosed by high mountains, which in winter limit considerably the number of hours of sunshine. It has this point of interest for those who are seeking treatment by hot sulphur baths in the winter, that it is one of the few sulphur baths available at that season, for Amélie is open all the year round. Its name is derived from that of the wife of Louis

Philippe. It lies at the extreme south-eastern corner of France, close to the Spanish frontier: it is thirty-eight kilometres from Perpignan on the railway from Elne to Arles-sur-Tech—a twenty-two hours' journey from Paris.

It has a mild winter climate, due to its protection from winds and its southern latitude, the average winter temperature being 46° F. Spring is the most disagreeable season there, owing to the prevalence of east wind. In the summer it is very hot; so that it is mostly a winter resort.

Its springs are numerous—twenty-two altogether—and they vary in temperature from 96° to 140° F. The characteristic ingredient is *sodium sulphide,* and this varies in amount from 0·025 to 0·039 grammes per litre. They are also rich in glairine and organic matter. The water is at first clear, but soon turns milky on exposure to the air. There are three establishments in which the springs are utilised. *One* is the great military hospital, which has accommodation for 66 officers and 379 non-commissioned officers and soldiers; the *second* is the Thermes Romains (built on the foundations of old Roman baths), and the *third* the Bains Pujade. These contain appliances for large and small baths, hot and cold douches, foot baths, vapour baths, massage, inhalations, and pulverisations. The apartments for inhalation communicate directly with the springs. *Buvettes* for supplying the water for drinking are numerous, the most frequented being the Source Pectorale.

The effect of the treatment is to produce a little excitement at first, but never so great as at the stronger sulphur springs; this is soon followed by a markedly sedative effect. The influences of the climate and water have been thus summarised—sedative to the circulatory system, stimulating to the nervous system, restorative of the nutritive functions. The alkaline, ferruginous waters of the neighbouring spa, Le Boulou, are often prescribed to be drunk at Amélie, together with the sulphur water.

Attacks of colic and diarrhœa are said not unfrequently to occur to visitors at Amélie even when not drinking the waters.

The principal diseases sent to this spa for treatment are, first, diseases of the respiratory organs, and especially torpid forms of phthisis; these latter deriving benefit both from the mild climate and the sulphur springs. Chronic laryngitis, bronchitis, asthma, and emphysema are also benefited. Like other thermal sulphur springs, these are applicable to cases of chronic rheumatism, to torpid skin affections, and to scrofulo-tuberculous disease of the bones and mucous membranes. A great many traumatic cases, especially amongst the military, are treated there—the consequences of gunshot and other wounds.

Patients are able to pass by covered ways from their hotel to the baths.

Apenta.—This, one of the most recently introduced of the Hungarian aperient waters, may be taken as the type of the so-called *bitter waters* which have, of late years, come into such general use as convenient and trustworthy laxatives.

Apenta, "like the whole group of those Hungarian aperient waters, is formed at no great depth—not more than 15 or 20 feet—its chemical composition being due largely to the solution in the water of the chemical salts of the stratum of the ground through which it spreads."

It is claimed for this water that, owing to the careful and scientific method in which its collection and bottling is supervised and carried out, its constancy of composition is maintained and can always be relied upon.

The chief active constituents of this water are the aperient sulphates of magnesium and sodium, and Professor Pouchet's analysis of Apenta water shows it to contain, per litre, magnesium sulphate 23·43 grammes, sodium sulphate 15·53, calcium and potassium sulphates 2·676, sodium carbonate 1·011, and sodium chloride 1·716. It also contains a small amount of oxide of iron, 0·046, and minute amounts of lithium and other less important constituents.

In the more generalised use of this water, as in the systematic treatment of hepatic and gouty troubles and for the cure of obesity, for which it has been extensively employed, the presence of sodium carbonate and chloride are not unimportant ingredients; while the presence of an appreciable amount of iron doubtless tends to counteract any lowering effect it might otherwise produce. The usual dose is from four to six fluid ounces taken in the morning fasting. It is often given warmed and mixed with an equal quantity of Apollinaris water, as a useful substitute for Carlsbad water in the treatment of gall-stones.

Apollinaris.—This, the most popular of *alkaline table* waters, may be taken as the type of that class of mineral spring. The dietetic value of such a water depends on its containing a definite and moderate (*not a large*) amount of sodium bicarbonate and sodium chloride and a considerable amount of free carbonic acid gas. According to the time at which it is taken, the first-named constituent is valuable for its antacid action in diluting and neutralising acid wines, for its solvent action on catarrhal mucus, for its stimulating action on the gastric secretion, and for its neutralising effect at other times on gastric hyper-acidity. The sodium chloride has a dietetic value as a promoter of gastric activity and of general metabolism, and the carbonic acid for its refreshing and agreeable as well as stimulating properties.

A water containing much alkali is counter-indicated as a "table water," as it might injuriously neutralise the needful acidity of the gastric juice when taken with meals, and a merely gaseous water with no alkali would obviously fail in one of its chief properties.

The Apollinaris springs rise in the Ahrthal in Rhenish Prussia, in close proximity to the celebrated springs of Neuenahr. These latter contain precisely the same constituents as the Apollinaris springs, only varying somewhat in the proportions of the constituents and in temperature. The chief of the springs at Neuenahr (the Grosser Sprudel) is a warm spring and has a temperature of about 96° F. It is interesting to compare the composition of this spring with that of Apollinaris. In the latest analysis of the latter (made by Th. Kyll, 1902), in a litre there is of sodium carbonate 1·248 grammes (Neuenahr 0·600), of magnesium carbonate 0·465 (Neuenahr 0·300), sodium chloride 0·421 (Neuenahr 0·100), sodium sulphate 0·247 (Neuenahr 0·083), calcium carbonate 0·250 (Neuenahr 0·200), iron protoxide 0·003 (Neuenahr carbonate of iron 0·012).

We see here a great similarity of composition. The Apollinaris water is richer in sodium and magnesium carbonates and in sodium chloride. The Neuenahr water contains a little more iron. It will be seen that the addition of a little hot water to Apollinaris makes it practically identical with the Neuenahr water.

This water is exported in bottles on a very large scale; about thirty million bottles, we are informed, are filled annually! For the purpose of enabling the water of the Apollinaris spring to be efficiently bottled to meet this enormous demand, without waste of time, and to prevent disturbance of the spring at its source, by an uneven method of pumping, the water is allowed to flow from the spring into tanks, from which it is drawn into cylinders; there it is re-combined with the carbonic acid, which has, meanwhile, been collected from the spring. A small proportion of common salt (one part per thousand parts) is added to prevent the reducing action of the organic matter of the cork on the sodium sulphate in the water.

Before this plan was adopted there was a risk of sulphuretted hydrogen forming in the bottled water. The bottled Apollinaris therefore contains *one per mille* more sodium chloride than at its source. The most minute care is taken, in all the details of bottling, to preserve the natural properties of the water.

Ashby-de-la-Zouch, a *cold salt* bath in Leicestershire, about three hours from London, is a town of about 5,000 inhabitants, at an elevation of 400 feet above the sea. Its chloride of sodium waters are moderately strong, and of a temperature of 62° F. It is said to be of about the same strength as sea water. It contains about 26·5 grammes of solids per litre, the chief of which is sodium chloride (18·7). Next in amount are calcium sulphate (2·5), and chloride of calcium and magnesium; there are small amounts of potassium chloride, carbonate of iron (0·05), lime, and manganese, bromide of magnesium, sulphate of alumina and silica. It also contains a small amount of dissolved carbonic acid and nitrogen (Paul, 1888). There is a small but well-equipped bath establishment standing in its own grounds, which are well laid out, and in which archery, tennis, and bowling can be carried on. There are six bath-rooms in each wing of the building, with drying-rooms and provision also for shower and needle baths and douches. It is heated throughout by steam, and so is the water for the baths, which are given at temperatures varying from 62° (the natural temperature of the water) up to 110° F.

Dr. Williams, consulting physician to the Bath Company, and medical officer of health, states that benefit follows treatment with these baths in the following maladies: gout, muscular rheumatism, sciatica, and chronic rheumatic joint affections; osteo-arthritis; scrofula; certain chronic skin diseases, as eczema, psoriasis, acne, etc. These are treated by internal as well as external administration of the water. In cases of debility and neuralgia, the internal use of the water seems to be serviceable as an iron tonic.

Askern Spa.—A *cold sulphur* bath in the West Riding of Yorkshire at an altitude of 25 feet, and about six miles to the north of Doncaster; four hours by rail from London. There are four wells, each containing sulphuretted hydrogen in varying amounts. The richest has about 3·5 cubic inches to a litre of water. They are feebly mineralised, for they contain only two grammes of solids per litre, consisting chiefly of calcium carbonate and calcium and magnesium sulphates; small amounts of sodium chloride and sulphate are also present. They are highly charged with organic matter derived from the peat, and have a yellowish aspect. "The village stands on the edge of an extensive plain, a large part of which is uncultivated and imperfectly drained peat bog."

Mr. Bothamly, F.C.S. (*Trans. Chemical Society*, 1893, p. 685), attributes the presence of H_2S to reduction of sulphates brought about in some hitherto undetermined way. Each of the four springs has a pump-room and set of baths attached to it, and in most the water is raised by means of steam to the temperature desired. Besides the baths the patients are directed to drink the waters cold in doses of eight ounces twice or thrice daily. They usually have a diuretic action, and are sometimes laxative.

The diseases treated at Askern with benefit are subacute and chronic gouty states; rheumatic and rheumatoid affections, especially when attended with pain and stiffness of joints; certain chronic skin diseases, *e.g.* eczema, psoriasis, pityriasis; some forms of dyspepsia, and liver troubles.

Ax les Thermes (Ariège), a rising and important Pyrenean Spa, containing a vast number of *sulphur* and other thermal springs, admitting of a great variety of applications. It lies between the Central Pyrenees and the Pyrénées Orientales on a branch line, 122 kilometres south of Toulouse and fourteen hours by express train from Paris. It is situated in a mountainous and picturesque country at an elevation of about 2,300 feet, and at the confluence of three mountain streams. Its climate is tonic and strengthening. As many as sixty springs are utilised in four bath establishments possessing every modern appliance. Their temperature varies from 65° to 170° F. They are used undiluted, and arranged in a graduated series, according to their activity. Some of these springs are, next to Luchon, the richest in sulphuretted hydrogen of the Pyrenean spas. Sodium sulphide is the characteristic ingredient of the majority, together with sodium silicate and a little sodium chloride. Some contain much nitrogen, no organic matter, and are of feeble alkalinity; others are alkaline and rich in *barégine*.

It is usual, for certain cases, to add to the baths some chlorides in the form of *eaux mères* or salts from *eaux mères*. What is known as the "degenerated waters" are those in which the sodium sulphide has undergone conversion into sulphate and hyposulphite, and so become changed from sulphur waters into simple, slightly alkaline thermal waters. These are regarded as having a sedative effect, while the sodium sulphide springs are stimulating.

The reputation of the waters of Ax is ancient, and it possesses a "lepers' bath," said to have existed since the reign of St. Louis (A.D. 1260).

The waters are both drunk and used as baths and douches. Gouty arthritis is especially treated by the sedative desulphurated water. The treatment at Ax can be so graduated as to extend from the mildest to the most energetic form, as desired by the medical attendant.

Painful joint affections and neuralgias, rheumatic and gouty, are specially treated at Ax. In the next order come scrofulous and superficial tubercular affections, some chronic skin diseases—certain anæmics, intolerant of iron, do well there. Chronic malarial cachexia, traumatisms, lead and other poisonings, chronic syphilis, uterine catarrh, chronic catarrhal affections of the respiratory organs, some neuropathic and neurasthenic cases, complete the list of patients claimed by Ax.

June, July, August, and September are the best months for treatment, but one of the establishments is open all the year. There is a civil hospital there with 120 beds. Many interesting excursions can be made into the mountainous district around.

Abano, in N. Italy, a few miles from Padua, on the line between it and Bologna. A highly *thermal* (temperature of hottest spring, 183° F.), somewhat feebly mineralised (6·5 grammes of solids per litre) *salt* bath with traces of free sulphuretted hydrogen; also utilises for local applications a *fango* or "mud," rich in organic substance, and saturated with the hot mineral water. Spring well known to the Romans (Aquæ Patavinæ).

The mineral ingredients consist of sodium (3·8) and magnesium (0·20) chloride, some calcium sulphate, a minute quantity of iodide of magnesium (0·02), and traces of H_2S.

The remedial agents employed are baths, inhalations of gases from springs, and local applications of *fango*. The diseases treated are chronic rheumatism and gouty affections, rheumatoid arthritis and surgical diseases of joints, skin affections, and certain forms of chronic paralysis. The season is from June 1 to Sept. 30.

Acquarossa possesses gaseous *chalybeate* springs, containing a large amount of calcium sulphate and carbonate, a small quantity of manganese, and minute amounts of arsenic and lithium. The temperature of this water is 77° F. A mineral mud is also deposited from this spring, which is said to be very rich in arsenic.

It is situated in Switzerland, on the Italian side of the St. Gothard mountains, and is approached from Biasca, a station on the St. Gothard line, from which it is an hour and a-half's drive. It can also be reached from Dissentis by the Lukmanier Pass. It is situated in the Val Blenio, at an elevation of 1,150 feet, and is surrounded by high mountains.

The amount of bicarbonate of iron per litre is 0·034 gramme; of manganese 0·019; and of arsenate of lime 0·00024; of chloride of lithium 0·0046; of borate of magnesia 0·0025. It is considered of value in anæmia, in scrofula, and in skin diseases. Together with climatic influences it is found restorative after acute illnesses; it is recommended also in glandular enlargements, scrofulous and syphilitic. In some obstinate skin affections the warmed mud is applied with benefit.

Acqui, in N. Italy, on the line between Alessandria and Savona, and 21 miles from the former place, has many feebly mineralised (1·5 gramme of sodium chloride per litre) but *very hot salt* springs, containing also free H_2S—La Bollende has a temperature of 158° F.—also a *fango* or mud, which contains much organic matter, is largely used, mixed with the salts of the mineral springs. Its application and virtues form the speciality of Acqui.

It has an altitude of 650 feet, and a climate which is moist and variable and very hot in summer.

The cases treated there are rheumatic, gouty, and traumatic joint affections, certain diseases of the skin, and certain neuroses, cases of chronic metallic poisoning (lead and mercury), and some forms of syphilis.

The season is from May 15 to Sept. 30.

Æsculap, an imported Hungarian "bitter" water, containing the aperient sodium and magnesium sulphates (31·1), and sodium chloride (2·9) and calcium sulphate (2·0 per mille).

Aibling, in Upper Bavaria, pleasantly situated at an elevation of 1,500 feet, a few miles from Rosenheim, has a speciality for the application of *mud*-baths—from the Aibling high moors—and the brine and *Mutter-lauge* respectively from Rosenheim and Reichenhall. The *mutter-lauge* is added to water, mud, and pine-needle baths.

Maladies treated there are chronic rheumatic and scrofulous exudations, rickets, chronic pelvic inflammations and deposits, and some forms of paralysis. Season, May 1 to Sept. 30.

Aigle les Bains, a hydropathic establishment (1,750 feet above the sea) about a mile from Aigle Station, on the Rhone Valley Railway. The water (similar to Evian water) is artificially charged with carbonic acid and drunk as a table water in stomach, renal, and bladder affections.

Aix en Provence, 30 kilometres north of Marseilles (line to Grenoble), elevation 590 feet, has *simple thermal* springs, the hottest 90° F. The baths are given with running water (*eau courante*), so that this temperature is maintained in them. The mineralisation is very feeble.

They are regarded as sedative baths, and are applied in cases of neurasthenia, rheumatism, neuralgia, stiff joints, and some skin and uterine affections.

Alet, a small French resort in the Department of Aude, 650 feet above the sea. It has *simple thermal* waters of very feeble mineralisation, chiefly of bicarbonate and phosphate of lime (0·520 in the litre). Temperature 86° F. It also has a cold iron spring (0·024 of oxide of iron). These waters do not contain free carbonic acid gas, and are therefore thought valuable to those whose stomachs cannot tolerate aërated waters. They are exported as table waters. There is a bath establishment for baths and douches.

Anæmic and chlorotic cases are treated with this iron spring. Other cases benefited by these waters are those of gastric irritability and painful digestion, flatulence, habitual vomiting, intestinal catarrh, dysentery, and the dyspepsia of convalescents from acute disease. They are given in moderate doses before meals, and sometimes mixed with wine.

It has a station, Limoux, distant 9 kilometres, on the line between Carcassonne and Quillan. It is a twenty-four hours' journey from Paris. At that distance from Paris and in a region so far south, and therefore so hot in the summer, it is naturally not much resorted to except by those in the locality.

The season is from June 1 to Nov. 1, but the bath is open all the year.

Alexandersbad, a *chalybeate*, highly gaseous spring (0·06 bicarbonate of iron) in Bavaria, lies on the north-eastern slope of the Luisenberg (Fichtelgebirge) at an elevation of 1,900 feet, surrounded by pine woods. The nearest stations are Markt-Redwitz on the Berlin-Munich Railway, and Wunsiedel. Besides drinking and bathing in the gaseous iron water, ferruginous mud baths are used, also pine-needle baths, and the usual methods of hydrotherapy. It is resorted to by cases of anæmia and chlorosis. There is also a sanatorium for nervous patients. It is not very far from Eger, and can therefore be conveniently visited as an "after-cure" by patients from Marienbad, Carlsbad, or Franzensbad.

Season, from June 15 to beginning of October.

Alexisbad (Germany), in the Selkethal, a valley of the Harz Mountains, 1,080 feet above the sea, has a *chalybeate* spring, to which carbonic acid is added for exportation. Pine-needle baths and artificial salt baths are also available there. It is resorted to also for its fresh forest air. It is a two hours' drive from the railway station of Gernrode.

Season, June 15 to Sept. 25.

Alvaneubad, a *cold sulphur* bath on the well-known Albula road to Davos and the Engadine. It is about midway between Coire and Davos, at an elevation of 3,150 feet. The spring is feebly mineralised (1·338 of salts), but contains a small amount of free H_2S and carbonic acid gas. The salts consist of alkaline and earthy sulphates, sodium chloride, magnesium carbonate, alumina, silica, and a very small amount of iron.

The sub-alpine climate is favourable to exercise, and the surrounding neighbourhood affords many interesting excursions. The water is prescribed internally in doses of four to eight glasses a day, and acts as a diuretic and laxative.

For the baths it is heated to 90° or 95° F., and they are often prolonged to an hour or longer in some cases. Douches, vapour baths, and fumigations are also employed. They are used in the same cases as other sulphur baths: chronic muscular and articular rheumatism and gout, skin diseases, especially eczema, chronic catarrhs of the respiratory and other organs, urinary gravel, some chronic affections of the female pelvic organs, anæmia, and general debility; in the latter the tonic climate counts for much. The season is from June 15 to Sept. 15.

Amphion les Bains. *See* Évian.

Andabre, in the department of Aveyron, France, has gaseous springs containing both bicarbonate of soda and bicarbonate of iron. It is a two hours' drive from the station St. Affrique, the terminus of a branch from the line between Clermont and Béziers. Its altitude is about 1,300 feet.

Its principal spring, La Buvette, has a mineralisation of 2·5 grammes per litre, of which 1·80 is formed of sodium bicarbonate, and 0·065 of bicarbonate of iron; the other ingredients are magnesium and calcium bicarbonates and small amounts of chlorides.

This water is used in baths and douches as well as drunk; it is also exported. It is adapted to the treatment of anæmic dyspeptics, chlorosis, and retarded convalescence.

Andeer-Pignieu, a Swiss resort, at an elevation of 3,200 feet, on the Splügen road, about three hours' drive from Thusis, which has a weakly mineralised *calcium sulphate* spring, arising at Pignieu and conducted to the bath establishment at Andeer. It contains 1·734 grammes of calcium sulphate in a litre, and 0·189 of calcium bicarbonate, 0·320 magnesium sulphate with smaller quantities of alkaline sulphates and a minute amount of iron. A ferruginous, vegeto-mineral *mud* is also utilised. The waters are drunk, and have a decidedly diuretic action. The dose is from two to five glasses daily. Douches are also given, and the water is inhaled in chronic catarrh of the pharynx and larynx.

The *mud* baths are made by mixing the mud with the water and heating the mixture by steam to 104° F. The bath lasts from thirty to forty minutes. The patient afterwards has a cleansing bath of water and a period of repose. The mud is also sometimes applied locally as a poultice, as hot as possible. Andeer is rather exposed to winds, and is distinctly bracing.

The mineral water is given in catarrhs of the respiratory organs, in pleural exudations, and in chronic cystitis. Chronic rheumatic and gouty affections, certain skin affections, chronic inflammatory exudations connected with the female pelvic organs, are treated with *mud* baths also. The season is from the middle of June to the end of September.

Antogast, a Black Forest resort with *gaseous chalybeate* springs; one of the "Kniebis Spas" in Baden. It is reached in half an hour's drive from the station of Oppenau. It has an elevation of 1,600 feet, and is surrounded by pine-clad mountains over 3,000 feet in height. It has three springs containing iron (bicarbonate of iron 0·04), together with the alkaline bicarbonates of sodium, magnesium, and calcium, a small amount of sodium sulphate, and free carbonic acid. The waters are drunk and used as baths; and as accessories "*mud ooze*" baths, pine resin baths, and brine baths are given, and the milk cure is also prescribed to some of the patients. The bottled water is exported. These springs have a reputation dating back to the middle ages. They are prescribed in stomach and intestinal complaints, in functional affections of the liver and kidneys, and in anæmia and certain diseases of women. Season, May to October.

Archena, a *hot sulphur* spring (temperature 131° F.) in the province of Murcia, Spain.

Argelès-Gazost, a *cold sulphur* water in the Hautes Pyrénées, conducted from Gazost to Argelès, a distance of ten miles. The springs are feebly mineralised, the strongest (Source Noire) containing 0·03 grammes of sodium and calcium sulphates to the litre, a small amount of sodium chloride (0·38), and, it is said, a small quantity of alkaline bromides and iodides. These waters are drunk, used as baths and douches, and inhaled in pulverisation. They are regarded as more sedative and less exciting than the *hot* sulphur springs. They are used in cases of chronic catarrh of the respiratory passages and in some female pelvic affections where sedative treatment is required, and in some skin diseases. These waters are exported. There is a suitable bath establishment, and good accommodation for visitors. The season is from June 1 to Sept. 30.

Argelès is beautifully situated and a charming resort on the line between Lourdes and Pierrefitte, 54 kilometres from Pau. It is surrounded by high mountains, which protect it from winds and assure it a mild winter climate; but it is *very hot* in summer.

Arnstadt, at the northern border of the Thuringian Forest, has a strong *common salt* spring used for bathing, and a milder one for drinking. Diseases treated there are scrofula, rickets, female pelvic maladies, etc. Season, April to end of September.

Assmannshausen, a pleasant Rhenish resort on the right bank of the river at the foot of the Neiderwald, has a weakly mineralised *warm muriated alkaline* spring (temperature 82·8° F.), having only 1 gramme of salts to the litre—sodium chloride, carbonate, etc. It is claimed for this spring that, owing to a small amount of *lithium* bicarbonate (0·028) contained in it, it is of much value in cases of gout, muscular rheumatism, chronic gastric and intestinal catarrh; functional renal and vesical affections and chronic catarrh of the respiratory passages are also treated there. The quiet, pleasant life, in picturesque surroundings, combined with the ingestion of much solvent tepid, though feebly mineralised, water, is calculated to be useful to sufferers from those maladies. Season, May 15 to Sept. 15.

Audinac, a warm (70° F.) calcareous earthy spring, containing a little iron, of no great importance, in the Pyrenees, about three miles from St. Girons Railway Station.

Auerbach, an agreeable summer resort, half an hour from Darmstadt, Grand Duchy of Hesse, has weak earthy mineral waters used as baths.

Augustusbad, a *chalybeate* spa in Saxony, an hour from Dresden, about half an hour from the railway station of Radeberg; has also a hydropathic establishment. It has an elevation of 718 feet. The chief constituent of the springs is protocarbonate of iron. Two of these are charged artificially with carbonic acid gas and used for drinking, the others are utilised for baths, inhalations, and gargling; *mud* (from the neighbourhood) baths and artificial carbonic acid baths are also employed. These remedial agents are applied in cases of anæmia, chlorosis, debility, rickets, digestive disturbances, some forms of cardiac disease, and female maladies. Season, May 1 to Sept. 30.

Aulus (Ariège, Pyrenees), reached by rail from Paris to Toulouse and Toulouse to St. Girons, then eighteen miles by carriage; it is situated in a valley about 2,400 feet above the sea, surrounded by high mountains. There are many charming excursions and mountain ascensions to be made there. The waters are of a temperature of 68° to 55° F., and contain *sulphate of lime* chiefly, a smaller proportion of sulphate of magnesia and chloride of sodium, small quantities of iron, manganese, and a trace of arsenic. The total mineralisation is about 2·8 grammes to a litre, of which 1·86 is sulphate of lime. It resembles the Contrexéville springs and belongs to the same class of *earthy calcareous* waters. It is drunk and used as baths and douches. It is also largely exported. These waters are said to be useful in debility of the stomach and intestines, with constipation, in vesical catarrh, anæmia, and chlorosis, and to exercise a specific effect in cases of inveterate syphilis. Their action is laxative and diuretic, and through their eliminative properties they may be regarded, in some cases, as tonic and anti-syphilitic.

As at Contrexéville, this cure is also indicated in uric acid, oxalic and phosphatic gravel. It is said to especially improve the abdominal circulation, and so to relieve hæmorrhoids and enlargements of the liver. There are two well-appointed establishments. The season is from June 1 to Oct. 1.

Aussee (Styria), 2,145 feet above the sea, is a popular Austrian watering-place in the Salzkammergut, about twenty miles by rail from Ischl. It is beautifully situated on the Traun, in the midst of charming mountain and lake scenery, and has extensive salt works, *salt baths*, whey cure, hydropathic establishment, etc. The season is from May 15 to Oct. 1.

Auteuil, a suburb of Paris, having a cold *chalybeate* spring and a bathing establishment. The iron is in the form of a compound sulphate of alumina and iron (0·71 grammes in a litre). It also contains calcium sulphate (1·70), sulphates of magnesia and soda (0·39), and traces of arsenic. The water is exported. It is used for drinking, bathing, and douches in cases of anæmia, chlorosis, and debility.

Baden-Baden is a well-known and popular health and pleasure resort, situated in the Grand Duchy of Baden, in the northern part of the Black Forest, at an elevation of 650 feet. It is reached by a short branch line from Oos, a station on the main line between Frankfort and Bâle. From London the most direct route is viâ Cologne and the Rhine, from Paris viâ Strasburg.

The situation of Baden-Baden is most picturesque and one of great natural beauty, surrounded as it is by forest-clad mountains, with pine trees of noble growth and magnitude, and presenting shady walks and drives of almost endless variety and distance, while the gardens and pleasure grounds of the town itself are laid out with remarkable skill and attractiveness. The hotel and other accommodation probably exceeds in comfort and luxury that of any other town in Europe, and amusements and distractions of all kinds are provided.

The climate is mild and sedative and the air still, on account of the height of the encircling hills, but it is somewhat humid. The mean annual temperature is from 48° to 50° F. It has an early spring and a protracted summer.

The number and attractiveness of the excursions

to be made from Baden-Baden into the adjacent regions of the Black Forest make it an admirable centre for exploring the northern part of that beautiful district.

The springs of Baden-Baden are *hot weak sodium chloride* springs, of which there are a great number—more than twenty—almost alike in composition and differing only in temperature (from 112° to 154° F.). They belong to the State, but some are leased to private hotels.

Their mineralisation is feeble, 2·7 grammes of solids per litre, of which, in the spring chiefly used for drinking, the Hauptstallenquelle, there are 2·0 of sodium chloride, 0·16 each of calcium chloride and carbonate, 0·053 of *lithium* chloride, and 0·0007 of *arsenate* of lime.

It is maintained that these minute amounts of lithium and arsenic are of importance in the treatment of gouty and cutaneous diseases, but this is at least doubtful.

The affinities of these feebly mineralised springs are clearly rather with the class of indifferent thermal waters.

The hottest spring and the one giving the largest outflow is the Ursprung. This has a temperature of 154° F. The springs have to be cooled, sometimes by the addition of common water, before they can be used for baths, inhalations, gargling, etc.

Drinking is rather secondary to bathing there, and it is often thought desirable to fortify the waters, when they are drunk, with other salts, such as those of Marienbad or Carlsbad, in order to render them somewhat aperient.

The bathing establishments are of the most luxurious and elaborate description — quite monumental edifices. The chief of them are the Friedrichsbad and the Kaiserin-Augustabad (for ladies only). Every kind of bath can be had in these institutions. Salt is often added to the ordinary thermal bath; what is known there as *Wildbad* is a bath with running water, so that the temperature is kept constant all the time; there are also vapour baths of the vapour of the natural springs (especially the Ursprung); hot air baths, general and local; mud baths made with the *fango* of Battaglia; electric baths; and all kinds of douches. A very complete installation of the Zander appliances for Swedish gymnastics exists at the Friedrichsbad. There are also arrangements for applying the Wassmuth and other methods of inhalation. All the methods of hydrotherapy can be carried out at Baden-Baden, and, at the proper seasons, the grape and milk cures. Compressed air chambers are also at the service of invalids suffering from chronic pulmonary affections, especially emphysema and bronchial catarrh.

Suitable walks have been marked out, for many years, for the application of the "Terrain-kur" for obese persons with cardiac feebleness; but this *very risky* method of treatment of chronic cardiac affections, risky owing to the inherent difficulty in diagnosing the precise conditions of the cardiac muscle in such cases, has rightly fallen into disuse.

As already stated, some of the hotels have thermal baths belonging to them, so that invalids can conveniently bathe without leaving their hotel. There is a State bath-house for the poor, the Landesbad, and there are several private sanatoria. Indeed, Baden-Baden, like Wiesbaden, is a sort of invalid's compendium, where various kinds of physical and other treatments can be applied in addition to the treatment by the thermal waters.

Finally, as to the cases suitable for treatment at Baden, first in order are rheumatic, gouty, and other affections of the joints; then *functional* disorders of the nervous system, hysteria, and other neuroses; loss of muscular power and certain forms of paralysis; the consequences of injuries to bones and joints; those chronic skin affections which are benefited by maceration in thermal water, or such as are associated with the gouty diathesis; catarrhal dyspepsia in feeble, nervous subjects; chronic catarrhs of the respiratory passages; and convalescents from malaria and other infective disorders.

The bathing establishments are open all the year round, but the best season for treatment is from May 1st to the end of October. It is sometimes very hot in July and August.

Baden, in Austria, a few miles from Vienna (one hour by train), is a *thermal sulphur* bath, and is highly popular with the Viennese as a summer resort. It is agreeably situated at an elevation of 700 feet at the entrance of the Helmenthal. The sulphur springs are of a temperature varying from 80° to 95° F., and they are used more for bathing than for drinking. Calcium sulphide is the characteristic ingredient, of which salt there is about 0·02 per litre. Besides thermal swimming baths there are *mud* baths (full baths and local baths) and the ordinary separate baths. The usual methods of hydrotherapy are also applied. The cases treated at this spa are chronic gouty and rheumatic joint affections, muscular rheumatism, and scrofulous affections of the glands, bones, joints, and skin. The thermal water, mixed with milk or whey, or some other mineral water, is sometimes prescribed in catarrhal affections of the gastro-intestinal and respiratory organs.

The baths are open all the year, but from May 15 to Oct. 15 is the best season for treatment. The hotel accommodation is good.

Baden, in Switzerland (canton Aargau), is a *thermal* bath on the line of rail between Bâle and Zürich, and only twenty-one kilometres from the latter town. It was known to the Romans as Aqua Helvetia. It is situated on the banks of the river Limmat at an altitude of 1,230 feet. It is in a picturesque, sheltered situation, surrounded by mountains and forests, and having a mild climate.

The waters, which spring from many different sources on both banks of the river, though smelling slightly of sulphuretted hydrogen, contain very little of that gas. Its total mineralisation is 4·0 grammes per litre, of which the largest portion is sodium sulphate (1·80) and calcium chloride (1·34); the remaining constituents being magnesium bicarbonate (0·35), sodium chloride (0·34), potassium sulphate (0·12), lithium chloride (0·02). Borates and a minute amount of arsenic have been found in these springs. Others regard them as containing a predominating proportion of calcium sulphate. But the published analyses have not always been in agreement with one another, and it is probable that certain variations in the composition of some of the springs occur from time to time. Their temperature varies from 100° to 120° F. The thermal water is chiefly used for baths, and drinking the water is quite subordinate to its external use. The water when drunk is often mixed with the laxative Birmenstorf water found in the neighbourhood. It is a great convenience to patients that the baths are to be found installed in the different hotels, and there is no separate bath establishment except a bath-house for indigent patients. Very prolonged baths used to be prescribed there, but now they are rarely ordered for longer than one hour.

The cases which are considered suitable for treatment at Baden are rheumatic joint affections, rheumatoid arthritis, atonic forms of chronic gout, traumatic stiff joints, neuralgia, sciatica, peripheral paralysis, lead poisoning, hæmorrhoidal affections, and certain affections of the female pelvic organs associated with abdominal plethora and of rheumatic origin.

The baths are usually taken in the early morning before breakfast, and sometimes, in order to increase the stimulating effect, they are fortified by the addition of salt from the neighbouring salt baths at Rheinfelden. Massage is freely applied, especially in cases of sciatica and lumbago. Chronic catarrh of the respiratory passages, when associated with gouty and rheumatic tendencies, is treated by inhalations of the water. The season is from May 15 to the end of September. A "terrain cure" can be carried out in the neighbourhood, if desired.

Baden possesses a casino situated in a tastefully laid-out park, and furnished with a theatre and convenient salons for the use of visitors.

Badenweiler, in the southern part of the Black Forest, has springs belonging to the class of *simple thermal* waters. The hottest of the springs has a temperature of only 80° F., and it is very feebly mineralised, having only 0·35 of solids per litre. These are reported to consist of sodium sulphate, calcium carbonate, and lithium chloride. The water is also said to contain much free nitrogen. There are large bathing pools, including the "marble bath," open to the air, in which the water is of the natural temperature, but for separate baths it has its temperature raised. There are remains of *thermæ,* which show that the Romans utilised these springs, The baths are used for their sedative properties, and if a more stimulating effect is desired, they are fortified by the addition of common salt, or *mother-lye* from some *Soolbad,* or other medicinal material. Vapour baths and mud baths—the mud being brought from Kaiserslautern—are also given there.

The cases sent to Badenweiler for treatment are those of neurasthenia, chronic gout and rheumatism in irritable and nervous constitutions, chronic neuralgia, convalescents from acute disease, and persons suffering from over-work and over-excitement.

Badenweiler is often prescribed as a climatic resort and *after-cure* for persons who have been taking more active mineral cures. It is well suited for this purpose by its beautiful and attractive situation at an altitude of 1,400 feet, in the midst of pine forests, and sheltered by a semicircle of mountains from all but westerly winds. It is often, on account of its equable, mild climate, recommended as a spring or winter resort for pulmonary invalids. There is a more bracing resort at hand—the "Haus-Baden"—at an elevation of 1,750 feet.

The ground on some of the surrounding slopes has been marked out for the "Terrain-kur." Good accommodation can be obtained both in hotels and private houses.

The nearest railway station is Mulheim, on the line between Frankfort and Bâle, from which Badenweiler is a short drive. The chief season is from May to October, but it has also a winter season.

Bagnères-de-Bigorre (Hautes Pyrénées) is a pretty little town of about 12,000 inhabitants, beautifully situated near the entrance to one of the most celebrated valleys of the Pyrenees. It has *earthy indifferent thermal* springs — some are reported to contain iron and arsenic—and also sulphur waters, which are imported from the neighbourhood. The sulphate of lime springs, however, are the *characteristic* waters of the place. Its baths were certainly known and esteemed by the Romans, and in the sixteenth century it was one of the most famous rendezvous of the Southern nobility. Montaigne describes it as at that time one of the best places he had discovered *de se laver le corps tous les jours* (*!*), on account of its agreeable situation, its comfortable quarters, good food, and good company.

It has two bath establishments, in which all the appliances are provided for baths, douches, vapour baths with massage, pulverisation, inhalation, gargling, etc. Its numerous springs are feebly mineralised, and of a temperature varying from 88° to 122° F.—the Source Salies is the hottest—and do not contain sulphur, a very exceptional circumstance in the Pyrenean springs. Their chief constituent is *calcium sulphate*, 1·80 grammes per litre. Some of these springs contain a little iron, *e.g.* La Reine contains, it is said, 0·08 of carbonate of iron. Some of the other cold springs are said to contain rather more iron, as well as sodium *arsenate*. The water of a *sulphur* spring eight miles off, at Labassère, is brought to Bagnères in covered vessels. It contains sodium sulphide 0·046, sodium chloride 0·20, and barégine 0·14.

These waters are used as baths and internally, and are thought to be especially valuable in cases of hyperæsthesia, in excited and feeble nervous systems; in such cases they are reported to produce remarkable calming and sedative effects. They are, in consequence, much resorted to by delicate ladies with hysterical and other disturbed conditions of the nervous system. Daily immersion for some time in thermal water has, no doubt, in many cases, a very soothing effect, and this influence must be aided and augmented by the calm, unexciting life, the mild mountain climate, and the agreeable surrounding scenery. The different *sources* employed there have, however, somewhat different indications. The Labassère sulphur water, in combination with the Salies spring, is used for catarrhal affections of the throat and respiratory passages, for torpid forms of rheumatism, and for eczematous, moist skin affections; but the dominant indication at Bagnères-de-Bigorre is neurasthenia—arthritic, cutaneous, uterine, gastro-intestinal, and anæmic states *in the neurotic*—including cases of over-work and insomnia.

The town lies at an elevation of 1,800 feet above the sea, on the Adour, in a charming situation, near the opening of the valley of Campan, and overlooking the rich plain of Tarbes (distant eighteen hours by rail from Paris). It is not *in* the mountains, like many of the other Pyrenean spas, but is situated just where the lesser elevations begin to rise from the plains. It is amongst the outposts of the great central chain. Its pleasant climate and attractive scenery, and its accessibility by railway, make it a much frequented resort of the permanent winter residents at Pau, anxious to escape the great summer heat of that town.

Bagnères-de-Bigorre is rich in Roman remains. "The Romans," says M. Taine, "a people as civilised and as bored as we are, came as we do to Bagnères. Rome has left her traces everywhere at Bagnères. The pleasantest of these relics of antiquity are the monuments which the patients who were cured there erected to the Nymphs, and the inscriptions upon which still exist. Reclining in their marble baths, they felt the healing virtue of the beneficent goddess spread through their limbs; their eyes half-closed, dozing in the soft embrace of the tepid water, they heard the mysterious spring falling drop by drop, in monotonous chant, from the bosom of its mother rock; they saw the surface of the effused water glisten around them with its pale green ripples; and there passed before them, like a vision, the strange look and the magic voice of the unknown divinity who visited the light in order to bring health to unhappy mortals."

Many highly attractive and interesting excursions can be made into the beautiful surrounding neighbourhood. The season is from June 15 to Oct. 1.

Bagnoles de l'Orne, a very feebly mineralised warm bath, which may be referred to the class of *simple thermal* waters, or *indeterminate* waters of French authors, is situated at an elevation of 750 feet above the sea in a well-wooded and picturesque part of Normandy termed La Suisse Normande, and its waters are specially applied to the treatment of inflammation of the veins, the various forms of phlebitis and their consequences. It has a station on a branch of the line between Paris and Granville, and is about five hours from Paris. It is the only important thermal bath in the west of France.

Its thermal spring, called La Grande Source, has a temperature of about 80° F., and is the one generally used, but it has also a *cold weak chalybeate* spring. The Grande Source is *very* feebly mineralised, having only ·0625 grammes of dry solids to the litre, and this is composed of sodium chloride (·0161) and sulphate (·0128), small quantities of silica and of bicarbonate of lime and iron. It has a peculiar unctuous feeling, which is referred to the presence of silicates and to a small amount of organic matter. It gives off gases composed mainly of carbonic acid and nitrogen with traces of *argon* and *helium*. It has a faint odour of sulphuretted hydrogen. The cold ferruginous spring has the same composition as the Grand Source, plus a little oxide of iron. Internally both these springs are used—the iron spring is often bottled and drunk as a table water at meals. For external use the Grande Source alone is used. Its temperature is increased by the addition of some of the mineral water heated in a closed vessel.

The special treatment at Bagnoles consists in drinking the Grande Source and bathing in *tepid* baths, but the fundamental part of the treatment is the bathing, associated with suitable, properly adapted movements, and massage. This is believed to act, first, by rousing and promoting the peripheral circulation by removing capillary and venous stasis, secondly, by stimulating vascular and visceral tone, and thirdly, by a sedative effect on the nervous system. Hence the value of the treatment in cases of diseases of the veins and especially of rheumatic phlebitis, as well as in the removal of the consequences of other forms of phlebitis such as the puerperal form; it is also of value in painful and congested varices, and it checks the tendency to recurrence in gouty phlebitis. In all affections of the peripheral circulation it is valuable. It is also recommended in convalescence from acute rheumatism, and is said to promote the retrogression of recent affections of the cardiac valves.

In other maladies in the neuro-arthritic it has been found of use, as in dysmenorrhœa, amenorrhœa, certain forms of metritis, in some atonic and gastralgic dyspepsias, and in some languid skin affections, particularly eczema and varicose ulcerations. Finally, excitable neurotics are benefited by the sedative baths and the mildly tonic forest climate. Caution must, of course, be observed so as not to send to Bagnoles cases of phlebitis in the acute febrile stage, or when there is still risk of embolism. "The cure of the consequences of attacks of phlebitis is," says Dr. Barrabé, "the triumph of our bathing station." He maintains that the water has a *special* vaso-constricting action on the smooth muscular fibre of the small vessels. The hotels are good and the charges moderate. The season is from June 1st to Oct. 1st.

Balaruc is a *thermal common salt* bath situated six miles from the Mediterranean port of Cette, from which town it is separated by the salt "Etang de Thau." It is from fourteen and a-half to seventeen hours from Paris by express train. Owing to its adjacency to the sea it combines the properties of a thermal salt spring with those of a maritime climate. It is, of course, very hot in summer.

It has three springs, the hottest of which (La Source Ancienne or Romaine) has a temperature of 118° F. Besides chloride of sodium (7·045 grammes per litre), magnesium (0·889), lithium (0·007), and copper (0·007), traces of bromides and nitrates are present, and some free nitrogen and carbonic acid gases. A colder spring (Bidon) is used to lower the temperature of the preceding. As the amount of chlorides in this water is not very great it can be taken internally with advantage, and, according to the dose, acts as a purgative, laxative, or alterative; it is said to exert at the same time a tonic effect. Externally as baths it exerts a stimulating action on the skin and peripheral nerves and promotes the superficial circulation.

It is administered as *local baths* (foot bath), as *general douches* to produce a stimulating effect on the nervous and circulatory systems, and as *local douches* to stimulate a particular region or organ. It is used also as a lotion (ophthalmias, ulcers), as injections in scrofulous affections (fistulæ), and for gargling. *Mud* from l'Etang, treated with the thermal water, is also used locally, and is found to be a very energetic stimulant.

The diseases especially treated at Balaruc are torpid diseases (paralysis) of the nervous system, scrofulous affections, rheumatism, uterine affections in the lymphatic and scrofulous—the use of the baths and uterine douches, together with the applications of the mineral mud, are reported to produce remarkable results in uterine fibromata. The water is used to promote healing in torpid traumatic conditions. Its application to paralytic states is limited to the period when all the acute symptoms have passed away, but must not be deferred until the case has become very chronic, when it is useless.

Owing to its nearness to large towns like Cette and Montpellier, living is commodious and cheap. Season, from May 1st to Oct. 1st. It is as well to avoid the great heat of July and August.

Barèges (Hautes Pyrénées) can be reached from Bagnères-de-Bigorre by a very beautiful drive through the valley of Campan and over the Col de Tourmalet—the highest carriage-road in the Pyrenees, and one of the highest in Europe, being nearly 7,000 feet above the sea—but this would take five hours, and it is therefore usually approached from Luz. It takes nearly an hour and a-half to mount the four and a-half miles of gradual and continuous ascent which leads from Luz to Barèges. In traversing this short distance we pass from a region of smiling pastoral beauty, of green pastures and wooded slopes, to one of almost dreary desolation. Barèges, which is situated at an elevation of about 4,000 feet above the sea, is a little town in a barren situation presenting nothing that is attractive or picturesque. "The landscape," says M. Taine, "is hideous, it looks like a deserted quarry." The climate is very variable, great heat alternating frequently with sharp cold. Cold mists from the surrounding mountains often collect over the valley, and it is tormented by violent winds. It is uninhabitable for five months in the year, when it is covered with fifteen feet of snow. "Il faut avoir beaucoup de santé pour y guerir," M. Taine pleasantly remarks.

Notwithstanding the dreariness of its situation, its *thermal sulphur* baths enjoy a very great reputation for the cure of certain maladies: especially of wounds received in battle, of chronic articular rheumatism, of certain forms of scrofula, torpid varicose ulcers, and of all kinds of diseases of the bones and joints, as well as some forms of skin disease (as at Luchon), and certain local paralyses. It is *especially* in the cure of scrofulous affections of the bones, joints, glands, skin, and mucous membranes, and particularly of affections of the bones, that it has gained so great a reputation. This curative influence is referred to its stimulating action on the circulatory and nervous systems, in which no doubt the bracing mountain climate has a great share. Syphilis in its secondary and tertiary forms is largely treated here in combination with the use of specific remedies, as at Aix la Chapelle. Its sulphur springs are amongst the strongest in the Pyrenees, or rather they are the *least changeable*, and this is probably the reason of their greater activity; they contain sodium sulphide (0·04), chloride, and silicate, and are rich in that peculiar organic substance to which the name of *barégine* has been given. This is especially the case at Barzun, a *source* a quarter of a mile below Barèges. It gives to the water a particular *unctuosity*. A minute amount of sodium arsenate is said to exist in the Tambour spring.

There are fifteen springs at Barèges, varying in temperature from 86° to 112° F. The waters are taken internally, and are also used as baths and douches. The fine bath establishment, built of marble from the Pyrenees, contains a very complete equipment—baths, douches, vapour baths, foot baths, swimming baths, gargling and pulverisation rooms, etc. There is also a much smaller establishment at Barzun. It is usual to begin with the springs of lower temperature and increase gradually to the higher ones, the highest being the Tambour (112° F.). Local douches of this temperature are sometimes given. This spring (the Tambour) is the one chiefly used for drinking, and the water is given in quite small doses, often mixed with milk or whey. The season begins early in June, and the place becomes so crowded in July and August that patients have sometimes to wait their turns at Luz until they can be taken in. July, August, and September are the best months.

Owing to the repute these baths have always maintained for the cure of injuries received in the field of battle a State military hospital has existed there since 1760. The place also possesses a hospital for the reception of nuns and priests, which also, from Sept. 1st to Oct. 15th, receives poor patients who are kept there at the expense of their *département*.

It is from Barèges that the ascent of the Pic du Midi de Bigorre is usually made, one of the finest points of view in the Pyrenees. Although about 9,300 feet above the level of the sea, the summit can be reached on horseback, and in about three and a-half hours from Barèges. An observatory has been established there. A small hotel, where food and beds can be obtained, has been built on a *col* about 1,600 feet below the summit.

It is fourteen hours from Paris to Barèges—rail to Pierrefitte—electric railway from Pierrefitte to Luz.

Bath, a city in Somersetshire, about two hours by express train from London, owes its name to the possession of mineral springs which may be classed amongst the *simple indifferent thermal* baths, but which have also some relationship, by their composition, to the group of earthy calcareous waters, represented on the Continent by such spas as Contrexéville. Weber observes that the Bath springs are "the only really hot natural waters of Great Britain," but the springs of Buxton are *warm*, although, with a temperature of 82° F., they certainly cannot be called "hot."

The history of the Bath thermal waters extends back into a remote and uncertain past, but we know from monumental evidences of the most remarkable and interesting nature that under the name of Aquæ Sulis it was a place of great resort of the Roman conquerors of Britain. The very perfect, extensive, and remarkable remains of Roman *thermæ* discovered at Bath testify to the importance that was attached to these waters by the ancient Romans.

Since those remote times Bath has undergone some singular vicissitudes, but if, in the present day, it is not quite the same fashionable resort it was in the days of Beau Nash, it is certainly a far better equipped health resort than it was then or at any former period of its history; while its usefulness to suffering humanity has been enormously increased in recent times; for, of late years, its resources have been intelligently and enterprisingly developed so as to bring it up to the standard of the most advanced and most perfectly equipped of Continental spas.

The situation of this city is a picturesque and attractive one, and the protection afforded it by surrounding hills gives it a mild and equable climate. The mean summer temperature is 61·1° F., and the mean winter temperature 46·4° F.; but it has a rather high degree of *humidity*, for while the dry north-east winds are "largely intercepted by the surrounding hills," it is exposed to the moist south-west winds blowing from the Bristol Channel; "the absolute humidity is greatest from November to March and least from April to August." The average rainfall is 32·064 inches. "Autumn is the wettest, and spring the driest season. January, September, and October are the wettest months." The spring and autumn are said to be the best seasons for the cure, the months of April, May, September, and October; but the baths are open all the year round.

Bath has three hot springs which are utilised for bathing, etc.; they are alike in chemical constitution, but differ in temperature. The "hot bath" has a temperature of 120° F., the King's Bath of 117°, and the Cross Bath of 104°.

With regard to the constituents of the springs, they appear to contain about 2·6 grammes per litre of solid constituents; the chief of these is calcium sulphate (1·3), there are smaller amounts of sodium sulphate (0·3), of sodium and magnesium chloride (0·2 each), of potassium sulphate and calcium carbonate (0·1). There is a minute quantity of silica and carbonate of iron (0·018 of the latter).

Some importance is attached by certain of the local authorities to the amount of free gases contained in the water, especially the nitrogen; there is also a small amount of *helium* and of *argon* in this as in similar springs.

The water of these springs is administered both internally and externally, and there are several establishments where the treatment can be carried out.

(1) The King's and Queen's Public and Private Baths, adjoining the Grand Pump Room. Here the Aix les Bains douche-massage methods are applied, as well as the ordinary reclining baths, vapour baths, etc., etc.

(2) The Royal Private and Hot Baths. Here also there are private reclining and immersion baths, douches, etc., and a tepid swimming bath.

(3) The New Royal Private and Swimming Bath, attached to the Grand Pump Room Hotel. Here, again, are reclining and douche baths, needle douches, and a large swimming bath.

(4) The Cross Bath, which is a cheap public bath. These establishments belong to the Corporation.

For *internal* use there is a fountain in the Grand Pump Room, which has a continuous supply of mineral water, coming straight from the spring at a temperature of 114° F. When this water is cooled the iron is precipitated, and this cooled water is considered more suitable to certain cases than the hotter water with the iron in it.

Large quantities of the water are not ordered to be drunk as was at one time the custom, four to eight ounces twice a day being all that is prescribed in many cases, but where a decided eliminative action is desired—especially by the kidneys in uric acid cases—larger quantities of the cooled water would certainly be advantageous.

For the *external* use of these waters, the arrangements are very elaborate and complete. Separate immersion baths of a temperature of 98° to 104° F., combined with what is known as a *wet* or *under-water douche* of a higher temperature, which can be directed upon any definite part of the body, are found to be a very efficacious method of treatment in some cases.

For patients requiring a *reclining* bath, arrangements exist whereby they can be lowered into the bath without any effort on their part.

Douches of various kinds—needle, ascending, rose, and spinal douches—varying in temperature from 100° to 105°, or colder, if thought desirable, can be applied generally or locally.

The Aix les Bains douche-massage method has already been described. This is very thoroughly carried out at Bath. Suitable "cooling" rooms are connected with this and other bathing methods.

Sprays and pulverisations for the treatment of catarrhal affections of the pharynx and respiratory passages are also provided in "the umbrella" spray chamber. Berthollet local vapour baths, the vapour coming direct from the springs, and what is known as the "bouillon" or general vapour bath, the vapour emanating also from the springs and common to many patients, are frequently used.

It is needless to enter here into further detail, as the application and selection of the particular method best suited to individual cases must necessarily be left to the experience, skill, and judgment of the local physicians.

The period of time during which the treatment should be applied must depend also on the nature of the case and the progress made; it is usually estimated at from three to eight weeks.

Certain forms of "medicated" baths are prepared at Bath, and prescribed in suitable cases, such as the sulphur bath for cutaneous affections, the "pine" bath for cases of neurasthenia, and the gaseous "Soolbad" (Nauheim bath) for some forms of cardiac debility. An artificial table water, the "Sulis water," is made at Bath by aërating the natural mineral water with carbonic acid gas.

Finally, as to the cases best suited for treatment: *Chronic gouty* and *rheumatic affections*, articular, muscular, or neuralgic, form the vast majority of the cases treated with benefit at Bath. The *eliminative* action of the waters, by stimulating the intestinal and renal excretions when taken internally, and by stimulating the cutaneous excretions by their *external* action, and the valuable effects of passive movements in restoring suppleness to stiffened and rigid parts and in promoting the removal of crippling exudations, afford an obvious explanation of the beneficial results obtained. In cases of irregular gout, and in gouty cases between the attacks, a course of treatment at Bath has been found most serviceable.

As to the treatment of cases of *osteo-arthritis*, or rheumatoid arthritis, at Bath, much difference of opinion exists, and this we think depends greatly on the variations in the manner of classifying the different forms of arthritis prevailing with different physicians. Those who limit the term "rheumatoid arthritis" to cases which we should be disposed to term cases of *true* osteo-arthritis, and which appear to have a *neurotic* origin, find the treatment by thermal waters, at Bath or elsewhere, of little use, and, indeed, sometimes injurious, especially in the more acute forms. (The *chronic* forms are, no doubt, more or less benefited by gentle douching and massage, and by such means a certain amount of movement may be restored, and muscular wasting checked.) Others who certainly include under the term "rheumatoid" arthritis cases which appear to us to be more or less distinct from *true* osteo-arthritic ones, and whose real affinities are with those of chronic gout and rheumatism, find, as we should expect, much better results from this treatment at Bath.

As to the treatment of rheumatic cardiac *valvular* affections at Bath, we are not ourselves convinced, by anything we have been able to see, that such cases obtain greatly better results from treatment at thermal baths than from other and more simple hygienic measures.

Certain dry forms of skin disease derive benefit from prolonged maceration in natural thermal waters. Such cases may find relief at Bath.

Cases of chronic lead poisoning and some other forms of paralysis, and some cases of multiple neuritis, are benefited. Traumatic joint affections are very suitable for treatment by the methods in use at Bath.

Other diseases have been mentioned as benefited by treatment with the Bath waters, such as anæmia, diabetes, some uterine affections, chronic gastritis, biliary colic, etc., but we have no authoritative information to convey under these heads.

Battaglia (in the province of Venice, Italy) is celebrated for its mud (*fango*) and feebly mineralised thermal springs containing a small amount of sodium chloride. They are usually classified amongst the *indifferent thermal* springs. The total mineralisation is 2·36, of which 1·5 is common salt; there are also small amounts of potassium and calcium chlorides, and traces of sodium iodide and magnesium bromide. Battaglia lies in a plain at the foot of the Euganean Mountains, and has a station on the line between Bologna and Padua, about thirty miles from Venice. The baths are open all the year, but the best season is from May to October.

It has grottoes, or caves, in part artificially excavated in the rocks, where natural vapour baths at a temperature of 110° to 116° F. can be obtained. There are four hot springs of a temperature varying from 136° to 160° F. Some resemblance has been thought to exist between these springs and those of Baden-Baden.

The mud or *fango* is collected from small steaming pools or lakes which "vomit a volcanic mud." This is collected and not only used at Battaglia, but exported to many other parts, and is especially utilised at Bex, in Switzerland, and in Berlin. In some cases the whole body is enveloped in a layer of hot mud—this usually produces profuse perspiration—in other cases only the limb affected is thus treated.

Cases of chronic gout and rheumatism, and cases also of rheumatoid arthritis, are treated there. Special arrangements also exist for the inhalation of the pulverised thermal water in cases of chronic bronchial catarrh.

Berchtesgaden, having *common salt* wells, is beautifully situated in the Bavarian Tyrol, close to the Austrian frontier, and only a short distance (omnibus or steam tram) from Salzburg. It is a well-known summer health resort much frequented by tourists on account of its natural beauties, pleasant situation, and good accommodation, and also for its nearness to the celebrated Königssee and the salt mines. It has a brine containing 26½ per cent. of common salt. Rachitic and scrofulous conditions are especially treated there, so also are chronic catarrhal conditions of the respiratory passages. It is also sometimes prescribed as a restful after-cure following treatment at the more active Bohemian and other spas. Its climate is mild, but not bracing, although its altitude is 1,890 feet, for it is much shut in by surrounding mountains.

Bertrich is romantically situated at an elevation of 530 feet in one of the valleys of the Moselle, a few miles from that river, and seven miles from the station of Bullay on the line between Trèves and Coblenz. It is sometimes spoken of as "the mild Carlsbad," because it has warm springs containing the same characteristic constituents (sodium sulphate and carbonate) as the great Bohemian spa, but of only about one-third the strength, and of much lower temperature than the hotter springs of Carlsbad.

Its two springs, the Gartenquelle and the Borgquelle, are conveyed into one channel and are used mixed. The temperature of the mixed springs is about 90° to 92° F. Their total content of solids is 2·24 per litre, of which sodium sulphate forms 0·886, sodium bicarbonate 0·728, and sodium chloride 0·218. There are also small amounts of carbonate of lime and magnesium, and minute quantities of iron and manganese. The water also contains free carbonic acid gas.

The waters are both drunk and used as baths. The baths are given either at the natural temperature of the springs, or raised to a higher temperature by means which are devised to prevent the loss of the carbonic acid gas. The baths are also given with *running* water, so that a constant temperature is maintained during a bath which may last for half an hour.

The affections considered most suitable for treatment at Bertrich are of the same nature as those treated at Carlsbad, but in delicate, nervous persons who require very mild remedies, and who prefer the very quiet and simpler life of the smaller spa. Cases of neurasthenia are found to be much soothed and benefited by the baths; cases of functional hepatic and gastric disorders, gallstones, lithæmia, obesity in the feeble and anæmic, diabetes—these are the chief maladies adapted for treatment at this spa.

Chronic gouty and rheumatic affections are claimed by every bath, and no doubt most such cases are benefited by eliminant springs and the free skin excretions which hot alkaline baths promote. Bertrich is very accessible, as it can be reached either from Coblenz or Trèves in two to three hours.

The season is from the beginning of May to the end of September.

Bex is a well-known resort, familiar to most visitors to Switzerland, situated at the opening of the Rhone valley, on the right bank of that river, a few miles from the east end of the Lake of Geneva, and with very grand and picturesque surroundings. It is a climate resort as well as a bathing station. At an elevation of 1,400 feet, its climate is mild and sedative rather than tonic. It is very hot in the summer months, and mosquitos abound. In winter, owing to the height and nearness of the neighbouring mountains, the hours of sunshine are very limited, during the shortest days not longer than from 11 a.m. to 2 p.m.; this, together with wide daily oscillations of temperature, renders the place unsuitable as a winter resort, although it is well protected from cold winds, except those coming from the north-west over the Lake of Geneva, and from the south (the Föhn). The spring (May and June) and autumn (September and October) are the best climatic seasons at Bex.

The adjacency of salt-works has provided Bex with a *strong salt* spring, St. Hélène "eau salée," and an "eau mère," which is derived from the evaporations of the former after as much of the common salt as can be is separated. It has also a *cold sulphur* water which is used as an auxiliary to the other sources. The mud (*fango*) from Battaglia near Padua has been added to the therapeutic resources at Bex. Admirable arrangements also exist there for the application of ordinary spring water in accordance with the usual methods of *hydrotherapy*. It is, further, a station in autumn for the *grape cure*. Bex is therefore a kind of invalids' compendium, where kinds of treatment suitable to a great variety of maladies can be applied.

The "eau salée" is rich in sodium chloride, = 156·668 grammes in a litre, and 3·731 of potassium and magnesium chlorides. It contains also calcium, magnesium and strontium sulphates, magnesium carbonate, and small amounts of lithium chloride and magnesium iodide and bromide. The "eau mère," by evaporation and the separation and removal of sodium chloride, is rendered much richer in the other less crystallisable ingredients—the sodium chloride is reduced to 33·92 grammes, whereas the other chlorides (magnesium, calcium, and potassium) are increased to 221·81, the calcium sulphate to 35·49, and the magnesium bromide and iodide to 0·73.

The baths at Bex are prepared by diluting in various degrees the "eau salée" with plain water and adding various quantities of "eau mère," according to the case. They are reported to have tonic and stimulating effects, and occasionally they prove too exciting to nervous persons and have to be suspended or modified. Children bear them well, especially when given in the warm season.

The "eau mère" is also used as compresses, inhalations, pulverisations, and nasal douches, and is given internally in small doses, beginning with one or two teaspoonfuls and increasing to two or three table-spoonfuls in soup, or in effervescing or plain water. The sulphur water is comparatively feebly mineralised, but contains sodium chloride (2·334 grammes in a litre) and is fairly rich in free sulphuretted hydrogen; it is given internally in doses of half a glass to two glasses, and is used for gargling, pulverisation, nasal douches, and baths.

Like other resorts of this class, Bex is especially indicated in scrofulous maladies—the torpid and the febrile forms are treated somewhat differently, careful medical direction and discrimination being all important to the success of the cure; scrofulous glands, abscesses, inflammation of the eyelids, diseases of the bones and joints, rickets, skin affections, are all adapted to this treatment Chronic pleuritic exudations and tendencies to bronchial catarrh, anæmia and chlorosis, nervous affections, neurasthenia, chorea, uterine affections, metritis, perimetritis, periuterine exudations, are all regarded as capable of amelioration by one or other forms of treatment applied at Bex. The Grand Hôtel des Salines is admirably equipped for the administration of these waters and baths.

Those who desire to try treatment by the mud (*fango*) applications from Battaglia will find Bex a convenient place for that purpose. It is suitable for cases of chronic rheumatism and articular gout, as well as to the other maladies treated at Bex.

Bormio is an Italian mountain resort situated at the foot of the celebrated Stelvio Pass, on its southern slope, at an elevation of 4,500 feet and at the head of the Valtellina. It has five hot springs belonging to the class of *simple thermal* waters, the hottest of which has a temperature of 104° F. The water is very feebly mineralised, containing only 1·0 gramme of solids to the litre, chiefly composed of calcium and magnesium sulphates and carbonates. A thin, dark-coloured, unctuous *mud* is deposited by the springs, and this is used for local applications and for mixing with the baths. The "new" bath-house is conveniently fitted up for baths, mud baths, douches, inhalations, etc. The "old" bath-house is situated 200 feet higher than the new one. The cases benefited by treatment at Bormio are those forms of chronic articular rheumatism and gout, and other manifestations of the uric acid diathesis, which require moderately bracing mountain air as an adjuvant to bath treatment. Some forms of chronic skin disease also are benefited. The treatment is especially useful when the above morbid manifestations are associated with neurasthenic conditions or a scrofulous constitution. Anæmic cases are often benefited by drinking, at Bormio, the waters of the neighbouring chalybeate spring of Santa Catarina.

Bormio is also a climate resort, and is sometimes of value, as a change, for those who find the climate of the Engadine too severe and yet require the bracing influence of mountain air. Sudden variations in temperature have to be provided against; hence the need of warm clothing.

The situation of Bormio is not very attractive—the immediately surrounding country has a barren aspect, and the background of reddish, bare, hot-looking mountains of uniform sugarloaf form is not picturesque. The place is, however, close to fine scenery, as it is only seven miles from Santa Catarina in the beautiful Val Furva. Bormio may be approached from the direction of the Lake of Como and the Valtellina. It is a nine or ten hours' drive from the station of Sondrio, the terminus of the Valtellina railway. Or it may be reached from Samaden or Pontresina in the Engadine by a long drive over the Bernina Pass to Tirano, and then up the Valtellina. It is usual to sleep on the way at Le Prese or Tirano. Finally it may be approached from the direction of Meran or Landeck by the fine road over the Stelvio Pass.

Boulou (Le) is situated in the Pyrénées Orientales, about twenty hours from Paris viâ Perpignan; its station is only a few miles from the Spanish frontier. It is about 270 feet above the sea, and has a very mild climate. It has four mineral springs varying in temperature from 60° to 67° F. They are somewhat analogous in composition to the waters of Vichy and Vals, one of the springs having nearly six grammes of bicarbonate of soda per litre. These are the only waters of that kind found in the Pyrenees. Iron and arsenic, in small quantities, occur in one or more of the *sources*. The waters are chiefly used for drinking, but baths and douches can also be obtained in the Établissement.

The maladies treated there are dyspepsias, gastric and intestinal ; gastralgias, chronic intestinal catarrh ; hepatic torpor, gallstones, uric acid gravel, gout, diabetes, malarial cachexia and enlargements of liver and spleen resulting from residence in the tropics, anæmia and chlorosis associated with dyspepsia. It has a military hospital.

There are many picturesque excursions in the country around. There is a hotel in the Etablissement. It may be frequented at any part of the year.

Bourbon Lancy (Department of Saone et Loire), in Central France, has weakly mineralised *thermal salt* springs. It is reached from Paris (226 miles) in seven and a-half hours by the Bourbonnais line viâ Nevers and Cercy la Tour. It has a station in the town. It is built on the slope of a hill, at an altitude of 780 feet, with steep granite rocks rising above it. It is protected from winds and has a temperate, moderately warm climate.

Fine views of the mountainous country around (mountains of Morvan) can be obtained from the summits of adjacent hills.

The springs, of which there are five, have a temperature varying from 105° to 136° F. Their mineralisation is feeble, the total amount of solids being only 1·80 per litre, of which 1·30 consists of sodium chloride. There is a small amount of mixed bicarbonates, and minute quantities of iodine, arsenic, manganese, and lithium. They also contain free nitrogen and carbonic acid gases.

These waters are taken *internally* (the Sources La Reine and Descures), 16 to 20 ounces daily, divided into three doses, taken at different times. But it is mainly their *external* use that is relied upon for their beneficial effect. They are given as baths, often followed by "submarine" douches; *i.e.* douches applied beneath the surface of the water; also as "Scotch" (hot and cold alternately) douches, as general and local vapour baths, irrigations, pulverisations, etc. These external applications stimulate the peripheral circulation and promote the eliminant action of the skin, setting up, as they usually do, profuse perspiration. They promote the disappearance of rheumatic (subacute or chronic) or other exudations in and about the joints; while they also exert a *sedative* or calming influence, which has been referred by some to the presence of free nitrogen in the springs and by others to the climate. Taken *internally* half an hour before food they improve the appetite, and taken an hour after food they quicken and facilitate digestion. They thus prove valuable in atonic dyspepsia. The Descures *source* has a slightly laxative effect.

The waters also promote *renal* elimination—uric acid and the acid urates—in the gouty and rheumatic.

The bath establishment is furnished with every convenience and appliance for carrying out the most modern methods of balneology, including a large swimming bath fed by the overflow of the thermal springs, and appliances for mechanical movements and Swedish gymnastics and the Herz apparatus for respiratory gymnastics, to promote chest development in children, and augment the cardiac muscular tone in others.

The following are the maladies treated with

advantage at Bourbon Lancy: chronic or subacute and still painful rheumatic arthritis in excitable, nervous patients, chronic articular gout, gouty neuritis and threatened arteritis, sciatica, rheumatoid arthritis (said to be much benefited by the sedative influence of these baths).

Some forms of *cardiac* disease are reported to be favourably influenced by treatment there, by its combination of resources — baths, "submarine" douches, the internal use of the waters, and dietetic and mechanical treatment.

The cardiac affections susceptible of amelioration by this treatment have been thus summarised: "valvular insufficiencies at their commencement, *i.e.* about six months after the beginning of the endocarditis; cardiac affections at the onset of failure of compensation; functional insufficiencies; mitral constriction, with or without arhythmic palpitations; arterial affections, at the period of heightened tension, and cardiac disturbances of renal origin with dyspnœa due to alimentary toxins; finally, functional troubles; fatty accumulations about the heart; palpitations of peripheral origin due to vascular spasm; cardiac disturbances during growth with malformed thorax; pseudo-anginas and the unstable pulse of the neurotic."*

The season is from May 15th to Oct. 15th. June and July are the best months. Bourbon Lancy has a hospital for the indigent, with 400 beds. There are excellent hotels at moderate prices, and accommodation can also be obtained in the bath establishment. Many interesting excursions can be made in the neighbourhood.

Bourbon l'Archambaut, with *thermal common salt* waters, is situated in Central France, about six and a-half hours by express train from Paris. It

* "Stations Hydro-Minérales de la France." Rédigé par La Société d'Hydrologie Médicale de Paris.

has a station on the line from Paris to Lyons by the Bourbonnais on the branch from Moulins. It is situated in a valley, in the Department of the Allier, between four steep hills, at an elevation of 800 feet above the sea. The Bourbon waters have a very ancient reputation, and were known and employed at the time of the Roman occupation. Louis XIV. often came to these baths, and Madame de Montespan passed the last twelve years of her life at Bourbon, and died there. Many other notabilities have been associated with it.

Its most important spring is the Source Thermale (temperature 125° F.). This spring contains 2·24 of sodium chloride per litre, 1·33 of mixed bicarbonates of sodium, potassium, manganese, and iron; minute quantities of silica, bromide and chloride of sodium; traces of arsenic, lithium, and copper, and free carbonic acid gas. It has also a cold spring, Jonas, used for drinking, which contains carbonate of *iron* and magnesium. A third spring, the Pardoux, silicated and containing much free carbonic acid, makes an excellent table-water.

The thermal water is taken *internally* in doses varying from one to four glasses daily. It is employed *externally* in baths of running water, varying in temperature and duration, the average temperature being 95° F.; also as tepid, hot, and *very* hot douches, general or local, following the bath, and with or without massage; also as "submarine," ascending, and irrigating douches. Applied in these ways, either for its general effects or for its local action, it exerts a powerful alterative, tonic, and stimulating influence on the nutritive functions.

There is at Bourbon a civil hospital for poor patients, and an important military hospital.

An admirable bath establishment has been provided by the State for carrying out these methods of treatment. It is one of the finest and most complete in France; having two large swimming baths and a department for vapour baths and pulverisations, besides the various other forms of baths and douches already referred to.

A speciality at Bourbon is a peculiar mode ot *dry*-cupping, used in addition to massage, and consisting in the application of small "cornets" or "horns," with holes pierced at the ends; these are applied to the skin by attendants, who suck out the air and then close the holes with wax.

The chief maladies treated at Bourbon are—Chronic rheumatism, following the acute affection, with stiffness or partial ankylosis of joints or effusion into them; also the effects of gonorrhœal rheumatism, all forms of muscular rheumatism or neuralgia. Recent rheumatic endo-carditic or pericarditic lesions are favourably influenced by the treatment here, as at Bourbon Lancy. The treatment is very useful also in neuralgias, intercostal and sciatic in particular. Excellent results are said to be obtained in cases of arthritis deformans, also in the joint troubles of atonic gout in the feeble and lymphatic, and in gouty diabetics with nervous depression and lowered vitality.

Bourbon has a traditional reputation for the treatment of scrofulous affections of the glands, joints, and bones. It also has an ancient reputation for the treatment of certain cases of paralysis; it is particularly useful in those following infective fevers and intoxications, and those of rheumatic origin. Cases of hemiplegia, the result of cerebral hæmorrhage, it is claimed, are much benefited if sent there for treatment *after* the inflammatory period and *before* muscular atrophies and contractures have set in; the same is asserted of paraplegias, rheumatismal, hysterical, or traumatic (concussions of the spinal cord), and of some forms of myelitis; it is said also to modify favourably the course of tabes, and to relieve its painful symptoms. If applied combined with the usual specific treatment it is found to exert a very favourable influence in syphilis of the nervous system.

The excellent results obtained in the military hospital testify to the value of this treatment in various forms of traumatism. Finally, many affections of the female pelvic organs are benefited at Bourbon; such as amenorrhœa, dysmenorrhœa, rheumatic metritis, and old thickenings and adhesions from perimetritis.

The season is from May 15th to Oct. 1st. There is a casino with theatre in the park. Hotel accommodation is good and prices are moderate. Many interesting excursions can be made into the surrounding forests.

Bourbonne les Bains, situated on the confines of the Vosges, is a very important spa, and is often spoken of as the French Wiesbaden. One of the largest military hospitals in France is established there, affording accommodation for 310 soldiers and 90 officers. Its springs are *hot sodium chloride* springs, and their special application is the treatment of chronic rheumatism; also the results of gun-shot and other injuries, and "scrofulous" affections.

Bourbonne is a small, pleasant town in the Department of the Haute Marne, about 800 feet above the sea-level, in a fine situation on an eminence abutting from Les Monts Faucilles, and surrounded by low hills covered by dense forests. It is about seven hours from Paris, and is connected by a branch line with Vitrey, a station on the Eastern Railway between Langres and Belfort. The little town is exceedingly French. The life there is simple and cheap. The inhabitants appear cheerful and prosperous; they manufacture lace and cutlery, and they hunt the wolf and the wild boar in their adjacent forests.

A small park, a casino, a theatre, a band of music, a *jeu de petits chevaux* are here, as elsewhere, essential distractions to a course of mineral waters.

The springs of Bourbonne are hot and salt—thermal and saline. The temperature of the principal springs is as high as 150° F., and there are others not quite so hot. The water has a very salt taste, and is considered to resemble that at Wiesbaden.

It is drunk only in small quantities, two to four small glasses a day; but is used chiefly in the form of baths and douches. They are very proud of their douches at Bourbonne, and consider them superior to *all* others. Mineral *mud* is also employed there.

The applications of electricity and of massage are used here as adjuncts to the thermal treatment, but they consider their strong douche (*douche de haute pression*) as a *douche de massage*, and that the vigour of its jets acts in the same manner as massage does. The baths and douches are prolonged ones; the former last from half an hour to an hour, and the latter from ten to fifteen minutes.

As the State has been to so much expense to establish a great military hospital at Bourbonne, we may safely conclude that the waters are found of great efficacy in the treatment of wounds and injuries received in battle. They are also applicable to all forms of chronic rheumatism of the muscles and joints, badly united fractures, and certain cases of paralysis and muscular feebleness. The number of persons that may be seen in wheeled chairs, or on crutches, or limping with sticks, or with deformed limbs, and also the number of pale, deformed, delicate, scrofulous children seen in the streets and in the hotels, point clearly enough to the uses of the Bourbonne springs. Chronic rheumatism in its many forms, chronic articular gout in its atonic forms, paralysis from muscular atrophy, sciatica and other forms of neuralgia, and the glandular and other affections of scrofulous children, certain chronic affections of the female pelvic organs—these are the chief maladies treated at Bourbonne. Affections of the nerves dependent on rheumatism are especially benefited, but ataxic cases are not suitable. Some torpid forms of constitutional syphilis are benefited there.

The time usually given to the cure there, as elsewhere in France, is the mystical twenty-one days, though at the military hospital, where "mystic" numbers are disregarded, two months and even longer are devoted to the cure! In obstinate cases it has been recommended that two periods, each of twenty-one days, should be allowed, with an interval of ten days, which may be spent in an excursion into the interesting country around or in Switzerland, which can be reached viá Bâle or Delle in a few hours.

Beside chloride of sodium these waters contain chlorides of lime and magnesium, carbonate and sulphate of lime, bromide of sodium, and the much-coveted chloride of lithium. In the published analysis as much as nearly nine centigrammes, about 1⅓ grains, of chloride of lithium is stated to be found in a litre of the water. If this statement be correct, then the water of Bourbonne contains more lithium than any other spring in France.

Bourbonne les Bains is no doubt an excellent spa for the treatment of severe forms of chronic rheumatism (not so useful in rheumatoid arthritis), obstinate neuralgia, slowly healing wounds, muscular atrophies, and all forms of scrofulous disease of the glands, bones, and joints. In this last class of affections it is probably no more efficacious than hot sea water would prove if applied systematically in the same manner, and associated with sea air.

There are two neighbouring springs which are used as auxiliaries in suitable cases—one, the Source de Larivière, is a tonic iron spring, and the other, Source Magnard, resembles in composition the springs of Contrexéville and Vittel, and can be employed, as they are, in cases of the uric acid diathesis.

The season is from May 1st to October.

Bourboule (La), in Auvergne, is specially famous for its hot *arsenical* springs, rich also in sodium chloride and bicarbonate. It is in the Mont Dore chain, and is situated only four or five miles from Mont Dore les Bains, the road thence following the course of the valley and the right bank of the Dordogne as it descends towards the north-west.

La Bourboule is not so high as Mont Dore, its elevation above the sea being only 2,770 feet. It is not so shut in as Mont Dore, but lies in a comparatively wide open valley, surrounded by hills of moderate height and very gentle slope. It is not, however, so well placed as Mont Dore for excursions into the interesting country around, most of the points of greatest interest being more easily reached from the latter.

It can now be reached from Paris by rail in about ten hours by express train. It has a subalpine climate well adapted to the cases sent there and the treatment applied. It possesses both hot and cold springs. The latter need not concern us as they are of altogether minor importance, both in mineralisation and in amount of outflow. The two hot springs are known as La Source Choussy-Perrière and La Source Croizat. The latter spring is of recent discovery. The Choussy-Perrière has a temperature of 136° F., and contains in a litre 3 grammes of sodium chloride, 3·8 of sodium bicarbonate, and 0·028 of sodium arsenate. The Croizat is not so hot, its temperature is 113° F.; it contains more sodium chloride (5·63), but less sodium bicarbonate (3·0) and less sodium arsenate (0·025).

It is maintained that the arsenic in Bourboule water has not the ill effects attributed to the use of arsenic in other forms, yet after its protracted use arsenic is found in all the tissues—the blood, the skin, and the hair. The baths are stimulating, and promote oxidation, tissue changes, and diuresis. On the skin La Source Perrière, at a moderate temperature, produces a soft, unctuous feeling, most calming and comforting in skin affections.

The *internal* use of the water is of main importance. It is usually drunk at a temperature of about 104° F., in doses varying from three to eighteen or even twenty ounces, divided into three portions, at different times in the day. When very large doses are thought necessary, a portion is often given by enema.

The *baths* are taken separately, or in a common bath, and in certain skin affections very prolonged baths are ordered, sometimes for several hours (macerations), but not very hot. In other cases the duration and temperature of the baths are greatly varied according to circumstances.

The *inhalation* chambers filled with the finely pulverised water are at the service of patients with respiratory affections. The temperature of these chambers is kept at about 90° F.

All the needful apparatus for naso-pharyngeal applications, for douches of all kinds, for vapour baths, for dry and wet massage, are found in a very perfectly equipped bath establishment.

Of the cases adapted to treatment at La Bourboule, *skin* affections stand in the first rank, especially those forms that have proved rebellious to other kinds of treatment, and although some of these prove intractable to this as to other methods of treatment, there are few that do not receive some benefit. The list drawn up by the local authorities is a long one, and includes ichthyosis, psoriasis, pityriasis rubra, eczema, lichen rubra, prurigo, erythema induratum, tuberculous affections, acne, boils, chronic urticaria, etc. The *chronic diseases of children* occupy the next place, especially the glandular and osseous affections of the lymphatic and scrofulous, particularly those children with whom the seaside disagrees.

Sufferers from *anæmia* and *chlorosis* not amenable to the usual treatment with iron benefit by the Bourboule course.

Certain affections of the *respiratory* organs, as chronic catarrhs of the pharynx, larynx, trachea, and bronchi in the arthritic, or neurotic and arthritic, especially when associated with some skin affections, are suitable for treatment there.

Infantile asthma, which often coincides with enlargement of the bronchial glands, is said to be generally cured at La Bourboule.

Early or very slightly advanced non-febrile cases of pulmonary tuberculosis, or persons apparently threatened with that disease, benefit by the climate and treatment.

Persons suffering from *malarial cachexia* (without serious hepatic trouble), from neuralgia of malarious origin, from *arthritis deformans*, from neurasthenia with anæmia, and some cachectic forms of syphilis, may derive benefit from the course combined with the tonic influence of the climate. Atonic forms of gout and rheumatism, especially if associated with cutaneous manifestations, do well there.

Finally, La Bourboule claims to be a suitable resort for the *diabetic* and for some forms of *albuminuria*. The cases of diabetes suitable for treatment at this spa are perhaps a little difficult to define; it is said that emaciating cases, with increased excretion of urinary solids (urates and phosphates), such as have failed to be benefited at Vichy, improve there, and that in other forms the results are sometimes good and at other times *nil.*

Nothing very definite seems to be known as to what cases of albuminuria are suitable for treatment at La Bourboule; it is suggested that cases of cyclic or functional albuminuria and those associated with phosphaturia are benefited there. But these cases can be dealt with very well by other means.

The season is from May 25th to Sept. 30th. The climate becomes often somewhat trying after September 20th. There are three bath establishments, one of which is a model of its kind.

The hotels are numerous and good. All the usu

distractions provided at French spas will be found at La Bourboule.

Brides les Bains and **Salins Moutiers** are situated in a charming valley in the Tarantaise, a part of Savoy exceedingly picturesque and Swiss-like in character. These two resorts are usually considered together, as they are only three or four miles apart, and in many cases the resources of both establishments are utilised for the same patients. Brides has *laxative* waters which are chiefly used internally, and Salins Moutiers has *strong gaseous salt* springs which are mainly used externally.

We shall now proceed to consider them separately; and first with regard to Brides les Bains.

Brides lies in the midst of very beautiful scenery, and few resorts of like importance medically can be found which present the same attractions for the lover of nature as this little Savoy village. It is situated in the valley of the Doron, which rushes through the village as a noisy, white, foaming mountain torrent, and joins the Isère at Moutiers. The valley runs deeply into those high Alps of the Tarantaise which lie, as the crow flies, about twenty miles south of Mont Blanc, and about one-half that distance north of Mont Cenis. Brides stands at an elevation of 1,800 feet above the sea, at the opening of two lateral valleys, the sides of which are thickly wooded, and afford many charmingly sheltered promenades amidst their woods and picturesque and primitive villages.

It can be very hot at Brides in the middle of a hot summer day, but the atmosphere is usually cool and fresh in the mornings and evenings.

A few years ago Brides was little known in England, and at that time it was somewhat difficult of access, but since the extension of the railway from Albertville to Moutiers and the recent connection of Brides with Salins by an electric tramway it receives far more English visitors than formerly.

Brides has been termed, from the action rather than the composition of its water, the French Carlsbad. The resemblance may not be very complete from certain points of view, but in one sense the term seems justified, for the Brides water is undoubtedly exceedingly well adapted to the treatment of many of the diseases in which the Carlsbad *source* is usually considered to be indicated. The springs are not so strongly mineralised as those of the great Bohemian spa, they are not of nearly so high a temperature, and they contain no sodium bicarbonate, which is a very important ingredient in the Carlsbad water. Of the 6·5 grammes of solids in the litre of Brides water the most active constituents are doubtless the sodium chloride (1·8318), and sulphate (1·1604), and magnesium sulphate (0·5288). Other ingredients in smaller proportions are calcium and magnesium carbonates, calcium sulphate, and minute quantities of lithium sulphate, ferrous carbonate, and sodium arsenate. The water also contains some free carbonic acid gas. Its temperature is 95° F.

It is a water better classified by its effects than by its composition. In small doses it promotes appetite and digestion, and is useful in certain cases of dyspepsia ; in larger doses it is distinctly laxative, but acts without causing any distress or exhaustion. "*Cela purge sans fatiguer*" is the local saying.

The Brides cure is chiefly a drinking cure, but the water is also used in baths and douches—in general douches, and in ascending douches. The water, when drunk, has a diuretic action and promotes the excretion of the urinary solids. It is decidedly eliminant, both renally and intestinally, and by its stimulating action on the intestinal secretions it indirectly promotes nutritive changes, and so has a tonic effect.

The bath establishment is very thoroughly equipped, and besides the usual arrangements for baths, douches, dry hot air and moist vapour baths, it has Swedish gymnastics, electric baths, and electric light baths, and an analytical laboratory and the necessary apparatus for radiography.

The following are the maladies in which the Brides course has been found useful. The first place is occupied by functional diseases of the liver, especially those occurring in persons of gouty constitutions. Biliary concretions and the tendency to attacks of biliary colic are favourably influenced by the free use of these waters; cases of hepatic engorgement, of catarrh of the bile ducts and jaundice; cases resulting from residence in the tropics, and as a consequence of malarial attacks—all these forms of hepatic or hepato-splenic disorders are benefited at Brides. Cases of hæmorrhoids are greatly advantaged. It is maintained that not only do these springs relieve congestions and restore healthy function by their laxative and eliminative influences, but that they are also tonic and eupeptic, and therefore assist in restoring strength to the enfeebled. Dyspepsias, dependent on chronic gastric catarrh, or on hyperacidity, or dependent on the preceding maladies, derive much benefit, so do the migrainous when their attacks are associated with disturbed hepatic functions, or appear as gouty manifestations.

These waters are also used in chronic intestinal catarrh, chronic dysentery, and in *obstinate constipation.* Chronic affections of the uterus of a torpid character, engorgements, hypertrophy, metritis, dysmenorrhœa, amenorrhœa, leucorrhœa, so often associated with anæmia and chronic constipation, are reported as very favourably influenced by treatment at Brides. In these cases the waters and baths of Salins prove valuable auxiliaries.

It has already been said that the treatment at Brides is especially beneficial in those disturbances of health which are ordinarily referred to the gouty constitution; it follows that certain forms of diabetes and of albuminuria are represented as suitable cases for this spa; the fat, gouty diabetics are generally benefited by combined treatment at Brides and Salins.

With regard to cases of albuminuria, much care and caution must be exercised in determining those which are and those which are not suited to treatment by mineral courses such as Brides. In cases of well-defined Bright's disease—of established nephritis—except in the very chronic form of obviously gouty origin, treatment at Brides is *not* to be recommended. The cases that are enumerated by Delastre as likely to derive benefit at Brides are those following infective fevers, the albuminuria of adolescents, that dependent on congestive conditions of the kidneys, the consequence of cardiac and circulatory feebleness, and especially when occurring in association with obesity, chronic alcoholism, and hepatic troubles.

The tendency to urinary concretions and deposits so common in the gouty is benefited by these waters. Combined treatment at Brides and Salins has been found very serviceable in those cases of anæmia and chlorosis associated with manifest torpor of the gastro-intestinal functions, and in which attention to the improvement of gastric and intestinal tone and activity by baths, exercises, and suitable laxatives is of chief importance.

Finally, Brides has a special reputation for the treatment of obesity. The combined treatment at Brides and Salins is most appropriate to many of such cases, including the anæmic form, and we can testify to the excellence of the results obtained there when combined with a suitable *régime.*

Salins Moutiers is now connected with Brides by an electric tramway, performing the journey in about a quarter of an hour. Its elevation is about 300 feet less than that of Brides. Its springs are rich in sodium chloride, containing over 13 grammes to the litre, and rich also in free carbonic acid gas; it also contains potassium chloride, calcium, and magnesium sulphates and carbonates and ferrous carbonate with minute quantities of lithium sulphate, sodium arsenate. and silica. Their temperature is 97° F. The new bath establishment is well equipped with baths and piscines and douches, two swimming baths, vapour baths, rooms for massage and Swedish gymnastics, etc. A ferruginous and arsenical *mud* is also collected from the deposits in the water conduits and used therapeutically. The baths, too, can be fortified by the addition of *eau mère.* Owing to the great amount of water proceeding from the springs the baths are given *à l'eau courante*, so that the water of the bath is continually renewed, and also maintained throughout of the same temperature. The gas in the water accumulates on the skin in little globules and is supposed to exercise a sedative action. The duration of the bath is determined by the medical attendant and varies according to the case. Patients express themselves as refreshed and invigorated by these hot gaseous salt baths in contradistinction to the languor complained of after hot baths in some other stations.

These baths are tonic and strengthening, improving the condition of the blood and the circulation, and are applicable to a variety of maladies, cases of slow convalescence, delicate lymphatic children, cases of overgrowth, of anæmia and chlorosis. In "scrofulous" manifestations affecting the glands, bones, and joints, ocular affections, ozæna; in uterine cases, combined with Brides waters internally, as already mentioned; in chronic rheumatism and old traumatic affections, the baths prove very useful. Owing to the resemblance of the waters to those of Nauheim, it was to be expected that certain forms of cardiac disease would be regarded as suitable for treatment here, but we are not aware that this suggestion has, so far, been widely adopted.

These waters are prescribed internally to children in moderate doses, and they appear to be easily digested. The season at Brides and Salins is from May 15th to Sept. 30th. The early and latter parts of the season are the most agreeable. The heat is often very great in July and August.

The journey from Paris to Moutiers Salins is performed in thirteen hours. Hotels are good and the usual amusements are provided. There are many suitable places in the neighbourhood for an after-cure: the nearest is Pralognan, about three hours' drive from Brides; it is in a beautiful and well-protected situation at an elevation of 4,600 feet.

Brückenau is a Bavarian spa not far from Kissingen, with a station on the Brückenau branch line from Jossa, between Elm and Gemunden, having weak *cold gaseous chalybeate* springs. Its situation is very picturesque, lying in the valley of Sinn, which abounds in beautiful scenery, at an elevation 980 feet above the sea. The village is built on the south-western declivity of the Rhön mountains, but the springs, with the Kurhaus and the handsome Kursaal, are two miles from the village.

The climate is mild and agreeable, the average summer temperature not exceeding 63° F.

The springs and the Kursaal, and the hotels and houses for the accommodation of the visitors, are situated in beautiful gardens and pleasure grounds, surrounded by hills covered with beech forests, through which there are picturesque walks and excursions of various distances.

The waters are very mild and contain iron only, in very small quantity; but they have an abundance of carbonic acid, which makes them very pleasant to drink. There are three springs, the chief and strongest of which is the Stahlquelle—it contains only 0·011 of carbonate of iron per litre. *Moor* baths from Gersfield Moor are used, as well as baths of the gaseous springs. Electrotherapy and hydrotherapy are likewise utilised. These waters are said to be useful as an after-course to Kissingen, and if, after three or four weeks of water-drinking at the latter place, one still has time and inclination for more, this inclination might, doubtless, be harmlessly and agreeably gratified by a week or two amidst the beautiful scenery around Brückenau, and the consumption of a certain amount of its sparkling and refreshing waters.

The medical authorities of the place claim that the waters are tonic and blood-restoring, and useful in many diseases associated with debility; that, combined with warm milk, they are beneficial in pulmonary affections, in chronic bronchitis, and in dyspepsia. The baths, no doubt, are stimulating to the skin, on account of the amount of carbonic acid they contain, and they are reported to be very useful in some female maladies. The patients are chiefly of the female sex. The season is from May 15th to Oct. 1st.

Builth Wells, a spa and health resort in Radnorshire, on the Wye, in a pleasant situation at an elevation of 400 feet. It is about a mile and a-half from the town of Builth, where visitors to the Wells usually stay. The springs resemble those at Llandrindod Wells—one, the chief, being a *saline* spring, another a *chalybeate* and saline, and a third a weak *sulphur* spring. The saline spring contains sodium chloride 12·5 grammes per litre, and calcium chloride 2·5. It appears to contain also *very* minute amounts of magnesium chloride and lithium chloride, and traces of iron, aluminium, and manganese.

The chalybeate spring is said to be a strong one, but we have not seen any detailed analysis published. These waters are served out in pump-rooms, all under the same roof. Hot and cold baths are also prepared with the saline and sulphur waters.

The therapeutic value of these springs cannot be said to have been precisely ascertained. Locally they appear to have a reputation for the relief of various maladies, especially gastric and hepatic disorders.

Bussang (Vosges).—Supposing you have finished your twenty-one or twenty-five days at Contrexéville or Plombières, it is an easy and pleasant change to go on for a few days to Bussang. An agreeable drive of an hour and a-quarter conveys you from Plombières to the railway station at Remiremont.

At Remiremont we take the railway to St. Maurice, an hour's journey through a most attractive valley, the line running along by the side of the Moselle, here a beautiful clear stream, nearly the whole way, amidst the greenest of pastures and surrounded by some of the highest of the Vosges mountains. At St. Maurice, which lies at the foot of the Ballon d'Alsace and the Ballon de Servance, the railway comes to an end, and you find a comfortable omnibus at the station waiting to take you on to Bussang, an uphill drive of three or four miles. Although Bussang has only had an *Établissement* for the reception of visitors in recent years, the water of its springs has long been known, and is so popular in France that upwards of a million bottles are annually exported. It is a very pleasant water to drink—it is gaseous and effervescent and at Bussang is taken with wine at meals. It is also mildly tonic. It contains small quantities of iron and manganese and minute amounts of arsenic and lithium, and it is slightly alkaline. There is about 1·5 of solids to the litre. The Salinade spring is richest in carbonic acid. It would seem to be an excellent mild tonic water, well adapted to cases of anæmia and anæmic dyspepsia, especially in the case of persons who cannot bear stronger iron waters. It must also be a good water for those persons to drink who, having finished the prescribed course at Contrexéville, still need to continue water drinking for some time; the *strengthening* constituents of the Bussang water should be altogether advantageous to them. The Bussang water is no doubt a really valuable as well as a pleasant spring. The mild mountain climate, combined with the mild tonic waters and the application of hydrotherapy, form an excellent treatment for cases of nervous exhaustion and overwork.

If favoured with fine weather, a visitor might easily become enthusiastic about the surroundings of Bussang. A quarter of an hour's walk from the hotel (2,170 feet above the sea) brings you to the top of the Col de Bussang (2,384 feet), where you find a long tunnel, in the middle of which is the boundary line between France and Germany. On going up to the Col you pass a little wooden shed erected to mark the spot where the Moselle has its source, for at Bussang this river is but a little trickling stream which a child can leap over. Passing through the Col, one looks down on the pretty little town of Wesserling, in Alsace. Close also to the hotel are several paths leading to beautiful walks and excursions amidst the highest of the Vosges mountains. The nearest and most readily accessible of these is the Grand Drumont, rather over 4,000 feet high, and reached from Bussang by an easy ascent of about an hour and a-half. From the summit, which is covered with soft green pastures (here called *chaumes*), a fine view is obtained of Alsace-Lorraine, of the Rhine valley, the mountains of the Black Forest, and on very clear days of some of the snow-topped mountains of Central Switzerland. The summit of the Ballon d'Alsace, a few feet higher, can be reached from Bussang in two and a-half hours—there is a hotel near the top, where those who require still more bracing air can reside, and the view is very fine and extensive.

A good hotel and a hydropathic establishment afford excellent accommodation for visitors. Altogether it would be difficult to find in the Vosges a more pleasant, quiet, mildly bracing mountain resort than Bussang.

The season is from June 15th to Sept. 15th.

Buxton, in Derbyshire, about four and a-half hours from London, has thermal waters which have enjoyed a well-merited celebrity for many centuries, and it is now one of the most popular baths in this country. It is said to have been a favourite resort of Mary Stuart. It has a large hospital, the Devonshire Hospital, where the efficacy and applicability of the waters have for many years been studied, a separate pump-room and bath establishment being at the service of the patients.

Buxton, being at an elevation of 1,000 feet above the sea, and in the midst of some of the finest scenery of Derbyshire, is a pleasant and cheerful place of resort and has fine, bracing air, which is not without its influence in the successes obtained there. It is, however, rather a rainy place.

The mean temperature for January, the coldest month, is 40·1° F., the mean minimum 30·0°; for July the mean maximum is 65·1°, and the mean minimum 48·4°. In 1893 the lowest temperature recorded, 9·4° F., was on January 5th, and the highest 83° F. on August 18th. The highest mean rainfall is in October and November, amounting to 10·93 inches for these two months; the lowest rainfall is in April, 2·48 inches. The yearly mean is 46·2 inches. Of hours of sunshine the highest mean is in June (151 hours), and the lowest in December (22 hours).

Buxton is a *simple thermal* spring, which may be compared to that of Ragatz or Wildbad on the Continent. The temperature of the water is 82° F., so that it is rather tepid than hot, and its peculiarity is the large amount of nitrogen gas it contains. The supply of water is very abundant. It is of very feeble mineralisation, containing only 0·4 grammes of mineral substance per litre, of which 0·2 is calcium bicarbonate, 0·1 magnesium bicarbonate, and about 0·05 sodium chloride. The usual dose prescribed internally is from 4 to 10 oz. There is a weak non-gaseous chalybeate spring sometimes drunk there, and especially used for bathing the eyes; it contains 0·015 grammes of carbonate of iron in a litre. A handsome new pump-room for drinking the waters was opened in 1894 by the owner, the Duke of Devonshire.

There are two separate bath establishments—one in which the water is used at the "natural" temperature, another the "*hot baths*" in which the water is artificially heated to any temperature desired. "The temperature is raised by mixing with the natural water a varying quantity of the same water heated in a tank by means of a steam coil to about 200° F."

The equipment of this bath establishment is very complete, with immersion baths having cranes and chairs for lowering cripples into the bath;

douches of all kinds, and vapour baths. A feature there is the "massage bath," in which massage is applied while the patient in the reclining position is treated with sprays and douches.

The baths are prescribed for comparatively short periods, the *natural* bath from four to seven minutes, the patient being instructed to keep moving about all the time; in the *hot* bath, which is preferred for patients with feebler powers of reaction, the period varies from four to fifteen minutes. A "brisk walk" is recommended after the *natural* bath, if, of course, the patient is capable of such a display of activity.

Some nervous or circulatory disturbances—giddiness, palpitation, insomnia—and occasionally slight febrile disturbances, occur to some persons at the commencement of the course.

Buxton is particularly celebrated for the cure or alleviation of chronic articular gout and rheumatism; "irregular" forms of gout are also benefited, and acute attacks are said to be warded off by treatment, in the intervals, at Buxton; the joint stiffness and painful conditions left by attacks of acute rheumatism are also relieved. Gonorrhœal forms are reputed as much benefited by the hot steam douches; its baths have also proved very useful in cases of hysterical paralysis and joint affections, in some forms of paralysis not dependent on central lesions, in sciatica, and other neuralgias of gouty or rheumatic origin, and in the removal of inflammatory thickenings of joints.

Massage in the baths, no doubt, contributes to the relief of many forms of chronic joint affections and neuralgias.

As to the value of the treatment at Buxton in cases of osteo-arthritis, some doubts may be permitted. Those cases which seem distinctly referable to a neuropathic origin are little amenable to thermal treatment of any kind; while those which are more closely allied to gouty or rheumatic states no doubt derive much benefit from the combination of massage and warm douching.

Many other morbid conditions have been mentioned as relieved by treatment at Buxton; but the specialisation of the treatment at this or similar spas must be referred to maladies connected with the rheumatic or gouty diathesis, and these are very numerous. The baths are open all the year round, but the summer is the best season for the course—from May to September.

Baassen, a *gaseous salt* bath in Transylvania, eight miles from the railway station of Mediasch.

Bagnoli, *hot springs* near Pozzuoli, Naples, together with the natural vapour baths ("Stufe") known as the Bagni di Nerone.

Bagnols les Bains, a thermal sulphur spring of feeble mineralisation (0·61 grammes per litre), temperature 95 to 105° F., situated at an altitude of nearly 3,000 feet in the narrow valley of the Lot, in the Department of Lozère, distant from Paris 628 kilometres, and 12 kilometres from Mende. The nearest railway station is Chadenet. The water contains a little sodium bicarbonate (0·226) and chloride (0·142), and 1·7 c.c. of sulphuretted hydrogen.

This spring has obtained a reputation in the treatment of chronic cardiac valvular affections dependent on rheumatism, where compensation is maintained. The good effects are not referred to any special or direct action on the cardiac valves, but to a modifying influence on the underlying rheumatic or gouty diathesis.

Scrofula, skin affections, and bronchial catarrh are benefited there as at analogous sulphur springs. The treatment is chiefly external, but the waters are also drunk. Baths, douches, dry hot-air baths, and especially foot baths of running water, are applied there.

The season is from June 15 to Sept. 15. It is hot there in summer, but somewhat wide oscillations of temperature are experienced on account of the elevation.

Bains (Vosges) is situated between Contrexéville and Plombières. It has a station on the East of France Railway, and is about fifteen miles from Epinal and ten hours from Paris. It has the advantage of being adjacent to the fine forest of Tremonsey, and is pleasantly situated in a valley, 1,000 feet above the sea, through which the River Sémouse flows.

It has several springs and two bath establishments. In the public baths the two sexes, appropriately clothed, bathe together. The temperature of these springs varies from 84° to 122° F. Their mineralisation is very feeble, about 0·20 of mineral constituents in a litre, consisting of sodium sulphate and chloride and a little silica. La Grosse Source is said to contain a little arsenic. The springs somewhat resemble those of Plombières, and may be classed among the *indifferent thermal* baths. Two of the springs are used for drinking, but the chief use of these waters is for hot baths. Like other baths of this kind they are used and found beneficial in cases of chronic rheumatism, muscular and arthritic, in chronic painful uterine and ovarian affections, in cases of want of tone and exhaustion with enfeebled digestion, and, as at Plombières, in cases of chronic enteritis. Residence in agreeable mountain scenery, and in fresh, pure air contributes to the good results obtained there. There is good accommodation at the Grand Hôtel, connected with which are a casino and a theatre. The season is from May 15 to Sept. 15.

Bakewell, in the Derbyshire Peak district, 400 feet above the sea, has springs somewhat resembling those of Buxton and Matlock, but having a constant temperature of 60° F. The supply is somewhat intermittent. So long ago as 1697 a bath-house was erected, and it has a large plunge bath (36 by 15 feet) reputed to be of Roman construction. The water is artificially heated to supply the warm baths.

Ballynahinch, a *cold sulphur* spring in Ulster, seventeen miles from Belfast by rail. One of the wells has about 3·6 vols. per 1,000 of H_2S. It has a local reputation.

Ballyspellan, a chalybeate spring in Kilkenny County, Ireland.

Barbotan, chiefly known as a "*mud*" bath, is situated in an out-of-the-way part of France, with a station on the line from Nérac to Mont de Marsan in the Department of Gers and the commune of Casaubon. It is situated at an altitude of about 400 feet, and has a mild climate.

It has several warm springs of very feeble mineralisation, containing a little sulphuretted hydrogen and sodium sulphide, and one, cold, contains a little iron. The waters are used to mix with the "vegetable muds" extracted from an adjacent marsh. These are used warm as baths, and are bathed in in common. Baths and douches of the thermal springs are also used, and the iron and sulphur springs are drunk.

The patients come chiefly from the locality itself, and are sufferers mainly from chronic rheumatism, stiff joints, neuralgias, rickets, scrofulous affections of the bones and joints, chronic uterine maladies, syphilis, intestinal catarrhs, and certain torpid skin diseases. The season is from May 1 to Oct. 1.

Bartfeld, a somewhat inaccessible Hungarian *chalybeate* spring in the Carpathians at the foot of the Kamenahola. It has several cold gaseous iron springs which contain also considerable quantities (the Doctorquelle) of sodium bicarbonate (4·8 per litre), common salt (1·1), and a minute amount of sodium iodide (0·001). There is a good bath establishment where hydrotherapeutic treatment is applied. The springs are prescribed for anæmia and scrofulous cases with dyspeptic symptoms. The combination of sodium bicarbonate and ferrous carbonate should be useful in such cases. At an elevation of 1,000 feet above the sea, Bartfeld has been suggested as an after-cure to Carlsbad, Franzensbad, etc. The nearest railway station, Eperies, is five hours distant, and the town of Bartfeld half an hour. Its distance renders it practically useless to English patients.

Barzun.—See Barèges, to which it is close. The water is conveyed to Lux.

Bauche, La, a cold non-gaseous *chalybeate* spring in Savoy, half an hour's drive from the stations of Lépin or Les Echelles, fourteen miles from Chambéry. The water is said to contain 0·14 bicarbonate of iron and 0·03 of *crenate* of iron. It is exported and also drunk and bathed in at a small establishment. La Bauche is situated in a beautiful district at an elevation of 1,640 feet above the sea. The water is said to be easily digested, and is given in cases of anæmia and chlorosis.

Bentheim, a small *cold sulphur* spa in Hanover, situated near the frontier of Holland at an elevation of about 300 feet. The spring contains H_2S calcium sulphate (1·3 grammes per litre) and sodium sulphate. It is on the Hanover-Salzbergen-Amsterdam line. It is mainly frequented by visitors from the Netherlands. The water is drunk and used for baths and inhalations. *Mud* baths are also prepared with mud brought from the neighbourhood and placed in reservoirs where it is saturated with the sulphur water. The diseases treated are gout and rheumatism, skin affections, respiratory and intestinal catarrh and syphilis.

Berg. *See* Canstatt, p. 132.

Berka, a weak *chalybeate* spa on the Ilm, in the Grand Duchy of Saxe-Weimar. It is a little town of 1,900 inhabitants, situated in a valley nearly 900 feet above the sea and surrounded by pine-clad hills. The season is from May to September. It is also a climatic winter resort.

The iron springs also contain lime salts. They are used for drinking and for baths. Other remedies applied are *mud* baths (the mud brought from the Ilm valley meadows), sand, and pine-needle baths.

The chief maladies treated there are anæmia and rheumatism. The station is on the Weimar-Berka-Kranichfeld line.

Bibra, a small *chalybeate* spa and summer resort with feebly mineralised springs, at an altitude of 410 feet, in Prussian Saxony. Railway station, Laucha, on the Naunberg-Artern line.

Bilin, in Bohemia, a few miles from Teplitz, is celebrated for its Sauerbrunn, a *cold alkaline* spring, rich in free carbonic acid and largely exported. It contains 3·3 grammes of carbonate of sodium to a litre, and 0·7 of sodium sulphate; the latter gives it a slightly aperient quality. It is also reported to contain a small amount of carbonate of lithium.

It is considered to be useful in the treatment of the following maladies: renal calculi and gravel—especially uric acid deposits; vesical catarrh and certain forms of chronic Bright's disease; dyspeptic states, stomach and intestinal catarrh; slight forms of hepatic congestion, sluggish flow of bile, and hepatic concretions with or without jaundice; catarrhal affections of the respiratory organs; also gout and diabetes.

There is a hydropathic establishment at Bilin, and vapour and electric baths, massage, inhalations, etc., can be obtained there.

The season is from May 15 to Sept. 30.

Birmenstorf.—At this Swiss village, near Schinznach, a purgative water is prepared by lixiviating fragments of gypsum rock, containing magnesium sulphate, in water until it has attained a certain strength. It is then bottled and exported, when it is found to contain 22 grammes of magnesium sulphate per litre and 7 of sodium sulphate, besides other ingredients in small proportions.

Birresborn has a station between Cologne and Trèves in Rhenish Prussia. It has a simple *alkaline gaseous* spring with about 2·8 grammes of bicarbonate of soda in a litre. It also contains some bicarbonate of magnesium and sulphate of sodium, so that it is slightly aperient. It has been prescribed in dyspeptic conditions associated with constipation. It is also used as a table water.

Bocklet is a prettily situated village, at an elevation of 680 feet, with *chalybeate* springs, about five miles up the valley from Kissingen. Ferruginous mud baths are also prepared. It has a pleasant, mild climate, and the accommodation there is simpler and living cheaper than at the popular neighbouring spa. It is completely surrounded by a Kurpark and a ridge of hills, except towards Kissingen, and these afford numerous agreeable walks for the visitors. Its principal spring, the Stahlquelle, contains 0·088 of bicarbonate of iron and 1·0 of sodium chloride per litre, and much free carbonic acid gas. It also contains some aperient constituents, in small amounts, such as magnesium sulphate and chloride and sodium sulphate.

It will be seen that it is a fairly strong gaseous chalybeate water, with some aperient constituents. It is used for drinking, bathing, and gargling.

It is admirably adapted for the treatment of cases of anæmia, associated with constipation, for which a calm, quiet life is desirable, and in such cases it has an advantage over those chalybeate springs in which the iron in them is associated with a considerable quantity of the astringent carbonate of lime. It has also a sulphur spring.

It is advised sometimes as an after-cure to Kissingen, where these iron waters are occasionally drunk. Besides cases of anæmia and debility, certain diseases of women and cases of rheumatism are treated.

The season is from May 15 to the end of September.

Boll, Bad-Boll.—There are two baths of this name; one is in the hands of an English fishing club, and is situated at an altitude of over 2,000 feet, near Bonndorf in the Black Forest; its station is Neustadt on the Baden-Höllenthal Railway. It has a spring containing sodium chloride and magnesium and calcium sulphates and carbonates, and some free carbonic acid. It is used for drinking, bathing, and inhaling, and mud baths (mud from Marienbad) and pine-needle baths are also applied. The water is exported after being artificially charged with carbonic acid.

It is reported to be useful in cases of rheumatism and gout, in catarrhal conditions of the mucous membrane, and in urinary affections and some forms of skin disease.

The season is from May 1 to Oct. 1.

The other Bad-Boll is in Würtemberg, in the Filsthal, at an altitude of 1,340 feet, about four miles from the station of Goeppingen. It has a cold sulphur spring containing free H_2S.

Borjom, a Russian spa (Tiflis) near Abbas-Tuman, in the Caucasus, has *warm simple alkaline* waters (temperature 84° F.) containing 5·0 grammes per litre of sodium bicarbonate and a small amount of bicarbonate of iron. It has been termed the Russian Vichy.

Borszek, a *chalybeate* bath in Transylvania, in the Carpathians, at an altitude of nearly 3,000 feet, near the frontier of Roumania. It has *cold iron* springs (0·09 of bicarbonate of iron), containing also alkaline-earthy salts, calcium, magnesium, and sodium bicarbonates (5 grammes of the mixed salts per litre). *Moor* baths are also prepared.

Bramstedt, a small *cold salt* bath on the Brame in Schleswig-

Holstein, on the Altona-Bramstedt road. It is surrounded by hills and close to a forest. The water is used exclusively for bathing in cases of gout, rheumatism, neuralgia, and scrofulous maladies.

Season, May 1 to Oct. 1.

Bremerbad, a *simple thermal* spring of comparatively low thermality at the summit of the Brenner Pass (4,360 feet) in Austrian Tyrol.

Bridge of Allan, three miles from Stirling, N.B., has a *cold salt* spring containing about 5·4 grammes per litre of common salt, 4·4 calcium chloride, and 0·5 calcium sulphate. It is usual to heat the water for consumption, and three glasses before breakfast is the ordinary dose. It is said to act as an aperient, and the spring has a local reputation as of value in functional hepatic and gastric complaints.

Bridge of Earn (Pit-Keathly), close to Perth, has weak *salt* waters, containing free carbonic acid gas. Artificial waters are prepared there and sold in bottles under the designation of "Pit-Keathly water" and "Pit-Keathly cum lithia."

Briscous (Biarritz) is the source of the *common salt* springs supplying the salt baths of Biarritz. These springs contain about 290 per mille of sodium chloride, and the *eau mère* is very rich in magnesium chloride. The water is heated to the required temperature for baths and douches.

Bukowine, a small *cold chalybeate* spa in Silesia. Railway station, Oels. Containing carbonate of iron chiefly. The Agnesquelle is used for drinking, the Luisenquelle is conducted to the bath establishment for the baths. *Mud* baths, from a moor near at hand, are also applied, as well as electricity and hydrotherapy.

Cases of chlorosis and anæmia, of rheumatism and gout, certain skin affections, and some chronic forms of paralysis are treated there.

Burtschied. *See* Aix la Chapelle.

Buzias, a Hungarian *chalybeate* and highly gaseous spring, three hours and a-half from the railway station of Temesvar, at an altitude of 420 feet.

Cambo (Basses Pyrénées), eleven miles from Bayonne, on the line between that town and Ossès, possesses a *tepid sulphur* spring (75° F.) which contains free sulphuretted hydrogen. Its mineral constituents are calcium and magnesium sulphates, and carbonates chiefly (1·83 per litre). It also has a cold *chalybeate* spring.

Cambo, no doubt, owes its growing popularity as much to its accessibility, especially from Biarritz, as to its pleasing situation and mineral springs. Those who have passed the greater part of the winter at Biarritz find it an agreeable change, when spring comes, to migrate for a few weeks to Cambo and exchange the Atlantic winds, sea air, and coast scenery of the former place for the soothing and sedative climate of this sub-Pyrenean station. The river Nive divides Cambo into two parts about half a mile distant from one another, *Le haut Cambo* and *Le bas Cambo.* The former, where the hotels and *pensions* are situated, is about 200 feet above the sea, on a steep terrace. It commands a charming landscape. At the foot of the hill the clear stream of the Nive forms a graceful curve, and from its right bank stretches away a vast extent of fertile fields and wooded country. On the other side rise the lower spurs of the Pyrenees, mountains of no great height, but giving variety to the landscape, which, although not grand, yet presents a pleasing, cheerful, calm and rusticity, full of freshness and delight.

The bath establishment has the usual appliances for the administration of the waters internally and externally. Very many charming walks and excursions can be made into the surrounding district.

The maladies adapted for treatment at Cambo are, as at all other sulphur baths, those of lymphatic and scrofulous origin, skin diseases, and catarrh of the respiratory passages. Hepatic congestions are also named as benefiting by treatment there.

The season used to be reckoned from the middle of April to the middle of November, but now, owing to the mildness of its climate, Cambo is open all the year round, and is resorted to in the winter as well as at other parts of the year.

Canstatt and Berg.—Adjacent towns connected with Stuttgart—of which they form a suburb—by a tramway. They are situated at an altitude oi 700 feet, with extensive park and wooded hills in the neighbourhood. Several springs are utilised, especially the Wilhelmsbrunnen at the Kursaal, and the Berger-Sprudel and Inselquelle between Berg and Canstatt, on a small island in the Neckar,

They are *tepid weak common salt* (2·0 per litre) and *carbonate of lime* (1·0) waters, containing much free carbonic acid gas. They also contain some carbonate of iron, and are termed "ferruginous" by some authorities. The Berger-Sprudel is largely exported in bottles, as well as used on the spot for drinking and bathing. Carlsbad salt is sometimes added to the water to increase its laxative action. The temperature of the springs is artificially raised for bathing purposes. Swimming baths, mud or *Moor* baths from Franzensbad, and electric baths also are provided. The cases treated there are catarrh of the respiratory organs, gastro-intestinal catarrh, anæmia, chlorosis, neurasthenia, and chronic scrofulous glandular affections.

The season is from May 15th to Sept. 15th.

The place has now rather too much the character of a manufacturing town to be very appropriate for spa treatment.

Carlsbad.—Of all the spas of Europe, Carlsbad may be regarded as perhaps the most important, if we have regard only to the activity of its mineral springs, and the gravity and seriousness of many of the maladies for which they are prescribed.

It is one of the oldest as well as one of the most frequented of German spas, and a vast concourse of invalids from every part of the world resort to it yearly.

Situated in the north-western corner of Bohemia, a few miles from the town of Eger, it is rather a long journey from this country, but this is now made easy by the luxurious express trains *en route* to Vienna viâ Nuremberg.

Carlsbad is situated in the valley of the Tepl, at an elevation of 1,200 feet above the sea. In hot seasons the air in this narrow valley gets close and oppressive. It is therefore desirable to procure lodgings on the hill, in what is called the English quarter, on the Schlossberg, an eminence situated just above the Schlossbrunnen.

There is no *table d'hôte* at the hotels or lodging-houses, and the meals are usually taken at the restaurants, which are many and good. The food at all these is subject to medical regulations and supervision, and this is considered a not unimportant part of the cure. The dinner-hour is from twelve to three, the supper-hour from seven to eight. Living is rather expensive there during the height of the season. As at most other resorts of the kind, there is a free concert every evening at the Kurhaus, a daily theatrical performance, and a dance once a week. The town of Carlsbad is to a great extent built on the crust of a vast common reservoir of hot mineral water, the Sprudel-Kessel. It stands on the lid of the kettle. The steam of this subterranean cauldron escapes through artificial apertures made in the rock, to prevent the natural boiler from bursting; and, notwithstanding these artificial vents, the water has been known to force new passages for itself. It is recorded as a curious fact that at the time of the Lisbon earthquake of 1755 the Sprudel ceased to flow for three days!

The narrow valley in which these springs are found is surrounded by pine-clad slopes, through which there are paths in all directions; and besides these agreeable shady promenades in the vicinity of the springs, there are many pleasant excursions, of various distances, into the surrounding country.

The springs at Carlsbad, nineteen or more in number, all contain the same constituents, and differ only in their temperature, which ranges from 48° to 162·5° F.

The well-known Sprudelbrunnen, situated on the right bank of the river, is the hottest; it rises to a height of about three feet from the ground, and every few minutes will suddenly leap to a height of twenty to twenty-five feet. The Sprudel, with some adjacent springs, is enclosed in a "colonnade"; and the Mühlbrunnen Promenade encloses that and several other springs. The remaining springs are in various parts of the town.

Of the bathing establishments at Carlsbad the first place must be given to the magnificent and monumental Kaiserbad, one of the most perfectly organised and equipped in Europe.

It provides all the most modern balneological appliances—douches and baths of all kinds, hot air and vapour baths, Franzensbad *Moor* or mud baths, pine-needle baths, electric baths, massage of all kinds, and a Zander institute for Swedish gymnastics, etc. Older bathing establishments are the Kurhaus, the Neubad, and the Sprudelbad.

The band plays at the Sprudel and the Mühlbrunnen from 6 to 8 a.m., and drinking begins at a very early hour. In the height of the season the crowd of patients at the latter spring is so great that they have to wait their turn *en queue* for a quarter of an hour at a time. To avoid this inconvenience, it is better to begin drinking a little later than the crowd, say 7.30 or 8 o'clock, and breakfast a little later.

We have said that the composition of all the springs is very nearly identical, and the selection of the spring suitable to particular cases is determined by its temperature and the amount of free carbonic acid it contains. The Sprudel, being the hottest (162·5° F.), contains the least carbonic acid. The two chief constituents of the Carlsbad springs are the aperient *sodium sulphate* (2·4 grammes per litre) and the alkaline *sodium bicarbonate* (1·2), and the next in importance is *sodium chloride* (1·0).

The springs in chief repute at Carlsbad are the Sprudel, the Marktbrunnen (104° F.), the Mühlbrunnen (124·5° F.), and the Schlossbrunnen (127° F.).

The Carlsbad cure is indicated in many serious

maladies, and great benefit often results from passing one or more seasons there. It is especially advantageous in diseases caused by defective oxidation and an insufficient elimination of effete matters.

It is particularly useful in certain derangements to which gouty persons and free livers are prone; in cases of "abdominal plethora," that is, of passive engorgement of the liver and of the intestinal vessels, with a consequent tendency to chronic gastric and intestinal catarrh, with or without diarrhœa. Such persons often suffer from a severe form of dyspepsia, with much stomach pain and flatulency, occasional vomiting in the morning, and obstinate constipation, with a disposition to hæmorrhoids; or there may be a tendency to frequent incomplete action of the bowels. Such cases derive much benefit from a carefully directed course of the Carlsbad waters. If there should be chronic intestinal catarrh (diarrhœa) it is usual to begin with quite small doses of the water, three ounces, or even less.

The Carlsbad cure is specially adapted to cases of jaundice, either catarrhal or dependent on the presence of gallstones; also to cases where there is a *tendency* to the formation and passage of gallstones, or biliary sand, or to the formation of thick, inspissated bile, although there may be no notable jaundice.

The Carlsbad course greatly diminishes the frequency and violence of attacks of biliary colic, even if it does not altogether arrest them. Gallstones are often passed during the course of treatment there, and it seems reasonable to believe that one of the effects of drinking the hot alkaline water is to stimulate a healthier secretion and promote the outflow of a thinner bile from the bile ducts. Enlargements of the liver, due to passive engorgement, from over-feeding and insufficient exercise, a condition frequently associated with hæmorrhoids, are suitably treated there.

Enlargements of the liver and spleen, induced by exposure to malaria in hot climates, and associated with constipation, find relief at Carlsbad. In short, the Carlsbad waters are indicated in all functional hepatic disorders and even in the early stages of alcoholic cirrhosis they may be found most useful.

Cases of gravel (uric acid deposits) and renal calculi, if connected with hepatic congestion and constipation and accompanied with catarrhal conditions of the bladder, are benefited by treatment there, but cases of uric acid deposit and renal calculi pure and simple, without any hepatic disorder and in feeble persons, are better suited to Vichy or Contrexéville.

No doubt the general gouty condition itself, apart from the particular modes in which it may express itself, is in most instances ameliorated by the Carlsbad course; this is strikingly seen in the case of the periodical headaches often associated with the gouty constitution.

The Carlsbad waters are great and powerful purifiers of the body, great eliminators. If bathing be associated with the internal consumption of the waters we submit the organism to a threefold purifying influence, for while the hot mineral baths stimulate the excretory functions of the skin, the internal use of the waters greatly promotes the discharge of effete substances through the evacuations of the intestinal canal and the kidneys; in this manner the blood and the tissues of the body become cleansed of retained effete and excrementitious substances.

Carlsbad, on account of this effect of its waters, enjoys the reputation of reducing corpulence, and it does, no doubt, lead to a moderate diminution of fat; but unless a very strict diet be followed, after as well as during the course, the fat readily returns.

Carlsbad has a special reputation for the treatment of *diabetes*, and there is no doubt whatever that it leads to a very great improvement in many cases, and to a temporary or permanent cure in others. It is in the gouty or fat diabetics that it is of such special service. It is of little or no value in the grave form as it occurs in *young* subjects.

The quantity of water necessary to be drunk will naturally vary with the nature of the malady and the constitution of the patient. Very large quantities of water such as were at one time taken are no longer prescribed. From two to six glasses a day are sufficient for all but quite exceptional cases; and any excessive aperient action of the waters should at once be taken as an indication for lowering the dose or suspending the course for a day or two. In some instances the water has no aperient effect, and it is a common practice to add some of the Sprudel salt to the water of the spring to give it a laxative action. It has also been observed that the hotter springs are less laxative than the cooler ones, and it has been suggested that for laxative purposes the waters of the Sprudel should be obtained the evening before and drunk cold in the morning.

As much exercise as possible in the open air is usually prescribed by the Carlsbad doctors, and this, together with the strict regulation of the diet there, contributes considerably to the good results usually obtained, but the prescription of much physical exercise must not be too universally given, as there are not a few patients for whom the Carlsbad course may be fitly ordered who need complete physical rest, and with whom the success of the cure would be seriously compromised by indiscreet efforts at physical exercise.

The springs at Carlsbad may be resorted to at any period of the year; the season, however, may be regarded as extending from April to October. Diabetic patients who might with advantage take the waters twice a year are advised to visit Carlsbad in April or May, and again in October. It is suggested that the more robust and vigorous patients should come in the cooler months of April, May, September, and October, and the feebler sort in June, July, and August.

The length of the course varies from three to six weeks, according to the nature of the disease, the age and strength of the patient, and the observed effect of the waters.

Much discredit is occasionally brought upon the Carlsbad course by sending patients there who are the subjects of undiagnosed malignant gastric, hepatic, or abdominal disease, or persons in very feeble, broken-down condition; when such patients succumb, as they are very likely to do, either at Carlsbad or soon after leaving it, the course there is given the credit of killing them!

It is considered important that those who intend submitting themselves to the Carlsbad cure should adopt a careful and rational diet some time *before*, as well as after the course. It is also suggested that a few bottles of Carlsbad water or a few doses of the Carlsbad salts should be taken, at home, for a week or ten days before setting out for the spa; and rest, mental and physical, is recommended during that period.

Although it is a rule at Carlsbad to drink the waters early in the morning, before breakfast, and only then, it is quite permissible and even advisable for persons who cannot digest the waters well on an empty stomach, to take a cup of tea, or coffee, or thin cocoa, or beef-tea half an hour before they commence drinking the waters. The warmer the spring the more slowly should it be drunk or *sipped*, and an interval of a quarter to half an hour should be allowed between each glass. After the last glass of water an hour's walk before breakfast is recommended; only, of course, when the patient is strong enough to take such exercise with advantage.

In those exceptional cases which require unusually large doses of the water, it is best to drink them at separate times of the day, at midday and from 4 to

6 p.m., as well as in the early morning. A glass may also be taken cold at bedtime.

Patients should clothe themselves warmly for the early dose of water, so that the action of the skin, which the warm drink promotes, may not be checked. The baths are best taken in the forenoon, about an hour and a-half or two hours after breakfast. Repose before and after the bath is desirable.

In many cases it is a decided advantage to take the course for two or three consecutive seasons.

The diet at Carlsbad is adapted by the physicians to each case; the following may be taken as an average one :—

Breakfast: Coffee, tea, or weak cocoa, and two or three small milk or water rolls, not more, to which may be added one or two soft-boiled eggs if required.

It is usual to call at the baker's for one's rolls, which are very well made, and take them in a little bag into the adjacent woods, where restaurants are placed at convenient distances.

Dinner: Soup, one or two light dishes of meat, or fish, or poultry, or game, fresh vegetables in small quantity, mashed potatoes or stewed fruit. Only the lightest kind of puddings, in small quantities, are allowable. One glass of claret, or one glass of Pilsener beer.

It is usual at Carlsbad to drink freely of a very excellent cold gaseous spring in the neighbourhood, which is bottled for table use and for exportation, the Giesshübler-Sauerbrunn.

A cup of coffee, with or without a small roll, is allowed in the afternoon.

Supper: Soup, or two soft-boiled eggs, or a small quantity of freshly roasted meat.

There is, of course, a special diet for diabetics.

It is by no means unimportant that the patient should, after the Carlsbad cure, continue more or less closely, for a few weeks, the *régime* which he has followed there, and it is often highly advantageous and in some cases really necessary to pass two or three weeks at some sub-alpine health resort in Switzerland or the Tyrol, or the Black Forest, where a quiet out-of-door life in pure air can be enjoyed.

Cauterets (Hautes Pyrénées), with its numerous *thermal sulphur* springs, is one of the most popular of Pyrenean spas when regarded from a purely medical point of view. It is not a resort of fashion and pleasure like Luchon, but most of the visitors to Cauterets come with a serious purpose. There is a business-like look about everybody at Cauterets. The patients look graver than usual, and more bent than usual on carrying out with business-like accuracy the details of the cure. "Nos eaux sont des eaux sérieuses," is the grave utterance of all the doctors and other people interested in and engaged at Cauterets. The atmosphere, too, seems a little heavy and business-like, and lacks that light and exhilarating tone observable at Luchon.

Cauterets is reached by an electric railway, which continues the regular line from its terminus at Pierrefitte. From Pierrefitte to Cauterets is a distance of about seven miles. The road ascends nearly the whole of the way, through a picturesque valley, dominated by lofty peaks, rugged and wild in parts. As we approach Cauterets the valley widens, and finally discloses the town situated at the bottom of a narrow basin, surrounded nearly on all sides by lofty summits frowning down from immense heights on the small town which lies crouched between their bases. Several mountain valleys open into this basin, and invite to wild and picturesque excursions into the very heart of the Pyrenees; none of them are carriage roads except that leading to Pierrefitte.

One of the most celebrated of these excursions is to the Pont d'Espagne and the Lac de Gaube, a three hours' walk from Cauterets. Cauterets is thus quite in the mountains, its elevation being a little over 3,000 feet; its climate, however, is scarcely so bracing as might be expected in a place of this elevation. It is so much shut in on all sides by high mountains that it is capable of becoming very hot and close in certain conditions of the atmosphere. The mornings and evenings are, however, fresh and pleasant, especially before the end of June and after August. The basin of Cauterets is very prone, like other places of this medium elevation, to become somewhat suddenly filled with clouds, which may linger long, and give rather a dull and sad aspect to the little town. The climate is also rainy, and subject to sudden changes of temperature.

The reputation of Cauterets as a health resort is very ancient. M. Taine tells us that Julius Cæsar is said to have been restored to health by the spring named after him "César," and Abarca, king of Aragon, by the spring on that account named "du Roi." It was here that Marguérite de Navarre, sister of François I., a distinguished example of the race of "superior women," wrote the chief part of the Heptameron. She came here with "her court, her poets, her musicians," interested in all subjects, reading Greek, learning Hebrew, and delighting in theological discussion; at the same time tender and simple: "Une imagination mesurée, un cœur de femme dévoué et inépuisable en dévoûments, beaucoup de naturel, de clarté, d'aisance, l'art de conter et de sourire, la malice agréable et jamais méchante." Such is the attractive picture M. Taine gives of Marguérite de Navarre at Cauterets.

The waters of Cauterets are *sulphur* waters, like those of Luchon, but they are considered to be milder in their action and more sedative. They are efficacious, like those of Luchon, in diseases of the skin, in scrofulous affections, in chronic throat ailments, and especially in chronic diseases of the respiratory organs. The testimony of the leading physicians there is so strong in favour of the great amelioration that certain cases of consumption undergo at Cauterets that it must, we think, take rank amongst the health resorts to which persons who are afflicted with chronic torpid forms of consumption may be sent.

There are a great number of mineral springs at Cauterets, and several bath establishments, some of which, notably the César, are most elaborately fitted with every appliance that modern science has suggested in the use of mineral springs—douches of all kinds, inhalation and pulverisation chambers, besides baths of every description.

The temperature of the stronger springs varies from 96° to 136° F., and their characteristic ingredient is sodium sulphide 0·02 per litre in the strongest. The hottest springs are used chiefly for the baths, and for inhalation and pulverisation chambers.

The *source,* however, which is especially valued for internal administration is La Raillière. It is really curious to encounter the long procession of drinkers coming away from the Raillière spring, which is situated at some little distance from the town; each, young and old, sucking a stick of "sucre d'orge à l'eau de Cauterets." It is said that ten thousand sticks of barley sugar are sold each day during the season! It is impossible to explain satisfactorily how the small quantity (sometimes only four or five tablespoonfuls twice a day) of this somewhat feebly mineralised sulphur spring can produce the remarkable curative effects that are claimed for it. But there seems no doubt that many chronic catarrhal conditions are greatly benefited or cured there.

Gargling with the Raillière or other springs is much practised at Cauterets, and its chief *speciality* is undoubtedly the treatment of chronic nasal, pharyngeal, laryngeal, and bronchial catarrhs. The Source Manhourat, close to the Raillière, only contains one-half the amount of sodium sulphide contained in the latter. It is only used for drinking, and is regarded as being of special value in some forms of dyspepsia and uric acid deposits.

The St. Sauveur spring is one of the feebler group, which are prone to undergo what is termed "degeneration" because of the tendency to oxidation of the sulphur in them and the formation of sulphites and hyposulphites. This spring is considered to have a more sedative effect than the members of the stronger group, and is therefore used in the treatment of dysmenorrhœal states as well as other female maladies—it is said with much benefit.

Many other diseases have been enumerated as suitable for treatment at Cauterets; amongst these are the common forms of rheumatism, and the douche-massage as practised at Aix is applied to the treatment of such cases. Myalgias, neuralgias, and painful visceral affections associated with or dependent upon the rheumatic diathesis are considered as suitable for treatment by these waters. We may add the scrofulous and cutaneous affections usually benefited by thermal sulphur baths, those at Cauterets being more especially adapted to cases requiring more sedative and less exciting treatment than they could find at certain other sulphide of sodium springs.

The season is from June 1st to Oct. 1st, but the best time for the treatment is between June 15th and Sept. 15th.

There are all the usual amusements and resources provided in a French spa. It is 876 kilometres from Paris.

Challes.—This important *source* is of comparatively recent discovery, and rises in a very picturesque district at an altitude of 900 feet, about three miles by steam tramway from Chambéry Station, and within an easy journey of Aix les Bains. It is sheltered by mountains from the north and north-east winds; while the south wind comes to it cooled by its passage over the glaciers of the Alps.

The Challes water is an exceptionally strong *cold sulphur water.* It is on this account largely prescribed by the physicians at Aix as an important adjunct to the treatment pursued there; it is also added to the baths there when it is thought desirable to increase the amount of sulphur in them. The sulphur in the Challes water calculated as sulphide of sodium amounts to 0·513 grammes per litre; it also has 1 gramme of bicarbonate of sodium, iodide (0·012), bromide (0·004), and chloride (0·155) of sodium.

The amount of water yielded by the spring is limited to 4,000 to 5,000 litres a day, so that its bathing establishment is necessarily restricted; it is, however, very well fitted up, and contains inhalation, gargling, irrigation, and pulverisation chambers in addition to the ordinary baths and douches. Treatment by pulverisation, inhalation, irrigation, and gargling of the nasal, pharyngeal, and laryngeal cavities for the various forms of chronic catarrh with which patients are liable to be affected is one of the chief specialities at Challes. It is also suitable for the treatment of some forms of chronic bronchial catarrh.

This water is especially valuable in *scrofulous* affections of the skin (eczema, acne, etc.) and other organs; in goitre, in chronic glandular enlargements, in chronic ulcers, in scrofulous disease of bones, in constitutional syphilis, and, as has been said, in chronic inflammation of the nose (ozæna) and throat, especially in tuberculous or scrofulous persons. The treatment of chronic rheumatism is also undertaken there. The water of the spring is usually diluted with ordinary hot water in the preparation of the baths. *Very small* doses of the Challes water are usually given at the commencement of the cure, about two or three ounces daily, which is gradually increased.

For all these purposes the Challes water can be taken at Aix alone or in combination with the Aix treatment; but those who prefer to reside at Challe can obtain good accommodation in the old château there, which has been converted into a hotel. It has a picturesque situation and commands a fine view of the Alps of Dauphiné and the surrounding country; many interesting excursions can be made from it.

The bath establishment is open from May 15th to Oct. 15th, but the best season is from June 10th to Sept. 15th. The place is growing in importance and reputation. The accommodation to be obtained is good, and the prices are moderate.

Châtelguyon (Auvergne), in the Department of Puy de Dôme, is a small town, picturesquely situated at an elevation of 1,300 feet above the sea, seven hours from Paris, about four miles from the railway station of Riom, which is within half an hour by train of Clermont-Ferrand. It has several warm mineral springs of a temperature varying from 82° to 95° F. Its climate is mildly tonic.

The water is rich in free carbonic acid gas, so that in the baths the skin becomes covered with bubbles of this gas, which have a stimulating effect on the surface. These baths are said to produce both a tonic and a soothing effect.

The mineralisation of these springs amounts to about 8 grammes of solids to the litre. *Magnesium chloride* (1·563) being regarded as the dominating and *characteristic* ingredient, sodium chloride (1·633), calcium bicarbonate (2·177) and sulphate (0·49), sodium bicarbonate (0·955), potassium (0·253) and lithium bicarbonate (0·0194), are present, as well as bicarbonate of iron (0·0685), a valuable addition. It will be noted that there are between three and four grammes of chlorides to the litre. It is upon the presence of these chlorides that the special application of the springs depends. There is but little difference in the composition of the different springs, but they vary in temperature. The Source Gubler is the only one bottled for exportation. The waters are given internally and used externally in a variety of ways; they are employed for *lavages* of the stomach, for intestinal irrigations, and as baths and douches. The doses drunk vary greatly, according to the effect it is desired to produce, but small quantities are preferred by most of the bath physicians—from five to fifteen or sixteen ounces daily, divided into three or four portions, and drunk at intervals of fifteen to thirty minutes.

The baths are given of "running" water, of a temperature of about 80° to 90° F., and as it proceeds directly from the spring, it preserves all its natural qualities, and its full amount of carbonic acid gas. There are very complete and convenient arrangements for hot and cold douches and for intestinal irrigations. *Lavages d'estomac* and intestinal irrigations are specialities of Châtelguyon. Massage and electrical treatment are also frequently employed.

These waters are said to increase all the intestinal secretions, and so act as laxatives and relieve congestion of the portal system and the organs tributary to it. It is especially employed in diseases of the gastro-intestinal canal and abdominal viscera, atonic dyspepsia and stomach dilatation, gastric catarrh, chronic constipation in anæmic and gouty subjects, and in cases of portal congestion, chronic appendicitis, and hæmorrhoids; in the atonic form of muco-membranous enterocolitis, accompanied by constipation; in functional hepatic disease, torpor, congestion, and biliary concretions; in lithiasis when the kidneys are sound, and in albuminuria, congestive or dietetic, and when not dependent on organic changes in the kidneys; in certain uterine affections, metritis, ulcerations of the cervix, and simple ovarian congestion; in gouty glycosuria, and other atonic gouty conditions, and in some forms of neurasthenia. The secondary effects of malarial fevers and of residence in tropical countries, such as anæmias, dysenteries, hepatic congestions, etc., do well there. Châtelguyon also claims to be of service in certain affections of children, *e.g.* anæmic children with faulty digestion, children of gouty antecedents, with feeble circulation and tendency to .constipation, convalescents from acute disease, and young girls at the approach of puberty.

The season is from May 15th to Oct. 15th.

There is good accommodation for visitors, and there are many pleasing excursions in the neighbourhood. There are the usual amusements—casino, theatre, club, etc.

Cheltenham, in the Severn valley in Gloucestershire, at an altitude of 150 feet, possesses springs containing the *aperient sulphates* of magnesium and sodium, combined with common salt. It has also chalybeate waters. It is about three and a-half hours from London, and is an attractive residential and educational centre. The Cotswold Hills afford it a protection from easterly winds. It is a favourite resort for those who have lived long in tropical climates, and who have families to educate. Being built on the level, it affords convenience for walking exercise for those who wish to avoid up-hill walks.

Cheltenham had a great popularity as a spa a century or more ago, when Continental resorts of the same kind were but little known in this country, and when travelling abroad was very costly and difficult. As facilities for travelling became developed, and the knowledge of the resources and attractions of foreign spas became spread abroad, the popularity of Cheltenham declined. A revival appears to be at hand, as local enterprise is being directed to the provision of those developments which the requirements of modern balneology and hydro-mineral therapeutics seem to necessitate.

Its climate appears to be fairly bracing. The mean annual temperature is 47·1° F. July is the warmest month with a mean of 61·3°, and

January is the coldest with a mean of 36·3°. The average number of rainy days is 189, of which October has the greatest number and March the smallest. The mean annual rainfall is 29·84 inches.

There are numerous wells at Cheltenham utilised for drinking.

The magnesia-saline wells (Chadnor Villa Well and the Cottage Well) contain the aperient magnesium sulphate (about 1·75 grammes per litre) and sodium sulphate (in rather less amount), and sodium chloride (0·4406 per litre). The other chief constituents are sulphate and carbonate of lime. There are also small amounts of potassium sulphate and sodium silicate, and minute quantities of other constituents. The soda-saline waters (the three Pittville springs) contain a small amount of sodium bicarbonate, a considerable amount of sodium chloride (up to 7·0 grammes per litre), and sodium sulphate (up to 2·2 grammes per litre), but *no* magnesium sulphate.

The chalybeate spring (Cambray iron water), according to an old analysis, contains about 0·1 carbonate of iron per litre.

The chief specialisation in the therapeutic uses of these springs is suggested to be their applicability to the treatment of the "deleterious effects of residence in hot climates, and the dyspepsia and renal and cutaneous affections attendant upon gout" (Wilson).

Contrexéville (Vosges).—The best known of the Vosges spas, Contrexéville, may be well taken as the *type* of the class of *cold earthy calcareous* waters. It has long enjoyed a European celebrity. Contrexéville has been described as "in the heart of the Vosges," but this is scarcely correct. The higher mountains of the Vosges are at a considerable distance from it. It lies on those western slopes of the chain which descend by a very gentle inclination towards Belfort and the plateau of Langres;

and a branch line connecting the latter town with Épinal and Nancy passes by it. It is easily accessible from all parts, and can be reached in about sixteen hours from London through Paris or Rheims.

The village and springs of Contrexéville are situated in a valley, or hollow, below the level of the surrounding country, although at an elevation of 1,100 feet above the sea. The village itself is altogether unattractive.

The Etablissement des Bains, with its hotel, casino, and theatre, is enclosed in a small park and surrounded by gardens and pleasure-grounds, prettily laid out and well arranged for the purposes it has to serve. The climate of the valley partakes of that of the Vosges generally in being subject to sudden changes of temperature, which must be guarded against by suitable clothing.

There is a considerable rainfall, and a good number of rainy days, and the sky is often overcast and cloudy. At other times, owing to the confined situation, the air is hot and relaxing.

The Pavillon is the chief spring, and it yields a very great quantity of water—200,000 litres a day. This is exported in enormous quantities, and its virtues give to Contrexéville its great reputation. There are other springs of nearly the same composition, which are used chiefly to supply the baths. A water possessing such remarkable virtues would naturally be expected to have a remarkable composition, but it is not so. Its chief characteristic is that it contains a great amount of lime, a property common to all "hard" waters! In 1,000 parts (a litre) of the Pavillon spring there are two and a-half parts of solid constituents, and of these, speaking roughly, no less than one and a-half consists of sulphate of lime, and one-half part of carbonate of lime. The remaining half is composed of minute quantities of sulphate of sodium, sulphate and carbonate of magnesium, and very minute quantities of carbonate of iron, carbonate of lithium, and chlorides of potassium and sodium. A French description of this water terms it "eau froide, sulfatée et bicarbonatée calcique, magnésienne, ferrugineuse, lithinée et silicatée"!

As so much, nowadays, is made of the curative influence due to the presence of lithium in a mineral spring, it is as well to realise clearly that in a quart of the Pavillon spring there is but one-seventeenth of a grain of bicarbonate of lithium!

The first thing that strikes one at Contrexéville, as compared with other spas, is the size of the glasses. Instead of holding about six ounces as elsewhere, they contain twelve ounces. And very large quantities of this water are ordered to be drunk: in many cases ten, twelve, and up to twenty glasses in the day, while over-zealous patients have been known, on their own responsibility, to take thirty glasses, *i.e.* ten quarts daily!

The water is clear, still, almost tasteless, of a temperature of 52° F., and neutral to test paper.

There is also a spring termed the Prince, which is richer in iron, another the Quai, containing more magnesia, and another, the Souveraine, which contains less iron and more magnesia than any of the others, and which is therefore thought better adapted to the treatment of constipation and liver affections.

The "cure" at Contrexéville formerly consisted exclusively in drinking the waters; now, following the fashion at other watering-places, the administration of baths, douches, and the application of *massage,* usefully fill up the time that otherwise would hang on the hands of the invalids still more heavily than it actually does.

Close to the Etablissement there has been erected a spacious promenade covered with glass, with a central dome surmounting an octagonal space in which is the Pavillon spring. In this promenade the visitors assemble and walk up and down, or lounge about on the seats, or examine the shops which line one side of it, or they stroll into the little park on the other side, and now and again come to the spring until they have drunk the prescribed number of glasses.

The young women who dispense the water have to begin their work very early in the day. At 4.30 a.m. the invalids begin to arrive, and they continue to come in increasing numbers until 7 a.m. At this hour the crowd is so great that it is only by great activity and constant good temper that the attendants are able to supply all the applicants. Before 9 a.m. the drinking ceases; it is renewed again, but on a smaller scale, between 2 and 5 p.m. From one to two and sometimes three quarts are prescribed daily, the dose being increased gradually.

In difficult cases as many as eighteen glasses a day are occasionally prescribed. Twelve of these are taken between 5 and 9 a.m., allowing an interval of a quarter of an hour between the doses, four more between 4 and 5 p.m., and two more before going to bed. But, except in special cases, some of the physicians of the spa set their faces against the afternoon drinking as not to be encouraged.

The consumption of this immense quantity of water has a decidedly diuretic and aperient effect.

The physicians at Contrexéville know that whatever special virtues these springs may possess, much of the success that follows the treatment there depends essentially on the *large quantity of water* which is daily passed through the system. "*Ce n'est pas précisément un lavage,*" say they, but the very form of the expression is three parts of an admission.

The waters are also applied externally as baths and douches; a douche to the loins being specially in favour. But great caution must be exercised in the prescription of baths for the gouty, as they are apt to provoke an acute attack. Massage is frequently combined with the other treatment, particularly in rheumatic cases. Pine, turpentine, and sulphur baths are also given when required,

But the point of chief practical importance is, To what cases are these waters applicable? What diseases do they cure or mitigate?

More than a century ago Bayard, the physician to King Stanislas of Lorraine, wrote as follows:—"Les eaux de Contrexéville sont souveraines dans les maladies des reins, des urétres, de la vessie, etc. . . . . souverainement efficace contre la pierre." This judgment, more than 130 years old, still holds good, and it is chiefly to the success with which calculous and renal and vesical disorders are treated there that Contrexéville owes its great renown. There is clearly one dominant idea in the minds of the physicians of Contrexéville, viz. that by far the greater proportion of maladies, to the treatment of which these waters are applicable, have their origin in gout, and are due to an excess of uric acid in the blood.

Briefly, *gravel* and *renal calculous disorders* are the *spécialité*—whether uric acid, oxalic, or phosphatic—of Contrexéville, and all the vesical troubles associated with the gouty constitution; pyelitis and pyelo-nephritis and catarrh of the urinary passages when dependent on calculous and gouty conditions. Nocturnal incontinence of urine in children is said to be cured there.

Further, congestions of the liver, gallstones, dyspepsias, and other disturbances of health, provided they are, in some way or other, associated with the gouty state, are, it is said, cured there. Diabetics, if also gouty, are benefited, but if the disease is what is known as *true* diabetes, and not dependent on gout, then it is not suitable. The rheumatic should not go there, unless the rheumatism is combined with gout, and then it is suggested that the gout should be first treated at Contrexéville, the rheumatism afterwards at Bourbonne or Plombières!

Finally, such skin affections as eczema, acne, or psoriasis, if dependent on the presence of uric acid in excess in the system, will be benefited by these waters; otherwise not. Gouty *iritis* and other *ocular* troubles of gouty origin are also benefited.

The words "gout" and "uric acid" give the clue to every condition that is cured at Contrexéville; though *alleviation* rather than *cure* would in many instances be the more appropriate term. The torpid, atonic forms of gout are those best suited to this treatment—what the French doctors term "*la goutte blanche.*"

As some doubts have often been expressed as to the mode of action of these waters, it may be as well to state the explanation put forth by the French physicians as to their *physiological* action. The water received into the stomach passes into the intestines, and is there rapidly absorbed by the mesenteric veins and passes by the portal vein to the liver and augments its secretion, thus causing bilious evacuations; an *excess* of the water may flow directly into the large intestine and cause watery stools; some of the water, not so disposed of, passes into the general circulation, washes the tissues, and is finally excreted by the kidneys. We can thus see that the water is cholagogue, laxative, and diuretic.

Patients do not feel debilitated by these purgations because of the tonic effects of the iron and certain other constituents of the water. In some few cases the water fails to have any purgative effect; it is customary then to have recourse to the Souveraine spring, or, if this fails, to give some aperient water, such as Apenta.

The purgative effect of the Contrexéville water is limited to the period before breakfast, and does not interfere with the occupations of the day, and the objection to drinking a portion of the water in the afternoon is that it may possibly cause some purging at night.

The water, then, *washes out* the liver and the

intestine and reduces venous engorgement. The stomach is cleansed and refreshed, appetite is improved and digestion stimulated. Hence the increase of strength and capacity for exertion so constantly observed to accompany the treatment. The diuretic effect of the water may be truly remarkable, and the patient is often led to imagine that he passes more water than he drinks. This, it is maintained, is the main object of the treatment, viz. to obtain a rapid current of water passing quickly through the organism, washing the blood and the tissues, and in its course dissolving and carrying away toxic substances and the less soluble salts needing elimination. At the same time this active current flowing through the urinary passages tends to carry away *mechanically* abnormal substances retained in them, as sand, gravel, mucus, pus, etc. At the end of the cure it is found that the daily excretion of urea is increased, whilst that of uric acid is diminished, from which it is inferred that the cure increases nutritive activity, eliminates nitrogenous waste, and promotes oxidation.

There are certain *counter-indications*, connected with the diseases for which Contrexéville may be prescribed, that it is desirable to mention. These are cases of pyelitis and renal gravel with *constantly* more than a gramme of albumin per litre in the urine; bladder cases in which there has been complete retention, or where there is a stagnant residue of more than 80 grammes of urine; or where there is a tight stricture; or where there is a stone in the bladder; cases of gout when an acute attack is threatening or has been just checked by specifics: such cases should not be sent for at least a month after the end of the attack; cases of hepatic cirrhosis; cases of diabetes with nephritis or cirrhosis, or with very large amounts of sugar, or in a cachectic state.

If such are the principal medical aspects of Contrexéville, what are its social attractions? The life is certainly monotonous and a trifle depressing.

Each day, from 6 to 9 a.m., there is the routine of water-drinking, the usual promenade and exchange of confidences as to the number of glasses you have been ordered to drink, and their effects. Occasionally the prescribed bath or douche, or the consultation with the doctor, varies the morning's employment. At 10 a.m. comes the very substantial *déjeuner*, and it is a point that the waters be drunk fasting, and that the drinking should be completed an hour and a-half before breakfast. Some of the patients after this long fast come to their meal famishing, and eat voraciously. Some English visitors prefer to postpone this heavy meal till their usual luncheon hour, and take only a light breakfast an hour after the drinking. The physicians at Contrexéville have been doing their best to get the *table d'hôte* made to conform more fitly to the objects of treatment there.

Shut in as Contrexéville is in a small, narrow valley, and at a considerable distance from any attractive scenery, there are but few possible excursions, within easy reach, possessing any great attraction. Such excursions as the surrounding country offers are most of them too far off to be consistent with due attention to the treatment, which is, after all, the end and object of being there; so that few visitors go beyond Vittel or Martigny, both rival spas, a few minutes' distance only by train.

Six o'clock is the dinner hour. After dinner on certain days in the week there are dramatic performances in the theatre, or concerts or other kinds of diversion. A certain amount of gambling can be obtained by means of baccarat or bridge in the *salle de jeu*, and in a milder form in the park by means of the highly popular *jeu de petits chevaux*.

Those who have to appear at the Pavillon spring at 6 a.m. naturally want to retire to rest early, and by ten o'clock most of the invalid visitors have withdrawn to their apartments.

The season is from May 20th to Sept. 20th.

Cadéac, a *cold sulphur* spring in the Hautes Pyrénées, of some strength, having 0·075 grammes of sodium sulphide per litre. It is in a picturesque situation at an altitude of 2,360 feet, 2 kilometres from Arreau. The nearest railway station is at Lannemézan on the line between Toulouse and Bayonne. There are two bath establishments. Chronic rheumatism and skin affections are the maladies treated there.

Capvern (Hautes Pyrénées). The baths, at an elevation of 1,360 feet, are about half an hour's drive from the little town and station, which is a few miles from Tarbes on the line between that town and Toulouse. The popularity of this station has increased rapidly of late years. There are two springs and two bath establishments. The springs are warm and have a temperature of 77° F.

In composition and uses they bear a strong resemblance to the Contrexéville springs. They are feebly mineralised, containing 2 grammes of mineral constituents to a litre. These consist chiefly of sulphate and carbonate of lime and sulphate of sodium and magnesium. There is a small amount of iron, and, it is said, of arsenic, copper, and lithium, The waters are said to powerfully stimulate digestion, to increase the renal, hepatic, and alvine secretions, and to be of especial value in gravel and catarrh of the bladder, in hepatic engorgements, and in gallstones, and in many uterine affections, also in gout and gouty diabetes.

Of the two springs the Hount Caoude is the one used for drinking and the Bouridé for the baths. This spring is described as "very unctuous," and as most soothing in cases of rheumatism, neuritis, and uterine affections.

Season, June 15 to Sept. 15.

Carabana, a spring rich in *aperient sulphates*, in the province of Madrid in Spain. Like Rubinat water, it is bottled and exported.

Carratraca, a Spanish *cold sulphur* spring, beautifully situated in the neighbourhood of Malaga. The waters are feebly mineralised, and are used in the treatment of syphilis and skin diseases.

Casamicciola. *See* Ischia, p. 214.

Castellamare di Stabia, a well-known resort in the Bay of Naples, has *cold alkaline-earthy* waters, containing about 5·0 grammes of sodium chloride and 1·0 gramme of calcium bicarbonate per litre. It also possesses chalybeate and sulphur springs.

Casséra-Verduzan, an important bath in an out-of-the-way part of France, 23 kilometres from the station of Auch in the Department of Gers, at an altitude of 320 feet. It has a *warm sulphur* spring (calcium sulphide) and a *cold iron* spring, and possesses a bath establishment for their employment both externally and internally. It is chiefly of local interest for cases of rheumatism, atonic dyspepsia, and anæmic forms of uterine and cutaneous disease.

The season is from May 15 to Oct. 15.

Castiglione. *See* Ischia, p. 214.

Castleconnell, co. Limerick, Ireland, has *chalybeate* springs.

Castro-Caro, province of Toscano, Italy, an hour's drive from Forli railway station, has *strong common salt* waters, containing also some bromides and iodides; there are 44·0 grammes of sodium chloride per litre, 0·197 of magnesium iodide, and 0·185 of magnesium bromide. They are applied in the cases usually treated with common salt springs.

Ceresole - Reale, in Piedmont, about five hours from Turin, has *arsenical* and *iron* springs containing 0·0057 grammes of arsenate of sodium, 0·17 of bicarbonate of iron, and 0·003 each of bicarbonate of lithium and manganese per litre. It is a high mountain resort 5,290 feet above the sea, with very beautiful surroundings, fine bracing air, and good accommodation. It lies between the Grand Paradis and the Levanna Mountains.

Charlottenbrunn, a small *weak gaseous chalybeate* spa in Silesia, on the railway line between Görlitz and Glatz.

Châteauneuf, a bath with somewhat primitive accommodation, in an out-of-the-way part of Auvergne, twenty miles by road from Riom station. It is in the midst of wild and picturesque mountain scenery.

There are as many as fifteen mineral springs scattered over this district, and varying in temperature from 59° to 100° F.; some are highly charged with carbonic acid.

Some are gaseous and cold, and contain a notable amount of iron; others are weak alkaline waters, while others have purgative properties. The reputation of this bath is chiefly local, and it is resorted to by two classes of invalids — first, the anæmic and dyspeptic; and, second, the rheumatic and gouty.

Chaudes Aigues, a small town of 2,000 inhabitants, taking its name from the possession of a great number of *hot* springs, said to be the hottest in France (180° F.), the water of which contains a small amount (0·471 grammes per litre) of carbonate of soda. It is situated at an elevation of 2,110 feet in a remote and out-of-the-way part of the mountains of Cantal, a very picturesque and wild country. It takes sixteen hours to reach it from Paris, first by rail to St. Flour, and then a mountain drive of three hours. The springs are brought by canalisation into the houses, and serve to warm them sufficiently even in that harsh winter climate. These hot springs yield more than a million litres of water per diem.

There is an Etablissement des Bains, with the usual provision of baths, douches, inhalations, pulverisations, etc.

The maladies treated there are rheumatism, swollen joints, visceral congestions, incomplete ankyloses, paralysis, and neurotic conditions. Its use is almost exclusively reserved to those living in the district.

Chaudefontaine, in Belgium, four miles and a-half from Liége on the line to Aix la Chapelle, in a fine situation in the valley of the Vesdre, has *simple thermal* waters, temperature 96° F., which are utilised in the same way as such springs elsewhere. These waters have been known for many centuries.

Chianciano, near Montepulciano, in Central Italy, has *thermal calcareous* waters of a temperature of 100° F., which are used chiefly for baths. They contain mainly calcium sulphate and carbonate. There are also gaseous chalybeate springs. It lies in the valley of Chiana, at an altitude of 1,800 feet, and is half an hour's drive from the station of Asciano.

Civillina, near Recoaro in Italy, has *strong sulphate of iron* waters, containing also sulphates of aluminium, manganese, calcium, and copper, some arsenate of iron, and a little free sulphuric acid.

Cività Vecchia, the seaport of Rome, has *weak hot sulphur* springs up to 132° F. Natural vapour baths can also be obtained there.

Condillac has a *gaseous alkaline* "table water," which is largely exported. The springs are situated a little distance from Montélimar, between Lyons and Marseilles. The water contains a small amount of iron. There is a bath establishment at Condillac, and the waters are drunk there in cases of dyspepsia, arthritism, uricæmia, intestinal catarrh, and anæmia.

Cours-les-Bains (Gironde) has a *cold* spring containing carbonate of lime and carbonate of iron (0·030), which is described as diuretic, tonic, and digestive, and is used in cases of anæmia, chlorosis, dyspepsia, and retarded convalescence. It is situated in a picturesque country, and has a station (Langon) on the Midi line 60 kilometres from Bordeaux. Season, May 15 to Oct. 15.

Court Saint Etienne, Brabant, Belgium, has an *arsenical* water (0·0263 of arsenate of sodium per litre), solely used for exportation.

Couzan, a French "table water."

Cransac, in the Department of Aveyron, France, with a station on the line between Rodez and Capdenac, has *cold earthy calcareous* springs. It is situated at the foot of a volcanic mountain at an altitude of 980 feet. The chief constituents of the water are calcium sulphate (1·5) and magnesium sulphate (1·9). It has a laxative action, and is prescribed in cases of dyspepsia, hepatic congestion and constipation, and cases of splenic enlargement from malarial poisoning. The water is exported. There are crevices or caves hollowed out of the mountain sides and filled with sulphurous vapours reaching a temperature of 118° F., forming natural vapour baths; they are used for the treatment of chronic rheumatism.

The season is from June 1 to Oct. 1.

Croft Spa, Yorkshire, a *cold sulphur* spring with a local reputation.

Csiz, in the Rima valley, Upper Hungary, has a *cold common salt* spring containing 18·0 per litre of sodium chloride and small amounts of magnesium bromide and iodide.

Cudown, in Silesia (Prussia), has well-reputed *cold alkaline gaseous chalybeate* springs. It is situated on pine-clad mountain slopes, at an altitude of 1,270 feet, close to the Bohemian frontier. Its nearest station is Nachod, on the line running from Hallstadt to Chotzen. The springs contain carbonate of sodium, lithium, and iron. The Eugenquelle, the richest in iron, contains 0·06 bicarbonate of iron, 1·29 bicarbonate of sodium, and 0·0025 arsenate of iron. They are all rich in free carbonic acid gas. They are heated for the baths by the addition of hot water. Ferruginous *mud* baths from Bohemia, and vapour and electric baths are also used. The diseases treated there are anæmia and chlorosis; some neuropathics; respiratory, gastric, and vesical catarrh, and some uterine affections. The climatic influences are favourable to the treatment of asthenic maladies.

Cusset. *See* Vichy, p. 359.

Dax, in the Département des Landes, about midway between Pau and Arcachon, is both a *mineral bath* and a *winter climatic resort*. As a bath it has two main resources—first, a *vegeto-mineral mud*, and second, *highly heated* natural springs.

This vegeto-mineral mud is produced by the circumstance that the river Adour (on the left bank of which the bathing establishments are built) is subject to frequent floods during the winter. Each overflow leaves on the surface, from which numerous hot springs arise, a thick, greasy, yellowish mud; this, with the thermal water mixing with it, forms the *mineral* part of the mud. In this a *vegetable* growth rapidly develops and forms a very complex *mud*, the mineral part being composed chiefly of calcium carbonate and sodium chloride. This medicinal mud changes to a *black* colour, owing to the mineral sulphates becoming converted into sulphides in contact with organic matter. It has a faint odour of sulphuretted hydrogen. Iron and copper sulphides are found in the mud, and in the cinders of the confervæ traces of iodine and bromine.

This mud is applied, in some cases, in the form of a *whole bath*, at a temperature varying from 95° to 115° F., lasting fifteen minutes. The mud is then washed off by means of a bath or douche. In other cases, when the lower extremities only are affected, it is applied as *half baths*, and as *local* applications to the hands and feet and to special parts of the body. These local applications are kept on from twenty minutes to an hour, and then washed off by a thermal douche or bath.

In whatever manner these mud baths may produce their effects, which is open to discussion, it is certain that they cause a great stimulation of the skin, together with excitement of the nervous system, capillary dilatation, and quickened cardiac action with free perspiration. It is maintained that nutritive changes are thus quickened, and waste products eliminated, congestive conditions are relieved, and the muscular system is stimulated.

The special therapeutic application of this thermal mud is for the relief of the various forms of chronic rheumatism, stiffened joints, joints with rheumatic exudation, sciatica, and other forms of rheumatic neuralgia, fibro-muscular rheumatism, rheumatoid arthritis, etc., etc.

The *thermal* springs of Dax are very numerous and yield a very large amount of water at a very high temperature (up to 147° F.). They are clear, tasteless, and odourless, with a slightly unctuous feeling and an alkaline reaction. Their mineralisation is feeble, about 1 gramme of solids to the litre; these consist mainly of sulphates of calcium, sodium, and potassium, carbonates of lime and magnesium, silicate of lime and traces of iron, manganese, iodine, and bromine. They belong to the class of "simple thermal waters." They are used as baths and douches; as *natural* vapour baths, the vapour coming direct from the hot springs; and they are drunk. The baths are sedative or exciting according to the temperature at which they are used. The water when drunk acts as a diuretic and stimulates renal elimination. Their diuretic effect is probably purely mechanical.

The cases in which these waters prove beneficial are those of neurasthenia, hysteria, "nervous rheumatism," and all cases requiring sedative treatment. In other cases, and at high temperatures, they prove stimulating, as in rheumatism, sciatica, chronic arthritis, etc. Some forms of uterine engorgements and periuterine exudations are treated at Dax.

The bathing establishments are most conveniently arranged in combination with hotel accommodation, and the charges are very reasonable.

They are open the whole year, but the spring and autumn are the best seasons for thermal treatment. Express trains from Paris perform the journey in ten or twelve hours.

Strong salt springs, sulphur springs, and sulphur and salt springs are found in the immediate neighbourhood of Dax, and are utilised there in suitable cases.

Dax has been advocated also as a climatic resort in winter, especially for invalids suffering from asthma and chronic bronchial catarrh, and who require a soothing rather than a bracing climate. It is said to have a higher temperature in winter than Pau, and a milder air. Its hot springs are said to raise the temperature of the air, and the surrounding pine forests to protect the place somewhat from cold winds.

Dax was known to the Romans as "Aqua Augusta"; this became shortened into "Aqua," and afterwards modified into Acq or D'Acq, and finally into Dax!

Driburg-Bad, in Westphalia, has a *cold gaseous earthy chalybeate spring*. It lies in a valley of the Teutsberg forest, at an elevation of 730 feet, in a pleasant situation. It has a station on the Altenbecken-Holzminden Railway, and is about twenty-four hours from London. It has several chalybeate springs rich in free carbonic acid gas. The strongest of these is the Hauptquelle, and contains carbonate of iron, 0·07 per litre, and carbonate and sulphate of lime, together 2·4 per litre, and much free carbonic acid. The other springs contain the same ingredients, but in smaller amount.

The stronger springs are used for drinking, the weaker ones for baths. The Gaspar-Heinrich-quelle is adapted to the same class of cases as the Wildungen waters.

Besides the gaseous iron baths, *sulphur mud* baths, made of sulphur-containing mud in the neighbourhood (Saatz-bad), pine-needle baths, artificial brine baths, and ordinary hydropathic treatment are utilised. The mineral water is warmed for baths (double-bottomed) by the Schwarz method. The cases suited for this spa are especially those of anæmia, chlorosis, hysteria, neurasthenia, and neuralgia, gastric and respiratory catarrhs, the same urinary affections as are treated at Wildungen; uterine affections also are specially claimed. Rheumatism and gout are included in the local list.

The season is from May 1st to Oct. 1st. Driburg is a very quiet, tranquil resort, with pleasant walks and drives, and living there is inexpensive.

Droitwich is a well-known *salt* bath in Worcestershire, 125 miles from London and seven miles from the city of Worcester. Beds of rock salt lie under the town, and as they undergo gradual solution by streams of pure water flowing over them, some very remarkable subsidences are observed there; and some of the buildings seem to be gradually disappearing! Partly on this account, the town has not an attractive aspect. But there is pleasant country in the neighbourhood, and the Malvern Hills are not far off.

It has been suggested that these salt beds are the remains of an inland sea or lagoon. Extensive salt works exist in the neighbourhood. The Droitwich brine, which is practically a saturated solution of common salt, is pumped up from a subterranean reservoir. The supply is unlimited. It contains 310 grammes per litre of common salt, and its specific gravity, and therefore its buoyancy, is so great that the body floats in it. Its other chief constituents are sodium and calcium sulphate. Its specific gravity has been found to be about 1,195.

The undiluted brine is quite unsuited for internal use, and is only used for bathing. Sometimes, largely diluted, a tablespoonful or two to a tumblerful of water is given as an aperient.

Two good and well-appointed bath establishments exist at Droitwich: the Royal Baths, which are connected with an hotel by a glazed corridor, so as to allow of patients residing in the hotel passing to their bath without going into the open air; and the St. Andrew's Baths, a modern building, also connected by a subway with adjacent hotels.

So great is the buoyancy of the brine that in some of the baths a wooden bar is fixed across the bath, at a suitable height, in order to keep the body submerged. The bath, at a temperature of 98° to 101° F., usually lasts about twenty minutes. The brine has to be diluted with about an equal quantity of hot water for the baths. Any attempt to heat the undiluted brine leads, on account of its concentration, to the deposit of salt, owing to the evaporation that takes place.

There are warm swimming baths for both sexes, which are much resorted to and appreciated. The water is of a temperature of 85°—88° F., and is heated by jets of steam from an iron pipe beneath the surface.

The St. Andrew's Baths are provided with douches and vapour and needle baths, which are given with diluted brine. Brine compresses are often applied to diseased painful joints with benefit. Electrical appliances are also made use of. The brine is often washed off with a spray of fresh water after immersion. The patient, wrapped in hot towels, is ordered to rest quietly for some minutes on coming out of the bath.

The course of treatment at Droitwich is found to be especially useful in *muscular rheumatism* and in *sciatica.* Cases of chronic gout are also often greatly benefited, but acute attacks are said to be occasionally provoked. In osteo-arthritis the results of treatment are uncertain. The joint stiffness following attacks of acute rheumatism is greatly benefited by the employment of douches and vapour as well as immersion baths.

Gonorrhœal arthritis, peripheral neuritic palsies, chorea, certain cases of tabes, and chronic congestive and inflammatory affections of the uterus are mentioned by local authorities as benefited by treatment at Droitwich. The baths are said to have a tonic effect in certain forms of debility and retarded convalescence from acute disease. Traumatic cases are also benefited.

The baths are open all the year round, but the summer months are most suitable for treatment there.

The Droitwich brine is conveyed to Malvern, and baths can be obtained there.

The Nauheim treatment of cardiac affections has been instituted at Droitwich.

Digne, Basses Alpes, France, has *thermal sulphur* and *common salt* waters. It is situated at an altitude of 1,960 feet.

Dinkholder - Brunnen, on the Rhine, near Braubach, has a *chalybeate* spring.

Dinsdale-on-Tees, not far from Darlington, Durham, has a *cold sulphur* spring.

Dirsdorp, a Silesian bath in the Lohe valley, at an altitude of 780 feet, has a *chalybeate* and a *sulphur* spring. The former contains carbonate of iron and carbonate of lime and free carbonic acid and nitrogen gas; the sulphur spring contains in addition sulphuretted hydrogen.

The waters are used for baths and drinking in cases of chronic rheumatism, gout, and anæmia.

The season is from May 20 to Sept. 15.

The nearest railway station is Gnadenfrei on the Breslau-Koberwitz-Gnadenfrei Railway.

Ditzenbach, in Würtemberg—the branch road, Geislingen-Ditzenbach - Wilsensteig, is in course of construction—lies in a picturesquely wooded valley at an altitude of about 1,600 feet above the sea, and has an *acidulous* (free carbonic acid) and *carbonate of lime* spring. As a health resort for drinking and bathing this place has only been acquired since May, 1900. It has two small public bath-houses. The water is exported.

Doberan, a small town in the Grand Duchy of Mecklenburg-Schwerin, with a station on the Rostock-Wismar Railway. It is connected by a steam-tram with the Baltic Sea resort Heligendamm. It has a *chalybeate* well containing protocarbonate of iron and carbonate of calcium. For drinking and bathing some carbonic acid is generally added to it artificially. Mud baths, artificial brine baths, pine-needle baths, hydropathy, gymnastics, and massage are all employed as accessory remedies. The cases considered suitable for treatment are those of gout, rheumatism, neuralgia, paralysis, anæmia, and chlorosis.

Season, from beginning of May to October.

Dürkheim, with *common salt* waters, is situated at the entrance of the Isenach valley, at an altitude of 380 feet, at the foot of the Hardt Mountains. Its railway station is Monsheim-Neustadt.

Its saline wells contain from 7·5 to 20·0 grammes of sodium chloride per litre; they also contain lime, and it is said a little lithium. They are used for drinking, but chiefly for baths and inhalations and gargling, and they are often increased in strength by the addition of mother-lye. The grape cure is also carried out there as an accessory remedy. The diseases treated are scrofula, rickets, skin diseases, rheumatism, gout, and female complaints.

The season is from May 15 to Oct. 15. The grape cure after Sept. 15.

Dürrenberg, a *common salt* bath, in the province of Saxony, with a station on the Leipzig-Korbeitha line. The salt water is diluted with hot river water for baths. Artificial carbonic acid baths and river wave baths with salt water douches are also given. The maladies treated are those for which salt baths are usually recommended.

The season is from May 1 to Sept. 30.

Dürrheim, a *common salt* bath and village in the Grand Duchy of Baden in the valley of the Baar, at an elevation of 2,300 feet. Its railway station is at Marbach, on the Baden Black Forest line. It has a saturated brine artificially produced by washings of a rock-salt stratum, and which is brought to the surface by pumps. It is warmed and diluted for drinking, and hot fresh water is added when it is used for baths and douches. It is also used for inhalation. Mud baths are given. These means are applied to the same class of cases as are usually sent to salt baths, and which have been repeatedly mentioned.

Eaux Bonnes (Basses Pyrénées), a well-known *thermal sulphur* spa frequented chiefly by persons suffering from affections of the throat and respiratory organs. "Chaque siècle," says M. Taine, "la médecine fait un progrès. Par exemple, au temps de François I. les Eaux Bonnes guérissaient les blessures: elles s'appellaient *eaux d'arquebusades;* on y envoya les soldats blessées à Pavie. Aujourd'hui elles guérissent les maladies de gorge et de poitrine. Dans cent ans elles guériront, peut-être, autre chose. Les médicaments ont les modes comme les chapeaux. Un médecin célèbre disait un jour à ses élèves: 'Employez vite ce rémède pendant qu'il guérit encore!'"

Eaux Bonnes is twenty-six miles to the south of Pau and three miles from the railway terminus of Laruns, sixteen hours by express from Paris. The omnibus takes three-quarters of an hour to drive from Laruns to Eaux Bonnes. As one enters the Vallée d'Ossau, about halfway between Pau and Eaux Bonnes, in the distance high above the other mountains one sees the Pic du Midi d'Ossau, easily recognised by its curious summit of two unequal peaks. The village of Eaux Bonnes, about 2,400 feet above the sea, is situated in a somewhat narrow gorge, stretching between the steep mountains which here bound on each side the Vallée d'Ossau. The chief part of the village consists of three rows of uniformly built houses and hotels, forming three sides of a quadrangle, and enclosing a space planted with trees, and called the Jardin Darralde, where the band plays, and where the visitors walk, or sit and talk, or read, or work, as they may be disposed. Beyond and above the Jardin Darralde is the Etablissement Thermal, and to the right, built in a conspicuous position on a terrace, is the handsome new church. Here also commences the remarkable and interesting carriage road, constructed through the mountains, which leads from Eaux Bonnes to Argelès.

A characteristic of Eaux Bonnes is the possession of a very fine promenade, which is called the Promenade Horizontale; it begins at the casino and is continued along the side of the mountain out of which it is cut, always on the same level, parallel to, but at a considerable elevation above, the road leading from Eaux Bonnes to Eaux Chaudes. It is planted with trees, under the shade of which many seats are placed commanding beautiful views of the Vallée d'Ossau.

Eaux Bonnes, with its excellent hotel accommodation, its pleasing site, and the numerous interesting excursions into the mountains which it commands, attracts every year a considerable number of the Parisian upper classes, who find a comparatively calm and unexciting and refreshing retreat there from the gay life of Paris. Its climate, too, is especially soothing; there is exceedingly little wind or dust there, and it is said that the air is often so still that one may pass days without seeing a leaf stir on the trees. It is, however, subject, like most other mountain stations, to thunderstorms and heavy rains.

Eaux Bonnes has three springs: one is cold, La Source Froide, another has a temperature of 72° F., La Source d'Orteig—this is merely tepid—and the third, the chief *source*, is known as La Source Vieille; this has a temperature of 90·5° F. and is the spring to which the place owes its reputation,

It has only 0·6 per litre of solid constituents, of which 0·02 is sodium sulphide, about 0·3 sodium chloride, 0·007 sodium iodide, with a small amount of calcium and other sulphides. It also contains certain gases, especially sulphuretted hydrogen and nitrogen. Its chemical composition has a certain stability and it does not turn milky on exposure to the air as do certain other of the sulphur waters of the Pyrenees. It is also rich in organic matter, glairine or barégine.

The quantity of water yielded by the springs at Eaux Bonnes is limited, so that it has never been the custom to use them, to any extent, as baths; the Grand Etablissement, however, contains a certain number of baths, as well as two rooms devoted to foot-baths, a chamber for gargling, another for throat douches and for *pulverisation.* There is also a smaller Etablissement d'Orteig, and a third, Le Châlet de la Source Froide.

It is to the use of La Source Vieille that the good results obtained in so many cases of throat and chest disease are attributed.

It is maintained by the medical authorities at Eaux Bonnes that these waters have "*une véritable affinité élective*" for affections of the respiratory organs; that when the water is drunk, sulphuretted hydrogen is exhaled through the lungs.

It is, then, for the cure of chronic affections of the nose, throat and chest—chronic granular pharyngitis, naso-pharyngeal catarrhs, and chronic laryngitis—that these waters are especially renowned, as well as for the cure of chronic bronchial catarrhs. It is also claimed for them—and this claim was advanced by that great physician Trousseau—that they are of unmistakable efficacy in certain cases of consumption; and this opinion is still maintained by those who have had many years of experience in treating such cases at Eaux Bonnes. It is, however, in the strictly local and limited manifestations of this malady, and not in those cases in which there is obvious general constitutional infection, or in which the disease is rapidly advancing, that it is suggested a cure can be effected at Eaux Bonnes. It is, says a local authority, not the disease phthisis that is cured, but a certain class of persons who have become tuberculous that can be healed, and especially certain subjects of protracted catarrhal pulmonary affections that are in danger of becoming tuberculous. In these the treatment exercises a restorative and immunising action on the lungs. There is much medical testimony forthcoming as to the efficacy of the waters of Eaux Bonnes in fitly selected cases of consumption, and many of those chronic cases which by careful management continue to maintain a feeble but tolerable existence, by passing the winter in the south, etc., come year after year to pass some part of the summer season at Eaux Bonnes. There are many consumptive French patients who, by the recommendation of their physicians, pass their winters on the Riviera, and their summers at Eaux Bonnes, or at one or the other of the Pyrenean health resorts, and this arrangement seems to suit them well, and if their malady does not become cured, at any rate its course is for a time arrested and retarded, and they obtain many years of agreeable existence which they could not insure in the north. The doses of the water prescribed internally are often quite small, eight to ten tablespoonfuls daily.

At the commencement of the course some general, as well as local excitement and stimulation is often observed, but this, as a rule, soon passes off.

In addition to the cases mentioned as suitable for this course, certain others are often benefited, such as cases of humid (not dry) catarrhal asthma, scrofulous tonsillitis and adenitis, enlargements of bronchial glands, often a sequel of whooping cough ; cases of anæmia and chlorosis not amenable to treatment with iron, certain moist skin diseases, as impetigo, and scrofulous fistulas and slowly healing wounds. The mildly bracing mountain climate is also suitable to convalescents from acute diseases, especially of the throat or lungs.

The season is from June 1st to Oct. 1st. There is excellent accommodation to be found at Eaux Bonnes, and residence there is cheerful though quiet.

Eaux Chaudes (Basses Pyrénées), like its neighbour, Eaux Bonnes, has *thermal sulphur* springs, which are more particularly resorted to for the treatment of female maladies. It is distant about six miles from Eaux Bonnes by a good carriage road; there is also a very interesting walk over the mountains between the two villages, commanding magnificent views of the grand surrounding mountain scenery. The carriage road for the first three miles is the same as that traversed in coming from Laruns to Eaux Bonnes. This road bifurcates within about three miles of Eaux Bonnes, the branch to the right going to Eaux Chaudes. When we reach this bifurcation we enter a narrow defile, sombre but picturesque, bounded on each side by enormous mountain walls, with a blue band of sky overhead. The road keeps to the left side of the gorge, often at a great height above the river—the Gave d'Ossau—which 500 feet beneath roars and foams along its steep and stony bed.

We come somewhat suddenly upon Eaux Chaudes, a simple village of a few houses and hotels, most charmingly situated at an elevation of 2,200 feet in the very bosom of the mountains. Eaux Chaudes is one of the most picturesque spots in the Western Pyrenees; within a short drive is the village of Gabas, most grandly situated amidst wild mountain scenery, the magnificent Pic du Midi of like composition to those of Eaux Bonnes, only closing in the horizon. There are seven springs, varying in temperature from 77° to 97° F. They are weaker. Their total solids are only 0·33 per litre, and the sodium sulphide is only 0·0088. The waters also contain alkaline silicates and glairine or barégine.

They are chiefly used externally—as baths, douches, irrigations, and pulverisations. Vaginal irrigations are a sort of speciality of this spa. They are applied with the water as it comes directly from the spring, which ensures its asepticity.

For throat affections the water is drunk and used for gargling.

Formerly the different springs were severally allotted to the treatment of different forms of disease, but this artificial distinction scarcely merits serious consideration. Generally speaking, these weak and tepid sulphur springs are regarded as more sedative than the stronger ones.

As has been said, female maladies are mainly the cases treated at Eaux Chaudes: vaginitis of indeterminate causation, metritis and perimetritis, as an aid to but not a substitute for appropriate local treatment; dysmenorrhœa, amenorrhœa, certain forms of sterility; hysteria, neurasthenia—all such cases, when requiring a sedative combined with tonic (climatic) treatment. In addition, rheumatic cases, articular, muscular, and neuralgic (sciatica), when occurring in the neurotic. Cases of slow recovery from exhausting disease may with advantage be sent to this quiet and mildly tonic station. The most suitable season is from June 20th to Sept. 20th; but the thermal establishment is open all the year round.

Elster (Bad Elster), in the kingdom of Saxony, is situated near the Bohemian frontier, with a station a few miles from Eger, on the line between that town and Leipzig. It lies in the Elster valley, at an elevation of about 1,600 feet, surrounded by pine-clad hills.

The principal springs may be termed *cold alkaline, saline, gaseous, chalybeate.* They are a combination of saline constituents and iron. There are five springs used for drinking—the Moritz, Marien, Koenigs, Alberts, and Salzquelle. There are other springs used only for supplying the various baths.

The Salzquelle is so called because of its richness in saline constituents; it contains 5·2 grammes per litre of sodium sulphate, 1·6 of sodium bicarbonate, 0·8 of sodium chloride, and 0·06 of bicarbonate of iron, and much free carbonic acid. The Moritzquelle is richest in iron. The Marienquelle contains the same amount of iron as the Salzquelle, about half as much sodium sulphate and bicarbonate, and twice as much sodium chloride. It also has much free carbonic acid, and is largely used for drinking. The Koenigsquelle is said to contain a "remarkable quantity of lithium."

It will be seen that they are fairly strong iron waters combined with alkaline and saline (aperient) constituents.

These springs are utilised for drinking, for gargling, for inhalations, and for mineral baths. The drinking waters are largely exported in bottles, after charging with artificial carbonic acid gas.

There is an elaborately equipped bath establishment, in which, in addition to the ordinary mineral baths, ferruginous mud baths, artificial carbonic acid baths, pine-needle baths, artificial salt baths, Russian vapour and Roman baths, hydrotherapy with massage, and electric light baths are administered. So that a great variety of therapeutic methods can be applied. The cases treated at Elster are those of anæmia and chlorosis, of gastro-intestinal and hepatic functional disorders, of gout, rheumatism, and obesity (especially the anæmic form), many female pelvic maladies, scrofulous disease of children, and some forms of neurasthenia. Briefly, such cases as call for a combination of tonic and eliminative treatment.

Elster has a hospital and charitable institution for the treatment of delicate children and the indigent. The season is from May 1st to Oct. 1st.

Ems, the well-known Bad Ems, is situated twelve miles from Coblenz, in the beautiful valley of the Lahn, and possesses celebrated *thermal* springs belonging to the *alkaline common salt* group. Its natural situation is very beautiful, and art has been liberally applied to aid nature in its embellishment.

Ems extends for a considerable distance along the right bank of the river Lahn. Along this bank, at the lower part, is the old Dorf Ems, where most of the poorer inhabitants dwell, while the upper part consists of handsome hotels and shops, and the fine Kursaal and the Kurhaus and the springs are all on that side of the river, together with some prettily laid-out, shady, park-like walks. On the left side of the river there are also bath-houses, and many fine villas and hotels, and many shady walks and drives extend up the wooded mountain side on this bank.

The pedestrian can find many attractive walks, with fine points of view, varying from half an hour to an hour and a-half's distance from his hotel. Or the woods on the summit of the Malberg, 1,000 feet above the town, can now be reached by a funicular railway.

A fine covered walk in the centre of the public gardens, near the Kursaal, affording shelter both from sun and rain, was erected in 1874, at the special request of the Emperor William, and is a real boon to the place. An historical monument, of which Ems is proud, is a small white stone let into the ground near where the band plays in the morning, with the simple inscription: "15 Juli, 1870, 9 Uhr Morgens"; this marks the spot where King William stood when he caused his memorable answer to be given to the French ambassador, Benedetti.

Ems has the reputation of being hot and relaxing, and no doubt it can be very hot at Ems during the height of summer. This probably assists in the cure of the cases of chronic bronchial and laryngeal catarrh that are sent here; but the early mornings and the evenings are cool, especially in the months of May and September, which are probably the pleasantest months in warm seasons, although by no means the most popular. Great pains have been taken, by cultivating trees in the public gardens, to afford as much shade as possible, and to provide cool retreats from the midday heat, while the abundance of water available enables the roads and the trees to be watered three times daily.

Ems is abundantly supplied with mineral springs; there are five or six principal ones, all having nearly the same chemical composition and differing only in temperature. The hottest is the Kesselbrunnen, 120° F.; then the Fuerstenbrunnen, 102°; the Augustaquelle, 101°; the Kraenchen, 90°; and the coolest, the Victoriaquelle, 80°. Those of the higher temperature are best suited to certain cases, those of the lower temperature to others. The Ems springs belong to the alkaline-saline group, and contain about 2·0 grammes of sodium bicarbonate per litre and 1·0 of sodium chloride. They also contain free carbonic acid in considerable amount and a little lime and magnesia. Ems possesses, too, a mild chalybeate spring. There are several public bath establishments well fitted up for the application of hot and cold douches, massage, and various kinds of baths. There are chambers for gargling and for inhaling the pulverised water, which may also be had medicated with pine oil or other substances. There are compressed air chambers and also apparatus (Waldenberg's) for inspiring compressed air and expiring into rarefied air—of use in the treatment of pulmonary emphysema. Artificial gaseous salt baths are given.

The chief uses of these waters is in the treatment of chronic catarrhs of the throat and air passages, and in the treatment of those affections they are drunk, used in the form of inhalations and sprays, and as gargles, and also bathed in. They are applied in certain forms of gout, especially in the acid dyspepsias of the gouty and those forms of gout that require gentle rather than active treatment, or that are associated with bronchial catarrh or urinary calculi or cystitis. In some forms of dyspepsia, with congestion of the liver, or inflammation of the bile ducts or chronic diarrhœa, the Ems waters often do good. Those chronic affections of the joints resulting from attacks of rheumatic fever are said to be benefited by treatment there. Ems is also very decidedly a "ladies' bath," and is found very serviceable in cases of leucorrhœa, uterine catarrh, and dysmenorrhœa in the neurotic. It is customary there to apply a vaginal douche in the bath. Ems has also a traditional reputation for the cure of sterility.

The climate of Ems is, as has been said, mild and relaxing, and from the beginning of July to the middle of August the midday heat is often very great. The town is, however, reported to be very healthy. It is not only abundantly supplied with water but well drained.

One of the great recommendations of Ems is its exceeding accessibility and the good hotel accommodation provided there. It can be reached viâ Cologne in sixteen hours from London.

Tradition still governs the method of drinking the waters at Ems, and the invalids, young and old, active or feeble, begin to consume their daily allowance between 6 and 8 a.m. The dose is repeated in the afternoon between four and six. The early morning hour is, no doubt, a good time for taking warm solvent water in many cases, but it does not admit of doubt that many feeble and delicate constitutions would do better to remain in their beds until eight or nine o'clock, and have their first glass of water brought to their bedside.

The season is from May 1st to Oct. 1st.

Enghien, a *cold sulphur* spa in the environs of Paris, from which it is distant only seven or eight miles, a journey of a quarter of an hour by quick trains on the northern line. It is a prettily built suburb, having a small lake and tastefully arranged pleasure-grounds. Pleasant walks and excursions can be had in the neighbourhood, especially in the adjacent forest of Montmorency.

Enghien has as many as eight springs, all of similar chemical composition and differing only in the proportion of the ingredients they contain.

The total solids in the stronger springs amount to 0·80, the chief in quantity being calcium carbonate and sulphate. But the characteristic ingredients are calcium sulphide and free *sulphuretted hydrogen*, of which there are 38 c.c. per litre; free carbonic acid and nitrogen gases are also contained in these springs. Traces of organic nitrogenous matters, too, are found.

A modern perfectly equipped bath establishment provides all the most recent methods of applying mineral waters—baths with general and local douches; douches of high pressure; nasal, pharyngeal, vaginal, and ascending douches; chambers for sulphurous inhalations and pulverisations; electric baths with sulphur water.

A recent installation is devoted to the application of warm sulphurous irrigations to the uterine cavity.

The waters are also drunk, besides being used for gargling.

There is an annexe in the park for hydropathic treatment.

The Enghien waters are employed chiefly in affections of the throat and respiratory organs, cases of chronic granular pharyngitis, laryngitis, bronchitis, and humid asthma in the rheumatic and herpetic. They are considered especially applicable to the treatment of catarrhal diseases of the nose and throat in public speakers, actors, singers, etc.

Chronic catarrhal affections of the genito-urinary organs, chronic metritis, especially when associated with anæmia, chlorosis, and lymphatism, are benefited by the internal irrigations referred to.

Chronic skin diseases, such as eczema, impetigo,

acne, lichen, cases of chronic rheumatism, muscular or articular, stiff joints, cases of sciatica, and some forms of neurotic paresis, are benefited. Special apartments are appropriated to the treatment of syphilitic cases.

As may be imagined, Enghien being a suburb of Paris, life there is characterised by much gaiety and brightness; concerts and balls in the casino, regattas on the lake, etc.

The season is from May 15th to Oct. 15th. June, July, and August are the preferable months.

Evian (Lake of Geneva).—The agreeable situation of the little town of Evian, 1,200 feet above the sea, just in the centre of the attractions of Lake Leman, its mild and genial climate, and its ready accessibility, by rail and steamboat, both from the north and from the south, have no doubt contributed greatly to its popularity. It is just opposite Lausanne, and the lake steamers cross in half an hour. From Geneva by express boat it is two and a-half hours.

It is said that the air of Evian and its vicinity is peculiarly favourable to those delicate, anæmic, hypersensitive young children who do not prosper at the seaside. It is assuredly not uncommon to meet with young feeble children who, if sent to the seaside, become bilious, languid, and irritable, lose their appetite, and become weaker instead of stronger. There is something in the air of the sea coast which seems to irritate instead of bracing them, and it would seem that such children obtain great benefit from the more mildly tonic air of Evian, and recover there their strength, their vivacity, and their colour.

Evian possesses five springs of nearly identical composition; the two chief are La Source Cachat and La Source Bonne-vie. They give their names to two distinct bath establishments. The Cachat has the greatest renown, and it is largely exported.

These springs are cold and very feebly mineralised; they contain, however, some amount of oxygen, nitrogen, and carbonic acid gases. It has been suggested that the springs act much in the same manner as distilled water would, and owing to great purity and the absence of solid mineral substances, their solvent and purifying properties are greatly increased; while, by their fresh and pleasant taste, they are rendered much more digestible and more readily absorbed than distilled water would be. Very large quantities of the Evian water can be consumed and absorbed daily, if some little care is taken to accustom the stomach to its use—"from four to twenty-five glasses a day"! When it is taken as a solvent of uric acid, it is considered that the possibilities of absorbing such large quantities of this very feebly mineralised water is altogether an advantage, because it possesses the important property of taking up more freely the less soluble organic salts encountered in its passage through the organism.

This water may be regarded, then, as washing the blood and the tissues, and removing from them any deleterious excrementitious substances that are difficult of solution; hence its value in the uric acid diathesis.

The published analyses of the Evian *sources* vary somewhat, but the following may be regarded as a fairly accurate approximation. In a litre (1,000 grammes):

	Grammes.
Sulphate of potassium	0·0052
Bicarbonate of sodium	0·0089
,, magnesium	0·1244
,, calcium	0·2822
Chloride of sodium	0·0030
Sulphate of sodium	0·0079
Free carbonic acid	0·03672

It will be seen by the above that it is a slightly alkaline and very feebly mineralised water. With regard to its properties, it is said to be remarkably diuretic. In the next place it promotes appetite, and in large doses it excites the processes of retrograde metamorphosis to such a degree that, notwithstanding the consumption of an increased quantity of food, many persons become much thinner. It has been said of Evian water that it acts "not by what it brings, but by what it carries away"!

Its property of increasing the urinary excretion renders it a valuable remedy in cases of gravel, renal calculi, etc.

The quantity taken varies from two to twenty-five glasses a day, according to the case and the object in view. It is usual to begin with small doses, and to take at least two-thirds of the total quantity between getting up and half an hour before the *déjeuner à la fourchette*. The dose of water must not be incautiously increased, but it must be first observed if it passes away freely by the kidneys, and if it is absorbed without any trouble or inconvenience. If it either purges or constipates, some medical treatment should be had recourse to, in order to modify this effect.

The baths generally have a soothing, sedative effect, relieving the pains of chronic cystitis, and nephritis, and restoring sleep to irritable nervous subjects. They, however, not unfrequently excite a return of subacute gouty attacks in those who are prone to them, and in some highly neurotic excitable patients they occasionally cause irritation and exhaustion. The alkalinity of the baths is of use in some skin affections, especially the lichenous and pruritic cases.

It is usual to drink one or two glasses of the water while in the bath.

Injections of the water while in the bath are useful in some uterine affections.

With respect to the maladies especially suited to treatment at Evain, the various forms of chronic dyspepsia must first be mentioned; and the cases of nervous and gouty dyspeptics, with tendency to great discomfort from flatulent distension, are treated in a special manner here by means of what is called the "dyspeptic douche." This douche is applied over the abdomen and stomach, and is accompanied by skilful massage. This method is said to yield remarkably good results, even in very inveterate cases. The douche is applied twice a day, together with massage, and from five to twelve glasses of the water are drunk.

In the next place must be mentioned renal and bladder affections, and amongst these certain forms of chronic albuminuria are said to be greatly benefited by treatment at Evian, especially the form due to catarrhal desquamative nephritis, and also the cases of parenchymatous nephritis. Speaking of the use of Evian water in this latter affection, the late Professor Noël Gueneau de Massy said: "This is the most easily digested water known, and it is voided easily on account of its eminently diuretic properties. It carries with it, without fatiguing the kidneys, all the epithelial and other débris which in case of inflammation encumbers the renal filter."

The cure at Evian is also recommended in cases of chronic pyelitis, especially when it has been induced by lithiasis and preceded by the passage of renal calculi.

But it is in cases of uric acid deposits and excess of urates in the urine, betraying the existence of a gouty condition, that the water of Evian is considered especially beneficial, and it is more particularly indicated in those individuals who are the subjects of asthenic gout, and who require gentle methods of treatment. It is desirable to begin with small doses of water, three to four glasses a day, which may be increased slowly up to twenty.

Cases of renal colic, due to the presence of urinary concretions (gravel and calculi), are fit subjects for the Evian course, and are often remarkably benefited thereby.

Cases of vesical catarrh not due to any organic cause but the result of chill, or of some temporary local or constitutional morbid condition, are said to be cured at Evian.

Cases of gouty or hepatic diabetes are benefited at Evian.

It is further claimed for the course of treatment and the *régime* pursued at Evian, that it is very beneficial and calming to persons of hypersensitive nervous organisation, who are suffering from overfatigue of the nervous system, sleeplessness, loss of appetite, etc.

Every recent development of hydrotherapeutic treatment can be carried out at the Institut Hydrothérapique, one of the most complete institutions of the kind in France.

The season extends from May 15th to Oct. 15th, but the best period for treatment there is from July 1st to Sept. 15th.

Accommodation can be obtained at Evian to suit all classes—rich and poor—in villas, hotels, and *pensions*. There is also a "hospice" for the reception and treatment of patients, with accommodation varying according to the price paid.

The life at Evian is, during the season, gay and cheerful, and a variety of amusements—balls, comedies, operettas, and concerts—are provided daily at the casino. There is a great variety of attractive excursions to be taken on the lake or into the surrounding country.

Amphion.—Within a twenty minutes' walk of Evian, and almost a part of it, is Amphion. Its situation on the border of the lake is very picturesque. The bath establishment is situated in its own grounds, which extend down to the lake. It is not one large building, but consists of three detached residences, and is specially suited to persons who need repose and prefer retirement. There is a landing-place and jetty for steamers and boats close at hand. The hotel and restaurant arrangements are excellent. Amphion lies at the foot of a hill which protects it, in the heat of summer, from the southern sun, and as the neighbourhood is well wooded the air is usually fresher and cooler than at Evian.

There are good arrangements for baths and douches, but on a much smaller scale than at Evian.

Amphion possesses three mildly *alkaline* springs almost identical in composition with those at Evian, and therefore it is appropriate to the treatment of the same class of cases. Amphion, however, boasts of the possession of a spring containing iron, and the use of this alkaline-chalybeate spring is recommended in cases in which anæmia and chlorosis play a predominant *rôle*.

For invalids requiring a quiet, picturesque, and cheerful summer residence in mildly bracing air, away from the excitement and gaiety of a fashionable spa, and yet with such a resort and its resources within ready access, Amphion presents exceptional attractions.

Eberswalde, in the province of Brandenburg, with a station between Berlin and Stettin, has a weak *chalybeate* water which is largely exported. Besides this there are utilised for treatment artificial carbonic acid baths and mud baths from the sea-water marshes at Britz, as well as hydropathy. Neurasthenic and convalescent cases are sent there.

The season is from May to October.

Eilsen, a *cold sulphur* bath in the principality of Lippe Schaumburg, and about an hour's drive from the railway station Bückeburg, between Minden and Hanover. There are seven springs. Those used for drinking are the Julianenbrunnen and the Georgenbrunnen. The former contains free H_2S (34 vols. per litre) calcium sulphate (2·0), and smaller amounts of sodium chloride, sodium sulphate, etc. The other springs are used for baths. There is also a weak chalybeate spring. Inhalations and gargles, sulphurous mud baths, massage, and electricity are utilised. The chief maladies treated there are gout, rheumatism, neuralgia, metallic poisonings, paralysis, skin diseases, and catarrh of the respiratory organs.

Season, May 15 to Sept. 1.

Elmen, one of the oldest salt baths in Germany, possesses *cold salt* wells, owned by the Prussian State. It is situated in Saxony, near Magdeburg, and it is connected by a tramway with the station Schönebeck-Elbe.

The Victoriaquelle contains 26·0 per litre of common salt. It is used for drinking (often mixed with seltzer water or whey) and for baths. It is diluted with fresh water for the baths, and *Mutterlauge* is sometimes added. Artificial sulphur baths and carbonic acid baths are prepared. Salt spray inhalations (produced by compressed air) are also administered. The diseases treated there include gout and rheumatism, scrofula, neurasthenia, catarrh of the air-passages, and female complaints.

The season is from May 1 to Oct. 1.

Elöpatak, in Transylvania, pleasantly situated in a valley at an elevation of 2,000 feet, about twelve miles from Kronstadt, possesses cold strong *alkaline gaseous chalybeate* springs. The principal springs contain 0·09 per litre of bicarbonate of iron, 1·0 bicarbonate of sodium, and 1·5 each of bicarbonate of calcium and magnesium, and much free carbonic acid gas. A valuable combination, but this spa is too far distant to be of any practical use to English patients. Hydrotherapy is applied. Gastric disorders, anæmia, and menstrual irregularities are treated there.

The season is from the middle of May to the end of September.

Encausse (Haute Garonne), in a picturesque and pleasant situation a few miles from St. Gaudens, on the line between Toulouse and Tarbes, possesses *sulphate of lime* springs containing also a little sulphate of magnesia and sulphate of soda. Like Contrexéville, it belongs to the class of earthy calcareous waters. They are slightly laxative and diuretic. They are said to act most efficaciously in the cure of the sequelæ of malarial fever. They are also used to cure obstinate constipation, and in hepatic and renal gravel. Uterine enlargements in the hysterical and nervous are also benefited.

The season is from May 15 to Oct. 1.

Erdöbenye is a Hungarian *chalybeate* spa three miles from the railway station Liszka-Tolcsva, in a wooded valley at an altitude of 780 feet. Its waters contain sulphate of iron, alum, and arsenic. It has little interest for English people.

Escaldas, Les, a *thermal sulphur* spa in the Pyrénées Orientales, in France, but close to the frontier of Spain. It is situated at an altitude of 4,400 feet. The Grande Source has a temperature of nearly 110° F., and contains sodium sulphide. It is somewhat difficult of access and out of the way.

Essentuke, a Russian spa in the Caucasus, ten miles from Piatigorsk, has *cold gaseous alkaline* and *common salt* springs, and also sulphur springs only used externally. The former belong to the same class as the Ems springs, but are more than twice as strong. The place is too difficult of access to be of use to English patients.

Euzet, a small *sulphur* bath (calcium sulphide) in the south of France, between Martinet and Tarascon, eighteen hours from Paris. The springs, which are cold, are characterised specially by containing some bituminous organic matters. They also contain some salts of magnesium and sodium and some free carbonic acid, which promote their digestion. They are taken internally in cases of gastro-intestinal dyspepsia with hepatic engorgement, and used externally in subacute forms of rheumatism, and as inhalations in chronic laryngitis, bronchial catarrh, asthma, and tuberculosis. It possesses a well-equipped bath establishment.

Season, from May to October.

Evaux, a French bath situated on the Orleans line of railway twenty-eight kilometres from Montlucon, in a retired and picturesque situation at an elevation of 1,400 feet. It is reached from Paris in six and a-half hours. It has several hot springs of feeble mineralisation, bringing it under the class of *simple thermal* baths. They vary in temperature from 80° to 130° F. The water contains 0·717 grammes of sodium sulphate per litre and a small amount of sodium chloride. Its speciality is the number of confervæ it contains, which float on the water as a thick greenish scum, termed *limon;* and it is used for local applications.

The waters are chiefly used externally in three well-appointed establishments. Their value depends mainly on their warmth and the mode of their employment. They are used in the treatment of cases of articular and muscular rheumatism and rheumatic neuralgia, especially in the lymphatic and scrofulous, also in respiratory affections and certain forms of scrofulous skin affections.

The season is from June 1 to Oct. 1.

Forges-les-Eaux, which has *cold chalybeate* springs, is conveniently situated, and easily accessible, on the line of railway between Dieppe and Paris, in the Department of Seine Inférieure. It has an elevation of 525 feet, in a highly cultivated, well-wooded, and picturesque country affording many agreeable excursions. It is protected from north winds, but its climate is somewhat variable, on the whole soft and rather humid, and is observed to have a sedative effect on the nervous system, which has been attributed to the influence of sea air modified by its passage over ten leagues of somewhat moist and wooded intervening country.

It has three iron springs, varying in strength and named, from the visit of Anne of Austria, Louis XIII., and Cardinal Richelieu in the seventeenth century, Reinette, Royale, and Cardinale. The iron exists in the water in the form of *protocrenate*, which is considered very assimilable. It is usual to begin with the weakest spring, Reinette, which contains only 0·03 grammes per litre, then to pass on to the next, Royale, with 0·07, and to finish with the strongest, Cardinale, having 0·10. It is usual to begin with quite small doses—one-third to half a glass —and to increase the dose gradually to five or six glasses a day.

The waters have very little mineral contents besides the iron—bicarbonate of magnesia (0·07), sulphate of lime (0·04), alumina (0·03), and a little free carbonic acid.

These springs are found to have a very diuretic effect, beyond what is usual with chalybeate springs.

An excellently fitted-up bath establishment, in a large park, provides all that is needed in the way of baths, douches, etc., as well as of amusement.

It is usual to give the baths at a temperature of 85° F., but douches are sometimes given in connection with hydrotherapeutic treatment at the natural temperature of the water, about 42° F. The duration of the bath is from fifteen minutes to an hour.

The cases treated at Forges-les-Eaux are, in the first place, those usually sent to chalybeate spas, chlorosis, anæmia, and their results; convalescents from acute disease; asthenic and atonic dyspepsias; in addition the local authorities mention chronic diarrhœa and dysentery, menstrual irregularities, uterine troubles arising from miscarriage or over-fatigue, chronic metritis and maladies causing sterility, and many neuroses. These waters were at one time much used in the treatment of vesical catarrh, gravel, and nephritic colic. The season begins June 15th and ends Sept. 15th. July and August are the best months.

Franzensbad is one of the three best known Bohemian baths, the other two being Carlsbad and Marienbad. They are all approached from England through the frontier town of Eger, from which Franzensbad is only distant five miles.

These springs resemble one another, more or less, in chemical composition, but vary in strength; but the distinguishing characteristic of the Franzensbad springs is that some of them contain a notable amount of *iron*, so that it is in a certain sense a *chalybeate* spa. It is also the chief and typical representative of the *Moor* or *mud* baths, the former being the appropriate name. Franzensbad is moreover distinguished as a "ladies' bath," since its waters and *Moor* baths have long been applied to the treatment of disease of the female pelvic organs.

The town is built on a plateau or depression and has a fine park for promenades, but its situation is less picturesque than that of either of its neighbours, Carlsbad or Marienbad. Its elevation above the sea is nearly 1,400 feet, and though hot in the midday in the summer, it is fresh and pleasantly cool in the mornings and evenings.

Franzensbad possesses twelve different cold mineral springs, and these may be arranged, according to their composition and uses, into three groups, one of which, the Salzquelle, may be taken as the type, and may be regarded as a *cold* Carlsbad water; another, represented by the Stahlquelle, which contains a notable amount of iron; and a third, perhaps the most characteristic and most resorted to, of the place, combining, as it were, the qualities of the other two, the Franzensquelle. The following table shows the relation in composition of these springs to one another and to the typical Carlsbad spring.

	Franzensbad Salzquelle.	Carlsbad Sprudel.	Franzensbad Stahlquelle.
Sodium sulphate ...	2·802	2·405	1·614
„ carbonate ...	0·677	1·298	0·574
„ chloride ...	1·140	1·041	0·612
Calcium carbonate ...	0·183	0·321	0·199
Magnesium „ ...	0·103	0·166	0·053
Iron „ ...	0·009	0·003	0·078

The Franzensquelle represents a group intermediate in composition between the Salzquelle and the Stahlquelle, having more sodium sulphate than the former (3·190 to 3·505) and less iron carbonate than the latter (0·017 to 0·030). They are all rich in carbonic acid gas. Franzensbad also possesses a simple gaseous acidulated spring resembling the ordinary "table waters."

It will be seen from the above table that all these springs contain sodium sulphate, carbonate, and chloride, like the two other great Bohemian spas, but some in smaller proportions; one, the Stahlquelle, has in addition a considerable proportion of iron, while its saline constituents are considerably less. The Neuquelle, one of the second group, is however now stated to contain more iron (0·127) than the Stahlquelle.

Some are disposed to call attention to a small amount of carbonate of lithium which some of the springs contain, the largest amount (0·010) being found in the Neuquelle and the Nathaliequelle. This means that there is about three-twentieths of a grain of carbonate of lithium in a quart of water! It can hardly be believed that this minute quantity can have any special therapeutic action.

In addition to the use of these mineral springs *internally*, Franzensbad is an important *bathing* spa, which employs several kinds of baths for therapeutic purposes, and has four well-equipped bath establishments (containing 460 rooms) in which they are applied. These baths are often spoken of as of three kinds—(*a*) the *mineral* baths, (*b*) the *steel* baths, and (*c*) the *Moor* baths. But as mineral water enters into the composition of all of them the classification is purely artificial. What are termed the "*mineral* baths," and sometimes the "Louisen baths," because the Louisenquelle is chiefly used to supply them, on account of its abundant yield of water, are ordinary mineral water baths, heated by steam, which causes the loss of a certain amount of the free carbonic acid. What are known as the "steel baths" are baths which are heated in a different manner, so that they retain much more of this carbonic acid; the method is that known as the Schwarz system, in which the baths, having a double bottom, are heated by a steam chamber or pipes at the bottom of the bath. These baths, rich in carbonic acid gas, are regarded as more stimulating than the "mineral" ones which are heated differently.

Finally, there are the celebrated *Moor* baths. The peat used in preparing these baths is obtained from moorland in the surrounding district, of which the supply is practically unlimited, so that *fresh* moor can be used for each bath. The moor earth is treated in a special manner, which need not be detailed here, but which comprises *a saturation with the salts of the mineral water.* In preparing these baths the moor earth, after having been exposed sufficiently long to the action of the air, is first saturated with mineral water, of which more is added, till the required consistency has been attained. The *mineral* water being charged with free carbonic acid, a certain amount of this gas enters into the composition of the bath. From Castellièri's analysis it appears that this peat, when prepared for the bath and ready for use, contains as much as 25 per cent. of substances soluble in water, of which 9·7 per cent. is sulphate of iron. These baths are usually given of a temperature of 90° to 95° F. The patient reclines in the bath, but not so as to allow the upper part of the chest to be covered, so that the bath acts practically like a large poultice to the lower half of the trunk and the lower extremities.

The bath can also be applied locally to a joint or limb or a definite portion of the surface of the body. A *cleansing* bath of *mineral* water is taken after the bath, and before entering it the moor earth covering the body is washed off by water taken from it.

There is still another kind of bath given at Franzensbad—viz. a *natural carbonic acid gas bath.* In a grove near the Franzensquelle a stream of carbonic acid gas, mixed with H_2S, ascends with some force from the ground. Over this a bath-house has been erected, and suitable arrangements are made for the general or local application of the dried and purified gas. The precise therapeutic value of these carbonic acid baths has yet to be determined. The late Prof. Frerichs thought well of them, and it is suggested that they are of use in certain affections of the peripheral nerves, neuralgia, hyperæsthesia and anæsthesia, reflex and hysterical paralysis, amenorrhœa, and impotence.

Possessing so many and various resources, it is

not to be wondered at that Franzensbad treatment is regarded as of value in a considerable number of maladies. It will, however, be convenient to consider, first of all, those cases which have acquired for it so great a reputation as a "ladies' bath"! We may mention, in the first place, the disorders of adolescence and the period of sexual development: amenorrhœa, dysmenorrhœa, and leucorrhœa, so often associated with anæmia and chlorosis and the strain of rapid growth. In older patients, chronic vagino-uterine catarrh, chronic metritis, uterine displacements, oöphoritis, and pelvic inflammatory exudations; a tendency to miscarriages and the exhaustion following profuse menstruation, repeated miscarriages, or too rapid child-bearing. Imperfect or retarded development at puberty, menstrual irregularities, vaginismus, ovarian neuralgia, sterility. In all these maladies the various mineral springs and baths and the *Moor* baths may be variously and discriminatingly applied with advantage by the experienced bath physicians.

The relative absence of constipating lime salts and the presence of laxative constituents in these springs render them very appropriate to many of those conditions in which constipation is so frequently a troublesome complication, and the iron in these springs is, in those circumstances, more likely to be assimilated.

To pass now to the consideration of other than special female maladies which may derive benefit from treatment at Franzensbad. The springs which resemble those of Carlsbad in composition may, when warmed, be applied to the same class of cases as are likely to be benefited by the Carlsbad waters, but who may require rather milder and more tonic treatment, more especially when an anæmic state coexists with other maladies. Several functional gastro-hepatic affections, habitual constipation, gallstones, catarrhal jaundice, lithæmia, obesity in the anæmic, the fat and gouty diabetics; certain forms of chronic gout, gouty neuralgia, and rheumatism in debilitated persons.

Simple anæmia, neurasthenic states, and other functional neuroses.

Certain chronic cutaneous affections, dependent on anæmia, scrofula, and depressed tone; purpura, lichen, prurigo, urticaria, psoriasis, chronic eczema, and slowly healing ulcers.

The life at Franzensbad is very quiet, and early hours are the rule. The waters are usually drunk between six and nine in the morning and again between four and seven in the evening. Walking exercise is usually encouraged. The hotels are good; quiet and comfortable lodgings are easily obtained at Franzensbad. The journey can be made from London in twenty-five hours by the Vienna-Carlsbad express viâ Nuremburg.

The season is from May to the end of September. Some moderately bracing place as an "after-cure" is very desirable.

Fachingen is situated on the Lahn between Ems and Limburg. It has a simple *alkaline* spring rich in carbonic acid gas and containing about 3·5 grammes of bicarbonate of sodium in a litre. It is only used for exportation, and may be ordered in much the same manner as the imported Vichy water.

Farnbuhl, a Swiss *chalybeate* spring in a pleasant sub-alpine resort, at an elevation of 2,310 feet, in Canton Lucerne, about an hour's drive from Malters railway station on the Jura-Berne-Lucerne line.

Faulenseebad, on the Lake of Thun, about twenty minutes above the village and landing-stage of that name, at an elevation of 2,600 feet, commanding a magnificent view of the lake and surrounding mountains; has a *cold calcareous* earthy spring containing a very small amount of iron and a faint trace of sulphuretted hydrogen. Its chief constituent is calcium sulphate (1·45 per litre), and next in amount is magnesium bicarbonate (0·197). This water is used in the treatment of a variety of maladies, and especially in catarrhs of the mucous membrane of the air-passages and in affections of the urinary tract.

Fideris in Switzerland, in the Canton Grisons, has very weak *chalybeate alkaline gaseous* springs. Fideris is in the Praettigau valley and has a station on the Landquart-Davos railway, and the baths are about an hour's drive from the station and half an hour from the village, at an altitude of 3,460 feet. There is only 0·016 of bicarbonate of iron per litre in the water, the other chief constituents being sodium (0·742) and calcium bicarbonate (0·973), and much free carbonic acid. The waters, combined with the mountain climate, have a tonic and stimulating action. Fideris is locally recommended for a great variety of maladies, but its usefulness is chiefly manifested in those which arise in connection with anæmia and loss of tone.

Fitero, a *simple thermal* bath (temperature 117° F.) in the north of Spain (province of Navarra) with a local reputation for the cure of chronic rheumatism.

Flinsberg, in Silesia (Prussia), has *cold gaseous chalybeate* springs. It lies at an altitude of 1,700 feet in the Queisthal at the foot of the Isergebirge, in a hilly district surrounded by pine forests, with walks planned out for Oertel's Terrain-Kur. It has a station (Friedeberg) distant an hour's drive, on the Friedeberg-Griefenberg Railway. Its climate is fresh and bracing. The springs used for drinking — the Ober- and Niederbrunnen—have about 0·04 of bicarbonate of iron per litre and much free carbonic acid. The other wells are used, diluted with ordinary hot water, for baths. Other therapeutic resources applied there are massage, mud baths, pine-needle and pine-bark baths and inhalations, and brine inhalations.

The maladies treated are anæmia, neurasthenia, respiratory and circulatory affections, and women's diseases.

The season is from May 1 to Oct. 1.

Flitwick, a *cold chalybeate* spring near Ampthill, Bedfordshire. It contains a considerable amount of ferric persulphate—an unusual constituent of mineral springs—and has a light yellow colour and a slightly acid taste. It appears from the *Lancet* analysis to contain 2·5 grammes of persulphate of iron per litre, with a little sulphate of alumina, about 0·41, and smaller amounts of sulphates of sodium and calcium. Its strength practically removes it from the class of ordinary chalybeate waters. It is given in one to three tablespoonful doses in the same class of cases as those for which the iron salts are usually prescribed.

Frankenhausen, with *common salt* wells, is in the principality of Schwarzburg-Rudolstadt, and has a station on the Bretleben-Frankenhausen branch line. It lies at an altitude of 370 feet. It has salt wells in connection with adjacent salt mines. It is used for the same purposes as other common salt baths, and has a sanatorium for scrofulous children.

Franz Joseph, one of the numerous Hungarian "bitter waters," owing its activity to the presence of magnesium sulphate.

Frienwalde, in Mark-Brandenburg (Prussia), on the Oder, with a station on the Frankfort-on-Oder-Angermünde line, has weak earthy *cold chalybeate* springs, containing a small amount of carbonate of iron (0·02 per litre), together with calcium and magnesium carbonate, and a small amount of carbonic acid gas. These springs are used for drinking and for baths and douches. Mud baths, artificial carbonic acid brine baths, pine-needle baths, and vapour baths are also prepared and applied there. Cases treated there are those of anæmia, retarded convalescence, rheumatism, and female maladies.

The season is from May 15 to Sept. 30. It is a summer resort of the people of Berlin.

Freiersbach, having *cold gaseous alkaline-earthy chalybeate* springs, is situated in the Baden portion of the Black Forest, in the commune of Petersthal, four miles and a-half from the railway station Oppenau. It is one of the Kniebis baths, and lies at an elevation of 1,260 feet in the Reuchthal, surrounded by pine-clad mountains. It has seven chalybeate springs. One of the strongest is the Friedrichsquelle, which contains 0·058 bicarbonate of iron per litre and 0·013 of chloride of lithium. It also has a Lithionquelle, containing more lithium (0·017 per litre); it has, in addition, a spring smelling of H_2S, and termed the Schwefelquelle. They all contain a considerable amount of calcium bicarbonate. The waters are drunk and used for baths. Mud baths and natural carbonic acid baths are also given. The usual maladies treated at chalybeate baths are treated there: anæmia, neurasthenia, female complaints, and those suitable to treatment by alkaline earthy waters, and which need also tonic remedies, as renal and vesical disorders, gout, etc.

The season is from May 1 to Oct. 15.

Friedrichshall, in Saxe-Meiningen, has a "bitter water" used only for exportation, contains much sodium chloride (24 grammes per litre) and magnesium chloride (12·0) as well as sodium sulphate (18·0).

Fuered, a distant Hungarian spa, having considerable local popularity, finely situated on the Platten-See, and reached by steamer in an hour from the railway station Sio-Fok.

Its waters are feebly mineralised and difficult of classification. The chief drinking well is highly gaseous — the Franz-Josephsquelle — and contains calcium (0·8 per litre) and sodium (0·11), carbonate and sodium sulphate (0·8), and bicarbonate of iron (0·01), as well as a large amount of carbonic acid gas. The lake water and mud are also used for baths.

The season is from May 15 to Sept. 15.

Fuscherbad, or St. Wolfgang's Bad, in Styria, at an altitude of over 4,000 feet, has very feebly mineralised springs, and is rather a climatic station. It is finely situated in the Fuscherthal, two hours distant from Brück railway station. Gastein patients are sometimes sent there for an after-cure.

Gastein or **Wildbad-Gastein**, to distinguish it from Hof-Gastein, from which it is distant four or five miles, is situated in Austria in the duchy of Salzburg, and possesses *simple thermal* springs. It is usually approached from Innsbruck or Salzburg. The nearest railway station is Lend-Gastein, four hours from Innsbruck. A drive of fifteen miles almost due south from Lend, through the Gastein valley, brings you to Wildbad-Gastein, passing through Hof-Gastein (four or five miles nearer Lend) on the way. Wildbad-Gastein, at the southern

[illegible]

[illegible] there are on an average sixty rainy days in the three summer months. But the rain often falls in sudden torrents with intervals of sunshine. August is usually the driest and the hottest month, the average temperature being 60° F. Rapid and considerable variations of temperature are not uncommon.

There are numerous thermal springs at Gastein, varying in temperature from about 80° to 120° F. The baths are generally given of a temperature of about 95° F., and the hotter springs are allowed to cool in reservoirs until they reach the temperature desired.

The thermal waters are supplied to the various hotels and lodging-houses, so that the patients are able to take their baths where they reside, a great convenience, especially to the many sufferers from diseases of the nervous system who flock to Gastein. These waters are also conveyed to Hof-Gastein in wooden pipes. The meals at Gastein are usually taken at restaurants *à la carte* and not at *tables d'hôte*, which is a decided advantage for invalids, and enables them to follow a diet suitable to their condition.

The water of these hot springs is *very feebly mineralised*, and contains only 0·3 of solids per litre, consisting of minute amounts of sodium sulphate and chloride and silica. There is nothing whatever in the composition of the water to account for any therapeutic results obtained by bathing in it—these have been referred to some mysterious hypothetical electrical condition of the waters. But the curative effects of the treatment at Gastein must probably be referred to the tonic and soothing effect of the climate and the influence of regular bathing in thermal water for half an hour or so daily. It is doubtless quite as much an air cure as a water cure.

There is exceedingly little *drinking* of the waters at Gastein, the physicians there trusting almost wholly to the baths; but the aid of massage and electrical treatment is constantly called in to supplement the thermal baths.

In considering the cases suitable to treatment at Gastein, it is well to remember that it has been termed an "old man's bath"—a resort for those who desire to retard the approach of senility. The baths have been described as "tonic and strengthening, giving new life to the organism; after a few baths a condition of nervous stimulation is produced, and the patient recovers his forces and his intellectual powers." It is certain that Gastein attracts great numbers of distinguished men, especially statesmen, politicians, and *literati*, who appear to be satisfied with the benefit it confers.

The chief speciality of Gastein is certainly the treatment of affections of the nervous system, functional and organic, as tabes dorsalis, paraplegias, hemiplegic contractions, and various forms of partial and peripheral paralysis, neuralgias, hysteria, and hypochondriasis, neurasthenia and overwork, insomnia, the loss of power associated with senility, impotence.

Other maladies are sent to Gastein, just as they are sent to similar thermal baths, such as cases of chronic gout and rheumatism and chronic affections of the female pelvic organs, especially when occurring in the neurotic.

The climate is well adapted to convalescents from serious disease and as an after-cure, after a course of such active waters as those of Carlsbad or Marienbad. Owing to its distance from England, other nationalities are more largely represented at Gastein than our own.

The season is from May to September, but July and August are the best months. The place is so crowded in the height of the season that it is necessary for visitors requiring comfortable quarters to engage them some weeks in advance of their visit.

Gleichenberg, in Styria, has *cold gaseous alkaline and common salt* waters belonging to the same class as those of Ems and Royat. An important and efficacious group of mineral springs. It is situated at an elevation, nearly 1,000 feet above the sea, in a pleasant and picturesque country, about three hours from Graz and an hour and a-quarter from Feldbach railway stations. The two principal springs are the Constantinquelle and the Emmaquelle. The former contains 3·6 grammes of sodium bicarbonate and 1·8 of sodium chloride per litre, and as much as 1·340 volumes of carbonic acid gas. The Emmaquelle is less gaseous. There is also in the neighbourhood a weak gaseous chalybeate spring, the Klausenquelle, and an alkaline chalybeate, the Johannisbrunnen, both of which can be utilised in anæmic cases requiring iron. Gleichenberg is a place of considerable local repute and resort, both for its pleasant mild climate and its waters, which are found very beneficial in cases of catarrh of the respiratory organs and certain forms of dyspepsia. The water is pulverised for inhalation, and also drunk. The processes of hydrotherapy, too, are applied.

The season is from May to September.

Gurnigelbad, a *cold sulphur* bath in Canton Berne, Switzerland, at an elevation of 3,783 feet above the sea. It is connected with Berne and Thun by a good carriage road, and is a drive of four to five hours from either town. A very fine bath establishment (with hotel) exists there in a commanding situation with very beautiful mountain views, and with spacious pine forests, affording charming sheltered and shady walks, immediately surrounding it. Many interesting excursions of varying distance can also be enjoyed.

The climate is bright and bracing with a rather high degree of humidity, due to the great extent of pine forest surrounding the place. These forests afford a protection from the north and north-west winds. Considerable variations of temperature must be expected even in summer.

Of its two springs, the Schwarzbrünnli is the stronger; it is rich in free sulphuretted hydrogen and free carbonic acid, and contains calcium sulphate 1·7, calcium and magnesium sulphide 0·0057 per litre, and minute quantities of other mineral substances of no special importance. The Stockquelle contains rather more calcium sulphate but much less sulphuretted hydrogen and no sulphides. An iron spring also exists in the forest, ten minutes distance from the baths.

These waters are administered internally and as baths and douches, and the most modern arrangements are provided for inhalations, sprays, and nasal irrigations. Hydropathy, electro-therapeutics, electric baths, massage, and milk and whey and diet cures are also available. These in conjunction with mountain and forest air are the remedial measures to be obtained at Gurnigel.

The sulphur water is said to be easily digested on account of the amount of carbonic acid in it.

The maladies especially suitable for treatment there are in the first place chronic gastric and intestinal disorders, catarrh, gastralgia, gastric dilatation and nervous dyspepsia (modern gastric methods of exploration and mechanical and electrical treatment are practised), chronic diarrhœa, constipation, hæmorrhoids, intestinal parasites—especially the tape worms and ascarides—functional hepatic disorders, congestion, catarrhal jaundice, biliary colic, catarrhal diseases of the nose, pharynx, larynx, and bronchi as at other sulphur spas, malarial cachexia, diseases of the female pelvic organs, certain skin affections, eczema, acne, furunculi, varicose veins, etc.

The season is from June to September.

Gandersheim, on the Gande, in the Duchy of Brunswick, with a station on the Magdeburg-Holtzminden Railway, has *common salt* springs, which are used in the treatment of rheumatism, gout, female affections, scrofula, etc.

Season, May to end of September.

Giesshuebl-Puchstein, in the valley of the Eger, Bohemia, about six miles from Carlsbad, has a bath establishment and a pleasant gaseous spring, which is largely exported as a table water.

Gilsland Spa, Cumberland, in a pleasant situation on the river Irthing, about twenty miles from Carlisle, possesses both *chalybeate* and *cold sulphur* springs.

Gmunden, in the Salzkammergut, Austria, lies, at an elevation of 1,370 feet, on the Traun-See, and has a station on the railway between Altnung and Ischl; it has a *common salt* bath prepared with brine from the Ebensee salt works, the strength of which is about 240 grammes per litre. Apparatus for artificial aërotherapy is also available.

Goczal Kowitz, in Upper Silesia, with a station on the Kattowitz-Dzieditz Railway, possesses a *cold common salt* well, which is used in the treatment of such cases as are usually sent to such spas.

Season, May 15 to Sept. 15.

Godesberg, a Rhenish resort with a station on the Cologne-Bingerbruck line, in a picturesque situation, has *alkaline-saline-chalybeate* springs.

The Stahlbrunnen contains sodium bicarbonate (1·4), sodium chloride (1·0), and bicarbonate of iron (0·029). Another spring, containing more iron, is only used for baths. Hydropathic treatment is also carried out there. The cases treated are those of anæmia, neurasthenia, and female complaints.

The season is from May 1 to Sept. 30.

Gonten, in Canton Appenzell, Switzerland, at an elevation of 2,900 feet, has *cold chalybeate* springs, having 0·043 of carbonate of iron per litre. It has a station on the Winkeln-Appenzell line. The water is more used for baths than for drinking. The climate is cool and the air tonic and pure. It is also a station for the milk and whey cures.

Season, June to middle of September.

Göppingen, in Würtemberg, has a *cold gaseous* (carbonic acid) spring, with a small bathing establishment, but it is chiefly used for exportation as a table water.

Gottleuba, in the kingdom of Saxony on the Gottleuba, has a *cold chalybeate* spring. The railway station is Berggiesshübel on the Berggiesshübel and Pirna Railway. Mud baths and artificial carbonic acid baths are also prepared. Cases of chlorosis, anæmia and retarded convalescence are treated.

Season, from May 1 to end of September.

Grau, a Hungarian spa possessing thermal earthy springs of a temperature 83-85° F., and also a strong "bitter water" containing 45 grammes of magnesium sulphate per litre.

Greifswald, a *common salt* bath on the Ryck, in the province of Pomerania. As it is a university town the baths are used in connection with the hospital and private cliniques.

Open all the year.

Grenzach, four miles from Bâle, on the Bâle-Constance line, has a *cold sodium sulphate* (3·2 grammes per litre) and *chloride* (1·9) water, containing also smaller amounts of calcium sulphate and bicarbonate. It is used chiefly for drinking. Artificial salt baths are also prepared. It is a small bath chiefly used for cases of gastric, hepatic, and renal disorders, gallstones, and obesity.

Season, April to October.

Gréoulx, France, Basses Alpes, a *thermal sulphur* bath, at an altitude of 1,140 feet, situated in a picturesque valley, about one hour and a-half's drive from the station of Mirabeau on the line between Grenoble and Marseilles. It has two springs, the hottest of which has a temperature of 102° F.; it contains 1·50 grammes of common salt per litre as well as free H_2S (4 c.c.) and much barégine—a valuable combination which would probably be more highly esteemed if this bath were not in so out-of-the-way a situation. The springs are used for drinking and for baths (swimming and ordinary), douches, and inhalations. The cases treated there are those of rheumatism, scrofulous, glandular and cutaneous affections, catarrhs of the pharynx, larynx, and bronchi; traumatisms, slowly healing wounds and ulcers, uterine affections.

The season is from April 15 to Oct. 15.

Griesbach, in the Baden Black Forest, one of the Kniebis baths, 1,850 feet above the sea, about seven miles from the railway station Oppenau, Appenweir-Oppenau line, has several *cold gaseous chalybeate* springs, of which the chief is the Antoniusquelle; it contains bicarbonate of iron (0·07), bicarbonate of calcium (1·6), and sulphate of sodium (0·7). This and other springs are used for drinking and for baths. Mud baths and several kinds of pine baths are prepared. Cases of anæmia, chlorosis, and female complaints are treated there.

The season is from May 15 to Oct. 1.

Hammam R'Irha, in Algiers, has *thermal earthy calcareous* waters used for baths, and a very weak *cold gaseous earthy chalybeate* spring, which is drunk there often as a table water.

It is also a winter climate resort, and will be

noticed in the second part of this work dealing with the subject of climate.

The hot springs are of a temperature of about 110° F. in the baths—they are large *swimming* baths. This is a high temperature for such baths, and they may feel at first uncomfortably hot, but the body soon becomes accustomed to the heat, and the sensation is said to become very agreeable. The Arabs drink the hot water while in the bath, which promotes free perspiration. The mineralisation of the water has probably little to do with its therapeutic effects. Its chief constituents are calcium sulphate and carbonate, forming together 1·510 of a total amount of solids of 2·330 per litre. It contains also a small amount of sodium chloride (0·439) and minute quantities of other salts. It much resembles the Bath waters and proves beneficial in the same cases, viz. chronic rheumatism (*especially*) and gout; some traumatic cases, as painful cicatrices; neuralgias, especially when of rheumatic origin; certain forms of paralysis, cases of vesical catarrh in the gouty, and some chronic affections of the pelvic viscera.

The climate is also suitable to cases of chronic bronchial catarrh.

The weak gaseous earthy chalybeate spring is used to mix with wine as a table water, and is also recommended to be drunk in cases of anæmia and chlorosis and in cases of malarial cachexia. It only contains 0·010 of bicarbonate of iron per litre. Its other constituents are mainly earthy sulphates and carbonates, and it is rich in carbonic acid gas, which makes it an agreeable drink.

There is a military hospital at Hammam R'Irha, and the results of treatment there show that cases of general chronic rheumatism are benefited in the proportion of about 80 per cent.; next in order are traumatic joint affections, then *articular* rheumatism, and the least benefited are joint affections referable to gout.

The warm, dry, and sunny climate has no doubt

a great share in the production of the beneficial results observed.

Hammam R'Irha is about sixty miles west-south-west of Algiers, and is reached partly by rail—to Bon Medfa in three to four hours—and then a drive of eight miles to the baths.

The hotel and bath establishment are very comfortable.

Harrogate, in Yorkshire, about six hours from London, has long been celebrated for its *sulphur* springs, of which a great number arise in the neighbourhood. There are said to be as many as 80 different mineral springs. They are all cold, and vary considerably in their strength. Most of them contain sodium sulphide and free sulphuretted hydrogen, as well as considerable but varying proportions of common salt.

The most popular of these, and the one generally used for drinking, is known as the "old sulphur spring" in the Royal Pump Room, and has about 0·07 of sodium sulphide and 37 volumes of H_2S per litre. It has also sodium chloride (12·7), and barium chloride (0·09). It has been suggested that the barium salt acts as a heart tonic, and corrects any depressing effect that the sulphur may tend to produce. But this is only a hypothesis.

Some of the sulphur springs are very strong—the Montpellier is estimated to contain 0·2 per litre of sodium sulphide, but has no H_2S—and others are very weak, as the Starbeck wells, and these are used chiefly for baths; while others are of intermediate strength; so that the waters present a sort of natural graduation adapted to the requirements of various cases. The strongest sulphur springs at Harrogate contain, as has been seen, a large proportion of common salt. Harrogate is also renowned for its chalybeate springs; these contain iron as well as sodium chloride. One of these, the celebrated "Kissingen well," contains 0·13 of carbonate of iron, 10·0 of sodium chloride, and 1·2 calcium chloride per litre. Another, the "chloride of iron well," contains chloride of iron 0·19, carbonate of iron 0·16, chloride of sodium 2·5, and chloride of barium 0·07 per litre.

Yet another iron water comes from the so-called "alum well" in the "bog-field." This is remarkable as containing ferrous sulphate and ferric sulphate, aluminium, calcium, and magnesium sulphate, about 1·0 per litre each. One of the milder chalybeate springs is artificially charged with carbonic acid, which not only makes it much more agreeable and refreshing to drink, but probably easier to digest.

Taken in large quantities these waters are purgative, like the common salt waters of Homburg and Kissingen, and in smaller quantities they are said to be alterative. Their use as aperients is not, as a rule, attended by any debilitating effect.

The chalybeate waters, when they are easily digested, are of service in anæmic cases, but they are not so digestible as those Continental chalybeate springs that are rich in free carbonic acid, the presence of which, in an iron water, seems to greatly favour its digestion and assimilation.

It has been said that it is an advantage, in some cases, to administer the sulphur waters, before giving the chalybeate springs, for the purpose of stimulating the excretory organs—liver, kidneys, and skin—thus getting rid of waste material, and so preparing the way for the absorption and assimilation of the iron. The stimulating influence on tissue changes of the sodium chloride in these waters is no doubt beneficial in many cases; in the debilitated and anæmic with "sluggish livers." It is also useful in the gouty bronchitic. Some of the waters are warmed before drinking by a special contrivance called the "Therma."

Treatment at Harrogate is recommended for the cure of chronic dyspepsias, constipation, congestion of the liver, and all functional hepatic disorders, also in conditions of abdominal plethora, and obesity, in short, in the same cases as the waters of Homburg and Kissingen. They are given internally and in the form of baths in cases of chronic gout and rheumatism. In certain forms of skin disease they lay claim to peculiar efficacy, as in chronic eczema, in psoriasis, lichen, acne, and troublesome syphilitic eruptions. (In constitutional syphilis the methods employed at Aix la Chapelle can be resorted to.)

These waters are also useful in the treatment of lead and mercurial poisoning, and the malarial cachexia. The chalybeate springs, besides being administered in cases of anæmia and chlorosis, and retarded convalescence, are found of much use in functional uterine disorders, when taken in association with the baths. They are prescribed also in scrofulous affections, and in chronic rheumatoid arthritis.

Unlike the physicians at Continental spas, those at Harrogate do not hesitate to employ other medicinal remedies as aids to the mineral treatment, and the free use of small doses of calomel is not uncommon with some of them.

The arrangements for drinking and bathing at Harrogate are good and complete, and the fine bracing air of the surrounding country no doubt contributes, in great measure, to the good effects obtained from treatment there.

Harrogate is in an open country, at an elevation of 260 to 600 feet above the sea. Upper Harrogate has a more bracing climate than the lower part of the town. There is a fine open common, the Stray, 200 acres in extent, around which the hotels and residences are built. The air at Harrogate is said to be very dry, owing to the absence of woods and of large river beds or lakes, and to the absorbent nature of the soil. "There are fewer rainy days than at most of the other English health resorts."

Phthisis is rare amongst the natives, but they are apt to suffer from rheumatism.

The New Montpellier Baths is a very fine building, and is furnished with every appliance which modern science has sanctioned in the application of mineral springs; baths and douches of all kinds (the Aix douche massage), electric light baths, etc.

Helouan les Bains, in Egypt, sixteen miles due south of Cairo, possesses *thermal sulphur and salt* waters, as well as a weak *common salt* spring containing iron, and another without iron. The thermal sulphur springs have a temperature of 90° F. at the source, and they contain 60 c.c. of sulphuretted hydrogen per litre, also 5·069 of common salt, 0·507 of magnesium sulphate, some calcium carbonate and sulphate, and a little potassium chloride. A water containing sulphur and salt like the Harrogate springs.

It has also a water which is termed "saline chalybeate," but the iron in it has been estimated, *together with alumina*, as 0·015 per litre; how much iron there is, apart from the alumina, does not appear to have been ascertained. We may assume that it is very weak iron water, but it also contains 4·705 of common salt per litre, and calcium carbonate and sulphate, together amounting to 1·249, and magnesium sulphate 0·361.

The New Bath establishment is very complete and is furnished with all the necessary requirements to make it equal to any European establishment of the kind. It contains immersion baths, combination baths, with needle baths, douches, and sprays of all kinds. Hot air and vapour baths, Aix massage, electric baths, inhalations, pulverisations, etc. A large swimming sulphur bath, with running water, adjoins the bath establishment. In addition to the baths, the dry, warm, sunny desert climate must be a very important therapeutic factor. The waters are used internally as well as externally, and have been found beneficial in the following maladies—dyspepsia, functional hepatic disorders, gout, lithæmia, and allied maladies, pharyngeal, laryngeal, and bronchial catarrh (aided greatly by the climate), certain affections of the female pelvic organs. Cases of sciatica and rheumatism, muscular and articular, cases of rheumatoid arthritis, are said to manifestly improve. Also cases of chronic skin disease, cases of overwork and neurasthenia. It must be difficult to apportion between the climate and the baths the precise amount of benefit derived.

The climatic characters and advantages of Helouan will be referred to in the second part of this work. Trains run from Cairo to Helouan hourly, in twenty-five to forty-five minutes. The best season for Europeans is from the beginning of November to the end of April.*

Heustrich, a *cold alkaline sulphur* bath situated in the vicinity of the Lake of Thun in Switzerland, is an important station for the treatment of catarrhal affections of the air passages and of the stomach, and merits to be better known in England. It is best reached from Spiez, a well-known steamboat station on the Lake of Thun, from which Heustrich is distant about five miles, or it is about an hour and a-half's drive from the railway station of Thun. It is picturesquely situated at the foot of the Niesen, on its eastern flank, at an elevation of about 2,200 feet, on the left bank of the Kander. It is close to the finest mountain scenery of the Bernese Oberland, and is immediately surrounded by a well-wooded and cultivated district. It has a sub-alpine climate, the air being fresh and mildly tonic, but hot in the mid-day in the summer. It is protected entirely from the winds coming from north and south, and as the baths are built away from the high road, it is very free

* "Helouan: Its Climate, Waters, and Recent Improvements," by Dr. W. Page May.

from dust. The air has a somewhat high degree of humidity, which the resident physician considers an advantage in the treatment of those suffering from catarrhal affections of the air passages, and these probably form the majority of the patients at this bath. It has a mild climate for a place of that altitude. Patients are, however, warned that they must come prepared for occasional sudden depressions of temperature, such as are common in all mountain stations like Heustrich.

There is a single spring which yields only a very moderate amount of water, about 1¾ litres per minute at a temperature of 43° F. It has a strong smell of sulphuretted hydrogen, and on exposure to the air it becomes cloudy from the deposit of sulphur.

It contains about 11 c.c. of H_2S per litre, which ranks it amongst the moderately strong sulphur waters—about one-third the strength of the Allevard water. But it has a great advantage over most cold sulphur waters in the absence of earthy salts and the presence of sodium salts. It is remarkable in containing no calcium sulphate, but as much as 0·671 per litre of sodium bicarbonate and 0·20 of sodium sulphate.

Much of the therapeutic action of this water is referred to its alkalinity—due to the presence of so much sodium bicarbonate—its stimulating effect on the appetite, and its notable diuretic action. It exerts a solvent effect on the urates and oxalates, and is therefore beneficial in vesical catarrh in the gouty. Its solvent action also renders this water useful in the treatment of chronic catarrh of the stomach and the respiratory organs. In the latter, expectoration is facilitated and cough relieved.

The utility of the *bath* in the cure of boils, of pityriasis versicolor, of varicose ulcers and other skin affections is probably largely due to the influence of the *alkaline* waters on the skin secretions; and the good effect of the baths in rheumatic cases is referred rather to the influence of the warmth of the bath than to its mineral constituents.*

Inhalation of the *pulverised* water is practised at Heustrich in the treatment of catarrhal affections of the respiratory organs, as it is at Ems and Allevard, the pulverisation being effected by means of compressed air. These inhalations are especially useful in catarrhs localised in the trachea and large bronchi. For deeper-seated affections aspiration of compressed air charged with vaporisable substances (pine oil, tar, turpentine) are used.

A *pneumatic cabinet* is available there for the treatment of cases of emphysema with chronic bronchitis.

For the many patients sent to this resort whose cases are complicated with neurasthenia the methods of hydrotherapy are available and prove very useful. Massage and electricity are also employed. Excellent provision is made for taking a milk cure.

Certain of the maladies suitable for treatment at Heustrich have already been indicated in a general sense: they may now be briefly enumerated more particularly.

1st. Catarrhs of the respiratory organs—chronic catarrhal rhinitis—treated by irrigations of the water at a temperature of 95° F.; and for this purpose a teaspoonful of sodium chloride is added to each litre of the water; ozæna, or fœtid rhinitis; chronic pharyngeal catarrh and catarrh of the Eustachian tube; chronic laryngeal catarrh, treated by inhalations of the pulverised water and its internal use; bronchitis and emphysema (in addition to pneumotherapy the internal use of the waters is necessary); cases of asthma dependent on nasal trouble.

2nd. Phthisis cases, in the early stages, or of the torpid form *without fever*, are benefited by the various therapeutic and tonic measures that can be applied, including the use of the water, which acts beneficially

* D. M. Neukomm, "Les Bains de Heustrich."

on the catarrhal symptoms. Febrile forms must not be sent there.

3rd. Dyspepsia and chronic gastric catarrh; dilatation of the stomach, in which case lavage and irrigation of the stomach are carried out as well as a careful regulation of diet; but much reliance is placed on the internal use of the water in these gastric cases.

4th. Chronic intestinal catarrh, disposition to habitual diarrhœa.

5th. Chronic catarrh of the female sexual organs: irrigations are applied in the bath.

6th. Chronic vesical catarrh, in cases associated with acid urine and deposits of urates or oxalates.

The season is from the beginning of June to the end of September. The months of June and September are very suitable for the treatment, and far less crowded than July and August. A vast number of interesting walks and excursions can be made into the attractive country around.

Homburg, or **Homburg von der Hohe**, in the province of Hesse-Nassau, Germany, is one of the most popular resorts in Europe. It possesses *cold common salt* springs rich in *carbonic acid gas*, and some of them contain iron, and these may be termed *gaseous chalybeate common salt springs.*

The possession of springs containing common salt is scarcely sufficient to account for the extraordinary popularity of Homburg.

But almost everything that art could do has been done to make the surroundings of the springs attractive; and pleasant shady avenues and covered walks, palm-houses, and parterres of flowers, and other attractions give to the neighbourhood of the mineral springs a very pleasing aspect.

There can be no manner of doubt that the attractiveness and the popularity of Homburg are quite as much dependent upon social considerations as upon medicinal ones. Something must be said in favour of the climate of Homburg. It is unusually dry and bracing for a place of such moderate elevation—650 feet above the sea. This is due to the absence of streams and rivers and to the absorbent nature of the soil, and to the position of Homburg, on a raised portion of a wide plain, the neighbouring mountains being sufficiently distant to keep the mists and clouds which frequently settle over them from influencing its atmosphere.

Owing to its somewhat exposed situation it suffers from the heating effect of the direct rays of the sun, but, as a compensation, cooling currents of air blow down from the distant forest-clad hills, and the mornings and evenings are fresh and exhilarating. There is a very general consent among those who have frequented the place for many seasons that "Homburg is bracing."

Homburg has several mineral springs; the chief of these, and the one that has obtained a world-wide reputation, is the Elisabethenbrunnen, and it is around this *source* that the gaily dressed crowd gathers during the early morning hours, from six to eight, when drinking mineral waters is presumed to have its greatest efficacy. The Ludwigbrunnen has also its patrons, but it has an afternoon popularity rather than a morning one. Then there are the Kaiserbrunnen, the Luisenbrunnen, and the Stahlbrunnen. A few words must be said about each of these. They all contain much carbonic acid gas, and they all contain salt, common salt, but in very different amounts. The Elisabeth spring contains about 10 grammes to the litre, the Ludwig about half, the Kaiser two-thirds, the Luisen about one-third, and the Stahl about half (5 grammes) that quantity. Then they all, in addition to sodium chloride, contain small quantities of calcium and magnesium and other chlorides, and bicarbonate of iron, in varying proportions; the Stahlbrunnen, as its name implies, contains much more than the others—0·09 of bicarbonate of iron per litre and 1·0 of bicarbonate of lime, which is also found in the other springs. The Luisen is the next strongest in iron, while the Ludwig contains scarcely any. Perhaps the next most important ingredient in these springs is carbonic acid gas. Here, again, there are considerable differences. The Kaiser contains the most—one-third as much again as the Elisabeth or the Luisen, and the Luisen contains the least. The presence of a small amount of sulphuretted hydrogen in the Luisenbrunnen and Stahlbrunnen undoubtedly detracts from their pleasantness as chalybeate springs.

Is it easy to determine what are the special uses of the Homburg springs from a consideration of their composition? It would seem not; there appears to be abundant room for differences of opinion. It is easy to dispose of the iron at once by admitting that it gives a tonic property *pro tanto* to all the springs into which it enters as an ingredient, and that according to the case or the constitution its tonic effects may be accelerated or hindered by the other constituents with which it is combined. It may also be said of the carbonic acid that its presence usually (not with all persons, however) aids the digestion of the water, and exercises a beneficial stimulating effect on the stomach, and also on the skin, when the waters are taken in the form of baths.

It must be borne in mind that it is next to impossible to decide altogether *à priori*—*i.e.* from a mere consideration of the component parts of a mineral spring—what will be its effect in all cases or in any particular case. In the final appeal experience must be the test. For it has been well observed that mineral waters are very composite remedies, and we cannot regard the combined action of a great number of substances merely as the sum of their separate actions, since they may partly aid and partly hinder each other in their effect upon the organism. In these very springs, for instance, we find the aperient chloride of magnesium counteracted by the astringent carbonate of lime.

Many gouty patients and sufferers from *uric acid* troubles are sent to drink the Homburg waters, but it is doubted by many authorities if Homburg is the best place to send gouty patients to indiscriminately. If Homburg, it is said, in addition to its Elisabethenbrunnen, had a mild, warm, alkaline spring, like the springs of Neuenahr or Ems, it would be worth all its other springs put together in the treatment of many forms of gout—forms of gout which are sometimes aggravated by drinking these exciting common salt waters. The best proof that a mineral water is doing good is the very practical one that the patient daily feels better and stronger. The appetite is better, exercise is less fatiguing, sleep is sounder and more refreshing, and there is a consciousness of returning and increasing energy, both intellectual and physical. He is a rash physician who, in the absence of any of these signs, relentlessly urges the unfortunate patient to persevere in irritating his stomach and his nerves with the promise of some far-off advantage.

The Homburg course is, no doubt, of great value in some cases, especially in certain forms of dyspepsia, where the organs of digestion require vigorous stimulation.

Many such cases have gouty and rheumatic tendencies, and then a combination of drinking and bathing in these salt and carbonic acid waters is of great service. But many rheumatic and gouty cases require a less exciting and more solvent alkaline water, and others a more decidedly laxative one. This is the point to be borne in mind, and it must not be overlooked that common salt waters, unless very weak, are irritating to certain constitutions, and quite capable of exciting gastric catarrh, which in others they may cure. The iron springs are useful to anæmic and debilitated persons whose gastro-hepatic functions may require stimulating;

and certain female pelvic affections appear to be benefited.

Much advantage no doubt attends the routine of rising early every morning and promenading, in cheerful society, for an hour or two in the fresh morning air; but some delicate persons are induced to do this who had better remain in their beds. No inconsiderable benefit is doubtless derived in many cases from the simple ingestion of a quantity of water, independently of and sometimes in spite of its mineral contents. The action of the chloride of sodium in these springs is believed to depend on its influence in promoting those tissue changes necessary to healthy nutrition. It helps us to get rid of the worn-out or half worn-out parts of our organism that linger in our bodies and clog and impede their mechanism, and interfere with their vital chemistry. It helps us at the same time to get rid of our somewhat ill-defined aches and pains and infirmities, which an artificial existence and a too busy or too careless life induces; and it would do this, perhaps, far more effectually if we did not find here too much of that very artificial and conventional life which brings these evils in its train. It is, indeed, certain that these social attractions induce many patients to visit Homburg whose maladies might be better treated elsewhere.

Scrofulous diseases of the glands, of the bones, of the skin—"torpid scrofula," as it is called—are treated advantageously with these salt waters, and especially with the salt baths. Many sufferers from chronic muscular rheumatism and chronic gout find great advantage from combining the use of these Homburg waters with that of the pine-leaf baths which are prepared here. An extract of pine-leaves is added to the heated salt spring, and a very grateful aromatic bath is thus produced. Mud baths, as well as pine-needle baths, electric and vapour baths, gymnastics, massage, and all forms of mechanical treatment can be obtained at Homburg.

The bath establishments are well equipped. Hotels and private apartments are comfortable or luxurious, and being only half an hour by rail from Frankfort, Homburg is very accessible from all parts of Europe.

Haarlem (Holland) has a *cold chalybeate* spring, containing also chloride of sodium (3·2 grammes per litre).

Hall (Swäbisch Hall) in Würtemberg, a small *common salt* bath picturesquely situated on the Kocher, in the Kocher valley, at an altitude of nearly 1,000 feet, and near extensive forests. It has a station on the Crailsheim-Heilbronn line. It has a cold salt spring, containing 23 grammes of sodium chloride per litre; a saturated brine is also brought from the Wilhelmsgluck salt works. A "mother lye" from the same source is also employed in the preparation of "sool" baths. Vapour baths, river baths, and artificial carbonic acid baths are used. The waters are employed for drinking, for baths, and for inhalation in the form of spray. The diseases treated there are scrofula, rickets, gout, rheumatism, paralysis, skin diseases, respiratory catarrhal affections.

Season, May to Oct. 1; also in the winter.

Hall, in the Austrian Tyrol, seven miles from Innsbruck, with which it is connected by railway and tram line, has a *cold common salt* bath, the strong brine (24 per cent.) being brought from the Salzberg, six miles off. There are also a chalybeate spring and a weak sulphur spring in the adjacent village of Heiligen-Kreuz.

Season, from May 15 to Oct. 1.

Hall (Bad-Hall), in Upper Austria, a *common salt* bath, has a station on the branch line of the Kremsthal. It has a well-known spring, the Tassilloquelle, which contains 12 grammes per litre of common salt and also bromide of magnesium (0·081) and iodide of magnesium (0·028); and other salt springs. It is a resort for scrofulous and rickety children, for syphilis, and for certain pelvic (female) maladies. It has a military and a civil sanatorium, and a hospital for scrofulous children.

The season is from May 15 to Oct. 1.

The water of the Tassilloquelle is exported under the designation of "Haller Iodwasser."

Hallein, an Austrian summer resort eleven miles from Salzburg, on the left bank of the Salzach, has well-known *brine* baths. It has a station on the line running south from Salzburg.

Hamm, in Westphalia—the bath two kilometres from the town—has *thermal gaseous brine* baths. It lies, surrounded by pleasure grounds, on the Lippe, and has a station on the Dortmund-Hanover and Unna-Hamm lines. The brine spring has a temperature of 94° F., and is diluted with hot water for baths and used undiluted for inhalation or spray. Mud baths and vapour baths are also applied. Rheumatism, gout, scrofula, and catarrh of the mucous membranes are the maladies treated.

The season is from May to Oct. 1.

Hapsal, in Esthonia, near the shores of the Baltic, has mud baths.

Harkany, in Hungary, has *thermal sulphur* waters of a temperature reaching to 145° F. An inflammable gas (sulphide of carbonyl = CO S) was found over the spring in considerable quantity by Karl von Than.

Harzburg (Bad-Harzburg), a *cold common salt* bath and a climatic summer resort in the Duchy of Brunswick, close to the Harz mountains and at the entrance of the Radan valley. The town lies at the foot of the Burg mountain, at an altitude of 850 feet. It is the terminus of the Braunschweig - Börssun - Harzburg line. It is surrounded by extensive forests of pines, beeches, etc., which provide a variety of attractive walks. It has two salt springs; one contains also magnesium sulphate and chloride, and the other sodium sulphate. Both are used for baths, diluted with fresh water. They are also used for drinking, gargling, and inhaling. Artificial carbonic acid baths are also used, and hot-air baths. Gout, rheumatism, neurasthenia, catarrhs of the respiratory organs, and gastro-hepatic diseases are the maladies treated there.

Season, May 15 to the end of September.

Heilbrunn (Adelheidsquelle), is a village in the Bavarian mountains, at an altitude of 2,620 feet, having a station on the Munich-Wolfratshausen-Klochl line. It possesses a spring, the Adelheidsquelle, which is a *cold common salt* spring (4·9 per litre), containing also sodium bicarbonate (0·9), bromide (0·05), and iodide (0·03). It claims to be the richest of the German salt waters in bromine and iodine. It is doubtful if these minute quantities exercise any special effect.

Season, May to October.

Heiligen Kreuzbad. *See* Rohitsch, p. 305.

Hercules-Bad, near Mahadia in Hungary, has *thermal common salt* and *sulphur* waters. It lies, at an elevation of 570 feet, in a beautiful situation at the foot of the Carpathian mountains, in the Czaona valley, and is a popular resort amongst the people of south-eastern Europe. It has a station on the railway between Orsova and Temesvar, three miles from the Danube. Its baths were known to the Romans. The thermal springs vary in temperature from 70° to 133° F., and, like the springs of Aix la Chapelle, contain sulphuretted hydrogen and common salt, and the same maladies are treated at this spa as at Aix la Chapelle. The waters are chiefly applied externally.

The season is from May to the end of September.

Hermannsbad, in Saxony, near Lausigk, has strong *sulphate of iron* waters unsuited for internal use.

Hermannsbad, at Muskau in Silesia, on the Neisse, at an altitude of 920 feet, has *cold sulphate of iron* waters. The drinking spring contains 0·19 per litre of sulphate of iron and 0·24 of carbonate of iron; the spring used for baths is much stronger. Ferruginous *Moor* baths are also prepared.

Honnef, on the right bank of the Rhine, at the foot of the Siebengebirge, with a station on the line from Cologne to Frankfort, and also a steamboat station, has a *cold gaseous alkaline salt* spring, called the Drachenquelle. Its chief constituents are sodium carbonate, chloride and sulphate, and magnesium carbonate. We are not in possession of the exact quantities, as its exploitation is of quite recent date.

It is used for drinking and inhaling and for baths and shower-baths. It is also exported charged with carbonic acid. There is a small new bath establishment. The mineral baths are warmed by the addition of hot mineral water, conducted through closed pipes. There is an inhalation room, the spray being produced by compressed air. It is much used by the patients at the neighbouring Hohenhonnef sanatorium. The grape cure can also be taken there in the autumn.

Hunyadi Janos, a purgative Hungarian "bitter water" containing sulphates of magnesium and sodium chiefly.

Ischia.—This historic and beautiful island in the Bay of Naples has been known for ages as possessing several important *thermal* springs. A melancholy interest attaches to those near Casamicciola, as the baths there and the patients dwelling in them suffered severely in the terrible earthquake which did so much damage in 1883. The Gurgitello spring, near Casamicciola, is probably the best known in the island. It is a weak *alkaline common-salt* spring of a high temperature, varying from 131° to 149° F. It is said to contain 2·7 of sodium chloride and 1·5 of sodium bicarbonate out of a total of solids amounting to 5·8 per litre.

There are satisfactory hotels at Casamicciola and others at Porto d'Ischia and Bagno d'Ischia, at a distance of three or four miles. Military and municipal thermal establishments are to be found at Bagno d'Ischia. At Castiglione and at other parts of the island natural vapour baths can be obtained. It is also a resort for sea baths and sand baths.

Ischl, 1,535 feet above the sea, most beautifully situated in the centre of the Salzkammergut, at the junction of the Traun and the Ischl, is one of the most frequented and fashionable of Austrian spas, crowded in the summer with visitors from Vienna, who visit it as a resort of pleasure, or for its climate as well as for its waters.

It possesses salt mines and salt works; and *Sool baths, i.e.* strong brine baths, are given there; also *mud* and *Moor baths*, sulphur baths, pine-cone baths, and *Sool* vapour baths are employed. The latter are produced by boiling the concentrated brine from the salt works, and residence in the steaming atmosphere thus formed is considered to be useful in cases of bronchial catarrh, and in some cases of phthisis.

The strong brine contains 235 grammes per litre of common salt. The Schwefelquelle has 17·0 grammes per litre of sodium chloride, and 4·0 of sodium sulphate, and a small amount of H_2S. The drinking springs (Klebelsbergquelle and Marie Luisenquelle) only contain about 5·0 grammes per litre of common salt. Other mineral waters are imported and often prescribed. Paths have been marked out for the "Terrain Kur" in the neighbourhood.

There is also a milk and whey cure; and, indeed, nearly every form of cure can be carried out at Ischl. Close to the town there is a well-arranged hydropathic establishment.

The climate of Ischl is peculiarly mild, equable, and soothing, and owing to its being surrounded by high mountains, covered with pine woods, the atmosphere is generally calm and moist; it is therefore well suited to delicate and irritable respiratory organs. Residence on the higher slopes, rather than in the town itself, is more bracing. Irritable conditions of the nervous system, and neurasthenia, certain disorders of the female pelvic organs, scrofulous affections, catarrhal disorders of the throat and air passages, and some chronic skin affections are benefited by treatment there.

It is also suitable as an after-cure to active treatment at other spas.

Ischl has a very fine Kurhaus, many first-class hotels (the Hôtel Bauer, on the hill, is considered to have the best situation), and every resource to make spa life pass pleasantly. It is connected by rail with the line running between Salzburg and Vienna.

The season is from June 1st to Oct. 1st, but it may be visited at an earlier or a later date.

Ilidze, in Bosnia, has *thermal calcareous sulphur* waters of a temperature of 124° F. They contain free sulphuretted hydrogen and about 1 gramme per litre of calcium carbonate and half as much sodium sulphate. It is in a fine situation, at an altitude of 1,600 feet, eight miles from Serajevo, the chief town of Bosnia.

These waters have a local reputation in the treatment of rheumatoid arthritis.

Imnau, with *cold gaseous chalybeate* springs, is situated in the principality of Hohenzollern, in a picturesque spot in the valley of the Eyach, and is half an hour's distance from the Eyach railway station, at an elevation of 1,140 feet. The strongest spring (Kasparquelle) contains 0·05 of bicarbonate of iron per litre, 0·03 of manganese bicarbonate, and 1·4 of calcium bicarbonate. A weaker spring (Fürstenquelle) has only 0·01 of bicarbonate of iron. Both are rich in carbonic acid gas.

Innichen, in the Austrian Tyrol --Wildbad Innichen — has two *cold sulphur* springs and a *chalybeate* one. It is finely situated, at an altitude of 4,370 feet, in the Passerthal. The bath is distant three-quarters of an hour from the railway station of Innichen.

Inowrazlaw is a considerable town in the province of Posen, Germany, and has a station on the Posen-Thorn line. Saturated *brine* from the salt mines is used there for baths. The principal constituents are sodium and magnesium chlorides. The baths resemble those at Droitwich. The brine and *Mutterlauge* obtained from it are diluted for the baths, and are also utilised for inhalation and gargling. Mud baths and artificial carbonic acid gas baths are also prepared. The cases treated there are those of chronic gout and rheumatism, scrofula, old inflammatory exudations, and female pelvic maladies.

The season is from May 15 to Sept. 15.

Inselbad, near Paderborn, in Westphalia, has a *cold weakly mineralised calcareous* spring, the Ottilienquelle, and a sanatorium, at an elevation of 520 feet, for the treatment of asthma especially, and chronic diseases of the organs of respiration. This spring is known for the amount of free nitrogen it contains (40 vols. per litre), as well as some carbonic acid gas. There is also a chalybeate spring, used for drinking, and a cold sulphur spring. The Ottilien water and the gases contained in it are used for inhalation. The water is also drunk. Mud baths, sand baths, and artificial carbonic acid baths are used.

The sanatorium is open the whole year. Railway station on the Soest-Holzminden line.

Ivonicz or **Ivonitch**, a resort in the Carpathians (Galicia), at an altitude of 1,340 feet, having *cold gaseous alkaline common salt* springs, also *chalybeate* springs and *naphtha* springs; the latter are used for inhalation. *Moor* and mud baths are also used. The Karlsquelle contains about 8·0 grammes of common salt per litre, 1·7 of sodium carbonate, and some sodium iodide and bromide (about 0·04 together). The bath establishment is about seven miles and a-half from the railway station.

Jagstfeld, Würtemburg, a few miles from Heilbronn, a *brine* bath on the Jagst, where it flows into the Neckar. It has a station on the Heilbronn - Osterburken line. Its elevation above the sea is 450 feet, and it is adjacent to extensive woodlands affording pleasant walks. It obtains a saturated salt solution from the Friedrichshall salt works; this diluted with water is used for bathing, inhaling, and gargling. The bath establishments are also hotels, so that patients have not to go out for their baths. There is a bathing sanatorium for children, the "Bethesda." Cases treated are scrofula, catarrhs of the air-passages, rheumatism, chronic inflammatory exudations, and female maladies.

The season is from May 1 to Oct. 15.

Jalcznovodsk, *thermal chalybeate* springs, in the Caucasus, said to resemble those of La Malou in the south of France.

Johannisbad, a Bohemian bath with *indifferent thermal* waters of a temperature of 85° F., is situated at an altitude of 2,300 feet in a mountainous district south of the Riesengebirge. There is also a weak chalybeate spring in the neighbourhood containing 0·01 of bicarbonate of iron per litre. The climate is said to be very exhilarating, and this combined with thermal treatment appears to have an excellent effect in cases of protracted convalescence and neurasthenia and general debility. Johannisbad is sometimes selected as an after-cure to Carlsbad and Marienbad.

The season is from May 15 to the end of September, but the best weather is usually met with at the end of August and through September. The place is a mile and a-half from Freiheit, the terminus of a branch railway from Trautenau.

Johannis water, an excellent *gaseous slightly alkaline* table water; the springs are at Zollhaus.

Juliushall. *See* Harzburg, p. 213.

Kissingen, in Bavaria, is one of the most popular spas in Europe, and justly so. It is not exactly fashionable, like Homburg, but it is better than that, it is useful and health-giving. It can be reached in twenty-seven hours from London viâ Aschaffenburg and Würzburg. It is situated in a pleasant open valley, through which flows the Franconian Saale. This valley is bounded on each side by picturesque wooded hills, and is 640 feet above the sea level. Terrain-Kur walks are marked out on these gently sloping hills. Kissingen was known as a health resort as long ago as the sixteenth century; but its great popularity is of modern growth, and the quiet village of former times has developed into a handsome, well-built town.

It possesses a fine, spacious promenade or Kurgarten, between the Kurhaus and the Kursaal, which presents an animated appearance between the hours of 7 and 9 a.m. and 6 and 7 p.m., when the band plays and the Kur-guests take their waters and gently exercise themselves. The two principal springs—the Ragoczy and the Pandur—are on the south side of this promenade; the Max-brunnen, the milder spring, is on the north side.

There are three bath-houses belonging to the State—the Kurhaus, the Saline, and the one formerly called Actienbad. The brine of the Schönbornsprudel is brought a distance of four kilometres to prepare the *Sool* baths. Mud baths are also prepared. There is provision for pine-needle inhalation, pneumatic treatment, gymnastics, massage, etc.

The usual daily life at Kissingen is to drink the waters from 7 to 9 a.m., breakfast in one's own rooms afterwards, and then those who bathe do so; one o'clock is the dinner hour, the dinner being, as a rule, plain and governed by medical orders; after dinner coffee is generally taken in the open air, and the time between this and 6 p.m. is devoted to exercise and amusement. From six to seven the waters are again taken, and there is a general promenade with music in the Kurgarten. Then supper and bed.

Kissingen is the type of a moderately strong *cold common salt spring*, with abundance of free carbonic acid. Compared with Homburg it contains but little more than half the quantity of common salt. The Ragoczy at Kissingen, the spring usually drunk there, contains six grammes of common salt to the litre.

The Pandur Spring scarcely differs in composition from the Ragoczy; it contains a little less common salt and a little more free carbonic acid. The Max-brunnen is much weaker—it is a very weak gaseous common salt spring, and is often taken merely as a pleasant beverage.

The Ragoczy contains, besides common salt and carbonic acid, a small quantity of the chlorides of magnesium, potassium, and lithium, as well as a moderate amount of the tonic carbonate of iron (0·03 per litre), and some carbonate of lime (1 gramme).

An artificial "Kissingen bitter water" is prepared from the *Sool* springs, and this is mixed, in certain proportions, with Ragoczy and Pandur waters when a more purgative action is desirable.

The Kissingen waters have proved beyond all others especially valuable in certain forms of atonic dyspepsia, in nervous as well as in gouty persons. In chronic gastric and intestinal catarrh, and the digestive troubles it involves, a course of Kissingen waters often proves more effectual than any other remedy. Many instances of this form of dyspepsia, which have resisted all forms of dieting and medication at home, recover completely at Kissingen. In some of these cases it is found advantageous to warm the water before drinking, in which process most of the carbonic acid escapes.

The moderate quantity of salt and the considerable amount of carbonic acid contained in the Ragoczy springs are sufficiently stimulating to the gastric mucous membrane to rouse it into greater activity; while the appreciable amount of iron gives tone to the debilitated and exhausted constitution, and the aperient ingredients promote the abdominal circulation, and tend to remove congestions of the liver and improve the functions of that too often erring organ. So that these springs act as aperients and hepatic stimulants.

They are therefore valuable in cases of constipation with hæmorrhoids, and in the constipation of anæmia.

By their aperient action and their tendency to promote tissue changes they are useful in the treatment of obesity, and are better borne by feeble persons, who have this object in view, than the stronger springs which are often prescribed for this purpose.

Painful gouty, rheumatic, and neuralgic conditions,

when they are obviously associated with digestive troubles, are suitable cases for treatment at Kissingen, and in the removal of these conditions the excellent baths available there afford important aid.

The warm mud baths prove exceedingly soothing to many cases of chronic muscular pains, chronic joint pains, and chronic neuralgias, especially when they are of rheumatic or gouty origin.

What are called "sool-spray baths" are also procurable here. These are a kind of vapour bath in which the atmosphere is kept at a temperature of from 78° to 86° F. saturated with vapour, and in which particles of salt are held suspended by means of mechanical pulverisation of the water. This is an excellent stimulant to the surface, and is not only useful in some forms of rheumatic and gouty pains, but is of value also in those chronic cases of bronchial catarrh which are met with in gouty persons. For these the moderately active aperient waters are also serviceable, as they tend to relieve the abdominal plethora from which such persons also suffer.

Persons affected with malarial cachexia are benefited by the Kissingen course. Cases of gouty glycosuria and early gouty nephritis also often do well there.

About a mile and a-half from Kissingen to the north, on the Saale, leading to which there are walks on both sides of the river, is a strong salt spring containing large quantities of carbonic acid; here there are salt works (the Saline and Gradirhauser), and the strong gaseous salt water is used for baths and douches of various kinds, and especially in the form of a *wave* bath: "a broad radiating sheet of water cuts the water of the bath at the point where it is brought in contact with it, lifting the surface into waves resembling those of the sea."

This bath is employed at a lower temperature than most saline baths, and is said to be very refreshing and invigorating.

There is also an arrangement here for collecting the carbonic acid gas as it rushes from the spring, and using it in various forms of gas baths in cases that are thought appropriate.

Chalybeate water from the neighbouring Bocklet spa is brought to Kissingen and drunk (usually later in the day) in addition to the other water in anæmic cases. Warm, gaseous Sool baths, like those at Nauheim, are prepared at Kissingen, and can be applied in the same cases as at Nauheim.

The season is from May 1st to Oct. 1st.

Kreuznach is situated in Rhenish Prussia in the valley of the Nahe, about ten miles from Bingen, on the left bank of the Rhine, at an altitude of 350 feet. It enjoys a pre-eminent reputation among *salt* baths for the treatment of all forms of scrofulous disease and of certain chronic uterine affections. The springs have been termed "bromiodduretted," and they contain a certain very small amount of compounds of iodine and bromine; but those who are most familiar with their use and application place but little reliance on the presence of these compounds, and regard them rather as strong salt springs, which they fortify in a special manner and apply also in a special fashion.

The Kurhaus is well equipped with hot-air and vapour baths and has excellent arrangements for massage and douches. It also has an inhalation chamber, the air of which is charged with pulverised mineral water by the Wassmuth method, as at many other spas. Patients sit in this chamber protected with a sort of loose frock and inhale the spray.

Artificial carbonic acid baths, mud, electric, and medicated baths are also used.

The springs chiefly used for drinking, the Elisabeth Spring and the Oranienquelle, arise in Kreuznach itself, quite close to the Kursaal; but the other springs used for bathing are found at some distance from Kreuznach, especially at Theodorshalle, a mile off, and at Münster-am-Stein, two and a-half miles distant. The Elisabeth Spring contains 10 grammes of chloride of sodium per litre, and small amounts of bromide and of iodide of sodium. Of chloride of calcium there is rather a large proportion—1·9 grammes per litre. It contains also minute quantities of other salts, and traces of arsenic. This is the only spring used for drinking, and it is drunk first in small quantities, and gradually increased to about a pint daily. It is usually drunk fasting in the morning. It is not sparkling, as it contains no carbonic acid; but it is not very unpleasant to drink.

It is chiefly, however, to the use of the baths that the physicians at Kreuznach trust for producing the good effects which they claim from the use of their springs; and these baths are administered in a special manner. Most of them are fortified by the addition of "mother lye," which contains about 200 grammes of calcium chloride per litre. This is prepared at Theodorshalle and Münster-am-Stein, in connection with the salt works at those places. Immense hedges of rough twigs and brambles are built up, termed "gradirhauser," and the water from the springs is allowed to flow over these, and by a great extent of surface being thus exposed to the air, it becomes concentrated to a certain degree; it is then collected and boiled in large pans, and after boiling it is kept at a high temperature for several days; in this process the chloride of sodium for the most part is separated by crystallisation, and the liquor left behind, after further concentration, forms the "mother lye."

This differs much in composition from the water of the springs from which it is derived. It is a yellowish-brown, oily-looking liquid, containing but a relatively small quantity of common salt; while the other chlorides, especially the chloride of calcium, are in larger amounts. It also contains an appreciable quantity of bromide of potassium. It is usual to add to a single bath about two litres of "mother lye" and two and a-half kilos of common salt; but this quantity of "mother lye" is largely increased in certain cases. In a bath of this kind the patients are retained for a long time, often for an hour, and a long period of repose is also needed after a prolonged bath of this sort. It produces much drowsiness and a feeling of exhaustion. The baths are given in wooden tubs owing to the action of the "mother lye" on stone and porcelain. The hotels and many of the houses are supplied with mineral water, which is very abundant.

Kreuznach is celebrated especially for the treatment of chronic catarrhs of the respiratory organs, nasal, laryngeal, and bronchial, of scrofulous, glandular, and other enlargements, certain diseases of women, as chronic catarrhal and inflammatory states of the pelvic organs and the residues of pelvic cellulitis and inflammatory exudations generally, certain forms of skin disease, especially syphilitic, and certain forms of gout and rheumatism. The system pursued there is regarded as the typical mode of applying strong salt springs, internally and externally, for the relief of chronic maladies.

Kreuznach possesses an abundance of springs, many of which belong to the salt works at Carlshalle, Theodorshalle, and Münster-am-Stein; and the large supply of "mother lye" and the salts extracted therefrom, always at hand, enables the physicians to use baths and local applications of any degree of strength they may require, and for any length of time. Such local applications prove most efficacious in promoting the absorption of scrofulous and other hypertrophies and deposits.

Munster-am-Stein, two and a-half miles higher up the river Nahe, also a bathing-station, where the same mode of treatment is carried out as at Kreuznach, is much more picturesquely situated. It lies at the foot of precipitous red porphyry cliffs—one, the Rheingrafenstein, rising to a considerable

constructed of white marble, the walls handsomely decorated with frescoes, and it is conveniently furnished with chairs and lounges and tables, supplied with a number of French and other newspapers.

In the next place, let us inquire what are the cases to which the treatment at Luchon is applicable. Rheumatic affections and all forms of disease associated with the rheumatic diathesis are suitable for treatment at Luchon. Respiratory diseases are considered especially suitable for treatment by *humage* of the natural sulphur vapours; tendencies to catarrhal attacks are removed—cases of nasopharyngeal catarrh, of rhinitis, of laryngitis and catarrhal otitis are said to be prevented and cured. Chronic bronchitis with emphysema and true asthma are also greatly benefited.

Some forms of tuberculosis do well there—the torpid, apyretic forms, with tendency to fibroid changes. The sequelæ of influenza and other acute infective diseases are benefited by the aseptic action of the sulphur vapours. Chronic diseases of the skin, and of these especially chronic eczema and parasitic dermatitis, do well. Other chronic skin diseases often improve considerably there, but they do not yield the same satisfactory result as cases of eczema. Certain diseases of the glands, and especially of the bones, often derive benefit in a marked degree at Luchon. The waters of Luchon are also reported to be, like those of Barèges, of great efficacy in the treatment of gunshot wounds. It is quite likely that they exercise a useful antiseptic action in such cases. Cases of lead and mercurial poisoning are said to be cured there. In some forms of nervous affections—*e.g.* of neurasthenia and neuritis—the treatment at Luchon exerts a calming and regulating influence, and cases of *tabes* have been greatly benefited. In syphilis, combined with specific remedies, the thermal treatment at Luchon proves of the greatest service. Bagnères de Luchon, then, is a thermal station of much importance and attractiveness.

The season is from June 1st to Oct. 1st. The most favourable period, especially for the treatment of respiratory affections, is from June 25th to Sept. 20th.

Luxeuil les Bains (France) is but a short distance from Lure, a station near Belfort. Although in the department of the Haute Saône, it is on the confines of the Vosges.

Luxeuil is not only picturesquely situated at an elevation of 1,000 feet above the sea, but it is a very interesting old town, with well-preserved quaint houses and buildings belonging to the fourteenth and fifteenth centuries, a magnificent church of the fourteenth century, and many remains of far greater antiquity preserved in the church and other buildings.

The waters of Luxeuil are hot, and resemble somewhat those of Plombières, but they are divided into two classes which differ in their physical appearances and chemical composition. One class, the *saline* springs, contains a small but appreciable quantity of chloride of sodium, about a gramme per litre, with minute amounts of lithium, arsenic, manganese, and iron, and has a temperature varying from 84° F. to 122° F.; the other contains much less chloride of sodium, but is characterised by the possession of compounds of iron (0·012) and *manganese* (0·07 per litre). The latter class, being also hot (temperature 80° to 84° F.), presents a rare form of spring, *almost unique in Europe.* The baths are prepared either of the saline water alone or mixed with the iron water.

The Etablissement des Bains, in a pretty garden and park, is well arranged, and contains all the baths and douches required for the treatment of the cases to which the waters of Luxeuil, and the methods employed there, are specially applicable; these are mainly diseases of women—those uterine affections so often found associated with anæmia and debility; also various rheumatic affections, and particularly cases of intestinal rheumatism and some functional nervous affections, neurasthenic and hysterical.

Cases of *periuterine adenitis—i.e.* chronic inflammation of the lymphatic glands and vessels surrounding the uterus—are reported to be frequently cured by the method of treatment adopted there. Ascending rectal douches and uterine and vaginal irrigations applied in the bath are amongst the most efficacious of the methods employed at Luxeuil. The former are employed in cases of chronic constipation, and in some forms of enteritis and intestinal dyspepsia, the latter in the uterine maladies just mentioned, in uterine or vaginal leucorrhœa, in uterine congestions and their consequences, dysmenorrhœa, metritis, etc. Uterine maladies complicated with neurasthenia, and the nervous disturbances of the menopause, are especially suitable to this spa.

The iron and manganese springs are considered of especial value in cases of anæmia. These are chiefly drunk, but treatment by baths predominates at Luxeuil.

Luxeuil is quite a small spa, and not very greatly frequented, but the surrounding country is attractive, and the ancient little town with its quaint houses and fine buildings is very interesting.

The season is from June 1st to Sept. 15th.

Ladis, in the valley of the Inn, Austrian Tyrol, two miles and a-half from the Landeck station, has *cold sulphur* waters containing H_2S. It is in a fine situation near the ruined castle of the same name, at an elevation of nearly 4,000 feet. About 600 feet above it is Ob-Ladis, which also has cold sulphur baths, and a gaseous spring, which is drunk.

Landeck, in the county of Glatz, in Prussian Silesia, on the branch line connecting Glatz, Landeck, and Seidenberg, has many *thermal* springs, which have been classed amongst the indifferent thermal waters; but as they contain minute quantities of sodium sulphide and H_2S they were at one time regarded as sulphur waters. They contain also sodium sulphate and free nitrogen. Their temperature varies from 66° to 84° F. Landeck is situated in a mountainous country, at an elevation of 1,470 feet, and in the vicinity of extensive forests. Two of the springs are used for drinking and gargling, the other for baths. The water of certain springs is collected in pools, in which twenty to thirty patients bathe together. Mud baths are also prepared, and hydropathic treatment is available. The springs of Landeck are said to have been utilised since the middle ages. The maladies treated are diseases of women, neuroses, rheumatism and gout, anæmia and catarrh of the respiratory organs.

The season is from May to the end of September.

Langenau, or **Niederlangenau**, in the county of Glatz, in Silesia, lies at an elevation of 1,130 feet in the Neisse valley, sheltered by surrounding mountains, and possesses *cold gaseous chalybeate* springs, containing 0·049 per litre of bicarbonate of iron. The water is used for baths and for drinking. Ferruginous *Moor* baths and hydropathic treatment are also provided. The chalybeate baths are warmed by the Schwartz method, the baths being double-bottomed.

Langenau has a station on the line between Breslau and Mittelwelde. Maladies treated there are anæmia, chlorosis, neurasthenia, gout, and paralysis.

The season is from May till the middle of October.

Langenbrücken, in the Grand Duchy of Baden, on the line between Heidelberg and Bâle, at an elevation of about 440 feet, has springs containing the *aperient sulphates* of sodium and magnesium, sulphuretted hydrogen, and free carbonic acid, "sulphated sulphur springs." The water is used for drinking and for baths, and the spray and vapour —in suitable chambers—is inhaled. The cases treated are those of catarrh of the respiratory organs, hæmorrhoids and abdominal plethora, chronic rheumatism and gout, and skin affections.

The season is from the beginning of May to the beginning of October.

Längenfeld, in the picturesque Oetzthal, Austrian Tyrol, at an altitude of 3,820 feet, has *cold sulphuretted hydrogen* waters.

Langensalza, in Thuringia, at an altitude of 660 feet, has *cold calcareous sulphur* springs, rich in sulphuretted hydrogen. The bath is at some distance from the town. The water is used for drinking, baths, and inhalations, in chronic catarrhal affections of the respiratory organs, and other diseases usually treated by sulphur baths.

Season, May 1 to Oct. 1.

Lauchstädt, in the province of Saxony, a very small bath with *earthy chalybeate* springs.

Laurvik, Norway, five or six hours by rail from Christiania, has *chalybeate* and *sulphur* springs and a thermal bath establishment. Sulphurous mud is also made use of, and living jellyfish are applied to produce counter-irritation in rheumatic and neuralgic cases.

Lausigk (Hermannsbad), in Saxony, has strong *sulphate of iron* waters.

Ledesma, a *thermal sulphur* spa in Spain, province of Salamanca, in a fine situation 2,000 feet above the sea.

Leixlip Spa, Ireland, two miles from Lucan, on the Liffey, weakly mineralised waters smelling feebly of H_2S.

Le Prese. *See* Prese, Le, p. 292.

Liebenstein, in the Duchy of Saxe-Meiningen, situated on the western slope of the Thüringer-Wald, at an elevation of 1,450 feet, has *cold gaseous chalybeate* springs, the stronger of which contains 0·104 per litre of bicarbonate of iron, the weaker 0·08.

There is also an establishment for hydrotherapy and Franzensbad *Moor* extract baths. *Fango* baths, pine-needle baths, artificial saline baths, and electric baths can be obtained. There are beautiful walks in the surrounding forests. The same cases are treated there as in other chalybeate spas. It has a great local popularity.

The season is from May 15 to Sept. 30.

Liebenstein is on the branch line Immelborn-Liebenstein of the Werra line.

Liebenzell, a *simple thermal* bath in the Würtemberg Black Forest, about eight miles from Wildbad and five miles from Pforzheim railway station. Its springs resemble those of Wildbad, but are of a lower temperature (72° to 82° F.), and are warmed for the baths.

The situation is picturesque, and the life is homely. The place is chiefly resorted to for female maladies, and by Germans mostly.

Season, from May to September.

Liebwerda, a *chalybeate* spa in Northern Bohemia, on the south-west slope of the Tafelfichte, at an altitude of 1,420 feet, three or four miles from the railway station Raspenau-Liebwerda. The iron spring is cold, and rich in carbonic acid, and contains 0·03 of bicarbonate of iron per litre. Ferruginous *Moor* baths are also prepared. It has another spring which is used as a table water, as it is weakly mineralised, and contains much carbonic acid.

Linda-Pausa, or **Bad Linda**, near Pausa, in the Vogtland, Saxony, has *chalybeate* wells containing carbonate of iron and sulphate of iron.

Lipetsk, Russia, picturesquely situated on the river Voronezh, has *cold chalybeate* waters and ferruginous peat baths.

Lipik, in Slavonia, has *hot weak alkaline* and *common salt* waters. The temperature of the hottest spring is 147° F, and this contains sodium bicarbonate 1·9, sodium chloride 0·6, and sodium iodide 0·02 per litre.

Lobenstein, in the Thuringian Forest, principality of Reuss, at an altitude of 1,650 feet, has *earthy chalybeate* springs and ferruginous *Moor* baths.

Lons le Saunier, picturesquely situated at an altitude of 840 feet, on the verge of the Jura chain in France, and on the line of railway between Lyons and Besançon, has *strong brine* baths, the brine coming from the "salines" of Perrigny. It contains as much as 305 grammes per litre of common salt, and the *eau mère* contains 6·9 per litre of bromides. Lons le Saunier has also a *saline chalybeate* spring, which is used for drinking, and in a litre contains sodium chloride 10·0, magnesium carbonate 1·6, and iron carbonate 0·09, with much free carbonic acid and a little of H_2S. It has a modern bath establishment, with brine baths, a small swimming bath, and the usual processes of hydrotherapy, together with external application of carbonic acid gas. The climate is somewhat variable, with rather brusque variations of temperature. The drinking spring is purgative in large doses, and in small doses is stimulating to the digestive organs and a general tonic. The cases treated there are scrofula and rickets, chronic rheumatism, and chronic uterine maladies. Interesting excursions into the Jura can be made.

Season, June 1st to Oct. 1st.

Lostorf, a Swiss bath on the southern slope of the Jura, one and a-half hour's drive from Olten, has *cold common salt* and *sulphur* springs, and a sulphate of lime spring.

Luhatschowitz, in a valley of the Carpathians (Moravia), a short drive from the railway station, Ungarisch Brod, at an elevation of 1,600 feet, has *cold gaseous alkaline common salt* waters, containing sodium carbonate 3·0 to 4·4, sodium chloride 2·4 to 2·5, sodium iodide 0·007 to 0·012, and sodium bromide 0·02 to 0·045 per litre, with much free carbonic acid. They are used in cases of uric acid gravel, and in gouty catarrhal affections.

Luz (Pyrénées). *See* St. Sauveur, p. 316.

Marienbad, like Carlsbad, is situated a few miles (eighteen and a-half) from the town of Eger, in Bohemia, and it is therefore reached in the same way as Carlsbad. It lies, however, in a different direction, being on the line of railway which runs from Eger to Pilsen and Vienna.

Marienbad has much in common with Carlsbad, but differs at the same time in some not unimportant particulars. It is situated in a beautiful broad, open valley, with pine-clad hills on three sides, and is at an elevation of 1,912 feet above the sea. This comparatively high situation gives it a fresh and somewhat bracing climate in summer.

The wooded hills around are intersected in every direction wtth footpaths, which afford delightful walks, and there are many fine points of view that are easily accessible.

The lower portion of the valley, where the wells are situated, is laid out in pleasure grounds, and these, with a fine Kursaal, colonnades for shops, a theatre, and excellent lodging-houses, render Marienbad a very agreeable place of residence.

The waters resemble those of Carlsbad, only they are *cold*, and they contain more of the aperient sodium sulphate and of the other sodium salts (bicarbonate and chloride), and more carbonic acid. Some of the springs also contain a notable quantity of iron—as much as 0·048 to 0·084 bicarbonate of iron per litre. The chief drinking springs are the Kreuzbrunnen, the Ferdinandsbrunnen, and the Waldquelle. The two former are brought by pipes, from about a mile distant, to the Promenaden Platz. The Ferdinandsbrunnen is the stronger of the two, having per litre 5·0 grammes of sodium sulphate, 2·0 sodium chloride, and 1·8 sodium bicarbonate. The Waldquelle, to the north of the town, is relatively poor in sodium sulphate (1·0), and rich in sodium bicarbonate (1·4) and carbonic acid gas.

The Marienquelle and the chalybeate waters of the Ambrosiusbrunnen and the Carolinienbrunnen are used chiefly for bathing. There is also an alkaline earthy spring, the Kronprinz Rudolfsquelle, applicable to the same cases as the Wildungen water.

Marienbad is celebrated for its baths as well as its drinking springs; and you can obtain there *Moor* or mud baths, pine-cone baths, carbonic acid gas baths, and ordinary alkaline and chalybeate mineral baths. The *Moor* or mud baths at Marienbad, as at Franzensbad, occupy an important place in the treatment. The Marienbad ferruginous peat, with which they are prepared, is said to be richer in iron than that of Franzensbad. These baths are applied in chronic female complaints, as at Franzensbad, and also as a form of thermal bath. The waters are taken in the early morning fasting, and again, if necessary, between six and seven in the evening. The dose is varied according to the case and the observed effects.

There being such a variety of springs, various ailments can be treated advantageously at Marienbad. In the first place, the waters are adapted to much the same cases as Carlsbad, but are better suited to those which require a more decidedly aperient effect, their aperient action being much more marked. Marienbad has acquired a great reputation for the reduction of corpulency and the treatment of cases of plethora and abdominal congestion in the overfed and sedentary. In many of these cases the liver is enlarged and the heart's action enfeebled. The waters of Marienbad appear to possess the property of diminishing the amount of fat accumulated in the body, without injuriously affecting the digestion or the processes of blood formation; so that while the fat is disappearing there is no loss of muscle, and the general health and nutrition are in many cases improved. Marienbad is the chief representative of these cold gaseous sodium sulphate waters, which are found so effectual in the treatment of obesity. The fat, however, soon re-forms if great care in diet is not observed *after* as well as during the course. Cases of gouty dyspepsia, periodical headaches, chronic constipation and intestinal catarrh, and hæmorrhoids are often greatly benefited by this course. Urinary maladies, catarrhal or calcareous, can be treated here by the Rudolfsquelle, as at Wildungen or Contrexéville.

Like the Carlsbad waters, those of Marienbad are also employed in cases of chronic enlargement of the liver and jaundice, gallstones, and the early stage of cirrhosis, and in glycosuria in the obese or gouty.

In cases of corpulency it is often thought desirable to allow some of the gas in the water to escape, lest it should be too exciting, and this is managed by pouring the water from one glass to another before drinking it. The presence of an appreciable amount of iron in these waters may impart to them a certain tonic effect.

Anæmic patients may drink the iron springs, if they find they can digest them; and the Waldquelle is prescribed in chronic catarrh of the respiratory organs.

Certain forms of cardiac disturbance are considered by some authorities well suited to treatment at Marienbad, even when there is valvular disease, such as cases of fatty *infiltration* of the heart in the obese, gouty disturbances of cardiac innervation, and the cardiac neuroses common at the menopause. But it must always be kept in view that it is not easy in many cases to estimate precisely the physical condition of the cardiac walls and valves, and that the greatest caution and discrimination are needed in submitting cardiac cases to thermal and mineral water treatment.

The invalid's life at Marienbad is much like that at Carlsbad. At 6 a.m. the band begins to play, either at the Kreuzbrunnen or the Ferdinandsbrunnen, situated at the opposite ends of a long, covered colonnade, and at this hour drinking begins, and continues until 8 a.m. At that time the band ceases playing, and the crowd of drinkers begins to disperse. It is the custom, as at Carlsbad, to proceed then to the baker's shop and select the *petits pains* quite hot and fresh from the oven that you intend to consume at breakfast. Those for the corpulent are baked hard and in long sticks. The patient departs with his bread in a little bag, and makes for the café of his choice. Most of these are situated at a little distance from the springs, in the adjacent woods, generally where there is a pleasant view. Here, at little tables in the open air, under the shade of the pine trees, the *café-au-lait* and the bread (without butter) are consumed; the addition of two lightly boiled eggs is the extent of indulgence allowed to the "cure-guests." Soon after breakfast the baths are taken, always followed by a period of repose. On non-bathing days it is usual to stroll into the pine woods after breakfast.

At 1 p.m. is the early dinner for the Germans, and a two o'clock dinner is provided at some hotels for the English. The afternoon is spent in promenades and excursions, and coffee or tea at the restaurants in the woods. A light supper between seven and eight concludes the invalid's day.

The season is from May to September. It is often cold at Marienbad until the middle of June.

Matlock Bath, Derbyshire, four hours from London, has simple *thermal* springs of a comparatively low temperature (68° F.), as well as several petrifying springs. It lies in the Derwent Valley, a dale in a picturesque and sheltered position. The thermal water is feebly mineralised, its chief contents being calcium carbonate 0·2 per litre, and magnesium sulphate 0·1, with minute quantities of sodium chloride and calcium sulphate, and a small amount of free carbonic acid gas. The mineral water is supplied to the "Fountain Baths," a private establishment where there are a swimming bath and slipper baths; to the Royal Hotel Bath Establishment, where there is a swimming bath also, and Turkish and various other baths and douches; and to the New Bath Hotel. The water is also supplied for drinking. Matlock is, however, chiefly frequented for its well-appointed hydros.

The mineral baths have been found useful in chronic gouty and rheumatic arthritis, and in lumbago and sciatica.

Pleasant excursions can be made from Matlock into the interesting Peak district.

Mont Dore (Puy de Dôme), France, at an elevation of 3,400 feet above the sea, is the highest mountain health resort in Central France, and certainly the most frequented. It can now be reached from Paris by express trains in about ten hours.

Mont Dore lies, with its houses closely packed together, in the bed of the valley of the Dordogne, surrounded nearly on all sides by high mountains, some reaching to nearly 3,000 feet above it. The surrounding country is very beautiful, abounding in richly wooded slopes, striking mountain forms, and pretty though small cascades, with many grand views from easily attained elevations. The Pic de Sancy, ovei 6,000 feet above the sea, the highest mountain of Central France, is easily reached from Mont Dore in a walk of about three hours. Horses can be taken to within ten minutes of the summit. A very extensive view is thence obtained.

Mont Dore possesses eleven warm springs and one (Sainte Marguérite) cold one. The latter is not looked upon as belonging to the same category. It is used as a gaseous table water. La Madeleine, Le Bardon, and the Ramond are those used internally. The Ramond contains more iron than any of the others. The other *sources*—the Cæsar, Caroline, St. Jean, Rigny, Boyer and Pigeon—are used chiefly for the baths. They have all very nearly the same composition, differing, however, in the amount of free carbonic acid gas they contain. The warm springs differ in temperature from 104° to 116·5° F.

They are feebly mineralised, containing only 2 grammes of solids per litre. They are weak alkaline waters, the chief constituents being sodium bicarbonate (0·53) and sodium chloride (0·36). There is also a small amount of bicarbonate of iron (0·02); the source Ramond is said to have as much as 0·05. Some appear to think the silica (0·16) an important factor. But the greatest stress is laid on the *sodium arsenate* the water contains, and it is often described as an "arsenical" water, although it only contains 0·0009 per litre, *i.e.* about $\frac{1}{70}$ of a grain in 35 ounces.

The waters at Mont Dore have been classified at different epochs under three distinct heads: 1, as waters containing a mixture of alkaline bicarbonates with iron; 2, as weak alkaline waters; and 3, at the present time, as arsenical waters.

Mont Dore has been provided of recent years with a very fine Etablissement Thermal—one of the most complete and well appointed in France. There the waters are administered internally and externally; in the form of ordinary baths; in the form of vapour and spray; in douches, local and general; in the form of gargles, and in other special forms. The waters are drunk fasting, in the morning, from three to four glasses a day, leaving an interval of half an hour between each glass or portion of a glass.

Some patients are also made to inhale the compressed vapour of the water in the *salles d'aspiration*, and Mont Dore claims for itself the credit of having first introduced this method of utilising such waters in the year 1833.

The *salles d'aspiration* are very extensive. It is a curious sight to enter one of these *salles*, filled with hot, dense, vaporous mist through which you dimly discern the forms of the patients, clad in a special flannel dress for the purpose, some sitting, some standing, some walking, some reading, some talking. Here every morning they are shut up for half an hour or longer to inhale the hot mist.

Great care is taken that a patient who is being submitted to this treatment does not take cold. He is brought to the bath from his hotel in a sedan-chair, and when he comes out of the vapour bath he is conveyed rapidly again in a sedan-chair to his hotel, and is expected to return to his warmed bed, and remain there for an hour. Thus it happens that, from the early hour of 4 a.m. at Mont Dore, the stairs and passages of the hotels resound with the clatter of wooden shoes and the hurrying to and fro of the sedan-chairs. Sometimes the patient is ordered a foot bath before entering the *salles d'aspiration*, and generally he drinks a little of the thermal water before and after the *séance*.

Other patients, chiefly those who suffer from throat affections, inhale the water in a state of pulverisation or spray, and also gargle with it. Douches of vapour applied locally are employed and thought of much value in muscular rheumatism and in rheumatic inflammation of the joints, as well as in sciatica and intercostal neuralgia. The patient is seated on a stool and an intermittent jet of vapour is directed upon the part affected. Douches of water, in the form of a jet, or a rose, and of varying pressure, are also used. They are applied to the spine as a stimulant to the nervous system, and in cases of lumbago and sciatica; to the joints when swollen and painful; to the chest in some chest affections, and, indeed, to any part which it is desired to influence specially. The ordinary baths are administered either at a high temperature, *i.e.* from 107° to 112° F., or at a moderate temperature, *i.e.* from 90° to 100° F. The latter temperature is considered more suitable to feeble, nervous persons, as well as to old people and children.

In some cases hyperthermal half-baths, or hip baths, are prescribed of the natural temperature of the particular spring used, viz., from 100° to 115° F.

Finally there are the hot foot or hand baths; which are thought of great importance there, and are believed to accelerate the circulation in the lower extremities and to prevent any tendency to congestion of the head which the rest of the course of treatment might possibly produce, as well as indirectly to relieve congestion of the respiratory organs. The patients sit with their feet and legs in hot water of the natural temperature, *i.e.* about 112° F. They remain in the bath from five to nine minutes and then walk for at least half an hour afterwards.

In the next place, what are the ailments to which the course of treatment instituted at Mont Dore is especially applicable? Chronic rheumatism of the joints and muscles, certain forms of neuralgia, chiefly sciatica and intercostal neuralgia, have already been referred to. To these must be added nearly all forms of chronic disease of the throat and respiratory organs, whether of the nose, pharynx, larynx, trachea, bronchi, or lungs; and it has quite a *special* and widely spread reputation for the cure of *asthma.*

The treatment of asthma at Mont Dore is considered fully in a special note.

The respiratory affections of the gouty and the diabetic are stated to be especially benefited by treatment there. Chronic rhinitis and pharyngitis, chronic recurring laryngitis and fatigue of the larynx, as it occurs in public speakers and others who may have to use their voice to excess, and nervous aphonia—such cases are common amongst the frequenters of this bath. Catarrhal and congestive chronic bronchitis and tracheitis, so often obstinate and recurrent in persons of gouty constitution; broncho-pneumonia in children, following acute infectious fevers, are especially suitable for this cure. Chronic pleurisy with adhesions improves greatly. As to the treatment of pulmonary phthisis there, much discussion of a somewhat heated nature at one time prevailed. The conclusion now generally adopted is that, in common with other mountain stations, early *afebrile* cases do well there, and in more advanced cases benefit may arise if the disease is limited and localised, free from fever and from serious constitutional disturbance.

The climate of Mont Dore is very variable, storms of rain and thunder coming on suddenly, and in some seasons frequently. Sudden and very localised gusts of wind are also commonly encountered. There is no doubt that the climate can be, and often is, exceedingly disagreeable. Owing to the situation and direction of the valley, the eastern slopes are in shade for a few hours after sunrise, but soon the sun mounts high above the eastern boundary and its rays stream down with great intensity into the deep valley, and it is often excessively hot during the whole of the day. The early mornings and the evenings are mostly fresh and bracing, and the pleasantest days are those on which the sky is covered with light clouds, without rain; then the air during the whole day feels fresh and invigorating. The atmospheric pressure at Mont Dore is considerably reduced, and the average height of the barometer is 26·6. The variations of temperature during the months of June, July, and August are sometimes very considerable, the maximum being 86° F. and the minimum 37° F. The average temperature in August is 57° F. The hygrometric condition of the air is, no doubt, favourable to most invalids; it is decidedly a dry air compared with the air of towns—as *e.g.* that of Paris, or of the seacoast. The relative amount of watery vapour in the atmosphere of Mont Dore as compared with Paris is as 9·94 to 15·46. Fogs and mists are, however, frequent, and the season of fine weather is often extremely short. July and August are the finest months, The season scarcely commences before the beginning of July, and is soon over after the end of August. There is an electric railway (*funiculaire*) leading to the "Parc du Capucin," which is about 800 feet higher than Mont Dore.

Note on the Treatment of Asthma at Mont Dore.

It was through a casual, and almost an accidental, observation that Dr. Michel Bertrand, a former celebrated inspector at Mont Dore, discovered that an attack of asthma would disappear under the influence of the emanations from the spring, and this observation induced him to attempt to procure a dense vapour of the water of Mont Dore in one of the douche chambers, by allowing the douche to flow for some time and break into spray by falling on a plank. He found that when asthmatic patients were admitted into the chamber and breathed this vapour, they found themselves rapidly relieved. This observation led to the construction of special chambers, into which the vapour of the Mont Dore water, obtained by special mechanical contrivance, could be forced in abundance, and in which patients could remain for some time, walking about or otherwise employing themselves.

This was the origin of those *salles d'aspiration* which have made Mont Dore celebrated. On chemical analysis of the vapours in these chambers, they are found to contain the same mineral and gaseous constituents as are found in the springs themselves, viz. carbonic acid gas, arsenic, and alkaline salts.

No doubt the atmosphere of these *salles* contains much suspended water in the form of hot spray, and it is not, strictly speaking, the *vapour* of the water that yields these matters on analysis.

It is maintained that through the breathing of these vapours, chiefly, the cure of asthma is effected; that the cure is greatly aided by drinking the waters, and by the use of the hot douche (98° F.) along the spine; also by means of foot baths, which divert the "congestion" towards the inferior extremities.

Asthmatic children do admirably at Mont Dore, especially

those in whom the attacks have appeared after the cure of scrofulous impetigo or eczema. In order to obtain a complete radical cure of asthma at Mont Dore it is held to be necessary to pass at least two consecutive seasons there, and more commonly three. The routine of the treatment is as follows :—

The patient is roused from his slumbers perhaps at 5 a.m., enveloped in suitable clothing, and carried off in a sedan-chair to the hot spring, where he drinks a glass of the water; he is then taken to the bath-room, where he may probably be ordered, as we have seen, to take only the foot bath and the hot douche on the spine, or a vapour douche, or he may take a half-bath, or in some cases the whole bath, the heat of which is occasionally raised even to 113° F. in refractory cases. After from ten to thirty minutes of the bath he is wrapped up in hot linen and dried, and next conveyed to the *salles d'aspiration;* he is here dressed in a loose, thick flannel dress, made for the purpose, as everything becomes rapidly saturated with moisture in these chambers filled with hot, dense vapour, which is forced into them under pressure. He remains breathing this hot, moist atmosphere, charged with vapours of the mineralised springs, from twenty minutes to an hour. After this he is again carried, warmly clothed, to the hot spring to drink another glass of water, and thence he is conveyed to his bed, which has been well heated by a warming-pan, and he is enjoined to remain there for an hour or more. Now it is easy to see that this is treatment of a very active kind, and when applied every morning for three weeks is very likely to have some decided result.

The most important, and perhaps almost constant, effect is a very decided determination to the skin; profuse perspiration, as a rule, appearing soon after the commencement of this treatment. In obstinate cases every effort is made to produce excessive action of the skin, and in this way both circulatory and nervous energy is directed to the cutaneous surface, for in proportion to the amount of function required of an organ will be the amount of expenditure of nerve force which presides over that function. Now the cutaneous surface is always in close and sympathetic correlation with the respiratory surface, and while wandering and irregular nervous energy in the nervous, spasmodic cases is thus diffused and dissipated at the surface of the body, the hyperæsthetic condition of the respiratory centre and its afferent tributaries is proportionately diminished.

An attack of spasmodic asthma may be regarded as a morbid manifestation of misdirected nervous energy often reflex in origin, just as some forms of hysterical and epileptic convulsions may be; by the diversion of such wandering nerve energy to the skin, and its diffusion and exhaustion in connection with a natural physiological process, the nervous equilibrium is restored, and the tendency to spasm relieved. It is thus that the spasmodic nervous element in asthma is attacked.

Let us look at the processes of the Mont Dore cure from another point of view. This daily ingestion of warm alkaline fluid taken together with the profuse "sweats" that are excited must have a very remarkable depurative influence. Retrograde tissue changes must be actively stimulated, and unstable irritating substances which may have accumulated in the organism from disordered assimilative processes, as in gouty conditions and the like, must be dissolved and eliminated, so that the treatment also attacks vigorously those states of blood contamination which are at the root of many spasmodic and vaso-motor nervous affections, in which category many forms of asthma may be placed.

Then again in those cases of asthma complicated with bronchial catarrhs, which form by far the greater proportion of all cases of asthma, those cases in which the morbidly increased secretions of the bronchial mucous membrane, especially when it is scanty and tenacious, act as excitants to the hyperæsthetic mucous membrane itself, just as a foreign body would—in such cases we have two obvious indications to fulfil, one to remove the catarrhal condition and free the air passages of accumulated mucus, the other to soothe and quiet the hyperæsthesia of the bronchial surface.

Both these indications appear to be fulfilled by the processes in use at Mont Dore. The use of pilocarpin in the treatment of catarrhal asthma has shown to what extent the catarrhal condition is relieved by excessive action of the skin, and here at Mont Dore we get excessive action of the skin without pilocarpin, a remedy far too dangerous and depressing for general use. Then there is the prolonged daily immersion, for immersion it practically is, in an atmosphere saturated with the hot vapours of the mineral water, which bathe the pulmonary mucous membrane, moisten and thin the secretions when dry and scanty, and in all cases promote their expulsion, while they must at the same time exercise a most soothing effect on the hyperæsthetic bronchial surface, and so tend directly to allay the nervous element which is a part of every form of asthma properly so called.

The action of the mineral and gaseous constituents of the water itself must not be overlooked; the carbonic acid, and the arsenic (the very small quantity which the water contains is said to be readily diffused in the vapour), and the alkaline salts may, and probably do, exercise a most important curative influence, but we can see that even without this the processes employed are energetic in their nature and physiological in their action. For no fact is now better established in therapeutics than the value of warm alkaline drinks in the treatment of bronchial catarrhs, and this always forms a part of the treatment at Mont Dore.

There is yet another condition, and that by no means an unimportant one, under the influence of which these processes are carried out. *Mont Dore is 3,400 feet above the sea.* The atmospheric pressure, as we have seen, is reduced, the average height of the barometer being 26·6. The air is much cooler and much drier than on the sea level; and though fogs and mists are frequent in bad seasons, yet the relative amount of watery vapour in the atmosphere of Mont Dore, as compared with that of Paris, is as 9·94 to 15·46. These processes, then, are carried out in a bracing air, in an atmosphere freer from permanent moisture than on the sea level. It is now a well-known fact that exposure to this kind of mountain air has the effect of greatly reducing that impressionability to cold which is so common in scrofulous subjects, and which is at the root of their catarrhal tendencies; while it is especially tonic to certain hyperæsthetic states of the nervous system. A climate like that of Mont Dore tends to diminish cutaneous and respiratory sensitiveness, and is therefore admirably suited for the application of the processes there in use to the cure of asthmatic and catarrhal conditions. The mountain air is an essential part of the cure. The climate itself is a nerve tonic, and exercises no small influence in the good results which are obtained there. We see, then, that the method of treatment pursued at Mont Dore answers many indications, and is applicable, from one point of view or another, to nearly all cases of asthma.

Monte Catini, province of Lucca, Italy, has several *thermal common salt* springs. It is a village in a picturesque situation in the Val di Nivole, at an altitude of 920 feet, and has a station on the railway line between Florence and Lucca. It has a mild climate, but is very hot in summer. It has four bath establishments. The temperature of the springs is not very high, and varies between 70° and 86° F. About a dozen of the springs have been utilised. The hottest of these are the Thermes de Leopold with a total mineralisation of 22·5 per litre, of which 18·5 is sodium chloride, 2·1 calcium sulphate, 0·7 magnesium chloride, with traces of iodides and bromides, and some free carbonic acid gas. These waters are used for drinking and for baths. Taken internally they are laxative and have a stimulating effect on the liver and the secretion of bile. They are used as *baths* in scrofulous affections and in rheumatism; and *internally* in gastro-hepatic disorders, congestion of liver and spleen, biliary catarrh, constipation and abdominal plethora, dysentery of tropical countries, gravel and vesical catarrh. The water is largely exported.

The season is from May 1st to Oct. 1st.

Mallow, in Ireland, 18 miles from Cork, with a station on the line between Dublin and Cork, has a *simple subthermal* spring of a temperature of 70° to 72° F. The place is beautifully situated on the north bank of the Blackwater. Baths were built there in the eighteenth century by the lord of the soil, Sir Denham Norreys. It was at one time much resorted to by invalids.

Marcols (France, Départetement Ardèche) has a *simple alkaline* spring, containing sodium bi-carbonate 2·6 per litre.

Marlioz. *See* Aix les Bains.

Martigny les Bains lies a few miles from Contrexéville, its elevation above the sea (1,200 feet) is some 160 feet greater, and it is well and pleasantly situated. It is a small spa which had fallen into comparative disuse until revived a few years ago by new proprietors. It now possesses a new and commodious *Établissement*, and is well equipped for competition with its better known neighbour. The number of visitors has therefore largely increased. Its springs have the same composition as those of Contrexéville and Vittel, *sulphate of lime* being the chief constituent, and are used in the same cases and in the same manner and have the same physiological effects. Martigny however claims as an especial recommendation of one of its springs (Source No. 1), that it contains much more lithium than the Pavillon, at Contrexéville, and is therefore better adapted to the treatment of the uric acid constitution. Some importance is also attached to the presence of silicates in these waters. It is usual to begin the cure with somewhat smaller doses of the water than those prescribed at Contrexéville and Vittel. The Source Savonneuse is reserved for external use in the form of baths, douches, pulverisations, injections, etc. Professor Jacquemin terms this spring the French Schlangenbad, and thinks it equal, if not superior, to the original. It is essentially a very quiet resort. The season is from May 20 to Sept. 20. It is often very hot in the months of July and August, and rather chilly in May and at the end of September. There are good hotels, and the usual amusements, theatre, casino, *petits chevaux*, etc. It is about the same distance from Paris and London as Contrexéville — six hours by express from Paris.

Meinberg, in the principality of Lippe, Germany, in the Werre valley, at an altitude of 680 feet, and having a railway station at Horn-Meinberg, on the Herford-

Altenbecken line, has several mineral springs. Two are simple "acidulous," *i.e.* carbonic acid, wells, which are used for drinking and exportation; it has also a gaseous common salt spring containing 5·5 per litre of sodium chloride, and this, aërated with carbonic acid, is also drunk; it has likewise special *sulphur mud baths* and carbonic acid dry gas baths, the gas being collected from the soil. This gas is also combined with vapour-douches, and used in making effervescent baths; artificial sulphur, salt, and pine-needle baths are prepared. The diseases treated at Meinberg are gout and rheumatism, diseases of the nervous system, and female maladies.

The season is from May 20 to Sept. 20.

Melksham, Wiltshire, thirteen miles from Bath, has springs resembling those of Cheltenham, *i.e.* containing *common salt* and the *aperient sulphates*. It also has a chalybeate spring.

Mendorf, Grand Duchy of Luxemburg, at an altitude of 650 feet, has a slightly warm *subthermal common salt* water (temperature 77° F.), which contains sodium chloride 8·7 and magnesium bromide 3·1 per litre. It is used for drinking, inhalations, and baths.

Middlesbrough brine wells. *See* Saltburn-by-the-Sea, p. 338.

Middlewich, Cheshire, has *brine* baths.

Mitterbad, in the Austrian Tyrol, at an elevation of 3,110 feet, in the picturesque Meran valley, three and a-half hours from Meran, has *chalybeate* springs containing sulphate of iron and small amounts of manganese, arsenic, strontium, zinc, and copper.

Moffat, in Dumfriesshire, eight and a-half hours from Euston, has *cold weak sulphur* waters and a *chalybeate* spring. The springs are some distance from Moffat, which is resorted to for its good air and fine situation. It has a well-known hydropathic establishment. The climate is rainy. Treatment there is said to prove useful in mild forms of anæmia and in cases of obstinate constipation arising from torpid liver in persons who have lived in hot countries.

Molitg.—A small *thermal sulphur* bath, twenty hours from Paris, in a fine situation in the Pyrénées Orientales, about 50 kilometres from Perpignan, and rather more than an hour's drive from the station of Prades. The bath establishments are situated at the bottom of a narrow gorge, at an elevation of 1,460 feet. The surrounding country is picturesque and mountainous. Molitg has a mild and pleasant climate even in winter. Its season extends from May 1 to Nov. 1. It has several springs, the characteristic ingredient of which is *sodium sulphide*, 0·093 grammes to the litre. They also contain a small amount of carbonate of sodium and silica and much organic matter (glairine), which gives the water a soft, unctuous feel. They vary in temperature from 70° to 99° F.

When drunk, the water is said to promote appetite, and to act as a diuretic, and to cause some slight stimulation of the nervous and vascular systems. The waters are also used as baths, douches, and pulverisations. The confervæ and organic mud deposited by the springs are applied locally. Skin diseases are the cases mainly treated there, catarrhal conditions of the mucous membrane are also benefited (vesical, gastro-intestinal and bronchial catarrhs), and chronic rheumatism in nervous and excitable subjects.

Monsumano, in the province of Lucca, Italy, in the Val di Nievole, about half an hour's drive from the railway stations Pieve and Monte Catini, possesses a *large cave* which is filled with steam arising from extensive surfaces of hot water, and forming a *natural* vapour bath. Garibaldi was healed there. It is resorted to by sufferers from rheumatic affections, sciatica, and certain neuroses. Patients find accommodation at Upper and Lower Monsumano and also at Monte Catini, which is near at hand. The season is from May 15 to Sept. 15.

Montegrotto and **Monte Ortone** belong to the "Euganean thermæ," in the neighbourhood of Padua, and have feebly mineralised but very hot springs, containing a little sodium chloride and sulphate.

Montemayor, a *thermal sulphur* spa in Spain, province of Caceres, in a fine situation at an elevation of 2,000 feet, is much frequented by native patients.

Montmirail, a bath in the south of France, possessing a *source* rich in the *aperient sulphates* of magnesium and sodium, a type of mineral water rarely found in France. It also has a cold sulphur spring containing calcium sulphide as well as a ferruginous *source*. The former of these waters is largely exported as a laxative mineral water. It contains 9·31 grammes of magnesium sulphate, 5·06 of sodium sulphate, and one gramme of calcium sulphate per litre. This water is an active purgative in full doses of three or four glasses. It is, of course, reserved for *drinking only*, on the spot, and for exportation. The sulphur spring is also drunk, as well as used for baths and douches. The purgative *source* has a green colour when seen *en masse* and hence it is known as *l'eau verte*. Montmirail, at an elevation of 580 feet, is situated at the foot of Mont Ventoux, Department of Vaucluse; it has a station, Sarrian Montmirail, about eight miles from Carpentras. A combination of the purgative and sulphur springs is used there in some cases of gastro-intestinal dyspepsias. The iron spring is used in cases of anæmia and chlorosis. Respiratory and skin affections, syphilis, and certain forms of dysmenorrhoea are treated there. The hotel and bath establishment are combined in the same building.

Montrond, France, Department Loire, has a *simple alkaline* spring (Source Geyser) containing sodium bicarbonate 4·5 per litre.

Morgins, in Switzerland, Canton Valais, a three and a-half hours' drive from the station of Monthey, on the line between Bouveret and St. Maurice, is situated at an elevation of 4,300 feet and has a weak *chalybeate* spring containing a large amount of calcium sulphate (2·5 per litre). This amount of sulphate of lime makes it difficult of digestion sometimes. The bath establishment provides baths and douches of all kinds.

It is resorted to by anæmic patients and sufferers from scrofulous disorders.

Munster-am-Stein is situated only a mile and a-half from Kreuznach, higher up the Nahe Valley. It has similar waters of rather higher temperature, which are used in the same manner for the same maladies.

Nantwich, in Cheshire, about four hours from London, has *brine* baths of the same character as those at Droitwich. It is a strong brine having a density of 1142·76. It contains, in a litre, sodium chloride about 210·0, magnesium chloride 2·30, potassium chloride 1·90, calcium sulphate 6·50, and sodium sulphate 5·0.

The Droitwich brine is stronger, but it is, there, diluted for its baths; at Nantwich the brine is heated by steam, and is used therefore undiluted, so that the baths are really stronger than those at Droitwich. They are, of course, diluted when necessary. They are given at a temperature between 98° and 104° F. The patient, after the bath, is wrapped in a large towel and directed to recline on a couch until dry; the salt is then rubbed off, the patient dresses and returns to his lodgings to rest for a few hours. There are at Nantwich "The Old Baths" and "The New Baths"—the latter provide better and more suitable accommodation than could be obtained before their construction. They are connected with the Brine Baths Hotel, and can be reached from that building through a corridor, so that patients need not go into the open air in passing to and from the baths.

The therapeutic indications are the same as those at Droitwich; cases of muscular rheumatism, lumbago, and sciatica appear to be most benefited there.

The joint pains left after attacks of acute rheumatism are usually relieved, but the presence of serious valvular lesions would counter-indicate this treatment.

The baths are open all the year round, but the best season for the cure is from the beginning of May to the end of September.

The climate of Nantwich is said to be mild, dry, and equable, with an annual rainfall of only 20·34 inches and 146 rainy days.

Nauheim, in the Grand Duchy of Hesse, is one of the most important *salt* baths in Germany.

It is situated at an elevation of 400 feet, at the foot of a fine wooded hill, the Johannisberg, one of the outlying spurs of the Taunus, at a distance of about twenty miles from Frankfort, an hour by rail.

Of its springs, three are used exclusively for bathing and two for drinking. The three bathing springs are hot, and issue from the ground at a temperature varying from 82° to 96° F. They also contain an abundance of carbonic acid, and one of them shoots out of the ground with great force and with much bubbling and foaming, and sometimes rises in a jet to a height of about 44 feet. This is the Frederick-William Sprudel, a very important spring, on account of the quantity of common salt it contains (its chief solid constituents are, per litre, sodium chloride 20 to 30 grammes, calcium chloride 2 to 3 grammes, and some bicarbonate of iron), and also of its warmth (96·4° F.), and of its richness in carbonic acid, 48,000 cubic feet of this gas escaping in twenty-four hours. The combination of these three properties — high temperature, richness in common salt, and carbonic acid—renders it unique among European mineral springs. The two drinking springs, the Kurbrunnen and the Carlsbrunnen, are weaker, though these are too strong to be drunk pure in most cases. They contain per litre 10 to 15 grammes of sodium chloride, and 1 gramme of calcium chloride, and enough free carbonic acid gas to make them effervescent. They are tepid or lukewarm. The Ludwigsbrunnen is a weakly mineralised water used as a table-water and for diluting the preceding. There is also another spring in the neighbourhood, the Schwalheimerbrunnen, which contains a little iron and only 1·3 of sodium chloride, and being gaseous is also used as a table-water; both these are bottled for use.

The bathing springs are used of their natural temperature and composition; very rarely they are made stronger, as at Kreuznach, by the addition of "mother lye."

The baths given are of different kinds. First, the *simple salt* bath at different temperatures, from which the carbonic acid has been allowed to escape; second, the effervescent bath, "sprudel bath"; and thirdly, the effervescent *wave* bath, or *sprudel stream* bath, fresh gaseous brine running directly from the spring into the baths at one end and a similar quantity running out at the other during the whole course of the bath. This kind of bath is highly stimulating and has to be employed with caution, for by constantly surrounding the body with fresh brine and fresh carbonic acid, a highly exciting effect is produced on the nerves of the skin. In some cases it is found necessary to dilute the mineral water before using it in the baths, on account of the irritating effect it produces on the skin; while in other cases, where it is thought necessary to produce very active stimulation of the skin, "mother lye" is added to make it stronger.

Rooms for inhalation are provided where the patients can inhale the spray of the pulverised brine.

The abundance of carbonic acid gas set free from the springs has led to the use of a gas bath at this spa. The patient sits enveloped up to the neck in an atmosphere of carbonic acid gas, and in some cases of gout it has proved serviceable.

There are "gradirhauser" at Nauheim, as at Reichenhall and Kreuznach, near which patients can sit to inhale the salt spray.

With regard to the diseases treated at Nauheim, it has been so much the custom recently to regard that spa as *specially* adapted to the treatment of heart disease that it has been to some extent forgotten that it may also be taken as a type of a strong salt spa—a *Sool* bath, as it is called in Germany—and from that point of view it will be interesting to inquire what are its uses and value, and especially in what respects it differs from hot and cold sea-water baths. First come the various

sceptical, and our doubts on this point are, we are aware, shared by many acknowledged authorities on cardiac affections. We shall have to refer in a later chapter to the general question of the treatment of heart disease by mineral baths. It will be well to state here how it is carried out at Nauheim.

In beginning the baths much care is needful. It is usual to begin with 1 per cent. simple salt baths *free from* carbonic acid, and at a temperature of 92° to 95° F.; the baths lasting at first only six to eight minutes. They should also frequently be omitted for a day. It is customary gradually to reduce the temperature at which the baths are taken, daily, until, in appropriate cases, a temperature of 85·5° F. is reached; at the same time the mineral strength of the water and the period of immersion are slowly increased. Later on the *Sprudel* bath is applied in cases that are judged suitable, and lastly, if the patient is thought to be in a condition to bear it, the highly stimulating "sprudel stream" bath. About six weeks, or even longer, is considered needful for the cure.

The "resistance" exercises* are applied by the medical or other skilled attendant.

Néris, a well-known bath of high temperature and feeble mineralisation belonging to the *indeterminate thermal* group (French classification), is situated in Central France, not far from Montlucon, in the department of Allier, and is *especially* applied in the treatment of diseases of the nervous system, and less specially to diseases of women and rheumatic affections.

Néris is built on a plateau in a pleasant situation, about five miles from Montlucon, at an altitude of about 1,200 feet above the sea. It has a mild and

* A detailed schedule of these exercises and directions for the preparation of artificial Nauheim baths will be found in the author's "Manual of Medical Treatment," new edition, vol. i., pp. 400-401.

equable climate. The springs are collected into six wells, all proceeding doubtless from the same sheet of water, and have a nearly identical chemical composition, but vary in temperature between about 110° and 126° F.

The Puits César is the one chiefly used. The water is clear, odourless, and tasteless, and has an unctuous feeling. It gives off bubbles of carbonic acid and nitrogen gases. Its unctuous feeling depends on the amount of organic matter it contains, and which forms a kind of gelatinous precipitate in the reservoirs, and gives rise to the growth of magnificent confervæ. The solids in this water are small in quantity, not amounting to more than 1·27 gramme per litre, and consist chiefly of sodium bicarbonate, calcium bicarbonate, sodium sulphate, and sodium chloride, and traces of fluoride of sodium. The chief characteristics of this water are its high temperature and its richness in nitrogen gas and organic matter. It has, however, been calculated that though it contains only about 6 grains of sodium bicarbonate in a litre, as there are 400 litres in a bath, such a bath would contain about 5 oz. of this salt!

Néris has two bath establishments, the smaller one being devoted to patients of the poorer classes. The waters are but little drunk; they are mainly used as baths, douches, irrigations, and vapours, and the confervæ are sometimes applied locally. Baths are the chief agents in the cure, and are given either in ordinary baths, or in large baths in common (*piscines*). Their duration varies greatly according to the case—from a few minutes to an hour, and in some special cases two or more hours. The temperature most frequently employed is from 92° to 95° F. Suitable apparatus are provided for applying irrigations, vaginal, rectal, nasal, etc. Vapour baths, general or partial, and vapour douches are also given. The local use of the confervæ is not so common as formerly, but they are sometimes used as poultices and frictions in rheumatic affections, and combined with local baths in certain diseases of the skin and especially of the nails.

Various auxiliary means of treatment are at the disposal of the physicians, such as the ordinary methods of hydrotherapy, massage, douche-massage, gymnastics, and physical exercises, electricity, etc.

The first effect of the baths is to produce, in many, some general excitement of the system—feverish discomfort, headache, prostration, sleeplessness, together with an aggravation of the symptoms of the patient's malady; this is termed by the local doctors "*la crise thermale.*" It comes on at varying periods from the third to the sixth or tenth day, and sometimes not at all, and is followed by the *sedative* effect looked for from the treatment. As already mentioned, it is in diseases of the *nervous* system that the cure at Néris is especially indicated: the *contractures* and hemichoreic symptoms following hemiplegia; *locomotor ataxia*, at the early stage, when the acute painful symptoms predominate, insomnia, gastric crises, lightning pains, etc. General paralysis at its onset, disseminated sclerosis, spasmodic paraplegia, myelitis from cold or injury, peripheral neuritis, toxic and traumatic; facial and other peripheral paralyses, all forms of neuralgia, muscular spasm, and professional cramps; the various *neuroses*, hysteria, chorea, neurasthenia, exophthalmic goitre in its early stages, migraine, etc. Amongst the *diseases of women* treated at Néris, special mention may be made of *genital neuroses*, coccydynia, pelvic inflammations, etc. Rheumatic cases are treated in the same manner as at other hyperthermal baths.

The season at Néris is from May 15th to Sept. 30th, but the most favourable part of the season is from June 15th to Sept. 15th.

Chamblet-Néris, the nearest railway station, is distant about three miles, and is reached in six hours by express trains from Paris during the season.

Neuenahr is situated in the valley of the Ahr, a small river which joins the Rhine at Sinzig, a little above Remagen, and about midway between Bonn and Coblenz. Neuenahr has a station on the railway that runs between Remagen and Altenahr. Remagen is an hour and a-half's railway journey from Cologne. The adjacent Apollinarisberg commands an exquisite piece of Rhine scenery.

The Ahr valley is wide and bounded by low and gently sloping hills; only one considerable hill, the Landskron, is remarkable, as it stands alone, a truncated cone of basaltic rock about 900 feet high, and forms a very prominent object. Near this rock we pass the Apollinarisbrunnen, the source of the Apollinaris water.

The baths at Neuenahr are in the Kurhaus, and are well organised, and furnished with the usual array of douches of all kinds. The springs at Neuenahr belong to the group of *simple alkaline waters.* They are warm, and contain a considerable quantity of carbonic acid. This gas is allowed to escape freely into the air from the principal spring, which is thus seen to seethe and boil and foam as it pours from its source into a basin, around which a well-shaped inclosure is built. Here the carbonic acid can be seen to form a dense and dangerous atmosphere over and around the spring. There are probably great quantities of this gas stored up, a little below the surface, in this part of the valley, and it is noticed in consequence that in many of the houses mice are never found. There are four springs in use—the chief of these are the Victoria- and the Grosser-sprudel. The temperature of the latter is 104° F.; the others are not so hot. A litre of the water contains about nine grains of bicarbonate of sodium and four and a-half of carbonate of magnesium, besides lime and small quantities of common salt and sulphate of sodium and a minute amount of iron—about 12 milligrammes in a litre.

These are the only hot simple alkaline springs found in Germany. They are analogous to the Vichy springs, although not nearly so strong.

The uses of these springs are various, depending on their mildly solvent alkaline action, so that they are especially applicable to cases of biliary and urinary concretions and their consequences; to cases of atonic gout, and especially those in which the stronger alkaline and saline springs are counter-indicated. Cases of gout which require very gentle treatment, and which support badly the depletory effects of stronger mineral waters — cases, for example, associated with a weak heart and feeble circulation—these are well suited to treatment at Neuenahr.

Cases of chronic rheumatism are treated there, and notably that which produces great deformity and crippling of the joints (*arthritis deformans*). Remarkably good results have been observed from the use of the Grossersprudel, followed by massage, in some of these distressing deformities. Of chest diseases, cases of chronic bronchial catarrh are much benefited, so are certain cases of chronic Bright's disease. There are suitable arrangements for inhaling the pulverised water in respiratory affections, as at Ems. Forms of dyspepsia with obesity, or fatty liver, and associated with a feeble heart, are better treated there than by the stronger courses of Marienbad or Carlsbad. But it is, above all things, to the successful treatment of *diabetes* that Neuenahr owes its great and increasing reputation. It does not pretend, however, to cure the grave forms. Some diabetic patients begin by drinking enormous quantities of the water, which they gladly do to quench the intolerable thirst from which they suffer.

The cases of diabetes best suited to treatment there are those associated with the uric acid diathesis. With regard to the climate of Neuenahr, it is said to be very dry and healthy, and to have a very even temperature; but, in common with much of the Rhine district, the place is subject at times to heavy morning mists. In summer there is generally a current of air blowing along the valley, but from the position of the town, with protection on the north by vine-covered hills and on the south by wooded heights, it is usually warm. The tortuous rocky defile below Altenahr closes the valley on the west, and there are no side valleys by which eddies and cold currents may be produced. During the spring and summer the wind is usually from the south-west or south, and, coming over great woodland districts, is pure and refreshing, but never cold.

The season is from May to October. There is very good hotel accommodation.

Nenndorf, near Hanover, and in the province of Hanover, adjoining the village of Gross-Nenndorf, has *cold sulphur* springs. There is also a salt well in the neighbouring village, Soldorf. Nenndorf is situated in a well-wooded country, at an altitude of 230 feet. The Trinkquelle, the richest in sulphur, is the only spring used for drinking, and contains, in addition to 1·0 per litre calcium sulphate, sodium sulphide 0·06 and H_2S 42 vols.

The brine from Soldorf. which is used for baths, contains 60·0 per litre of sodium chloride and a trace of H_2S. It is often fortified with *Mutterlauge*.

A Nenndorf sulphur soap is made from the precipitate of the Badequelle. Sulphurous mud baths are also prepared from large mud beds near at hand. Inhalation of the gases emitted from the sulphur springs is also prescribed.

The cases treated there are chronic rheumatism and gout, skin diseases, catarrhs of the respiratory passages, asthma, scrofulous affections of the joints and other organs, metallic intoxications, female maladies. The season is from May 1 to Oct. 1.

Neuenhain, close to Soden, near Frankfort-am-Main, has a *gaseous chalybeate* spring, containing 0·04 per litre of bicarbonate of iron.

Neuhaus, Bavaria, in the valley of the Saale, near Neustadt railway station, and at the foot of the Salzburg, has *cold gaseous common salt* wells containing 9·0 to 1·5 per litre of sodium chloride. There are also simple gaseous springs used as table waters; mud baths are prepared there. It is a small bath, chiefly of local interest. Season, middle of May to end of September.

Neuhaus, in Styria, in an agreeable situation at an altitude of 1,200 feet, near Tüffer and the railway station of Cilli, has *indifferent thermal* springs of a temperature of 98° F., and a chalybeate spring.

Neu-Ragoczi, named after the well-known spring at Kissingen, is situated in the province of Saxony, at an hour's distance from the railway station of Halle-on-the-Saale, and possesses *common* *salt* waters (sodium chloride 10·0 per litre) containing a little iron and much *nitrogen* gas. The waters are used for drinking and for baths, and the nitrogen is collected for inhalations.

Neustadt-Eberswalde, beautifully situated in Mark Brandenburg, Germany, at an altitude of 100 feet, is a summer resort, with *chalybeate* waters poor in carbonic acid gas.

Niederbronn, in Alsace, on the eastern slopes of the Vosges mountains, at an altitude of 620 feet, with a station on the Strassburg. - Hagenau - Saargemund railway, has *common salt* wells, only one of which is used, the Niederbronner - mineral - wasserquelle, of a temperature of 64° F. It contains sodium chloride 3·0, calcium chloride 0·6, and bicarbonate of iron 0·01 per litre. It is said also to contain a small amount of lithium. There are baths in the hotels and private houses. The water is also used for drinking, inhaling, and gargling. Niederbronn has an ancient reputation for the treatment of gastro-hepatic and intestinal troubles, catarrhal jaundice, hæmorrhoids, renal and cutaneous affections, scrofula and female maladies. The season is from May 1 to Oct. 1.

Niederlangenau. *See* Langenau, p. 251.

Niedernau, in the Würtemberg Black Forest, having a station on the Suttgart-Tübingen-Horb line, is situated in a side valley of the Neckar valley, at an elevation of nearly 1,200 feet, and has several *cold chalybeate* springs, rich in free carbonic acid, of which the Stahlquelle is the strongest. Franzensbad *Moor* baths and carbonic acid baths are also provided. It is a small spa, in which are treated cases of anæmia, chlorosis, neurasthenia, and female maladies.

Oeynhausen, or **Rehme-Oeynhausen**, now generally known by the former name, is a well-known *warm gaseous common salt* bath in Westphalia, having much in common with Bad Nauheim. It is situated on the river Werre at an altitude of 230 feet and has a station on the line from Cologne to Berlin, four and a-half hours from the former city.

It has three warm common salt wells, to which must now be added a fourth, bored in 1898 and named the Kaiser-Wilhelmsprudel. These wells are very rich in free carbonic acid, and vary in temperature from 77° to 92° F. They contain per litre 31 to 34 grammes of sodium chloride, also sodium and calcium sulphate, about 3 grammes of each, and nearly 1,000 volumes of carbonic acid gas. There is also a cold salt spring, the Bülowbrunnen, containing a large quantity of sodium chloride, which is used for baths and for the extraction of salt and the preparation of *Mutterlauge.* Very complete bath arrangements exist there, and by blending together the waters of the different wells and by artificial heating, baths can be given of various strengths, in salt and gas, and of different temperatures.

The diseases amenable to treatment at Nauheim can also be treated as advantageously at Oeynhausen, where springs of precisely the same composition exist and the same methods of applying them prevail; therefore the same therapeutic indications apply to both these spas; but while Nauheim has been diverted to the *special* treatment of cardiac affections, Oeynhausen has been specialised in the direction of the treatment of diseases of the *nervous* system. The season is from May 15th to the end of September, but there is also a winter season.

Oberlahnstein-am-Rhein has a gaseous spring, the Victoria-brunnen, containing small amounts of sodium bicarbonate and chloride. It is exported as a *table-water*, a part of the carbonic acid which has escaped being added to the water on filling the bottles.

Obersalzbrunn (Bad-Salzbrunn) is situated in Silesia, about two hours by rail from Breslau and six from Berlin. It lies on the River Salzbach, at an elevation of 1,320 feet. Its chief spring, the Oberbrunnen, is a *cold alkaline* spring containing 2·15 grammes of bicarbonate of sodium in a litre, 0·01 of bicarbonate of lithium, and 0·45 of sulphate of sodium, and a considerable amount of free carbonic acid gas. Its mild, mountain climate, dust-free air, and forest walks are considered to augment the value of the mineral water. Milk and whey cures are also carried out. Baths, mineral and medicated, massage, gymnastics, and a pneumatic inhalatorium will likewise be found. The diseases treated there are catarrh of the respiratory organs, bronchial asthma and emphysema, stomach and intestinal catarrhs, gallstones, disease associated with the uric acid diathesis, gout, chronic renal disease, diabetes, obesity. The season lasts from May 1 to Sept. 30. The much advertised Kronenquelle is a proprietary spring in this resort. It is used chiefly for exportation, and claims to be especially rich in lithium. It is really but feebly mineralised, and only contains 0·01 gramme of bicarbonate of lithium in a litre.

Obladis. *See* Ladis, p. 250.

Offenbach-am-Main, four miles from Frankfort, has a *cold alkaline common salt* spring, containing sodium bicarbonate 2·4 and sodium chloride 1·2, and lithium bicarbonate 0·019 per litre. It is exclusively exported.

Oldesloe, in the province of Schleswig-Holstein, has *cold common salt* and *sulphur* springs and mud baths.

Olette (Pyrénées Orientales),

reached by rail from Perpignan to Prades, thence by carriage drive of about ten miles, is a *sulphur* spring containing sodium sulphide. There is a good bath establishment, 2,300 feet above the sea-level, with all the appliances usually found in such institutions. The springs, of which there are many, are warm, and vary in temperature from 80° to 170° F. They are of feeble mineralisation, and resemble in their properties and uses the other numerous sulphur springs of that region. Interesting walks and excursions abound.

The climate is like that of mountain districts generally, there being a considerable difference between day and night temperature. The waters are drunk and used as baths, douches, and inhalations, and are applied in all forms of rheumatism, in respiratory catarrhal affections, and in gastric and vesical catarrh; also in surgical cases, especially the consequences of injuries, and in certain neuroses.

The season is from June 1 to Sept. 30.

Ontaneda, a *thermal sulphur* spa in Spain, in the province of Santander.

Orb, a *cold gasc us brine* bath in the Prussian province of Hesse-Nassau, five kilometres from the railway station of Wichtersbach, on the Frankfort and Bebra line. It is applied in the same diseases and by the same processes as other waters of the same kind.

Orezza, in Corsica, has two *cold gaseous strong ferruginou s* springs, the water of which is largely exported. The village of Orezza is situated in the mountains in the interior of Corsica, at an altitude of nearly 2,000 feet, thirty-two kilometres from the railway station, Ponte alla Leccia, on the line from Bastia to Ajaccio. The patients lodge in localities near the springs. These springs are rich in bicarbonate of iron, 0·128 per litre, together with small amounts of the bicarbonates and sulphates of lime and magnesia and a very large quantity of free carbonic acid. Notwithstanding this large amount of carbonic acid in the water, a portion of the iron is very prone to precipitation. Orezza is resorted to by natives of the island in summer.

Oriol, a *gaseous alkaline earthy chalybeate* spring, near Grenoble, in France.

Pierrefonds, a *cold sulphur* bath eight and a-half miles' drive from Compiègne station and sixty from Paris (Northern line), lies at the foot of a hill surmounted by a castle and near a small lake. It is pleasantly situated at an elevation of 275 feet on the borders of the forest of Compiègne. Its mineral springs resemble those of Enghien in composition, and contain sulphydrate of calcium (0·015 per litre) and a small amount of earthy salts. The waters are used in the same cases as other sulphur springs. Treatment by the application of pulverised water (introduced here in 1856 by Dr. Sales Girons) is especially popular; and a special room in the well-appointed bath establishment is devoted to *pulverisation.*

Pierrefonds possesses also a chalybeate spring containing 0·139 of bicarbonate and crenate of iron per litre, a little earthy salts, and traces of manganese and arsenic. The cases treated there are those of chronic pharyngitis, laryngitis, bronchitis, and asthma, also herpetic skin affections, rheumatism, and functional uterine disorders associated with anæmia and chlorosis.

The neighbourhood of Pierrefonds offers many attractive walks and drives, and it has the advantage of being adjacent to the magnificent forest of Compiègne.

The climate is rather humid. The season is from June 1st to Oct. 1st. The waters are exported.

Plombières, in the Department of the Vosges, with *indifferent thermal* springs, is a small, clean, well-built town of 2,000 inhabitants, situated at an elevation of 1,300 feet above the sea in a beautiful green valley, surrounded by gently sloping hills covered with dense forests of beech and pine.

It is useless to speak of the antiquity of these baths. Wherever there were hot springs the Romans were certain to turn them to account, and numerous remains of Roman baths are to be found at all these thermal stations. But we find Montaigne visiting Plombières in the sixteenth century, and since his time it has had many distinguished guests; some of the family of Louis XV., Stanislas, Duke of Lorraine, Voltaire, Maupertuis, Beaumarchais, la Reine Hortense, Napoleon III., etc.

The possession of several springs—thirty in number, furnishing an enormous quantity of water, and varying in temperature from 55° to over 165° F. —has led to the creation of several bathing establishments not far from one another in the town, as well as the new one connected with the Grand Hotel.

In one of these, which is partly subterranean, the remains of an old Roman *piscine*, some feet below the level of the ground, is used as a vapour bath (*étuve*), and here one may witness some of the characteristic treatment of the place in operation.

The hot vapour from the natural spring is admitted into this old Roman chamber, and the patient (who is, we will suppose, the victim of chronic rheumatism) is placed in this moist and superheated atmosphere until he perspires freely; he then passes out and up again into an apartment with several cabinets each containing a couch or bed on which he reposes, well wrapped up, until his perspiration is pretty well over, then he passes into the hands of the *masseur*, and is submitted to the process of massage; this over he passes into another apartment devoted to douching, and is finally finished off with a general douche.

All these springs are very feebly mineralised, the hottest, which are also the strongest, do not contain more than 0·39 of solids per litre. Some of them have an unctuous feeling due to the presence of silicate of aluminium and hence termed "*sources savonneuses.*" They have a faintly alkaline reaction, due probably to the presence of a small amount of sodium bicarbonate. All the springs contain traces of arsenic. There is also a cold ferruginous spring, La Bourdeille, at Plombières. But the cure there consists essentially in the *external* application of the water; the internal use is quite secondary and subordinate.

The methods of applying the thermal waters are numerous, viz. the single bath and the *large* bath, or both, with or without douche or massage; the hot douche during the bath; the so-called "submarine douche" (*i.e.* applied under the surface of the water); the cold douche or the Scotch douche; the vapour bath (*étuve*) followed by "sudation," with or without massage; ascending douches; large intestinal "lavages"; vaginal irrigations; inhalations, etc.

In the next place, what are the diseases especially suited to treatment there and by these methods ?

First and foremost are all the many painful conditions associated with the name chronic rheumatism or dependent on the inherited rheumatic constitution. Sciatica and other forms of rheumatic neuralgia, muscular and articular rheumatism, migraine, and especially those forms of *gastralgia,* chronic nervous dyspepsia, and gastric and intestinal catarrh, associated either with constipation or diarrhœa, especially when connected with the rheumatic constitution, "*enteralgia névralgique et arthritique.*" The physicians who have been long in practice there claim great success in the treatment of these troublesome affections. Neurasthenia and other functional disorders of the nervous system, particularly when associated with arthritism, uterine neuralgia, irritable uterus, and especially chronic metritis in the neuropathic or rheumatic, are also advantageously treated at Plombières. So also are some cases of dysmenorrhœa, amenorrhœa, and sterility when due to faulty development of the uterus. Most of these maladies fall under the denomination in use there of "*rheumatisme névropathique,*" a mixture of nervous, neuralgic affections with rheumatism ; and under this head are comprised, besides the maladies already mentioned, certain forms of vertigo, spinal irritation, nervous palpitations, and superficial neuralgias.

The successful treatment of habitual constipation is another claim put forward by the physicians at Plombières ; such cases are treated by daily hot baths of half an hour to an hour and a-half, followed by the rectal douche.

But of late years it is *specially* in the treatment of *chronic diarrhœa,* and particularly of *muco-membranous enterocolitis,* that Plombières has become celebrated. "Two new establishments and more than sixty special compartments have been exclusively reserved for the application of *enteroclyse* (intestinal lavage) in the recumbent position."

The season is from June 1st to Oct. 1st. The Bain Romain remains open all the year round.

The duration of the *cure* is from 21 to 25 days; in exceptional cases, 30 days.

Plombières can be reached from Paris viâ Belfort in seven hours, and from London in sixteen hours viâ Calais and Chaumont.

Pougues les Eaux is about four hours from Paris on the Lyons Railway, on the right bank of the Loire, at an elevation of 650 feet, and only eight miles from the interesting town of Nevers. Pougues has been termed the "Paradise of the dyspeptic," and appears to have recovered the popularity it possessed some three centuries ago, when it was much resorted to by some of the chief persons in France. In the reading-room of the casino the walls are covered with portraits of some of its ancient patrons. Its waters may be classified as *cold gaseous alkaline earthy* springs.

There are altogether seven springs, but three only of importance—the Sources St. Leger, Saint Léon, and Elisabeth. But the interest and importance of Pougues is really concentrated in the Source St. Leger. The chief constituents of this spring are bicarbonate of lime and magnesia, together 2·1 per litre. It also contains sodium bicarbonate 0·78, small amounts of sodium chloride and sulphate, and minute quantities of bicarbonate of lithium (0·003) and iron.

These waters are considered to be especially suitable to cases in which the waters of Vichy are too powerful. In atonic dyspepsia and chronic diarrhœa in delicate, nervous subjects; in the gouty diathesis, with uric acid deposits in the urine; in feeble persons; in diabetes, and in some forms of chronic vesical catarrh and renal disorders.

The presence of a small amount of iron in these

waters makes them valuable in the treatment of chlorotic anæmic states associated with menstrual irregularities, and with gastric feebleness.

It is usual to begin with small doses of the water —a quarter, a half, or a whole glass taken in the morning fasting. This is sometimes repeated in the afternoon. The average daily dose for the dyspeptic oscillates between twelve and twenty-four ounces. In certain cases much larger doses are given—up to forty ounces even. The methods of hydrotherapy are almost always combined with internal treatment.

These waters are said to increase the digestive secretions, and therefore improve gastric tone and function; they are highly diuretic, and promote renal excretion.

At first, and in small doses, they tend to constipate, but in large doses they often prove laxative. In anæmic persons the proportion of oxyhæmoglobin in the blood is said to be increased. At Pougues douches and baths of all kinds can be obtained, as well as massage and Swedish gymnastics. The "Terrain-Kur" and air cure are practicable at Pougues-Bellevue, situated at an altitude of nearly 1,000 feet, on the western slope of Mont Givre, about three-quarters of a mile from the St. Leger spring. It has a fine terrace dominating the valley of the Loire, and charming walks in the surrounding woods.

The season is from June 1st to Oct. 1st, but the casino does not open till June 15th, and closes on Sept. 15th. All the amusements and distractions usual at French spas are to be found in the casino at Pougues. The waters are *exported*.

Pyrmont is situated at an elevation of about 400 feet, in a well-wooded district in a deep valley of the Weser Mountains, in Waldeck-Pyrmont, near Hanover, and is well known for its *gaseous chalybeate* springs. It is one of the oldest and most celebrated spas in Germany. Besides its iron springs, it also possesses common salt springs. It likewise utilises a *ferruginous mud*, obtained from near the chalybeate spring, which is said to have the same composition as the Franzensbad mud.

The chief iron spring is the Hauptquelle, a decidedly strong one—stronger than those at Schwalbach and St. Moritz—but it is not so agreeable to drink, as it contains a small quantity of the bitter sulphate of magnesia. It contains, per litre, bicarbonate of iron 0·077, bicarbonate of manganese 0·0062, and carbonic acid 1,476 c.c., besides chlorides in small amount and sulphates, chiefly the sulphate of magnesia (0·453).

There are also three chief salt springs, one of which, with much carbonic acid, is used for drinking; it contains, per litre, sodium chloride 7·06, sodium sulphate 0·12, magnesium sulphate 0·96, and carbonic acid 954 c.c. The bathing springs contain more sodium chloride, the strongest as much as 32 grammes per litre. There are very complete bath arrangements for (1) the chalybeate, (2) the salt, and (3) the mud baths. Besides these there are wave baths, pine-needle and other medicated baths, and massage, gymnastics, electrical treatment, and the whey cure are available.

Owing to the possession of two distinct groups of mineral springs, the *cure* at Pyrmont is applicable to a great many morbid conditions, while it admits of a *combined* treatment very appropriate to many cases.

For patients requiring chalybeate waters Pyrmont offers an alternative to such resorts as Schwalbach or St. Moritz; for those suffering from gastric and hepatic troubles it may take the place of Homburg or Kissingen; and for many female maladies it offers much the same remedial measures as may be found at Kreuznach. In addition, then, to cases of anæmia, chlorosis, retarded convalescence, functional nervous affections, and scrofula, Pyrmont has been *specially* advocated for the treatment of certain *female* complaints, particularly with its *Sool* and *mud* baths—

chronic pelvic, periuterine exudations, and those the result of chronic perityphlitis, the cachectic states associated with menstrual disturbances, uterine and vaginal catarrhs, non-malignant uterine tumours; *obesity*, especially in chlorotic women and associated with *sterility*—in such cases the combined use of the iron and salt waters has been found of much value.

Pyrmont has a healthy, mild, and agreeable climate. It is rarely too hot in the daytime in summer, but the nights are cool, and warm clothing is always needed. The soil is porous, and the ground dries quickly after rain. The air is very pure and free from dust.

The season is from the beginning of May to Oct. 1st. Accommodation is good, the prices are moderate. The quickest route is by Queenborough and Flushing, eighteen hours from London.

Panticosa (Spanish Pyrenees).—This Spanish mountain spa must be classed with the *weak sulphur* springs, its several *sources* being very feebly mineralised. It would be an extremely interesting excursion for the hardy and enterprising pedestrian and balneologist, to visit this Spanish mountain health resort from Cauterets, and return by Gabas and Les Eaux Chaudes. From Cauterets to Panticosa is an arduous mountain walk of eight hours, crossing a steep *col* about 8,000 feet high; a horse can be taken for about the first half of the way; and a guide is necessary, as the first part of the descent on the Spanish side is rather difficult. It is usually, however, approached on the French side from Les Eaux Chaudes, a twelve hours' journey on horseback. On the Spanish side it is approached from Huesca, but it is a drive of forty-four miles by carriage from that town, so it is a place difficult of access. It is picturesquely situated in the mountains, at an elevation of 5,600 feet, near a lake and some waterfalls. The climate is harsh and very cold at night. We have very little reliable information about this Spanish Pyrenean bath. It possesses several springs, which are somewhat quaintly named, according to their uses: "Del Higado" (for the liver), "De los Herpes" (for eruptions), "Del Estomago" (for the stomach), "De la Taquara," etc. Their temperature is about 84° F. Their mineralisation is very feeble, Estomago contains only 0·15 grammes to the litre—chiefly sodium sulphide and sulphate, with some free sulphuretted hydrogen gas. Higado and Herpes contain much free nitrogen. The springs are used for drinking and for baths. Nitrogen inhalations are also prescribed. Cases treated at Panticosa comprise chronic catarrhs of the respiratory passages, phthisis, dyspepsia, rheumatism, and skin diseases. The high mountain climate must be an important therapeutic factor.

Parad, in Hungary, on the line of rail from Kis-Terenne to Kaal-Kapolna has *strong sulphate of iron* waters. An alkaline gaseous sulphur spring arises in the neighbourhood and a bicarbonate of iron spring at some distance off.

Passugg, in Switzerland, about an hour's drive from Coire, at an elevation of 2,710feet—the carriage road turns off from that to Churwalden — has *cold gaseous alkaline* and other springs of some local renown. The most strongly mineralised of these, the Ulricus, is said to contain as much as 5·669 grammes per litre of bicarbonate of sodium, 1·026 of bicarbonate of lime, and 0·0837 of chloride of sodium, and a minute amount of bicarbonate of iron. It has also a cold gaseous and calcareous chalybeate spring, much richer in iron, and a highly gaseous weak alkaline *source*, suitable for a table-water. The springs are situated at some distance (twenty minutes) from the bath establishment, where carbonic acid baths are prepared. These waters should prove of much therapeutic value; they are resorted to chiefly by cases of dyspepsia and anæmia. The subalpine climate must favour the cure. Season, from June to September.

Peiden, a Swiss bath in the Grisons, about four miles from Ilanz (between Coire and Dissentis), in the Lugnetz valley, has *cold calcareous* waters, containing 3·6 grammes of solids per litre, chiefly carbonate and sulphate of lime (together 1·952), and a little iron, 0·023 of bicarbonate of iron, and free carbonic acid. It also contains some sodium sulphate (0·948) and chloride (0·219) and magnesium bicarbonate (0·378). May be prescribed in the same cases as other earthy springs. The season is from June 15 to Sept. 15.

Pejo, in the Pejo valley in the Tyrol, south of the Orteler range, at an elevation of 4,430 feet, possesses an *alkaline chalybeate* spring said to contain 0·05 per litre of bicarbonate of iron.

The nearest railway station, San Michele, is a twelve hours' drive.

Pestrin, Le, France, Department Ardèche, near Vals, has *chalybeate* waters.

Petersthal, in the Baden Black Forest, has *cold gaseous chalybeate* springs, containing bicarbonate of iron about 0·045, bicarbonate of calcium 1·5, and sulphate of sodium 0·7 per litre. It is situated at an elevation of 1,330 feet, in the Reuchthal, on the western slope of the Kniebis mountains, and is five miles from the railway station of Oppenau.

Pfaeffers. *See* Ragatz-Pfaeffers.

Piatigorsk, in Russia (the Caucasus), has *thermal common salt* and *sulphur* waters, of a temperature varying from 83·5° to 117° F. Diluted mud baths are also prepared, the mud coming from the neighbouring lake Tambukan. The scenery is said to be very beautiful—the place has an elevation of 1,685 feet. The season is from May to September. The Maria Theresa purgative spring arises at Karras, five miles off; it is known as "the bitter water of the Caucasus."

Pietrapola, in Corsica, in a picturesque situation, has *thermal sulphur* springs at a temperature of 90° to 137° F., and containing 0·02 per litre of sodium sulphide.

Pitkeathly. *See* Bridge-of-Earn, p. 131.

Poretta, in the province of Bologna, Italy, with a station on the railway line from Bologna to Pistoja, has *thermal common salt* and *sulphur* waters. It lies amongst the Apennines, at an altitude of 1,100 feet, in the valley of the Reno, These waters have been known from very ancient date, partly because of the remarkable circumstance that an inflammable gas (carburetted hydrogen, or marsh gas) is disengaged from the surface of the spring and has been utilised for illuminating purposes. There are as many as nine springs, varying in temperature from 91° to 95° F. Besides the mineral constituents, some of them contain an oily or bituminous substance. They have an odour of H_2S, and a disagreeable bitter taste. They are used for drinking, for douches, baths, and inhalations. The Leone, one of those chiefly used for drinking, has 8·0 grammes of sodium chloride per litre, with minute amounts of iodides and bromides, traces of arsenic, and a small quantity of free H_2S, and "marsh" gas. These waters are laxative and diuretic, and are given *internally* in cases of hepatic congestion, gallstones, hæmorrhoids, and abdominal plethora, and as *baths* for skin diseases (moist eczema, psoriasis, acne) and rheumatism. Season, June 30 to Sept, 30.

Pouillon, near Dax, France, has weak *common salt* waters.

Pozzuoli, on the Bay of Naples, between that city and Baiæ, has weak *thermal alkaline common salt* waters of ancient historic repute. A half-extinct crater in the neighbourhood, the Solfatara, yields sulphurous fumes and a little carbonic acid gas, and in the time of the Romans was used as a natural vapour bath. Above the Solfatara are the hot Pisciarelli springs containing sulphate of iron and alum.

Preblau, in the Lavanthal, Carinthia, has an *alkaline* spring, in a beautiful Alpine situation, at an elevation of more than 3,000 feet above the sea. The water is alkaline, containing 2·2 grammes of bicarbonate of sodium per litre. It is cold and gaseous, and is largely exported as a table water. It is also drunk at the source, and prescribed in cases of chronic catarrh of the bladder and urinary tract, in renal calculi, and in certain forms of Bright's disease. This resort is, however, too distant to have any great interest for English patients.

Préchacq-les-Bains, a French resort, having *thermal* waters and *mud* baths identical with those at Dax, from which place it is only a short distance. Like Dax, it is in the valley of the Adour. The nearest railway station (seven kilometres) is Laluque, on the line between Bordeaux and Bayonne. The chief constituent in the thermal springs is calcium sulphate; they also contain some free nitrogen, oxygen, and carbonic acid gases, and an abundance of confervæ. They are of a high temperature (140° F.) and of almost unlimited amount. Their action, taken internally, is diuretic, and they have been found very useful in cases of gravel, renal colic, and vesical catarrh. As baths they produce a marked sedative effect on the nervous and muscular systems, and are valuable in many forms of rheumatism, neuralgia (sciatica), gout, and neuritis. The *vegeto-mineral mud* is used in the same way and for the same cases as the mud at Dax—as full baths, half-baths, and as local applications. These baths promote greatly elimination by the skin, and are powerful sudorifics. *Chronic* rheumatism is the malady for which they are specially employed, and rheumatic sciatica, lumbago, and muscular paresis. Uterine enlargements are also benefited, as by the Moor baths of Franzensbad. *Acute* conditions are not suitable for this treatment.

Préchacq has also a *cold sulphur* spring, which affords an additional resource in certain cases.

The fine bathing establishment is open from May 1 to Nov. 1.

Pré-Saint-Didier, near Courmayeur, in North Italy, at an altitude of 3,000 feet, has *simple thermal springs* feebly mineralised, and of a temperature of 95° F. They are used for baths only.

Prese, Le, in Switzerland (Canton Grisons), on the southern or Italian side of the Bernina Pass, close to the Lake of Poschiavo, and about six hours by carriage from Samaden, has feebly mineralised *cold sulphur* waters, and is in a picturesque situation, at an elevation of 3,100 feet. Its total solids only amount to 0·202 per litre, the chief of which is calcium sulphate 0·125, and magnesium carbonate 0·094. They also contain 6 c.c. of H_2S per litre. They are used for drinking and for baths. Le Prese has a well-arranged bath establishment and comfortable hotel accommodation. Its moderate elevation and its protection from winds make it a suitable summer resort for many cases. The waters are applied in the same manner and in the same cases as similarly constituted and similarly situated springs. The season is from the beginning of June to the end of September.

Preste, La, a *thermal sulphur* bath in the narrow mountain valley of the Tech, at an elevation of 3,700 feet, in the Pyrénées Orientales, a drive of four and a-half hours from Céret, a railway station thirty-eight kilometres from Perpignan. Owing to its southern latitude and protected situation, the baths are enabled to be kept open all the year round.

There are four springs, containing sodium sulphide, at a temperature of 112° F. The total mineralisation is small, 0·13 grammes per litre. These waters are allowed to remain exposed to the air before use, when they undergo "degeneration," the sodium sulphide being converted into sulphate and hyposulphite. They are chiefly used internally, but baths, douches, pulverisations, and inhalations are given. From ancient date these waters have been employed in the treatment of urinary affections—painful catarrh of the bladder, phosphatic and uric acid gravel, chronic nephritis, and nephralgia. They are also used in respiratory affections, in dry skin eruptions, and in rheumatism. The bath establishment contains the hotel and casino. The water is exported.

Pullna, near Teplitz, has "bitter" *purgative* waters containing sodium sulphate and magnesium sulphate and chloride, chiefly exported.

Purton Spa, in Wiltshire.—The water contains *aperient sulphates.*

Puzzichello, in Corsica, possesses cold H_2S springs, which have a local reputation in the treatment of skin diseases.

Pystjan, or **Pöstyen,** in Hungary, on the river Waag, at an elevation of 490 feet, and sheltered by the Carpathian mountains from north-east winds, has *thermal sulphur* waters varying in temperature from 135° to 146° F., chiefly used for baths. Sulphurous mud baths are also prepared, and applied generally and locally. The cases chiefly treated there are those of injuries to bones and joints, rheumatoid arthritis, and syphilis.

Ragatz-Pfaeffers, a well-known Swiss bath with *simple thermal* waters. Ragatz is 1,628 feet above the sea, and Pfaeffers 2,130 feet. The water from the hot springs at Pfaeffers is conducted in wooden tubes to the baths of Ragatz, a distance of about two and a-half miles. The baths of Pfaeffers, situated near the source, a building capable of accommodating 200 persons, is so inconveniently placed, shut in as it is in a deep and dark gorge, that most visitors prefer to take these baths at Ragatz, the position of which is far more attractive and convenient, and where there is excellent hotel and bath accommodation. The temperature of the water at its source at Pfaeffers is 98·6° F. It loses a few degrees in its transit to Ragatz, where the temperature of the baths is 93·5° F. It is an *indifferent thermal* spring, producing its effects mainly by its warmth, and resembling, in this respect, Teplitz and Wildbad. It is, like the Wildbad waters, rich in nitrogen gas. The cases suitable for treatment here resemble those sent to other "Wildbäder," such as Wildbad or Gastein—viz. cases of chronic rheumatism, of rheumatoid arthritis, of sciatica, of chronic gouty exudations, of tabes and certain other paralytic conditions, of hysteria and hypochondriasis; cases requiring careful management on account of their occurrence in persons of sensitive nervous organisation, certain special female maladies, cases of retarded convalescence, in which the mildly tonic climate and quiet life are advantageous. There are excellent new baths, with a swimming bath, at Ragatz, and appliances for douches, electric baths, hydrotherapy, and Zander's Swedish gymnastics. A continuous flow of the hot mineral water is kept up in the baths, so that they are maintained at an equable temperature. The bath usually lasts half an hour. It is more a bathing than a drinking cure, but some patients are ordered two to four glasses of the water daily. Ragatz has a station on the line between Zürich and Coire, within a few miles of the latter town.

The season is from the beginning of May to the end of October. July and the first part of August can be very hot at Ragatz. The cure is therefore better taken either before or after this period.

Reichenhall is an important health resort in the Bavarian highlands, close to the Austrian frontier, at an elevation of 1,571 feet above the sea, fourteen miles by rail from Salzburg, and four hours from Munich, in the midst of the finest scenery, and within a few miles only of Berchtesgaden and the Königsee. It possesses a variety of curative means. These include treatment by variations of air pressure in the pneumatic chamber, the whey cure, waters of other well-known spas, pine-cone baths, an elaborate inhalatorium for the inhalation of the brine spray, etc. Its subalpine climate is fairly bracing, mild yet invigorating. It is enclosed on three sides by an amphitheatre of mountains, from 4,400 to 6,400 feet high. It is the great centre of the Bavarian salt works, and the surplus brine of the Berchtesgaden salt mines is conducted there. It has sixteen salt springs, the chief of which are the Edelquelle (with 220 grammes of salt per litre) and the Karl-Theodorquelle. These are mixed together for the baths, which are sometimes fortified by *Mutterlauge* containing much magnesium chloride. It also has spacious salt works and graduating-houses (*Gradirhauser*). The patients promenade near the latter so as to inhale the salt-impregnated air. There are also *Gradirwerke* in the Kurgarten for the same purpose, with a salt water fountain forty feet high.

In the inhalatorium it has been calculated that a cubic metre of air contains from six to forty grammes of salt, according to the distance from the apparatus. The inhalation of this brine-spray is found very useful in promoting expectoration in cases of chronic bronchial catarrh. It is also a resort for cases of chronic stationary phthisis, on account of its mild subalpine climate. It is, however, sometimes very hot in summer. Like other salt baths, this is suitable to chronic, lymphatic, and scrofulous affections; also cases of asthma and emphysema, as well as chronic catarrhal cases, are treated there by inhalation of compressed air and expiration into rarefied air, and in the pneumatic chamber. Indeed, the cases chiefly and specially treated at Reichenhall are chronic catarrhal affections of the respiratory organs.

The water of the salt springs has to be diluted for drinking. A laxative "bitter" water has been prepared from the *Mutterlauge*, and, for drinking, the brine can be obtained impregnated with carbonic acid, diluted and bottled. Artificial gaseous Sool baths are prepared there, in imitation of those at Nauheim, and artificial gaseous chalybeate baths also. Altogether Reichenhall is a very important health resort.

The season is from May 1st to Oct. 1st.

Rheinfelden, in Canton Aargau, Switzerland, on the left bank of the Rhine, nine miles from Bâle, is a *strong brine* bath. The town is charmingly situated, at an elevation of 870 feet, on the northern frontier of Switzerland, separated only by an old wooden bridge from the Grand Duchy of Baden. It is protected to the north by the Black Forest mountains, and to the west and south by the Jura chain. Its climate is mild and temperate, rather hot in summer, but on the whole very suitable for a bathing-station of this kind.

More than half a century ago a vast deposit of salt was discovered a little distance from the town, at a depth of 120 metres, and this led, in course of time, to the establishment of a manufactory of common salt and the formation of a mineral water spa.

The Rheinfelden brine is practically a saturated solution of salt, and contains 311·6 grammes per litre of sodium chloride, as strong as it is possible to be, and in this respect it resembles the brine of Droitwich.

The *Mutterlauge* obtained from it resembles it closely in composition; it contains 310 per litre of sodium chloride, 3 of magnesium chloride, and 2 of calcium chloride. It therefore differs much less in composition from the brine than the *Mutterlauge* of weaker salt waters. Indeed, the salt water and the *Mutterlauge* have very nearly the same composition, and of all the sodium chloride waters Rheinfelden is the strongest.

It is used in baths of various strengths and of various degrees of temperature—as compresses, as lotions, gargles, pulverisations, and nasal and vaginal injections. It is very rarely taken internally, and then very diluted. The soft water of the Rhine is used for diluting the brine for the baths. The methods of hydrotherapy are also employed, and especially the various forms of douches. Other therapeutic measures employed are vapour baths, massage, electricity, *hydro-electric baths*, pine-extract baths, the use of other mineral waters, especially of the chalybeate group, and the milk cure.

The cases best suited to treatment there are retarded convalescence from infective fevers; general debility following nutritional disturbances or exhaustive discharges; anæmia and chlorosis; *scrofula in all its forms and manifestations;* chronic affections of the bones and joints unsuitable for surgical operation, and wounds and fistulas the result of such operations; rickets; *chronic rheumatism;* gout, *with certain precautions; skin* affections allied to scrofula, psoriasis, and hypersensitiveness of the surface; functional affections of the nervous system, neurasthenia and certain forms of paralysis (in those cases a combination of electricity with the salt baths proves very useful); those female maladies usually submitted to treatment by salt baths, etc., including *obesity*.

The season is from the middle of May to the end of October. The accommodation is good, and there is a well-managed hospital for poor patients. The railway station is on the line between Bâle and Zürich.

Rippoldsau, a *chalybeate* bath in the Black Forest, in the Grand Duchy of Baden, is one of the Kniebis spas. It is situated in a beautiful, thickly wooded Black Forest valley—the Wolfthal—at an elevation of nearly 2,000 feet, and is highly esteemed both for its invigorating subalpine climate and its mineral springs. It lies at the southern foot of the Kniebis mountains. There are numerous and charming promenades and excursions into the surrounding forests and mountains. It is usually approached from Wolfach, a railway station on the Black Forest line, viâ Strasburg or Cologne and Offenburg. From Wolfach it is a drive of nearly three hours. It has three cold gaseous springs, utilised for drinking, and one for baths. They all contain iron, much free carbonic acid, and much bicarbonate of lime, and a certain amount of sodium and magnesium sulphate, which distinguishes them from a simple chalybeate water like that of Schwalbach.

The strongest of the springs in bicarbonate of iron (0·094 per litre) is the Wenzelsquelle, and this also contains sulphates of sodium and magnesium amounting together to 0·952. The Josephsquelle contains much less iron but more of the aperient sulphates (1·117). It is usual at Rippoldsau to prepare from some of the mineral springs—the Josephsquelle and the Leopoldsquelle—artificial mineral waters, by the addition of sodium sulphate and carbonate and carbonic acid gas to the former, and the same salts, with a little sulphuretted hydrogen, to the latter, in imitation of the Kreuzbrunnen at Marienbad, and the Schwefelbrunnen at Weilbach. The first of these is termed Natroine, and the second Schwefelnatroine. This, of course, extends considerably the range of applicability of the Rippoldsau waters. The chalybeate waters are prescribed in the various maladies associated with anæmia and chlorosis, and the Natroine is used as a purgative in cases usually treated by such waters, while the artificially produced "sulphur" water is used in such cutaneous, catarrhal, and other affections as are usually sent to sulphur spas. The baths are prepared from one of the weaker iron springs, which is, however, specially rich in free carbonic acid.

Moor baths are also prepared from moor-earth, obtained directly from Franzensbad, mixed with the iron water. Hydro-electric baths, pine-needle baths, all kinds of douches, massage, hydrotherapy, gymnastics, and the whey and milk cures can be obtained at Rippoldsau. The season is from May 15th to Sept. 15th.

Roncegno, in the Austrian Tyrol, is a three hours' drive, or about 20 miles, from Trent, on the Brenner line to Venice. It is situated in the picturesque Val Sugana, watered by the river Brenta, at an altitude of 1,750 feet, and now possesses a railway station on the new Val Sugana line, which brings it within an hour of Trent. It has a Kurhaus capable of accommodating 150 guests, and four or five small hotels.

The water is remarkable among mineral waters for its large proportion of metallic sulphates. It contains sulphates of iron, *copper*, manganese, aluminium, nickel, cobalt, etc., together with a notable amount of arsenic. It is obtained from a mine in the adjacent Mount Tesobo; it is cloudy at its source and has to be allowed to stand in reservoirs until the sediment is deposited and the clear upper stratum can be removed. It is easy to understand why strong mineral springs like these should enjoy a great *local* reputation, but they hardly come under the category of ordinary mineral waters such as foreign visitors might be attracted to, as "water" enters little, if at all, into such a cure, owing to the strength of the spring. The water is exported.

The water is employed as baths, largely diluted

with fresh water, and is also taken internally—one or two tablespoonfuls for a dose. Owing to the large amount of arsenic in the water (0·109 of arsenate of sodium and 0·115 of arsenic anhydride) any increase of these small doses must be carefully watched. The muddy sediment from the water is also applied locally like a poultice. The cases considered most amenable to treatment at Roncegno are those of anæmia, neurasthenia, many cutaneous affections, malarial cachexia, chronic muscular and articular rheumatism, chronic bronchial catarrh, early phthisis, and cases of protracted convalescence from acute disease.

The season is from May 1st to the end of September.

Royat les Bains. — The volcanic district of Auvergne is, as might be expected, rich in *thermal* springs, many of which rise in mountain regions, where picturesque scenery and fine bracing air contribute no unimportant addition to the effects of these mineral *sources*. It is said that there are no less than 500 distinct mineralised springs in Auvergne, while the department of Puy de Dôme alone contains over 200. Of the better known and more frequented sources, Mont Dore, La Bourboule, and Royat are the chief.

Royat has, of late years, attained great popularity and importance. It is finely situated not far from Clermont-Ferrand, 1,460 feet above the sea-level. It has an agreeable refreshing climate, and possesses several springs which in their constitution somewhat resemble those of Ems.

As to the composition and uses of the waters at Royat, they are described by French authorities as "thermal, alkaline, gaseous, chloride of sodium, iron, arsenical and lithiated," and in other works they are included in the class of "alkaline common salt" waters, of which Royat and Ems may be taken as types.

At Royat, however, much importance is attached to the presence of *arsenic*, *iron*, and *lithium* in its springs.

But, apart from the presence of lithium and arsenic in the waters of Royat, they contain other important constituents in considerable quantity. The alkaline bicarbonates predominate, as in most of the mineral springs of this district—those of soda, lime, and magnesia chiefly—and to these must be added chloride of sodium. The Source Eugénie is the most richly mineralised, and contains of solids 5·62 per litre; of this 3·46 consists of alkaline bicarbonates, 1·72 of sodium chloride, 0·035 of lithium chloride, 0·056 of salts of iron and manganese, and in the Source St. Victor 0·0045 of sodium arsenate. The Sources St. Mart and St. Victor are somewhat less richly mineralised, and the Source César is but very feebly mineralised, and as it contains a considerable amount of free carbonic acid, it is the best suited for use as an ordinary drinking water. It is by no means unimportant to bear in mind that three of these springs—viz. the Eugénie, the St. Victor, and the César—contain an appreciable quantity of bicarbonate of iron. There are thus four principal springs at Royat: Eugénie, St. Victor, St. Mart, and César. These are all thermal springs; the Eugénie is the hottest, and has a temperature of 96° F.; the St. Victor the coolest, its temperature is 68° F.

At Royat, as in most other large spas in France, the waters are utilised in every possible manner; the well-appointed *Établissement* provides douches of all kinds. To each bath there is a douche, and douching and massage "*sous l'eau*"—*i.e.* under the water in the bath—are applied. Baths and douches of carbonic acid, hydro-electric baths, and baths with *running water* (*à eau courante*), in which the water is admitted directly from the spring, and by being kept flowing through the bath a constant temperature is maintained—these are highly valued methods of treatment at Royat. There are also *salles d'aspiration*, in which the patient sits, fitly attired, and breathes the vapour driven into the chamber from the hot springs themselves, and, after being steamed in this fashion for half an hour, is hurried off to his hotel in a sort of sedan-chair and ordered to repose for an hour. There are also well-appointed *salles de pulvérisation*, in which jets of water are pulverised by being driven with great force against metallic discs, or the water is driven into spray by means of steam. These jets of spray and pulverised water are inhaled, and are the chief treatment employed in affections of the throat and nose. Royat also possesses a fine swimming bath, one of the largest of its kind, furnished with a gymnastic apparatus, and very popular with the French ladies.

The chief *buvette,* or drinking fountain—that of the Source Eugénie—is situated in the tastefully arranged park, and the water is ladled out from the bubbling source itself by female attendants. Before breakfast in the morning — the serious *déjeuner* is at eleven o'clock—and again between three and four in the afternoon, are the times appropriated to drinking the waters, the dinner hour being six. It is usual to begin with quite small doses of the water, half a glass twice a day gradually increased.

The treatment at Royat is *specially* applicable to what the French authorities term "*des arthritiques anémiques,*" which corresponds with the group of patients who in England are said to suffer from "*atonic gout*"—a combination of joint troubles with anæmia and debility. The arsenic and the iron combined in the Royat waters render them decidedly tonic. It may here be said that they prove less successful with the rheumatic than with the gouty. Atonic dyspepsia in the gouty is also a condition adapted to treatment there. Certain forms of skin disease—indeed, nearly all forms having direct relation to the gouty constitution—are very greatly benefited by this course.

Acne, it is said, is very amenable to the Royat waters. Gouty eczema—*i.e.* patches of eczema, limited and localised—belong also especially to the list of ailments cured there, as well as those cases of troublesome local *pruritus* connected with the gouty constitution. Diabetes and certain forms of Bright's disease, when associated with gout, especially in the debilitated and anæmic, are suited to Royat; so are cases of biliary and renal colic of moderate severity in the anæmic.

Anæmia and chlorosis, and other *diseases of women* similar to those treated at Ems, are also treated at Royat with success. Diseases of the throat and respiratory organs, chronic bronchial catarrhs, catarrhal asthma, especially when they occur in the gouty, are sent in considerable numbers to Royat for treatment; and its climate is considered very suitable to such conditions. Cases of chronic laryngitis and pharyngitis in gouty people are greatly benefited there. In these cases the treatment by inhalations proves of much service. Finally, the neurasthenic, the migrainous, the over-worked, and sufferers from those neuroses which are dependent on cerebro-spinal anæmia, may derive benefit from the Royat course.

The climate of Royat depends partly on its adjacency to the great central mountain chains of Auvergne, the Monts Dômes, and the Monts Dore, partly on the porous volcanic soil, and partly on its own particular situation. Lying as it does in the floor of a somewhat narrow valley, surrounded on all sides by mountains, and only open to the east, running, moreover, in a direction exactly east and west, and facing the east, it is particularly exposed to the direct heat of the sun. From the moment the sun rises in the east above the mountains of Forez until it sets in the west behind the gigantic mass of the Puy de Dôme, Royat lies exposed to its rays; and it is therefore exceedingly difficult to find any kind of shady walks in the immediate vicinity of Royat when the sun is up and the sky is cloudless. Generally, however, when the sun goes down, the cooler upper strata of air rush down from the higher plateaux into the valley, and thus you get cool refreshing currents of air playing through the valley on the evenings of even some of the hottest days in summer.

The invalids and visitors at Royat are well provided with amusements; the presence of two regiments of artillery at Clermont, with a permanent band, provides very good orchestral music. At the casino there is a concert or ball or dramatic performance every night, and some of the eminent singers who are following the course of treatment at Royat often take part in these entertainments.

The season is from May 25th to Sept. 30th.

Rabbi, in the Val di Rabbi, a branch of the Val di Noce, Tyrol, possesses two *strong alkaline chalybeate* springs. This small spa is situated at an altitude of 4,100 feet and is distant ten hours from a railway station (San Michele). Its stronger spring is said to contain 0·18 bicarbonate of iron and 1·0 bicarbonate of sodium per litre. The season is from June 15 to Sept. 15.

Radein, a bath in Styria, too distant to be of much value to English patients. It has a *cold gaseous alkaline* spring, and also a *chalybeate* spring. The former is said to contain three grammes of carbonate of sodium and 0·3 of carbonate of lithium in a litre. It is exported as well as drunk at the source. Vapour baths, douches, massage, etc., are applied there. Urinary affections, gravel, catarrh, associated with uric acid (gout), also acid and catarrhal dyspepsia, are treated there.

Rajecsfürdö, one hour from the railway station of Sillein, in Upper Hungary, at an elevation of 1,374 feet, has *indifferent thermal* waters of a temperature of 91° to 95° F., which are said to contain minute amounts of iron and alum.

Rappoltsweller, in a valley of the Vosges, Upper Alsace, at an elevation of 920 feet, connected by tram line with its railway station (two and a-half miles off), on the Strasburg-Bâle line, has a feebly mineralised *calcareous* spring, of a temperature of 62° to 65° F., the Carolaquelle. The Carolabad, at a little distance from the town, is prettily situated in its own grounds, and here the water is utilised for drinking, for inhalation, baths, and douches. It has a large, open swimming bath. It is a pleasant quiet, summer resort.

Rastenburg and **Finneck**, in the

principality of Saxe-Weimar, on the Lossa—the terminus of the Weimar-Rastenburg branch line —is a small *chalybeate* spa with weak iron springs.

Ratzes, in the Austrian Tyrol, between three and four hours from the railway station Atzwang, is situated at an altitude of 3,900 feet, close to the Schlern mountains, and has a *sulphate of iron* spring (0·3 of sulphate of iron to the litre), and a cold, sulphur spring.

Recoaro, Province of Vicenza, Italy, twenty-six miles from Vicenza station, and connected with it by steam tram to the south of the Alps of Tyrol, has several *chalybeate* springs, rich in carbonic acid gas. The most used is the Lelia, and this contains 0·046 per litre of carbonate of iron together with a small amount of lime salts (carbonate and sulphate). Recoaro is situated at an elevation of 1,400 feet, in a picturesque neighbourhood, and has good accommodation.

Rehburg, Germany, Province of Hanover, with a station on the Steinhuder-Meer line, has cold feebly mineralised *earthy* springs, used only for baths in cases of rheumatism, etc.

Rehme. *See* Oeynhausen, p. 280.

Reiboldsgrün, Saxony, has *chalybeate* waters and a sanatorium for consumptive patients.

Reinerz, in the county of Glatz, Silesia, seventeen miles from the town of Glatz, with a railway station at Rückers-Reinerz, and at Nachod (Austria), has nine *cold gaseous alkaline earthy chalybeate* springs, one of which contains 0·05 per litre of bicarbonate of iron. They also contain sodium, calcium, and magnesium carbonates. Three of the springs are used for drinking, and six for the baths. The Laüquelle is used for gargling and inhalation. Iodised, ferruginous mud baths are also prepared. Walks adapted to the "Terrain-Kur" are marked out in the pleasant, wooded, hilly country around the spa. The cases treated there are catarrhal affections of the respiratory, gastro-intestinal, and renal organs, anæmia, neurasthenia, retarded convalescence, etc.

Remoncourt, France, Department of Vosges, *earthy calcareous* waters, resembling Contrexéville.

Renlaigue, Saint Dierry, Department Puy de Dôme, France, a pure *strong gaseous chalybeate* water, with 0·08 per litre of bicarbonate of iron.

Rennes les Bains, France, Department Aude, at an elevation of 1,040 feet, in a narrow valley on the river Salz, about an hour's drive from the station of Coneza, on the line from Carcasonne to Quillan, has *weak thermal* springs, the hottest of which has a temperature of 124° F. It is usual to speak of some of these as chalybeate, but the amount of iron is very small, only 0·002 per litre. There is, however, a cold spring, Du Cercle, said to contain 0·015 of sulphate of iron, and others more than this. The water of the river Salz is also utilised, as it contains much sodium and magnesium chloride, and sulphates of sodium, calcium, and magnesium, derived from salt springs which flow into it. One of these springs is said to contain as much as 56·0 grammes per litre of sodium chloride.

Cases of anæmia, scrofula, and rheumatism are treated there.

Reutlingen, Würtemberg, on the Echaz, at an elevation of 1,110 feet, nine miles east of Tübingen, has *cold sulphur* waters containing small amounts of sodium and magnesium bicarbonates.

Rietbad, a Swiss *cold alkaline*

sulphur bath, at an altitude of 2,790 feet, in the Lautern valley, connected with the Toggenburg valley, in Canton St. Gall. About three hours' drive from Ebnat station.

Rio (Elba), has a *sulphate of iron* spring.

Rohitsch, or Heiligen-Kreuzbad, in Styria, about an hour and a-quarter's drive from the railway station of Pöltschart, has *cold alkaline gaseous* springs, containing sodium sulphate chiefly, and so allied to such waters as those of Marienbad, only much weaker. Other constituents of these springs are sodium, calcium, and magnesium bicarbonate and sodium chloride. They are employed in cases of dyspepsia, with constipation and gastro-intestinal catarrh. The season is from May 1 to Oct. 15.

Römerbad and **Tüffer**, Styria, Austria, on the railway from Graz to Trieste, are close together, at an altitude of about 800 feet, and have *simple thermal* springs.

Römerbad is specially noted for the treatment of hysteria and chronic uterine affections.

Roncas-Blanc, near Marseilles, with which it is connected by a tramway, has a *warm common salt* spring (as well as sea-baths) at a temperature of 70° F. It contains 20 grammes per litre of sodium chloride and 2 each of magnesium chloride and calcium, magnesium, and sodium sulphates. It is used for drinking and for baths in the same cases as other common salt springs. Roncas-Blanc has the further advantage of the Mediterranean climate.

Ronneberg. — A small *chalybeate* spa in the duchy of Saxe-Altenburg.

Ronneby. — A Swedish *chalybeate* spa, with an "old" and a "new" spring—the latter contains 2·5 of sulphate of iron and 1·5 of sulphate of aluminium per litre. The "old" spring is much weaker. The stronger spring is used for baths only, the weaker one is sometimes drunk.

Rosenheim, Upper Bavaria, on the line between Munich and Salzburg, at an altitude of 1,640 feet, has *brine* baths, prepared with brine from Reichcahll (240 grammes of sodium chloride per litre). It has also a weak chalybeate spring.

Rothenbrunnen (Switzerland).— A *weak alkaline chalybeate* spring, on the right bank of the Rhine, about midway between Reichenau and Thusis, said to contain a little iodide of sodium. Its elevation above the sea is about 2,000 feet. Spoken of specially as a *children's* bath.

Rothenfelde, in Hanover, with a station on the line between Osnabrück and Bruckwede, has a *Soolbad* The *cold salt* springs are rich in free carbonic acid gas and contain 56 grammes per litre of sodium chloride, and also some calcium bicarbonate and magnesium chloride, and, it is reported, some iodides and bromides. A *Mutterlauge* and "bath salt" are prepared at the salt works, and used to fortify the baths. A weaker water is used for drinking. The brine, besides being used for baths, is also employed for gargling and inhalations.

These waters are used in the same cases as other thermal *Sool* baths.

The season is from the beginning of May to the middle of October.

Rouzat, Department Puy de Dôme, France, a few miles from Riom, at an elevation of 1,300 feet, has *cold earthy* and *common salt* springs, containing a little iron.

Rubinat - Llorach, a Spanish *purgative* water, coming from a village of the same name, is rich in sodium sulphate (96 grammes per litre), and has a much smaller quantity of sulphates of magnesium, calcium, and potassium, together 5·3 grammes, and 2 grammes of sodium chloride. It is chiefly exported.

Saint Amand (Department du Nord), France, celebrated for its *mud baths*, is situated between Lille and Valenciennes and about 160 miles from Paris. It is in a flat country at an elevation of 100 feet. It has the advantage of being near a large forest. Fontaine-Bouillon is the nearest railway station to the well-organised Grand Hotel and Etablissement Thermal, about two miles from the town, accommodating about 100 patients or guests; in one part of the building the "mud" baths are given, while the other part is devoted to private baths and douches. The springs, of which there are five (three only are utilised), are moderately warm (79° F.) and feebly mineralised (1·35 of solids per litre). The chief constituents are calcium sulphate (0·612) and magnesium sulphate (0·324); there are also present small amounts of chlorides and bicarbonates. They have been classed amongst the *indeterminate thermal springs*. Some authors term them "weak sulphate of lime waters." They have a slight sulphurous smell. They are drunk and applied in the form of baths and douches.

These waters are readily tolerated by the stomach, and when drunk in large quantity aid the action of the mud baths as eliminative agents, by causing very free diaphoresis and diuresis. They augment the discharge of uric acid and urates.

They exercise a sedative action on the stomach, and are useful as table-waters for gouty and acid dyspeptics.

In the form of very hot douches and with douche-massage they also aid the action of the mud baths.

The vegeto-mineral ferruginous *mud*, which is collected on the spot, is saturated with sulphur water, which it encounters in the soil.

Patients are immersed in this black mud from half an hour to five hours at a time, in separate compartments so arranged that they can read, write, and feed in the bath. After the mud bath the patient is conveyed to the ordinary baths and washed. The mud is also applied in partial baths and as local applications. The mud baths and local applications are given at temperatures varying from 85° to 130° F.

The cases benefited by treatment by the mud baths at St. Amand are those of atonic gout, chronic rheumatism of the muscles and joints, rheumatoid arthritis, obstinate sciatica, some forms of paralysis, chronic diseases of the bones and joints, sprains, gunshot wounds, and some forms of uterine disease (hypertrophy and ulceration). The thickenings and infiltrations associated with chronic phlebitis and varicose veins are greatly benefited; also those associated with appendicitis. Nervous affections with trembling and inco-ordination and the lightning pains of the tabetic are greatly relieved; so are certain skin diseases, especially the dry forms associated with the rheumatic and gouty constitution.

Cases of neurasthenia are especially benefited by the combined mineral water and mud treatment. It must be remembered that at St. Amand a threefold curative agency is applied—the hot vegeto-mineral sulphurous mud, the thermal springs, and the forest air. There are beautiful shady walks in the adjacent forests.

The season is from May 15th to Sept. 30th. The warm months are most favourable for the mud treatment.

Saint Christan, in the Basses-Pyrénées to the south of Pau, is situated at the entrance of the narrow valley of Aspe, at an elevation of nearly 1,000 feet. It is approached from the station of Oloron, the terminus of a branch line from Pau, and is distant about six miles from the station. Its climate is mild, and is said to be particularly sedative.

It has five cold springs· (three only are utilised), which must be classed amongst the *weakly mineralised* cold earthy waters—as there are only 0·2 to 0·5 total solids per litre. The peculiarity of the Source des Arceaux is that it has a very small amount of copper—0·0003 per litre of sulphate of copper; it also has a little carbonate of iron and manganese (0·001). Another spring, Source du Prieuré, is tepid, its temperature being about 75° F., and it has a slightly sulphurous smell; it is more strongly mineralised, and contains more copper than the preceding. Finally, there is the Source du Pécheur, a small spring, cold and sulphurous, and only used for drinking.

The water is drunk in large quantities, two to ten glasses daily, including that taken *at meals*. Externally it is employed as general and local baths, fomentations, irrigations, *douches*, and *pulverisations*. The latter are especially popular, and form the chief treatment applied to many cases. They are modified and adjusted in every possible way.

The internal use of the water is attended with very free diuresis, and in gouty subjects with a free elimination of uric acid.

A speciality of this spa is the treatment of affections of the *mouth* and *tongue*: leucoplasia, leucokeratosis, ulcers, fissures, and indurative glossitis often associated with the preceding. Also leucoplasia vulvo-vaginal, chronic blepharitis and conjunctivitis are advantageously treated with the warm, fine pulverisations.

Certain skin affections, especially eczematous and lichenous forms and acne and psoriasis, are greatly benefited.

Besides certain forms of glossitis, atrophic or catarrhal, rhinitis and pharyngitis are suited to this treatment. Neurasthenia from overwork is beneficially influenced by the sedative action of the waters and climate.

The establishment is open all the year, but the

most favourable season is from the beginning of June to the end of September.

St. Gervais, in the Department of Haute-Savoie, France, is situated amidst grand and picturesque scenery in the immediate vicinity of Mont Blanc. It now has a station on the line which connects Geneva with Chamouni. The bath establishment is picturesquely placed in a gorge, about 2,000 feet above the level of the sea. The old bath was situated in the narrow gorge of the Bonnant, and was swept away by that torrent in July, 1892, with tragic results. The new establishment has been constructed in a more suitable situation.

As might be supposed, in an attractive mountainous district like this the number of interesting excursions amongst the surrounding valleys and mountains are numerous, and of all varieties of length and difficulty. The climate is said to be very mild and particularly sedative.

The village of St. Gervais lies higher than the spa (2,680 feet) and gets more sun, and the visitors to the baths can obtain good accommodation there. It is a more suitable place of residence during the heat of midsummer than the baths. Patients who come from Aix les Bains for an after-cure of mild mountain air at St. Gervais should choose the village to reside in rather than the baths.

The waters at St. Gervais have been described by some as *common salt* and *sulphated* waters, and by others as common salt, sulphated, and *sulphurous* waters; but only one of the three springs can correctly be termed sulphurous, and that is the Source du Torrent, which contains H_2S. The other two, the Sources de Goutard et de Mey, contain sodium sulphate 1·7 per litre, sodium chloride 1·7, calcium chloride 0·9, sodium bromide 0·032, and lithium sulphate 0·102. The proportion of *lithium* is relatively large.

The temperature of these springs varies from 102°

to 108° F. As they contain aperient sulphates and chlorides, they are mildly laxative in large doses.

They are employed internally and also externally in the various forms of baths and douches now usually found at all such establishments. They are adapted to the treatment of certain chronic *skin diseases*, especially those occurring in the neurotic, eczema, psoriasis, lichen, prurigo, etc.

They are given in *dyspepsia* associated with intestinal atony and constipation, in the gastro-hepatic affections of the gouty, in muco-membranous entero-colitis, in functional nervous disorders, as neurasthenia, neuralgia, and especially sciatica. The sulphur water is also useful in catarrh of the respiratory organs, in hepatic and uterine congestions, hemorrhoids, and phlebitis.

The baths at St. Gervais are especially indicated in those cases in which it is desired to combine with bath treatment the tonic and soothing influences of a mild mountain climate.

The season is from June 1st to Oct. 1st.

St. Honoré, a *thermal sulphur* bath in the Department of the Nièvre, is about 190 miles from Paris and is best reached viâ Nevers. Its station is Vaundenesse, from which it is distant about six miles.

It is situated at the foot of the mountains of Morvan at an elevation of about 900 feet above the sea, between two wooded hills, on one of which stands the Château de la Montagne. The country around is picturesque and is covered with magnificent woods of great extent most suitable for promenades and gentle excursions. The springs, of which there are four, vary in temperature from 80° to 88° F.

Their mineralisation is extremely feeble; they contain, however, free sulphuretted hydrogen, nitrogen, and carbonic acid gases, and a very small amount of sodium sulphide (0·002) and arsenate (0·001 to 0·004) They have a distinct though slight odour of sulphuretted hydrogen.

The waters are administered in various ways, but the chief methods employed at St. Honoré, besides drinking the waters, are *pulverisations* and *hot douches to the feet*. The latter are much prized there. The natural gases from the waters are also inhaled. Besides the application of the natural thermal springs, courses of hydrotherapy can be followed with ordinary water coming from the mountains.

The bath establishment has recently been remodelled, and provides all the most modern developments for mineral treatment.

The action of these waters is described as, ultimately, a local sedative action on the skin and mucous membranes, and a like general effect on the processes of nutrition, circulation, and on the nervous system. Its therapeutic effects are manifested in the treatment in the first place of diseases of the respiratory organs, especially in feeble and excitable patients, chronic catarrhs of the nose, pharynx, larynx, and bronchi, bronchial (humid) asthma, and the susceptibility thereto.

The treatment and the climate, the purity and sedative action of the air, are considered to be especially serviceable in cases in the early stage of *pulmonary tuberculosis*, if there is not much fever, and if the *cure* is a *prolonged* one.

It is useful, too, in certain skin diseases, especially eczema and impetigo; also in uterine catarrh.

Diseases of children are reported to be very favourably influenced by the climate and waters of St. Honoré—feeble, lymphatic children, with scrofulous tendencies, with chronic tonsillitis, adenitis, chronic bronchitis, or asthma. Every precaution is taken to prevent the spread of tuberculous infection. The best season for treatment is from June 15th to Sept. 15th.

St. Moritz-Bad, in the Upper Engadine, Switzerland, at an elevation of 5,800 feet, has *chalybeate* springs of undoubted value and importance.

Although these springs do not contain as much iron as some other well-known chalybeate spas, their richness in free carbonic acid, their digestibility, and the advantage of the fine bracing climate, impart to them special activity as tonic and restorative agents.

The St. Moritz springs have an ancient reputation, and in the sixteenth century were recommended in the writings of Paracelsus, after whom the principal spring is named; but they were practically unknown in this country until about the year 1860, when the Upper Engadine began to attract attention on account of its climatic advantages, and in a very short time became a fashionable resort, the popularity of which has gone on steadily increasing until, at the present time, it is one of the most frequented health resorts in Europe. Of its climatic character we shall have to treat fully in Part II. We must now restrict ourselves to an account of the waters of St. Moritz.

Until about twelve or fifteen years ago there were only two springs utilised at St. Moritz, situated near the Kurhaus. One, the weaker, was termed the Altequelle, and was used chiefly for the baths, and the other was named the *Paracelsus*, or the Neuequelle, and was and is the spring chiefly used for drinking.

In the year 1886 another spring was discovered situated not far from the others—the "Fontana Sarpant"—rather stronger in iron than the other two. In 1892 a new hotel was opened close to it—the Hotel Neues Stahlbad—and since then this spring has been utilised both for drinking and for baths.

The Paracelsusquelle, the one most commonly drunk, contains per litre 0·038 of bicarbonate of protoxide of iron, the Altequelle 0·033. Of sodium bicarbonate the former has 0·181, and the latter 0·272; of calcium bicarbonate the Paracelsus has as much as 1·301, and the Altequelle 1·226; and of magnesium bicarbonate the former 0·202, the latter 0·197. They also contain small amounts of sodium sulphate and chloride, and minute and unimportant quantities of various other ingredients. The springs are very rich in free carbonic acid.

The baths supplied chiefly from the Altequelle are heated by steam, after Pfriem's system, by which the water loses but little of its carbonic acid. Their chief effect is due to the action of the carbonic acid on the skin. For the douches ordinary water is used, flowing down at high pressure from adjacent slopes. This is heated by steam. The St. Moritz water is a pleasant refreshing water to drink, owing to the amount of free carbonic acid it contains. The water of the Altequelle is said to prove rather more digestible, with some invalids, owing to the amount of sodium bicarbonate in it.

The best time for drinking the water is about 10 or 11 a.m. Some—Germans chiefly—drink it early, before breakfast; but this plan does not suit delicate persons, and those who attempt it should warm the water, as drinking this cold water on an empty stomach has produced very depressing effects on some persons. If a glass is drunk at 10.30, another may be taken after a fifteen or twenty minutes' walk. Between 4.30 and 5.30 in the afternoon is another favourite time for drinking—between the afternoon walk and the dinner hour.

The Kurhaus and the baths are situated at a much lower level than the village of St. Moritz (an electric tramway connects them), on the flat ground that extends from the St. Moritz Lake to the Campfer Lake, and many patients prefer living at the hotels on the higher ground at St. Moritz-dorf. The Kulm, rather more than a mile from the baths, has an elevation of 6,100 feet. Many patients also stay at Campfer, which is about the same distance on the other side of the baths, and not quite so high as St. Moritz-kulm.

The course of waters at St. Moritz is well adapted to the treatment of anæmic neurasthenics who have adequate capacities of reaction to the vigorous stimulation of the climate. Anæmic patients, with very feeble circulation, and little or no latent power of reaction, get chilled and depressed there, and should be sent to lower levels. It is often needful to take aperients while drinking the St. Moritz waters, as the amount of lime they contain is apt to cause constipation.

For the same reason these waters often prove useful in cases of chronic diarrhœa, dependent on an irritable condition of the gastro-intestinal mucous membrane, and associated with nervous excitability. In such cases they should be warmed before drinking.

Cases of chlorosis and anæmia in young females, which fail to improve with ordinary ferruginous tonics administered at home, often recover rapidly at St. Moritz under the combined influence of the iron water, the gaseous baths, and the invigorating climate. Menstrual irregularities and catarrhal affections of the pelvic organs are often benefited by treatment at St. Moritz. Sterility due to such causes is said to be often cured. Persons who suffer from functional hepatic disorders, sluggish liver, hæmorrhoids, and constipation should avoid the St. Moritz waters.

It is sometimes advisable, especially with feeble, nervous, and excitable patients, to test their capacity for living in a climate of this kind by directing them to remain a few days at an intermediate station, such as Tarasp-Schuls or Vulpera (where good accommodation can be had), or at Churwalden or Bergun, or at Soglio in the Val Bregaglia. As the railway between Thusis and the Engadine is now open, it will be easy to stop at an intermediate station for a few days when good accommodation is provided.

The season for taking the waters at St. Moritz is from June 15th to Sept. 15th. The month of August is generally very crowded, and accommodation should always be secured beforehand.

St. Nectaire (Auvergne, Puy de Dôme) is situated at an altitude of 2,500 feet, about half-way between the towns of Issoire and Mont Dore, and about two and a-half hours by road from either place. It is usually approached from the railway station of Coudes or from that of Issoire, a drive of about two hours. It is close to some of the finest and most interesting mountain scenery in Auvergne. The romantic and imposing ruins of the Château de Murols are only three or four miles distant.

The numerous springs are divided into two groups — those at St. Nectaire le Haut (Mont Cornadore), and those at St. Nectaire le Bas, about three-quarters of a mile from one another. Twelve springs are utilised, having much the same composition, but three are hot, with a temperature of 103° to 120° F., and the rest are cold. These springs belong to the class of *alkaline and sodium chloride* waters. They contain about 2·5 grammes of sodium chloride, 2·2 of sodium bicarbonate, and 1·0 of calcium bicarbonate per litre. Some of the springs contain a little *iron*, especially La Source Rouge, and some are said to contain small amounts of lithium and arsenic.

These waters are used internally, in very varying doses, according to the case. They are also employed as baths of the natural temperature of the springs, or at a lower temperature by admixture of the water of the cold springs. Douches of all kinds are given, including carbonic acid gas douches. An *intermittent* spring at St. Nectaire le Haut, very rich in carbonic acid, is used as a vaginal douche, for the effect of an alternating gas and mineral water douche.

Other measures employed are massage, hydrotherapy, and the air cure on the neighbouring mountains.

A variety of maladies are treated at St. Nectaire, such as chronic rheumatism and neuralgia, and especially sciatica (after the acute period has passed), by the hot douches, etc.; atonic forms of dyspepsia and chronic gastric catarrh in rheumatic subjects; functional, uterine, and ovarian troubles in torpid, anæmic, and scrofulous persons. Latterly cases of albuminuria have been claimed as suitable for treatment at St. Nectaire, especially cases dependent on gastric and nutritional disturbances, as well as in certain forms of nephritis. The season is rather a short one, from June 20th to Sept. 15th, as the weather is apt to be boisterous and unsettled in the mountains of Auvergne earlier and later in the year.

St. Sauveur (Hautes Pyrénées, France), a *thermal sulphur* bath, situated in the valley of Luz, only a mile from the latter place. Luz is a charming little town ; the meadows around it are remarkable for their greenness, owing to being irrigated by numberless little mountain streams. It has been called "the most Pyrenean spot of the Pyrenees" ; it is the spot from which the tourist visits the Cirque de Gavarnie, the great show-place of the Pyrenees. A drive of three hours along a road of extraordinary wild and savage grandeur leads to the mountain village of Gavarnie ; but it is still a walk of two hours more before you reach the very depths of the magnificent cirque.

A good road, planted with trees, connects St. Sauveur with Luz. St. Sauveur is *par excellence* the ladies' bath of the Pyrenees, and it enjoyed for a time the personal patronage of the Emperor Napoleon III. and the Empress Eugénie. The springs are of comparatively feeble mineralisation ; but, like those of other Pyrenean spas, are characterised by containing sulphide of sodium, which gives them their characteristic odour.

St. Sauveur has a hot spring, La Source des Dames, of a temperature of 95° F., and a cold one, "La Hontalade." The former has sodium sulphide 0·022 per litre, and the latter 0·019. The cold spring is chiefly used for drinking. La Source des Dames contains much *barégine*, and feels soft and unctuous.

These waters are applied especially to the treatment of uterine maladies, and sterility dependent thereon, in neurotic, irritable constitutions, which need above all things soothing and sedative measures. They also prove useful in cases of inveterate muscular rheumatism in hypersensitive patients; in gastralgia and dyspepsia of a neurotic type; in cystitis, when not of uric acid origin. It has a mild mountain climate, being at an elevation of 2,360 feet above the sea. It has rather a high degree of humidity, and is rather subject to mists, but very free from winds. It is considered sedative, and is regarded as specially adapted to females who suffer from pelvic and other maladies into which nervous irritability enters as an important element. The season is from June 1st to Sept. 30th. St. Sauveur is about seven miles from Pierrefitte, which is about fourteen hours by rail from Paris. There is an electric railway between Pierrefitte and Luz.

Barzun, with a more exciting sulphur water, is only distant three-quarters of a mile (at Luz), and can be used by residents at St. Sauveur if desired.

Salies-de-Béarn.—This is a *strong salt* bath in the Basses-Pyrénées, twelve hours from Paris by express train. It lies at an elevation of 200 feet amongst the wooded hills that separate the *gave* of Pau from that of Oléron. Twenty miles to the south is the chain of the Pyrenees, and at the same distance to the west is the Atlantic, so that its climate is said to partake of the characters both of the mountain and of the seacoast—soft, temperate, sedative, and tonic. It is sheltered from the cold winds both to the north and east. It has an early spring, a hot summer, and a protracted autumn. The bath establishment is open all the year, but the spring and autumn are the best seasons for the cure.

The two springs generally used are the Bayaa and the Griffon. Two wells termed Oraas and the *eau mère* from the neighbouring salt works are also used.

The Bayaa is highly mineralised, having 256

grammes of salt to the litre; it also contains much vegetable organic matter, which imparts an unctuous feeling to it. The Griffon is less highly saturated.

A natural bath at Salies contains about 80 kilos of alkaline salts, 76 kilos of which are chlorides, 4 kilos sulphates and carbonates, 200 grammes bromides and iodides, and the rest silica, alumina, and organic substances.

The predominating bases are sodium, magnesium, and calcium. Of the *eaux mères*, the richest contains 487 grammes of salt per litre, 10 grammes of which are bromide and 1 gramme iodide of magnesium. The Source Oraas has 301 grammes of salt per litre.

Baths and douches, general or local, cold, tepid, or hot, and nasal irrigations, all of the pure water, are given. By mixture with ordinary water, in various proportions, baths of various degrees of strength are provided. Or they are modified in their action by the addition of *eau mère;* this is also used for compresses and lotions. Massage and out-of-door exercise in this picturesque country are additional means favourable to recovery.

These waters are regarded as exercising both a sedative and stimulating action on the peripheral nerves and vessels, and thereby producing an improvement in general tone—intestinal congestions are relieved, elimination is promoted, and nutrition is improved.

The cases most suitable for treatment at Salies are lymphatic children with scrofulo-tuberculous affections of the joints, bones, glands, skin, and mucous membranes. Young persons of nervous and lymphatic temperament with scoliosis, incontinence of urine, amenorrhœa, dysmenorrhœa, anæmia, and chlorosis. Women with uterine troubles causing sterility—atony, displacements, chronic inflammations, fibromata, and related nervous troubles. Pelvic and sciatic neuralgias.

There are numerous hotels of all kinds and prices, and furnished apartments. There are the usual amusements.

Salins-du-Jura.—A *cold salt* bath in the French Jura, not far from the Swiss frontier at Pontarlier, and approached by a branch line from Mouchard, between Dijon and Pontarlier, 402 kilometres from Paris. It is situated at an elevation of 1,170 feet, in a valley running north and south amongst mountains of about 2,000 to 3,000 feet high, and has a subalpine tonic climate. The nights are cool, and the north-east wind is sometimes troublesome. It has a dry soil, is supplied with an abundance of pure water, and is surrounded by vast forests.

Its salubrity is reported to be remarkable. Only one spring is utilised (Puits à Muire), and that contains 27 to 30 grammes of solids per litre, of which chloride of sodium forms 23 grammes. It also contains chlorides of magnesium and potassium, sulphate of lime, and a small amount of bromide of potassium (0·03). It has a slightly sulphurous odour.

The treatment at Salins consists mainly of baths of the salt water, raised artificially to a suitable temperature, and fortified by the addition of *eaux mères* in varying proportions, according to the nature of the case. The *eaux mère* obtained, after removal of the sodium chloride, at the salt works, in the usual way, has a total of 317 grammes of salt per litre, 158 being chloride of sodium and the rest composed of chlorides of magnesium and potassium, and 2 to 3 grammes of bromide of potassium. The water is occasionally prescribed internally to children in doses of a quarter to half a glass mixed with syrup. Salins has the usual bath establishment, with appliances for hydrotherapy, douches, irrigations, etc.

The *eaux mères* are also applied as compresses.

These waters have the physiological effects

usually experienced in the application of waters of this type; they are tonic, and stimulating, and promote the absorption of inflammatory exudations. If drunk they are diuretic and slightly laxative.

The purity of the air and the salubrity of the climate aid in no slight degree the tonic and remedial action of the waters.

As at like stations in France, "lymphatism and scrofulo-tuberculous" affections are the maladies specially adapted to treatment at Salins: scrofulous affections of the joints, bones, glands, mucous membranes, and skin; rickets; infantile paralysis; torpid chronic uterine affections; fibromata; old inflammatory exudations; and certain forms of chlorosis. The treatment at Salins is said to be better tolerated by sensitive and excitable patients than at some of the stronger salt baths. The best part of the season is from June 20th to Sept. 15th.

There are also good hotel accommodation and the usual amusements.

Salins Moutiers.—*See* Brides les Bains, page 116.

Salso Maggiore, in the province of Parma, Italy, is approached from the station of Borgo San Donnino, on the main line between Milan and Florence; from that station it is distant about five miles, and is connected with it by a steam tramway, which traverses the distance in half an hour. The whole journey from Milan to Salso Maggiore occupies about two and a-quarter hours.

Salso Maggiore is a small Italian town of about 1,200 inhabitants, situated at an elevation of nearly 500 feet above the sea at the extreme northern limit of the Apennines, where the foot hills join the plain of Lombardy. From the low hills behind the little town there is an uninterrupted view over this vast plain. The surrounding country can hardly be termed picturesque, although some of the visitors take a delight in driving to certain old castles which are to be found on the neighbouring hills.

Salso Maggiore has become widely known as a health resort on account of the remarkable wells which are found there. They are quite unlike those to be found at any other spa with which we are personally acquainted. It is scarcely correct to term them wells of mineral water, simply, because they are also wells of mineral oil and inflammable gases.

From these wells, which lie at a considerable depth below the surface, there is pumped up a mixture of strong brine and petroleum, and from this mixture an inflammable gas is given off, so abundantly that it pays to collect it and use it for illuminating purposes.

The fluid thus pumped up is allowed to flow into reservoirs, where it separates into two strata—the upper one consists of a dark brownish liquid, which is petroleum, the lower stratum consists of a strong brine.

The petroleum is collected and disposed of in commerce, and much of the brine is used, as at other brine wells, in the production of common salt. This is separated from the brine by boiling and evaporation. The less soluble sodium chloride is deposited, collected, and sold, and the more soluble salts remain in the residual liquid, which is termed *aqua madre*, and corresponds with the mother *lye*, or *Mutterlauge*, or *eaux mères* of other salt baths.

The gas given off from the mixture of brine and petroleum is collected and stored in gasometers, and used for lighting and heating purposes. "It contains two-thirds methane and one-third ethane with heavy hydrocarbons and carbonic acid gas" (*Lancet* Commissioner).

For *therapeutic* purposes the medical men at the baths used the *brine* pure, or concentrated, or diluted with plain hot water, or sometimes treated with carbonate of soda before concentration for the purpose of getting rid of the iron and some of the salts of lime and magnesium ; they also make use of the *aqua madre* in various ways, and they likewise use a *mud*—that is, a soft clay deposit formed in the reservoirs—for local application.

The natural brine, strongly smelling of petroleum, the *aqua madre,* and the deposited "mud" are, then, the three mineral agents used in the treatment of the cases that come to Salso Maggiore.

The *special peculiarity* of the place as a spa is the presence of petroleum in the brine, which renders it unfit for drinking, however much diluted. To what extent the *antiseptic* properties of the petroleum may promote or enhance the curative effects of the brine it is difficult to estimate. We are disposed to think it is not inconsiderable.

The analysis of the water recently made in the *Lancet* laboratory shows it to contain 169·31 grammes of solids per litre, 146·29 of which are sodium chloride, and 22·06 other chlorides—calcium, magnesium, ammonium, strontium, and lithium. The lithium chloride amounts to about 0·64, or "5 grains per pint," a relatively large proportion of this salt, but in a water that *cannot be drunk* the presence of this constituent is, of course, of minor importance.

The same remark applies to the presence of salts of strontium, of which there are 0·5 of the chloride and 0·48 of the sulphate.

The brine is also comparatively rich in compounds of iodine and bromine, as it contains per litre 0·066 of magnesium iodide and 0·30 of magnesium bromide. Its natural temperature is 68° F., and its specific gravity 1120.

The brine, as it is collected from the well, is turbid and brownish from precipitation of ferric oxide.

The composition of the *aqua madre,* which has become concentrated by evaporation, and relatively much richer in certain constituents from the separation of much of the sodium chloride, has been thus estimated:—In the strongest, having a density of 1270, there were found, per litre, 369·4 of solids, of which only 45·86 consisted of sodium chloride, while the calcium chloride had increased to 221·55, and the other chlorides (magnesium, strontium, ammonium, and lithium) to 96·15; the magnesium iodide to 1·0, and the magnesium bromide to 4·835.

Compared with other waters of the same type, it is exceptionally rich in compounds of lithium, bromine, and iodine. It has been calculated that there are in a pint of this *aqua madre* 80 grains of lithium chloride, 37 of magnesium bromide, and 8 of magnesium iodide. "They are also saturated with gaseous hydrocarbons, and these contain impurities of a bituminous nature and sulphur" (*Lancet* Commissioner).

As already mentioned, these waters are only suitable for external use, or for absorption, to whatever extent is possible, by the *inhalation* of the fine spray and vapour.

There are three chief bath establishments, the largest and most perfectly equipped being the "Terme Magnaghi." The baths are prepared of graduated and varying strength, according to the case; the average strength is obtained by diluting the natural brine, which has a density of 1120, till its specific gravity is reduced to 1096. These baths are ordered to be taken daily or on alternate days, and they can be obtained in the Grand Hôtel des Thermes, thus saving the residents the inconvenience of going out for them. The course lasts usually about three weeks. If it is thought desirable to increase the strength of the bath in iodine and bromine this can be done by adding *aqua madre.*

In the bath establishment special provision is made on an elaborate scale for treatment by *inhalation.* This is carried out in two ways; one is the inhalation of the spray by means of Seigle's steam atomisers, and the other is by admitting the patients into a special chamber (after the manner at Mont Dore), which is filled, by means of special apparatus, with the vapour and fine spray of the water. In this chamber the patients, enveloped in a suitable covering, sit, or promenade, or engage in gymnastic exercises, as exercise is regarded as promoting the absorption of the saline vapour. "The odour in this room is strongly suggestive of an iodo-organic compound, as well as oily" (*Lancet* Commissioner). A new building has recently been opened for the extension of this method of treatment. The *mud*, of which we have spoken, is saturated with the salts of the water, and also contains petroleum, and is applied locally in suitable cases as a kind of poultice, when a powerful local effect is desired.

Accessories to the mineral-water treatment are provided in the form of an X-ray room, a high-frequency apparatus, and an apparatus for the application of the ultra-violet rays; there is also adequate provision for skilled massage and for mechanotherapy. Special care is taken to maintain the baths, the linen, and everything used in the bath establishments perfectly clean and aseptic.

It must be admitted that the authorities have taken remarkable pains to give to Salso Maggiore the most complete possible equipment as a modern spa.

It only now remains to mention the class of cases that are best suited to treatment there. As in all spas of this type, scrofulous or tuberculous maladies stand in the foremost place, whether affecting the bones, the joints, the glands, or the skin. It was in such cases that the beneficial action of these waters was first noted, and also in cases of secondary and tertiary syphilis. It is the custom now to send parties of poor scrofulous patients to be treated at the sanatorium for three weeks at a time.

The sequelæ of gonorrhœal infection—especially of the pelvic organs in women—and arthritic troubles are also treated successfully. Chronic inflammatory exudations, peritoneal, pleural, and periarticular, are especially amenable to treatment there. It is believed that there is a considerable absorption of the saline and other substances contained in the water by the mucous membrane of the air passages from the inhalations, and these are found very serviceable in chronic catarrhal affections of the nose, throat, and upper air passages. Chronic bronchial catarrh and catarrhal asthma are also reported as benefited. The treatment of throat affections occupies a special prominence, and an eminent throat specialist resides there.

It is doubtful if these baths have any special advantage over others in the treatment of chronic articular affections dependent on gout and rheumatism. Every bath, or nearly every bath, claims credit for curing such cases. Doubtless the hot application of the mineral waters and the mineral mud are calculated to relieve some of the joint affections associated with these constitutional states.

There seems to be a general consent as to the value of this treatment in certain gynæcological cases, such as pelvic peritonitis and cellulitis, endopara- and endoperimetritis, and in menstrual troubles. It is also said to remove the causes of sterility in certain cases.

Certain anæmic, chlorotic, and neurasthenic cases are said to improve there.

Traumatic cases—old painful cicatrices—dislocations, fractures, etc., are reported as particularly benefited, especially by the local application of the *mud* or *fango*.

With regard to some of these maladies it may perhaps be said that, as in many similar resorts, the net has been cast rather too widely, and that the tendency has been to over-estimate the extent of applicability of this spa.

Excellent accommodation can be obtained at the Grand Hôtel des Thermes, which is under very capable management.

The season is from April 1st to the end of October, but the most suitable time for English visitors is the spring and autumn—April, May, June, September, and October. In July and August, and sometimes in the early part of September, it is unpleasantly hot.

Salzschlirf.—A spa situated in Hesse-Nassau, near Fulda, with a station on the Giessen-Fulda Railway. It lies at an elevation of 820 feet, in an agreeable valley, between the wooded heights of the Vogelsberge and the Rhön mountains.

It has a *cold gaseous common salt* spring, the Bonifaciusbrunnen, and some importance is attached to the amount of *lithium chloride* it contains, 0·21 grammes per litre, and to the presence of minute amounts of magnesium bromide and iodide, 0·005 of each. Of sodium chloride it contains 10·0 per litre, of calcium sulphate 1·5, and of magnesium chloride 1·0.

It is also fairly rich in carbonic acid gas.

Of the other springs, one, the Templebrunnen, has less lithium but more of the other salts, the Kinderbrunnen is much weaker, and the Schwefelbrunnen also has much less solids, but it contains H_2S, six volumes per litre. A *purgative* water obtained from the neighbouring village, Grossenluekler, is also used there. Besides sodium chloride (15·4) it contains magnesium sulphate (1·3), and calcium sulphate and carbonate (1·6 each), and a little carbonate of iron. The springs are used as baths, and the Bonifaciusbrunnen is drunk and used for gargles and inhalations. Mud baths are also available.

The drinking is usually done early in the morning, between 7 and 8 a.m., and you are directed to sip the water, taking a quarter of an hour to drink each glass. More water is taken again at 5 p.m.

The baths are taken at first for ten minutes at a time, and this period is increased by five minutes daily, until the full period of thirty-five minutes is reached.

These waters are reported as of remarkable value in the treatment of chronic gout and the various manifestations of the uric acid diathesis, and in impaired metabolism and nutrition generally.

They are also useful in rheumatism, renal and biliary calculus, cystitis from uric acid, gastro-intestinal catarrh, obesity, and some female complaints. The St. Boniface spring is said to be the richest of all the spas in Germany in lithium. The water is largely exported.

The season is from May 1st to the end of September.

Schinznach is a popular Swiss *thermal sulphur* bath, in a very accessible and pleasant situation, being on the Bâle-Olten-Zürich Railway. It lies at an altitude of about 1,100 feet, in the valley of the Aar. The rapid current of this river flows along between the bath and the line of railway, and imparts a refreshing movement to the air, even during the hottest seasons.

The bath establishment is distinct from the village and is surrounded by its own grounds, and has been sometimes termed the "Habsburger-Bad," from the circumstance that the ruined castle of Habsburg is on a neighbouring height. Extensive woods are in the immediate vicinity of the spa. Schinznach has a mild and temperate climate, but it can be hot in summer; the adjacent woods, however, afford cool and shady retreats.

The temperature of its warm sulphur spring seems to be variable, and to range between about 83° and 95° F. It is rich in sulphuretted hydrogen, and of its solid constituents of 2·1 per litre, calcium sulphate forms nearly one half (1·0), and sodium chloride 0·6; there is also a minute amount of *sulphide* of calcium (0·008).

. The bath establishment, which also serves as a hotel, is well provided with the appliances needed to give ordinary baths, or vapour baths, or nasal and local douches, and for the inhalation of the pulverised water, or of the gases given off by it. It has a special building devoted to pulverisation, inhalations, and gargling.

It is sometimes found necessary to heat the natural water for the baths, which are occasionally ordered of very long duration, especially in certain chronic skin affections requiring long *maceration*—those baths may be prolonged to one and a-half or two hours. The waters are also taken internally before the baths.

This spa has recently been much recommended in cases of chronic gout and rheumatism, but its established reputation is chiefly in connection with the treatment of chronic, obstinate *skin affections*, especially eczema.

The inhalations, etc., are also found useful in chronic catarrh of the respiratory organs, in naso-pharyngeal catarrh, and chronic bronchitis. In syphilis and in metallic intoxications the treatment is also useful. In scrofulous affections and in leucorrhœa and other female maladies it has proved serviceable. The bromo-iodide water of the adjacent Wildegg spring is also employed there.

The season is from May 1st to Oct. 1st.

Schlangenbad (in Nassau) is beautifully situated about midway between Eltville, a port on the Rhine, and Schwalbach. Steam trams run to it from Eltville. It is difficult to imagine a more picturesque spot for a watering-place than Schlangenbad—a winding valley, turning upon itself with a sharp bend, so that one end of the village is brought nearly on a line with the other, surrounded by high wooded hills, their lower slopes covered with scattered villas surrounded by flower-gardens and bright green lawns —such is Schlangenbad. A pretty, quiet, peaceful retreat. It has a Kursaal, with shady walks and seats around, nice clean hotels and three bath-houses, one quite modern, where the patients can live in apartments, some of which are even elegantly furnished, at a fixed price. On the ground floor are the baths; these are extremely well arranged. Those in the modern bath-house are really luxurious. Reclining in one of those sumptuous baths, the water, with its delicious softness and pleasant temperature, seems to envelop the whole body with a sort of diffused caress; while, from some peculiar property in the water, it gives a singular lustrous beauty to the skin, which seems to be suddenly endowed with a remarkable softness and brilliancy. It certainly tends to put one upon the best possible terms with oneself, and one can readily understand the calming influence which these baths are found to exert over irritable and disturbed states of the nervous system.

Schlangenbad, 900 feet above the sea, belongs to the group of so-called *indifferent earthy* baths, and is very feebly mineralised, having only 0·4 of solids per litre, and thus resembles Gastein, Pfaeffers, and Wildbad; the natural temperature of the water ranges from 81° to 89° F.; it is raised in the baths to from 87° to 92°. Less stimulating than the same kind of water at higher temperatures, as at Teplitz and Gastein, it is therefore more suitable to those sensitive organisations whose nervous systems above all things need a soothing treatment, and its comparatively slight elevation above the sea accords with this indication, for its climate is mild, though fresh and equable. The surrounding woods afford every opportunity for open-air exercise and lounging, and the quiet yet pleasing life there makes this place the type of cheerful repose. It produces a calming and at the same time refreshing effect upon the invalid requiring gentle management, and is therefore particularly suited to irritable forms of neurasthenia. Delicate ladies who suffer from hysterical and other forms of nervous excitability and exhaustion and chronic uterine maladies, and who need repose, are especially suited for this spa.

Painful forms of spinal disease, with loss of muscular power, unable to bear the stimulating treatment of the thermal salt baths, are often soothed and benefited by treatment there. Milk and whey cures can also be had.

The season is from May 1st to Oct. 1st.

Schwalbach, or Langen-Schwalbach (Hessen-Nassau), is perhaps the most renowned of all European *chalybeate* spas. Although Schwalbach is nearly 1,000 feet above the sea, it is much hotter than might be expected in a place of that elevation, owing to its being so much protected by the hills around, so that it becomes very hot in the floor of the valley, during the middle of the day, in the months of July and August. As the visitors to Schwalbach are for the most part anæmic patients, the life there is, as may be imagined, very quiet, and devoted chiefly to drinking the waters and bathing in them. Schwalbach possesses a good Kursaal. The hotels are good, and situated close to the springs and the bath-house, but many persons live in lodging-houses, which are numerous and comfortable, and in some cases moderate in price. Schwalbach is especially an iron cure. It is *the* iron cure of Germany. Its water belongs to the class of simple iron springs in which the iron exists as the chief constituent, unassociated with any ingredients which can complicate or interfere with its action. It is one of the strongest and purest iron waters in Europe. It also has the advantage of possessing a very large proportion of free carbonic acid, which makes it sparkling and pleasant to drink, increases its digestibility, and renders it valuable as a medium for bathing in.

There are only two springs that are used for drinking—the Weinbrunnen and the Stahlbrunnen. The Stahlbrunnen contains much more iron than the Weinbrunnen and rather more carbonic acid. The former contains per litre 0·08, and the latter 0·06 of bicarbonate of iron. Minute amounts of manganese are said to be also found in these springs. There are many other springs, the water supplied by which is used for the baths, and others which are not utilised at all.

The bathing arrangements at Schwalbach are good. The chief benefit of the bath being believed to consist in the action of the carbonic acid, which the water contains, on the skin, it is so contrived that as little as possible of this gas shall escape in the conveyance of the water to the bath, while the bath itself is of copper, and is provided with a double bottom. Between the two bottoms is a chamber, into which steam is conveyed for the purpose of heating the water to the required temperature. As the water in the bath becomes heated it gives off myriads of bubbles of carbonic acid gas, and the contact of this gas with the skin is considered to have a beneficial effect upon the superficial vessels and nerves. There can be no doubt that the gas does exercise a distinct influence on the skin, which becomes red and experiences a diffused tingling sensation.

Peat baths are also given at Schwalbach. The peat is obtained in the neighbourhood, and is mixed with the mineral water and heated by steam in wooden tubs to the temperature required. It is thought best in some cases to commence the treatment with the peat baths and follow on with the chalybeate baths.

The temperature of the iron baths is generally lowered, if the patient can bear it, as the course advances. A period of repose is advisable after the peat bath. Abdominal massage has been found useful in some cases that are constipated by the iron waters.

The course at Schwalbach is considered especially applicable to cases of bloodlessness, arising as a consequence of hæmorrhages, or of any exhausting disease, or in retarded convalescence from acute maladies; also in anæmia, so often associated with disturbances of the nervous system—hysteria, etc. In these latter cases, the use of the tonic water, the soothing baths, and the influence of the calm but, at the same time, cheerful surroundings of the place should exercise an undoubtedly curative effect. In leucorrhœa and chronic uterine affections which are often treated with advantage at Schwalbach, vaginal douches of the mineral water are found serviceable.

The season is from May 1st to Oct. 15th. Those who suffer much from heat had better choose the earlier or later parts of the season.

Soden is one of the several *common salt* spas which are found on the southern slope of the Taunus mountains. It is connected with the Taunus railway by a branch at Höchst, and so is brought within half an hour of Frankfort. It is about nine miles from Homburg, and is prettily situated, at an elevation of about 450 feet, in a valley bounded to the north by wooded hills, which form, as it were, the base of the two highest peaks of the chain, the Alt König and the Feldberg. It lies open to the south, but is protected also by hills of gentle elevation to the east and west. From its protected situation the climate of Soden is essentially a mild one, the air is balmy and soft and still, though the close vicinity of the mountain chain often causes a freshness in the evening air which is grateful and invigorating. It is possible there for invalids to spend much time in the open air with advantage, and this they often do, extended in hammocks suspended from the branches of trees. It is found that persons with chronic catarrhal conditions of the throat and air-tubes, and cases of consumption that require soothing rather than bracing treatment, do well at Soden.

Cases which require bracing are not suited to it. Cases of purely nervous asthma do not do well there, while the catarrhal cases improve. Soden has a great number of mineral springs, twenty-four altogether, and, although they vary scarcely at all in the nature of their ingredients, they vary greatly in their quantity and in temperature. Their temperature ranges from 52° to 86° F., and their contents of chloride of sodium from 2·4 to 15 grammes per litre. They vary much also in their richness in carbonic acid gas; some contain scarcely any, others, such as the Champagnerbrunnen, a great deal. There are springs as strong as those of Homburg and Kissingen; there are others which are as pleasantly mild and gaseous as seltzer-water. The milder springs have been found of great use in cases of chronic bronchial catarrh. Such are the Warmbrunnen and Milchbrunnen, containing only 2 to 3 grammes per litre of common salt; these are largely drunk in catarrhal affections of the respiratory organs. Some of the springs contain an appreciable amount of iron.

There is one—the Soolensprudel—used in the preparation of gaseous thermal *Sool* baths which, besides being very rich in carbonic acid gas, contains also a little H_2S. A chalybeate spring can be drunk, a short distance from Soden, at Neuenhain. Soden possesses a conveniently arranged bath-house, where douches and many varieties of baths can be given, including salt baths and gaseous salt baths; it also has inhalation rooms for the treatment of chronic laryngitis and bronchitis. Scrofulous children are said to do well at Soden. Dr. Dettweiler's Kuranstalt Falkenstein is only about three miles off.

The season is from May to the end of September.

Spa, in Belgium, close to the German frontier, is agreeably situated in a valley of the Ardennes, at an elevation of about 1,000 feet above the sea. Having been a popular European resort for centuries, it has had the distinction of giving the name of "spa" to all places resorted to for the purposes of treatment by mineral waters.

Spa is very fortunate in its surroundings. The town itself is beautifully and tastefully laid out, but it is in the beauty of the drives and walks on the hills and high ground around that its real charm is to be found. The country roads are lined with avenues of tall trees, which afford pleasant shade at all times of the day and in the hottest seasons; and although Spa itself lies in a hollow, the air on the hills around is most fresh and exhilarating.

The climate, then, of Spa may be said to be that of the surrounding forests and hills or high plateaux; that is to say, bright and fresh, without being subject to great heat in summer, but, as in all hilly countries, subject to sudden and great changes of temperature occasionally.

Its springs belong to the class of pure, or almost pure, *gaseous chalybeate* waters, and contain much free carbonic acid gas. There are eight or nine altogether, but only two are found in the town; the rest are scattered about in picturesque spots on the adjacent hills. The springs situated in the town, and which are chiefly used, are Ponhon Pierre le Grand, and Ponhon Prince de Condé. It is maintained that these springs contain more iron than any of the other European iron waters, and this may be the case, although the available analyses do not all agree as to the exact amount found in these *sources*.

Ponhon Pierre le Grand, the strongest, is said to contain, per litre, 0·112 grammes of bicarbonate of iron; the others to contain 0·08, 0·06, and 0·04 per litre. They contain also small quantities of sodium bicarbonate and chloride. But more recent and authoritative analyses are to be desired. The water is ordered to be sipped, or drunk slowly through a glass tube, in order that the stomach may not be chilled by a large, hasty draught of the *cold* water. The waters are prescribed in doses of two to five glasses daily of six ounces each, and for persons who are strong enough, and who find it agrees with them to do so, they are ordered to be taken in the early morning, between 6 and 8 a.m.; but this hour rarely suits English patients, and it is by no means desirable to disturb feeble anæmic persons at that early hour. For such patients about an hour before lunch is a good time; and again in the afternoon, about an hour and a-half or two hours before dinner.

Those who drink at the more distant springs can take their second dose of water in their afternoon drive at the Tonnelet, the Marie-Henriette, or the Géronstère.

There is a well-arranged bath establishment in the town, having a special spring of its own, the Nivèze, which arises about a mile and a-half from Spa. These baths, as at Schwalbach, are believed to produce their tonic effect mainly by the action of the carbonic acid on the nerves of the skin.

At Spa much value is placed on the use of the hip bath of *warm running* water, so that the temperature is kept constant during the bath. It is prescribed in cases of leucorrhœa and female pelvic diseases, the local action of the water being ensured by the use of a wire vaginal speculum during the bath, which the patient can herself introduce.

The methods of hydrotherapy, and especially the use of cold water douches, are much in vogue at Spa, and contribute, no doubt, greatly to the tonic effect of the iron waters.

Mud baths are also in use there. They are made by mixing a turf which abounds in the neighbourhood with the mineral water.

If the chalybeate waters cause constipation, it is usual to give an imported Hungarian bitter water, such as Apenta, to act as a laxative.

Next, as to the class of cases treated at Spa: Spa is particularly adapted to the treatment of the many disturbances of health in women more or less closely associated with *anæmia* and *chlorosis*, *e.g.*

menstrual irregularities, menorrhagia and tendency to abortion; vaginal and uterine catarrh and sterility depending on these conditions and on general debility; in some forms of atonic dyspepsia, with a tendency to diarrhœa, the treatment proves of value; also in cases of depressed health from prolonged residence in hot climates; in neurasthenia, migraine, and neuralgia, and other nervous affections connected with anæmia. The baths are usually given hot in neuralgic and rheumatic cases.

The *mud* baths are found specially useful in chronic gouty and rheumatic affections—in cases of stiff joints, in muscular atrophy (combined with massage); in tabes; in the removal of pelvic exudations; and in some cases of gouty kidney.

Spa is a very suitable place for an after-cure for patients returning to England from a course of treatment at many of the German baths, such as Kissingen, Carlsbad, and Marienbad.

The season is from May to October.

Strathpeffer, a Scottish Highland *cold sulphur* bath in Ross-shire, has come into considerable repute in recent years. Though situated in the north of Scotland, it has a comparatively mild climate owing to its position in a very sheltered valley. Evergreens grow there luxuriously, and plants bloom out of doors as freely as in some mild south of England districts. Indeed, in certain seasons the climate may appear somewhat relaxing.

There are two kinds of water utilised at Strathpeffer—a *cold sulphur* water, the principal therapeutic agent of the spa, and a *cold weak chalybeate* water.

The sulphur water is feebly mineralised, but contains potassium and sodium sulphide amounting together to ·027 per litre, and a variable amount of H_2S. It also contains sulphates and carbonates of lime and magnesia in small amount, and a little sulphate of sodium. The chalybeate water ("Saint's"

Well) is very feebly mineralised, and contains about 0·035 per litre of carbonate of iron. The recently utilised Lady Cromartie Well is said to be a stronger sulphur water than that whose composition has just been stated.

The bath establishment is not a large one, but baths and douches of various kinds are prepared and given there. For the sulphur baths the sulphur water is usually warmed by the addition of one-third of hot rain water.

Peat baths are prepared from peat brought from adjacent hills, and mixed with warm water to the temperature required. Pine baths are prepared with pine extract obtained from Germany. Brine baths can also be obtained. Friction, massage, and packing are used in suitable cases. The most important part of the treatment is, however, the internal use of the waters. The usual time for drinking the waters is about 8 a.m., and again about 11.30 a.m.

The cases mainly treated at this spa are those of chronic gout and rheumatism, and patients are recommended not to rest content with a single visit, but to repeat it for at least two seasons. Caution is needed in dealing with cases of gout, as acute attacks are occasionally induced during, or shortly after, treatment there. Cases of sciatica are said to be rarely benefited by treatment at Strathpeffer. Certain cases of skin disease do well there, especially those of eczema and psoriasis, particularly if associated with a gouty constitution, or dependent upon gastro-hepatic disorders. Dyspeptic symptoms in the same class of patients are also benefited, and for them the mildly bracing climate is a valuable auxiliary. The hotel accommodation is simple but good. Comfortable lodgings can also be obtained. The season is from May to October, but the spa is open all the year. It is about twenty miles from Inverness and five from Dingwall. The journey from London takes about fifteen hours.

Sacedon, or La Isabella, a *simple thermal* spa in Spain, Province of Guadalajara, temperature 84° F.

Sail les Bains, Department Loire, France, has *simple thermal* feebly mineralised springs, temperature 80° to 95° F., also a weak chalybeate and a sulphur spring. It is situated at an altitude of 800 feet, forty minutes' drive from the railway station, St. Martin d'Estréaux, between Moulins and Lyons. The water is exported.

Sail sous Couzan, a French table-water, largely exported under the name of "Couzan" water. The spring is situated in the Department of the Loire—railway station between Clermont and St. Etienne. It contains bicarbonates of sodium, calcium, potassium, and magnesium, and a small amount of iron and much free carbonic acid.

Saint Alban, a French table-water, largely exported; the springs are situated in the Department of the Loire, about two hours' (driving) from Roanne, on the line between Moulins and Lyons; the waters contain bicarbonates of sodium, calcium, and magnesium, with much free carbonic acid – the Source César contains 0·023 per litre of bicarbonate of iron. In the bath establishment *special* use is made of the carbonic acid gas collected from the springs for inhalations, baths, and local douches.

Saint Antoine de Guagno, in Corsica, forty miles north of Ajaccio, has *thermal sulphur* springs, temperature 124° F. The Grande Source contains 0·02 per litre of sodium sulphide. It is used in the treatment of old gunshot wounds and skin affections. There is a military hospital there.

Saint Boès, a *strong cold* (Pyrenean) *sulphur* spring, only used for exportation. It contains sodium sulphide and H_2S, and is bituminous. It is reported to act beneficially in catarrhal affections of the respiratory and intestinal mucous membranes, and in pulmonary tuberculosis.

Saint Galmier, a French table-water, largely exported. The springs, of which La Source Badoit is the chief, contains mixed alkaline and earthy bicarbonates, two grammes per litre, and small amounts of sulphates and chlorides and much free carbonic acid.

Saint Laurent les Bains, in France, Department Ardèche, has *simple thermal* springs, of a temperature of 128° F. It is picturesquely situated, at an altitude of 2,700 feet, six miles from La Bastide railway station.

Saint Olafs, Norway, close to Modum, a popular resort, with a *chalybeate* spring and *mud* baths, picturesquely situated, at an altitude of about 500 feet.

Saint Pardoux. *See* Bourbon l'Archambaut, p. 107.

Saint Vallier, in the Vosges, has *earthy* waters, like those of Contrexéville.

Saint Yorre, near Vichy, has *strong cold alkaline* springs used for exportation.

Salies du Salut, France, Haute Garonne, with a railway station on the branch line between Boussens and Saint Girons, lies on the Salut stream, at an altitude of 960 feet, and has *cold common salt* waters, containing 30 grammes per litre of sodium chloride and 3 of calcium sulphate. It also has a cold sulphur spring containing calcium sulphide 0·11 per litre. There is a children's sanatorium, connected with the hospital at Toulouse.

Salins Moutiers. *See* Brides les Bains, p. 116.

Saltburn by the Sea, Yorkshire, has a bath establishment in which *brine* baths are given, the brine being brought from the brine wells at Middlesbrough. This brine has 250 grammes per litre of sodium chloride. In the same establishment there is provision for various kinds of douches, electric and vapour baths, and sea-water swimming baths.

Salvator spring in Szinye-Lipocz, near Epiries, in Hungary. It is exported, and belongs to the *simple alkaline* group. It is cold and gaseous, and is reported to contain 0·3 grammes of bicarbonate of sodium in a litre, 0·9 carbonate of magnesium, 0·9 borate of sodium, and 0·2 of bicarbonate of lithium. It has been recommended in renal affections associated with the uric acid diathesis, in gout and rheumatism, and in gastric and bronchial catarrh.

Salzbrunn. *See* Obersalzbrunn, p. 281.

Salzburg, in Transylvania, is a popular *brine* bath, with brines of various strengths—from 50 to 150 grammes of common salt per litre — containing also sodium iodide 0·8 to 0·25 per litre. It is situated at an altitude of 1,600 feet.

Salzdetfurth, in Hanover, in the valley of the Lamme, amongst the foot hills of the Harz mountains, at an elevation of 500 feet, has *common salt* wells which are used, more or less diluted, for baths, inhalations, gargling, and drinking, in the various maladies in which such waters are applied. Season, May 1 to Oct. 1.

Salzerbad, Lower Austria, has waters containing *common salt and sulphate of sodium* : 14·1 per litre of the former and 4·6 of the latter, and 2·8 of calcium chloride. It is situated at an altitude of 2,000 feet.

Salzhausen, a small bath in the Grand Duchy of Hesse, possessing *cold salt* wells and wells containing iron, lithium, and sulphur, in addition to sodium chloride. The salt wells are weak, containing about ten grammes per litre of sodium chloride and 1·0 of magnesium chloride, and some free carbonic acid. They are concentrated, and often fortified by *Mutterlauge* for baths.

It is at the foot of the Vogelsberg, at an elevation of 470 feet, and is close to Nidda railway station.

Salzuflen, in the principality of Lippe-Detmold, with a station on the Herford-Detmold line, has three *salt* wells, used for baths and drinking—for the latter purpose one of the springs is diluted and artificially aërated with carbonic acid.

Salzungen is in the Duchy of Saxe-Meiningen, Germany, finely situated in the Werrathal, at an elevation of 780 feet, on the south-western slope of the Thuringian Forest. It has a station on the Eisenach-Lichtenfels line, and has *salt* wells varying in strength from 30 to 250 grammes per litre. The *Mutterlauge* obtained from the salt water is available for fortifying the baths. It contains much magnesium, chloride, and small amounts of magnesium bromide and iodide. Inhalations of the salt-water spray, *Moor* baths, and douches are also given, and the water of the weaker springs is drunk.

San Bernardino, in Switzerland, on the southern side of the Bernardino Pass, between Splügen and Bellinzona, about equally distant from Thusis and Bellinzona stations, has *cold gaseous earthy chalybeate* springs with 0·035 per litre of bicarbonate of iron, 0·01 bicarbonate of strontium, and 1·2 sulphate of calcium,

Its altitude is 5,320 feet. Cases of anæmia and chlorosis, cases of convalescence, and all such as require bracing mountain air in combination with iron waters, are suitable for this resort.

Sanct Lorenz, in Upper Styria, with a station on the Rudolfsbahn, has two *gaseous alkaline common salt* springs, largely exported. The principal spring contains sodium carbonate 1·0 gramme per litre, sodium chloride 2·7, bicarbonate of iron 0·5, etc. The weaker spring contains only 0·03 of bicarbonate of iron, and is known as "Austrian Selters" water.

Sandefjord, in Norway, situated on a small fjord on the North Sea, four or five hours by rail from Christiania, has *cold gaseous common salt* and *sulphur* springs used for drinking and bathing; also a cold *weak* salt spring, and a *chalybeate* spring said to contain 1·29 per litre of sulphate of iron. Cold and hot sea-water baths can also be had. A sort of sulphurous slime, collected from the fjord, is used for frictions and as hot applications in chronic articular rheumatism. There is also a practice there of applying live jelly fishes as counter-irritants to the skin in neuralgias and chronic rheumatism.

Sandrock, Isle of Wight, near Blackgang Chine, has a *chalybeate* spring.

San Marco, in Central Italy, three miles from Castiglione della Pescaja, has a *gaseous alkaline* water, largely *exported*, usually after the addition of more carbonic acid gas. It is reported to contain, per litre, sodium bicarbonate 1·3, magnesium bicarbonate 1 6,and lithium bicarbonate 0·26.

San Pedro do Sul, a Portuguese *thermal sulphur* bath of high temperature, about 159° F.

San Pietro Montagone, one of the "Euganean Thermæ," in the neighbourhood of Abano, Italy, has very *hot* waters, of the same character as those of Abano, and feebly mineralised.

Santa Agueda, in the North of Spain, Province of Guipuzcoa, has *cold earthy sulphuretted hydrogen* waters, and an *iron* spring.

Santa Catarina, Italy, about seven miles fron Bornio, through the picturesque Val Furva, possesses a *strong chalybeate* spring. It is 5,700 feet above the sea, in an exceedingly beautiful situation, surrounded by a semi-circle of magnificent snow mountains. Being on the southern side of the Alps, its climate is doubtless less bracing than the same elevation on the northern side (like St. Moritz) would be.

Santenay, France, the Côte d'Or. A *cold sodium chloride* water, containing also lithium chloride and sulphates of sodium magnesium and calcium. Its total mineralisation amounts to 9·2 grammes per litre, of which 5·2 is sodium chloride. The lithium salt amounts to 0·092 and the sodium sulphate to 2·15. It is chiefly a drinking cure, but baths, douches, and massage are also employed. It is recommended in cases of gout and gravel, and biliary and renal calculi; also in functional hepatic and gastro-intestinal affections attended with constipation. It is reached by a branch line from Chaguy, between Dijon and Macon. An automobile conveys patients from the station to the baths. It is distant about seven hours from Paris.

Saxon, a Swiss bath in the Rhone valley, with a station on the line between Lausanne and Brigue, at an elevation of 1,560 feet. Its *earthy* waters are cold and very feebly mineralised—less than one gramme of solids to the litre. They are reputed to contain small amounts of calcium and magnesium bromides and iodides, but they are found to be absent, intermittently, for short periods—the intermittances not exceeding two or three days. Whatever popularity these waters may have had at one time has almost wholly passed away. The place is very hot in summer, and mosquitoes are very active. The water is exported.

Schandau, on the Elbe, in Saxon Switzerland, at an altitude of 400 feet, has a *weak chalybeate* spring containing, per litre, 0·015 bicarbonate of iron and some bicarbonate of lime, used only for drinking. Various accessory remedies are applied, as Franzensbad *Moor baths*, artificial brine and carbonic acid baths, pine-needle, electric, vapour, and hot-air baths. Hydrotherapy, *fango*, massage, and gymnastics. The place is frequented by tourists, and has a station on the Dresden-Bodenbach line. The season is from May 1 to Oct. 1.

Schimberg, a Swiss *cold alkaline and sulphurous* bath of the same character as Heustrich, but with rather less sulphur. It is situated on the western slope of the mountain of the same name, at an elevation of 4,670 feet, and about two and a-half hours' drive from the station of Entlebuch, on the Berne-Lucerne line. It has a relatively humid climate for a place of that altitude. Somewhat sudden changes of temperature and a certain amount of fog must also be looked for. It is protected from the north-east winds. It would not seem to be quite a typical resort for chronic catarrhal affections of the respiratory organs, for the treatment of which its waters are regarded as specially suitable. The sulphur spring is feebly mineralised, containing sodium bicarbonate chiefly – this salt forms 0·683 out of a total of 0·773 of solids per litre—it also contains sodium sulphide 0·03, and H_2S 6·7 c.c. For the baths a spring termed "ferruginous" is utilised. It contains the same ingredients as the sulphur spring without the sulphur. Season, June 10 to September 20.

Schmalkalden, a small bath with a weak *common salt* spring, in Hesse-Nassau.

Schmiedeberg, a small town with *iron-mud* baths, in Saxony, with a station on the Wittenberg-Eilenberg line.

Schwalheim, dietetic table-waters. *See* Nauheim, p. 269.

Schwarzbach, a *weak earthy chalybeate* spring in Prussian Silesia.

Schwefelberg, Switzerland, two and a-half hours from Gurnigel, at an altitude of 4,570 feet, has the same kind of *cold sulphurous* waters as Gurnigel.

Schweizerhalle, a Swiss *brine* bath in Canton Bâle, near Pratteln railway station.

Sciacca, in Sicily, twenty-two miles from the railway station Castelvetiano, has *hot common salt* and *sulphur* springs, temperature 125° F., also hot springs (100° F.) containing iron. Here were the ancient "Thermæ Selinuntinæ." Near at hand are the natural vapour baths (*stufe*) of San Calogero.

Segeberg, a *salt* bath in Schleswig-Holstein.

Selters—Niederselters.—Natural seltzer water, an alkaline table-water containing 2·0 grammes per litre of common salt.

Serneus, a Swiss *cold sulphur* spring, containing H_2S. The bath establishment is at an elevation of 3,240 feet, in the Praetigau valley on the Landquart-Davos line.

Shanklin, Isle of Wight, has a

chalybeate spring with 0·068 per litre of carbonate of iron.

Shap Wells, three miles from Shap, in the centre of Westmorland, and some distance from a railway station—waters containing alkaline and earthy chlorides and sulphates, and a little iron and silica, with similar properties to those of Leamington.

Siradan, Sainte Marie (Hautes Pyrénées), in a pleasant valley with a lake, a short distance from Saléchan, on the line of railway from Toulouse to Luchon, is about twelve miles from the latter place. It has four springs, two of which are *ferruginous* and cold, and two warm; the latter resemble greatly in composition, character, and uses those of Contrexéville, but they are more feebly mineralised. They belong to the class of *earthy* or calcareous waters. They enjoy considerable local popularity. The iron springs are used for cases of anæmia, chlorosis, and general debility. Siradan is well sheltered by mountains, at an elevation of 1,350 feet. It has a soft and temperate climate, and its season is unusually long—from April 1 to Nov. 30.

Soden - Salzmunster, *gaseous common salt* wells, and *Sool* baths, in Hesse-Nassau, with a station on the Bebra-Frankfurt-am-M. Railway.

Sodenthal, in northern Bavaria, near Aschaffenburg—a small bath with *cold common salt* wells, which contain a little magnesium bromide and iodide.

Soden a Werra, a *cold salt* well in Hesse-Nassau.

Solis, near Tiefenkasten, Grisons, Switzerland, a *cold alkaline gaseous* spring, containing chiefly sodium sulphate, chloride, and bicarbonate, with a small amount of bromide and iodide, and a little iron.

Soulzmatt, in a valley of the Vosges, Alsace, between Bâle and Strasburg—a *cold alkaline gaseous* table-water, largely exported, as well as used for bathing and drinking at the source—chiefly in dyspeptic states.

Srebernik, in the east of Bosnia, has a cold spring containing arsenic—0·006 per litre of arsenious acid; it is also reported to contain sulphuric acid and sulphates of iron, zinc, and aluminium. Dose at starting, one ounce.

Stachelberg, Canton Glarus, Switzerland, in the Tödi district, in a beautiful situation, at an altitude of over 2,000 feet, has a *cold sulphur* spring of feeble mineralisation containing a small amount of H_2S and sodium sulphide. It is used at the bath establishment in the same cases as are amenable to sulphur treatment elsewhere, with the additional advantage here of a fresh, subalpine climate. It is near the railway station of Linththal.

Stafford has *brine* baths similar to those of Droitwich.

Steben, an old-established *cold gaseous chalybeate* spa and ferruginous *Moor* bath in Upper Franconia, Bavaria, at an altitude of nearly 2,000 feet, the terminus of the Hof-Steben line. The iron springs, containing 50·05 and 0·06 per litre of bicarbonate of iron and much carbonic acid, are drunk, used as baths, and exported. Mud baths, artificial salt baths, and pine-needle baths are also prepared.

The cases treated are chiefly those of anæmia, chlorosis, neurasthenia, and female diseases.

Stoney Middleton, Derbyshire, has waters similar to the Bakewell waters.

Suderode, a *brine* bath in Prussian Saxony.

Sulza, Grand Duchy of Saxe-Weimar (Thuringia) between

Weimar and Naumburg, on the Ilm, at an elevation of 480 feet, has *common salt* springs containing, besides sodium chloride and sulphate, small quantities of magnesium chloride and sodium bromide and iodide. Its reputation is almost exclusively local.

Sulzbach, in the Baden Black Forest, with railway station at Hubacker, on the Appenweier-Hubacker line, has *simple thermal* or tepid waters of a temperature of only 70° F. They are given in gout, rheumatism, and nervous affections.

Sulzbrunn, near Kempten, in Upper Bavaria, a small bath, at an elevation of 2,800 feet, has *weak salt* springs, containing a little magnesium iodide.

Swanlinbar, a small village in county Cavan, Ireland, possesses *cold sulphur* springs, popular in former times.

Sylvanès, Department of Aveyron, France, has *thermal* waters which have been classed amongst the *simple thermal* and also amongst *arsenical* waters. Its railway station is Ceilhes-Roqueredonde, on the line between Arvant and Béziers, It is situated in a mountainous country, at an elevation of 1,300 feet. The springs vary in temperature from 88° to 97° F. It is one of the rare instances of a *hot* iron water. The water contains 1·0 gramme of *solids* per litre, of which 0·02 is carbonate of iron, and 0·016 of arsenates of iron and magnesium; it also contains manganese carbonate, calcium carbonate, and sodium chloride.

The *simple gaseous alkaline* water of Andabre (1·8 gramme of sodium bicarbonate to the litre), only two to three miles off, is sometimes drunk at Sylvanès, whose waters are chiefly used for baths. The cases treated there are those of anæmia, neurasthenia, general debility, affections of the respiratory organs, chronic metritis.

Szczawnica, on the northern slope of the Carpathians, in Galicia, at an elevation of 1,700 feet, has *cold gaseous alkaline common salt* springs. One of the springs contains as much as 8·4 grammes of sodium bicarbonate and 4·6 of sodium chloride. These waters are valuable in the treatment of chronic catarrhal affections of the respiratory passages, the spray being inhaled, in addition to drinking the waters. It is often combined with the whey or koumiss cures. The nearest railway station, Alt-Sandeck, is six hours distant.

Szkleno, in Hungary, has *thermal calcareous* waters varying in temperature from 100° to 128° F., containing 2 grammes per litre of calcium sulphate. The situation is picturesque, at an elevation of 1,130 feet. The nearest railway station is Guram-Berzenscze, a drive of two and a-half hours.

Tarasp-Schuls, in the Lower Engadine, Switzerland, has *alkaline aperient saline* springs of much the same character as those of Marienbad, being, however, more alkaline and less aperient. If Tarasp be approached from St. Moritz or Samaden, in the Upper Engadine, it is about a five hours' drive from the latter place, descending the valley of the

Inn through, for the most part, interesting scenery. It has been more usual to travel by rail to Davos and then drive over the Fluela Pass (about six hours) to Tarasp or Schuls, but with the completion of the railway from Thusis to St. Moritz, the route viâ Samaden in the Upper Engadine is more likely to be adopted. The Kurhaus of Tarasp is built close to the principal springs, and the baths are within the building itself. It is situated at an elevation of 3,890 feet on the northern bank of the Inn, which flows close by it.

A fine Trinkhalle with a covered promenade and a row of shops is built on the right bank of the river close to the principal spring.

The springs which give Tarasp its chief reputation are its alkaline-saline *sources*, which rise close to the river, and in the immediate vicinity of the Kurhaus. They are the St. Lucius and St. Emerita springs, which are used for drinking, and the Ursus and New Bath springs, which are weaker, and are only used for baths. The St. Lucius is the most richly mineralised, and, according to the latest analysis (1900), contains, per litre, sodium sulphate 2·245 grammes, potassium sulphate 0·334, sodium carbonate 3·045, sodium chloride 3·890, calcium carbonate 1·567, and small amounts of other constituents, such as carbonate of *iron* (0·012), of magnesium (0·659), sodium *borate* (0·884), sodium bromide (0·037), and lithium chloride (0·055).

The St. Emerita contains precisely the same constituents, but while the total solids in the St. Lucius amount to 12·834 per litre, in the St. Emerita they are only 11·339. The former is also richer in free carbonic acid. As compared with the strongest of the Marienbad springs they contain less than one-half the amount of sodium sulphate, but much more sodium bicarbonate and sodium chloride. Compared with the Carlsbad springs they contain rather less sodium sulphate and much more sodium bicarbonate and chloride, and being cold they contain more free carbonic acid gas. When *warmed* the Tarasp springs have much the same characters as the Carlsbad springs, only they are richer in the alkaline sodium bicarbonate and in sodium chloride. They are nearly as rich in sodium bicarbonate as the Vichy springs.

Owing to the carrrying out of a "new encasement" of these springs in 1899 the amount of free carbonic acid gas is said to have increased by more than one-third.

Tarasp possesses also weak gaseous chalybeate springs; the one chiefly drunk is the St. Bonifacius spring, situated a little distance from the Kurhaus on the right bank of the Inn. This spring has recently received a "new encasement," and the most recent analysis (1900)* shows that it now contains less iron than it used to, and that its characters rather tend to group it with such alkaline earthy springs as Wildungen and Antogast; but it is much richer than either in lime salts and in free carbonic acid. It is now used more for its beneficial action on the digestive and urinary organs. The Wyquelle, situated above the neighbouring village of Schuls, is another mild chalybeate spring, and there is a still weaker gaseous iron spring at Schuls, the Sotsass, which is often drunk as a table-water.

The mineral springs of the neighbouring Val Sinistra are also brought to and utilised at Tarasp. These are gaseous alkaline saline springs, which also contain iron and *arsenic*, and it is the possession of the latter constituent which confers upon them their chief importance. In a litre of the strongest spring—the Ulrichsquelle—there is 0·007 of sodium arsenate. It also contains 0·020 of carbonate of iron, and 0·023 of chloride of lithium. In Tarasp a combination of the Val Sinistra waters with the Lucius spring is often prescribed.

At the Kurhaus *gaseous alkaline saline* baths

* By Professor Treadwell, of Zürich.

are prepared with the waters of the Ursus and the New Bath springs, and the overflow of the Lucius and Emerita springs, and *chalybeate* baths with the water of the Carola spring.

Other curative agencies applied at Tarasp are the Battaglia *fango* (mud) baths, the baths prepared with Rheinfelden brine added to the ordinary warm gaseous effervescent baths, massage and medical gymnastics, and the Terrain-Kur.

The waters are usually drunk early in the morning, beginning with two or three glasses (six ounces each), and increasing gradually to five or six, according to the case, at intervals of a quarter of an hour, gentle walking exercise being taken all the time. Persons who cannot take the water cold before breakfast can have it warmed, or may take a light breakfast two or three hours before drinking.

Many of the visitors to Tarasp prefer to reside in a higher and more open situation than that of the Kurhaus, and this can be done either at the village of Schuls, in an open situation on the north side of the valley, about twenty minutes distant from Tarasp Kurhaus, or, better still, at Vulpera, a village above Tarasp, on the south side of the valley, at an elevation of about 4,200 feet. At Vulpera two large new hotels have been opened, the Hôtel Waldhaus in 1897, and the Hôtel Suisse in 1900. These are both finely situated, and patients by living at Vulpera can combine the advantages of an Alpine climate with treatment by mineral waters.

The therapeutic affinities of Tarasp are with such mineral waters as those of Marienbad, Carlsbad, and Vichy; and in certain cases the course at Tarasp may be presented as an alternative to either of these. When warmed the waters of Tarasp may answer the same purpose as the Carlsbad waters, and would be especially suitable to those who find Carlsbad too hot and relaxing. For those who require a rather milder course than that of Marienbad, less purgative and more alkaline, Tarasp is available, and for patients who, besides the alkaline property of the Vichy springs, need an aperient, the combination is found at Tarasp, while the climate is bracing, and not hot and relaxing, as Vichy is apt to be in the summer months. In suitable cases at Tarasp the use of the chalybeate springs can be associated with the alkaline-saline waters.

The diseases chiefly suitable for treatment at Tarasp may be thus enumerated: chronic gastro-intestinal catarrh, constipation, hæmorrhoids, chronic diarrhœa, dyspepsia in the anæmic, congestion and hypertrophy of the liver, commencing cirrhosis, catarrhal and obstinate jaundice and gallstones, obesity and related conditions, diabetes, the same class of cases as are benefited at Carlsbad and Vichy, gouty and uric acid states, renal catarrh and gravel (the earthy alkaline Bonifacius spring is especially adapted to the treatment of these states), chlorosis and anæmia in certain persons, and especially when the consequence of malarial infection and associated with splenic enlargement (the combination of iron and arsenic in the Val Sinestra waters proves valuable in some of those cases); catarrhal affections of the respiratory organs in obese persons are also said to be benefited. The season is from June 1st to October.

Teplitz, or Teplitz-Schönau, as it is now called, since it has been united with the neighbouring village Schönau, is the oldest spa in Bohemia. It is usually approached from Dresden viâ Bodenbach and Aussig, in about four hours and a-quarter. It is celebrated for its *hot* springs, of which it possesses many.

It is situated in a somewhat open valley, 750 feet above the sea, between the Erzgebirge, which shelter it on the north, and the Mittelgebirge on the south, with a somewhat variable climate.

There is a hill, the Mont de Ligue, between

Schönau and Teplitz, commanding a fine view; and to the east of Schönau there is another admirable point of view, the Schlossberg, 1,280 feet above the sea, easily ascended in half an hour. Teplitz is surrounded by pleasing country, into which many attractive excursions of various lengths may be made.

There are excellent hotels and lodging-houses there, some of the best being on the road which connects Teplitz with Schönau.

The thermal waters are supplied to quite a large number of bath-houses, the most luxurious of which is the Kaiserbad, which belongs to the town, and in nearly all of these bath-houses patients can obtain apartments. The water is pumped up from the springs.

The springs, on account of their feeble mineralisation, are usually classed amongst the *simple thermal* waters, but it is also claimed for them that they are *alkaline* waters; and so indeed they are, as out of a total amount of 0·7 of solids per litre (the Stadtquelle), 0·4 consists of sodium carbonate. There are also small amounts of sodium sulphate and chloride, and calcium carbonate, and very minute quantities of lithium and strontium carbonates. It is therefore a weak alkaline thermal water of a temperature of 115° F.

There are public baths for the gratuitous use of the poor, and there are also military hospitals for invalid soldiers. Besides the mineral-water baths, Teplitz has also *Moor* or peat baths. The peat is found in the neighbourhood, and is said to be less stimulating than the Franzensbad peat, as it contains less iron. The Teplitz peat bath is given at a temperature of 99·5° F., and is said to have a very soothing effect.

Teplitz is the warmest of the "indifferent" thermal baths, and in some cases the baths are given at a high temperature, but this is less the custom than it was formerly. They are also in some cases given tepid. Although bathing is the chief part of the treatment at Teplitz, it has become the practice recently to prescribe the water to be drunk also in certain cases. In the Kurgarten, mineral waters from all the chief European spas are kept, and are supplied to the patients according to the remedy required.

The more active thermal treatment is intended to promote the absorption of morbid exudations in persons suffering from chronic gout, rheumatism, and certain forms of paralysis.

The tepid baths are better suited to sensitive and delicate persons suffering from functional nervous affections, upon whom they often produce a soothing and alleviating effect.

The cure at Teplitz is recommended in the following cases: chronic gout and rheumatism, and related affections, as sciatica, lumbago, and other neuralgias and myalgias; certain nervous diseases, especially those related to gouty or rheumatic or traumatic conditions or overstrain, and those associated with *metallic* poisoning; also hysterical forms; in some chronic skin diseases, especially eczema, psoriasis, prurigo, and pruritus, and some forms of secondary syphilis. The mild alkaline water of the baths has an excellent effect in some of these cases. The season is from May to the end of September, but treatment can be obtained there at any part of the year.

Tunbridge Wells, in a fine situation, at an altitude of 420 feet, on the borders of Kent and Sussex, and surrounded by most attractive and picturesque country, is resorted to largely, and is a popular health resort, not, as formerly, on account of its *chalybeate* spring, but for its pleasant situation and its tonic and mildly bracing air. It has also the great advantage of being within a very short railway journey of London, about an hour.

At one time "the Wells" were much frequented by fashionable visitors, who came to "take the waters";

but that was in the seventeenth and eighteenth centuries.

The mineral spring is situated at one end of the Pantiles, an old-fashioned paved promenade, having on one side a covered way for protection in bad weather, and a row of shops. The water is dispensed from basins at the springs by persons who are known as "dippers," and at the other end of the Pantiles it is also procurable in a reading-room provided for visitors.

The water is only used for drinking purposes; its defect as a chalybeate spring is the absence of any amount of free carbonic acid, the presence of which, in large quantity, gives to the best known Continental iron springs their chief value. We doubt also whether the amount of water obtainable from the springs would be large enough for the constant supply of a large bath establishment.

An analysis made by Stevenson in 1892 gives the amount of carbonate of iron per litre as 0·06. This is a fair amount of iron for a chalybeate spring. The other constituents are of little or no importance. There is a little sulphate of lime and chloride of sodium, and minute amounts of other sulphates and chlorides.

These waters are prescribed for patients suffering from anæmia and debility, but the local practitioners consider it needful in severe cases to give ordinary preparations of iron in addition to the waters. Only small quantities of the water are usually prescribed—two half-glasses—with a short walk between—about eleven or twelve in the morning. There is no particular season.

Tabiano, Italy, three miles from Salso Maggiore and four from Borgo San Donnino railway station, in the Province of Parma, has *cold sulphur* waters.

Teinach, a small bath and summer resort, situated in a protected valley in the Würtemberg Black Forest, at an elevation of 1,300 feet, in the neighbourhood of pine woods, about one and a-half miles from its railway station on the Stuttgart - Calw - Horb lines, has cold, feebly mineralised gaseous springs, some containing a small amount of iron, and therefore termed *chalybeate;* others weakly *alkaline* (small amounts of sodium and calcium carbonate) are used and exported as table-waters. There is a hydro-therapeutic establishment there, and the natural springs are used for drinking, gargling, and inhalations, also for baths and douches. *Moor*-bath-extract, pine-needle, and electric baths are prepared. The maladies treated there are anæmia, dyspepsia, catarrh of the mucous membranes, neurasthenia, gout, female disorders. The season is from May 15 to Oct. 15.

Tennstedt, a very small *cold sulphur* bath in Saxony, on the Schambach (main line Gotha-Leinefelde).

Termini-Imersee, on the north coast of Sicily, has *hot* springs (108° F.), said to contain common salt and aperient sulphates. It is a small bath, and little accurate information about its springs is obtainable; it was the Roman "Thermæ Himerenses."

Thale, a *common salt* (Sool) bath in Saxony, at the entrance of the Bodethal, in a beautiful situation, at an elevation of 740 feet, in the Lower Harz Mountains. Terminus of the branch line Halberstadt-Thale. The saline spring, the Hubertusquelle, arises in an island on the Bode, where the hotel and bath establishment are also found. It is also a summer climatic resort.

Thonon, a steamboat station on the southern shore of the Lake of Geneva, in Haute Savoie, has *cold feebly mineralised* waters, like those of Evian, and used in the same cases. The water is said to contain some organic-resinous substances.

Tiefenkasten, Grisons, Switzerland, has *sulphated alkaline chalybeate* springs—"St. Peter's Well." The chief constituents are sodium sulphate and chloride, magnesium sulphate, and calcium carbonate, and about 0·03 of bicarbonate of iron. Used chiefly in gastro-hepatic disorders associated with anæmia.

Tobelbad—a *simple thermal* bath in Styria, at an altitude of about 1,000 feet. Temperature of springs 77° to 84° F.

Tölz, or **Krankenheil-Tölz**, in Upper Bavaria, on the right bank of the Isar, at an elevation of about 2,100 feet, finely situated on the northern slope of the Blomberg, has cold *weakly mineralised* springs of indeterminate classification. It has a station on the Munich-Holz-Kirchen-Tölz line. It has six springs, which have been termed "iodine, alkaline, common salt wells," containing per litre 0·19 to 0·33 of sodium bicarbonate, 0·03 to 0·29 of sodium chloride, and about 0·001 of sodium iodide and a little sulphuretted hydrogen gas. The springs are so far from Tölz that the waters are brought in bottles for drinking, and through galvanised iron pipes for the baths. A great deal of commercial enterprise is associated with these weak springs, and "Krankenheil Soaps," "Spiritus Saponaris," "Krankenheil Pastilles," as well as the waters, are prepared and exported. Various auxiliary remedies are also employed, as brine and mud baths, pine, vapour, chalybeate, sulphur and other baths, milk and whey cures, and "extracts of mountain herbs." The fresh mountain air is probably as efficacious as any of these.

The diseases especially treated are scrofulous affections, skin disorders, chronic metritis, catarrh of the respiratory organs.

Törmisstein, or the **Heil-**

brunnen, near Brohl, on the Rhine, in Rhenish Prussia—a *highly gaseous alkaline* spring—sodium bicarbonate 2·5 per litre, magnesium bicarbonate 1·6, and *common salt* 1·4. Used and largely exported as a dietetic table-water.

Topusco, *simple thermal* springs, temperature 122° to 135° F., in Croatia.

Traunstein, in Upper Bavaria, at an altitude of about 2,000 feet, on the Traun, with a station on the line between Munich and Salzburg, has several *cold earthy calcareous* springs connected with the Kurhaus Traunstein and the Wildbad Empfing, which is near at hand, containing magnesium and calcium carbonate and sodium chloride. It also has *brine* baths, the brine being brought by pipes from Reichenhall, and mud baths and pine-needle baths are available. The Empfing water is considered valuable in the treatment of certain renal and vesical affections. There are pleasant walks around.

Trefriw, North Wales, in the valley of the Conway, two miles from the railway station of Llanrwst, has *strong iron* springs, containing "large quantities of protosulphate of iron and sulphate of aluminum," but "the water varies much in composition from time to time" (Leech).

Trencsin Töplitz, a Hungarian *thermal sulphur* spring, with sulphur-mud baths.

Trillo, a Spanish (Province of Guadalajara) *thermal common salt and iron* water, with a smell of H_2S. Temperature of springs 77° to 86° F. Used in rheumatism and skin diseases.

Tusnad, a *chalybeate* spring in Transylvania.

Uriage is a celebrated French spa, with a spring containing, as its chief ingredients, free sulphuretted hydrogen and sodium chloride—a *sulphur and salt* spring.

Uriage is situated in the Department of the Isère, in a beautiful valley of the mountains of Dauphiné, and may be regarded almost as a suburb of Grenoble, It is between seven and eight miles from that remarkable town, the situation of which is certainly one of the most picturesque and striking in Europe.

The baths of Uriage are situated at an elevation of 1,358 feet above the sea, and although this is not a considerable elevation, it is quite enough, owing to the open character of the valley, to give a distinct freshness to the air, which, even in August, is at times quite cool in the early mornings.

Uriage also has a *chalybeate* spring of no great pretensions, but, as we have said, its chief mineral *source* is characterised especially by the presence in considerable quantity of sulphuretted hydrogen and common salt. The temperature, at the *source*, is about 80° F., but it gets colder before it reaches the *buvette*, and it has to be heated artificially for the baths. It has a strong smell and taste of sulphuretted hydrogen, and a strong taste of salt also; but it is not so unpleasant to drink as might be imagined, and one quickly gets accustomed to it. It contains rather more than 10 parts of solid constituents to the litre: of sodium chloride 6 grammes, of calcium, magnesium, and sodium sulphates 3 grammes, and of sulphuretted hydrogen 7 volumes per 1,000. It is taken in very variable quantities, according to the nature of the case and the constitution of the patient; and whereas several glasses daily may be ordered to be drunk by some patients, half a glass twice a day is as much as is permitted to others: its alterative or tonic action being especially needed in some cases, its eliminative action in others. In the larger doses it is purgative.

The cases especially suitable to treatment by the waters of Uriage are those associated with what the French term *lymphatisme*--what used to be termed "scrofula"—as well as some forms of chronic rheumatism and gout, and particularly certain skin affections, the existence of which may be dependent on these constitutional states. The various forms of chronic eczema, especially the moist forms; the different kinds of acne, boils, chronic urticaria, herpes of the genitals, and tubercular or scrofulous skin affections, are benefited by these waters. Some very chronic forms of skin disease, as *prurigo* and *psoriasis*, are greatly benefited and sometimes cured.

Treatment at Uriage has been found very beneficial to delicate, scrofulous, and anæmic overgrown children, and is said to act like a "sea bath in the mountains."

Many other affections of children are reported as suitable for treatment at Uriage, such as *scrofulous* inflammation of the eyelids and similar diseases of the eyes and ears; chronic nasal and pharyngeal catarrh, glandular swellings, scrofulous diseases of the bones and joints, etc. In all such cases the curative influence of the waters is greatly aided by the healthy, open-air life in this mildly bracing mountain air.

Chronic rheumatism, as Dr. Doyen, the well-known specialist of Uriage, so well observes, is benefited by the judicious use of almost all mineral waters, and he therefore claims no *special* influence over this malady on the part of the waters of Uriage, but he maintains that they are just as useful as those of many other spas in muscular and articular rheumatism, rheumatic neuralgias, and chronic sciatica.

Chronic uterine inflammations, when associated with *lymphatisme*, are benefited by treatment there.

Douche massage is applied in a special manner at Uriage, and was introduced there so long ago as 1838. The patient lies on an inclined table, and a single attendant only is needed. Such applications last about fifteen minutes.

Finally, the treatment of constitutional syphilis is undertaken there in the same manner as at Aix la Chapelle, and with good results.

The chalybeate spring is occasionally used as an auxiliary remedy, and only for drinking.

The season begins on May 25th and finishes Oct. 15th. June is the best month, July and August the next best. A steam tramway now connects Uriage with Grenoble (twelve kilometres) in thirty-five minutes. Grenoble is 634 kilometres from Paris. The journey takes ten to eleven hours.

Ueberlingen, in the Duchy of Baden, on the Ueberlingen Lake, a bay of the Lake of Constance, has an *earthy chalybeate* spring, which is conveyed to the Bath Hotel for drinking and bathing, in cases of chlorosis, neurasthenia, and female maladies.

Urberoaga de Alzola, a Spanish bath a few hours' drive from San Sebastian, in the Province of Guipuzcoa, with picturesque surroundings. It has feebly mineralised *thermal alkaline earthy* waters, of a temperature of about 87° F., which are used as baths and drunk, especially in affections of the urinary organs.

Ussat (Ariège, Pyrénées), situated at an elevation of 1,460 feet, in a picturesque valley, through which the river Ariège flows, within half an hour's drive of Tarascon station, is a popular "ladies'" bath, and is annually resorted to by a great number of invalids suffering from uterine and allied nervous and hysterical affections. There is a fine "Etablissement Thermal," situated in a spacious park, and the bathing arrangements are exceedingly good. There is a small hospital for the reception and gratuitous treatment of poor patients. The temperature of the springs is from 90° to 100° F. Their mineralisation is feeble (1·27 grammes to a litre), and consists chiefly of small amounts of the carbonates and sulphates of lime, magnesia, and soda. It is classed amongst the *indifferent thermal* springs.

These baths, when employed at a moderate temperature, are said to be exceedingly soothing to the nervous system, and of great value in the treatment of chronic metritis, dysmenorrhœa, and pelvic neuralgias, especially in the neurotic. The baths are also found useful in nervous dyspepsia, in cutaneous hyperæsthesia, in chorea, and some forms of paralysis of doubtful causation. One of the specialities of Ussat is the administration of baths of *running* water, a stream always running through the baths and keeping the water continually fresh and of the same temperature, which can be varied according to the distance of the bath from the source. Season, June 1 to Sept. 15.

Vals in Ardèche (sta. Vals les Bains), between Lyons and Marseilles, sixteen hours from Paris and five from Lyons, on a branch line between Vogüé and Nieigles-Pendes, is one of the most important spas in France, and were it not for its distance from the capital (434 miles), it would probably be as much frequented by foreigners as Vichy is. Its waters, as exported, are of world-wide reputation, and its popularity as a watering place has grown greatly of late years. The little town is picturesquely situated on the right bank of the river Volane, in a valley of the Cevennes, and is surrounded by an amphitheatre of volcanic mountains. It consists of little else than a long street of hotels (twenty or more in number), *cafés* and *maisons meublées*. Vals is surrounded by vast and shady parks and most interesting country, rich in picturesque sites of wild and savage beauty. It is situated at an elevation of about 800 feet above the sea. Its climate is temperate, and intermediate between that of the Mediterranean and that of the mountainous region in the centre of France. Average summer temperature, 70° F.

The springs, of which there are fourteen principal ones, are *cold*, and contain large but varying proportions of *bicarbonate of soda* and large quantities of *free carbonic acid*.

Vals possesses two bath establishments. The larger of the two possesses the following *sources:* Rigolette, Précieuse, Magdaleine, Désirée, Saint Jean, and Dominique: the smaller one has the *sources* Marquise, Souveraine, Pauline, Chloé, des Convalescents, Saint Louis, and Constantine. All these contain considerable but varying quantities of bicarbonate of soda, except the Dominique, in the larger establishment, and the Saint Louis in the smaller one; these two are ferruginous and arsenical springs.

Owing to the large amount of carbonic acid in these springs, even the strongest of them are not unpleasant to drink. The water of some of the *sources* is largely exported, especially Précieuse, Magdaleine, and Rigolette.

We may take the Source Magdaleine as a representative of the stronger springs, containing, as it does, over 7 grammes of bicarbonate of soda per litre; and the Source Pauline as a representative of the weaker springs, as it contains only about 1½ gramme of bicarbonate of soda per litre; and we have between these several degrees of mineralisation, as, for instance, the Source Désirée, with 6 grammes per litre; the Source Rigolette, with rather more than 5 grammes; the Source Souveraine, with 2½ grammes (this spring also contains a small amount of lithium); and the Source Chloé, with 2 grammes.

The Rigolette is often *warmed* for use in the same cases as those suitable for treatment with the hot springs of Vichy.

The following is the detailed analysis of the

Sources Constantine and Pauline (per litre — 1,000 grammes):

	Constantine.	Pauline.
Bicarbonate of soda	7·05300	1·6117
„ potash	0·07109	traces
„ lithia	0·01075	„
„ lime	0·43700	0·0288
„ magnesia ...	traces	0·0083
Carbonate of iron	0·00670	0·0090
Silicate of alumina, potash, and soda	0·15900	0·1824
Chloride of sodium	0·28000	0·0414
Sulphate of soda	0·20400	0·1696
Phosphate of soda	traces	traces
Organic matter	traces	traces
Free carbonic acid gas ...	2·10000	1·0820

The Vals waters are richer in bicarbonate of soda than any other known mineral waters, and the graduation in quantity presented by the different *sources* is of great convenience in their therapeutic application.

The Vals waters have a large range of applicability. They are useful in the various forms of acid dyspepsia, nervo-muscular atony of stomach and gastric catarrh, in hepatic congestion, jaundice, and gallstones; in diabetes of the fat and gouty type; in gravel and renal and vesical calculi, and in prostatic enlargement and irritability of the bladder (in cases with much painful cystitis the cure must be applied with great caution, and only the mildest springs employed); in some forms of chronic gout and rheumatism; in splenic enlargements as a sequel of malarial fevers, and in certain anæmic and chlorotic conditions associated with functional uterine and gastric disturbances, or the consequence of chronic malarial cachexia. The combination of the alkaline with the iron and arsenic springs renders the cure valuable in such cases.

The selection of the particular spring and the doses of the water must be adapted to each individual case. The alkaline and the iron and arsenical baths have their appropriate indications. Inhalations and vaginal douches of carbonic acid gas are also prescribed in suitable cases. An establishment for giving vapour baths is also available.

Alkalinity of the chief sources of Vals estimated as bicarbonate of soda per litre.

	Magdaleine	... ...	7·25 grammes
(*a*)	Désirée ...	... ...	6·04 „
	Rigolette ...	... ...	5·80 „
(*a*)	Précieuse ...	... ...	5·80 „
(*b*)	Impératrice	... ...	1·66 „
(*b*)	St. Jean ...	... ...	1·48 „

(*a*) Contains also a considerable amount of bicarbonate of magnesia.
(*b*) Used as table-waters.

Season: May 15th to Oct. 1st.

Vernet les Bains, a *thermal sulphur* bath in the Pyrénées Orientales, on the river Cady, at the foot of the Canigou, on its western side. It has an elevation of 2,100 feet and a mild, dry, and tonic climate. It is one of the most southerly of French spas, being twenty-one hours from Paris and only a short distance from the Spanish frontier. It is half-an-hour's drive from the station Villefranche de Conflent, the terminus of the line between Perpignan and Prades. Vernet possesses as many as twelve springs varying in temperature from 100° to 140° F., the dominant ingredient of which is sodium sulphide, 0·0188 gramme per litre. The water also contains some free nitrogen and sulphuretted hydrogen gases. Some of these springs contain a large amount of *glairine*, which gives them an unctuous feeling. They have been found very useful in some skin affections and in certain forms of gastro-enteritis. They have also been given, in very small doses, in cases of early phthisis.

The hotter springs are especially reserved for baths and douches, and are chiefly used in cases of chronic rheumatism and other chronic joint affections, as well as in certain cases of perimetritis.

The weaker springs are drunk and applied as gargles and inhalations, with benefit, in chronic pharyngitis and laryngitis.

The three bath establishments are perfectly equipped with all the most modern appliances for the application of thermal waters, and in addition possess special apartments devoted to massage, gymnastics, fencing, boxing, etc. The hotel accommodation is good, the amusements are varied.

The best season for treatment is from May to October.

Vernet, besides its thermal establishment, is well known as possessing a *sanatorium* for the treatment of consumption on hygienic principles. It is known as the Sanatorium du Canigou. It is quite independent of the baths.

Vichy, one of the best known spas in Europe and perhaps the most frequented of all the French spas, is situated on the right bank of the river Allier in the Department of that name, about 240 miles from Paris, between seven and eight hours by fast train. It is situated at an elevation of about 850 feet above the sea. Its immediate surroundings cannot be said to be very picturesque, but agreeable and attractive scenery lies close at hand.

The buildings devoted to the reception of visitors are of the most elaborate kind. The New Etablissement Thermal, only recently opened, is one of the most magnificent buildings of its kind, elaborately fitted up and admirably adapted to all the purposes it has to serve. There is provided every kind of bath and douche, all kinds of massage, and all forms of "mécanothérapie." There are several smaller bath establishments.

Inhalations of oxygen and of carbonic acid are provided. A *carbonic acid bath* is also employed, and is regarded there as a valuable remedy in certain forms of neuralgia and in cases of gouty irritation of the skin, while inhalations and douches of this gas are said to give relief in some forms of dry asthma, of angina, and of chronic coryza. Other accessory methods of treatment—such as the curative application of heat, light, electricity, and mechanical appliances—are provided.

The casino is an elegant and luxurious building, providing every imaginable resource to prevent the visitors at Vichy from falling victims to that most terrible of maladies, *l'ennui.* Balls, concerts, and excellent operatic and dramatic performances, in which some of the most distinguished actors and singers in France frequently take part, are daily provided.

Vichy may be regarded as the *type* of *simple alkaline* springs, its richness in bicarbonate of sodium being its chief characteristic.

Its immediate neighbourhood is extraordinarily rich in mineral springs. Wherever a shaft is sunk within a distance of six or seven miles in the basin surrounding the place, alkaline gaseous springs analogous to those of Vichy are certain to be found. Hence it is that many of the springs are private property and bear the names of their proprietors — such, for example, as the Source Lardy, the Source Larbaud, and others, each proprietor naturally claiming special virtues for his own spring. But the springs chiefly employed belong to the State. Now, although all these springs are of the same general character, they differ, many of them, from one another in obvious physical qualities. Some are cold, most are hot; some contain a considerable quantity of free carbonic acid, some contain very little; some are clear and sparkling, some are slightly cloudy.

Moreover, some of the Vichy springs contain iron in appreciable quantity, while others do not, and this fact is made use of to classify these springs into two groups—the simple alkaline waters and the alkaline iron waters. It is to the possession of the former, however, that Vichy owes its great reputation. The predominating ingredient in all the *sources* of Vichy is bicarbonate of soda, and it is the chief one in its simple alkaline springs. Of these there are three which are commonly drunk. Two are hot springs—viz. the Grande Grille, having a temperature of 106° F., and L'Hôpital, having a temperature of 81·5° F.); the third is a cold spring, the well-known Célestins, so called because of the existence of an ancient convent of that name close to the *source*. It is a very pleasant water to drink, and has none of the disagreeable alkaline taste which an ordinary solution of bicarbonate of soda has. Its taste is, moreover, quite different from that of the other two springs, although their chemical composition is nearly identical. The difference of temperature and of relative proportions of free carbonic acid in each may, to a certain extent, account for this.

The mineral constituents found in the Vichy springs amount to about 8 grammes in the litre. Besides bicarbonate of soda, these *sources* contain bicarbonates of potash, magnesia, strontia, and lime, chloride of sodium, and small quantities of sulphate and phosphate of soda. Some of the springs at Vichy contain as much as 5 grammes of bicarbonate of soda to the litre; this fact, together with the relatively high temperature of some of its springs, gives to these waters a very high degree of importance medically. It is worth noticing that these springs contain also a minute quantity of arsenic, two or three milligrammes of arsenate of soda in a litre. This ingredient increases in quantity, and assumes great importance, in some of the neighbouring spas of Auvergne.

The spring at Vichy which contains the largest amount of iron is the Source Mesdames. It arises about two miles from Vichy, and is conveyed to the town in pipes. Another spring, the Hauterive, which contains a notable amount of iron, and is richest of all in free carbonic acid, arises at a distance of three miles from Vichy, and is, on both these accounts, largely used for bottling and exportation. Four springs have been conducted to the "Trink-hall" of the new establishment—the Grande Grille, the Mesdames, the Chomel, and the Lucas.

It need scarcely be pointed out that serious treatment by an active agent such as the mineral waters of Vichy imperatively demands constant and experienced medical counsel and supervision. Where there are so many *sources* having only slight shades of difference in quality and composition, the advantage of prolonged study and experience in determining the selection of one in preference to another is quite obvious. Then there is the question of the quantity of water suitable to each case, the question of baths and of the length of time during which such baths should be taken, the propriety of using douches and the kind of douche to be employed, the length of time the cure should last: these and many other minor questions must be left to local authority and experience to answer.

Speaking generally, the *source* prescribed for stomach affections is L'Hôpital, that for hepatic disorders the Grande Grille, and that for gout and renal maladies the Célestins. But in each case the temperament, the constitution, and the habits of the individual have to be considered, as well as the nature of the malady. These traditional indications are not, however, always applicable—*e.g.* when the liver is very irritable and readily congested, the Grande Grille should be used with much caution or altogether avoided, and the Célestins must not be given in cases of old-established renal lesions or cases of irritable bladder. L'Hôpital is said to be less exciting than any of the other springs, and best suited to feeble and irritable stomachs. The Grande Grille is hotter, more stimulating, more rapidly digested, acts more quickly and energetically, and is especially indicated in cases of hepatic torpor and congestion and in cases of gallstone, with or without jaundice. It is to be preferred in lymphatic and debilitated constitutions, and is of especial value in the malarious cachexia often engendered among the French colonists in Africa, taken either alone or mixed with one of the ferruginous springs.

The Célestins, much preferred for its agreeable taste and sparkling quality, is said to be highly stimulating and exciting to the nervous system. The iron springs, the Source Lardy and the Source Mesdames, are especially serviceable in the case of women and children suffering from the after-effects of malarial fevers, and are also well borne by dyspeptics who require iron. The quantity of water to be taken daily varies of necessity with the malady and the individual; it is no longer the fashion to prescribe the large quantities which were at one time consumed. Indeed, the tendency has sometimes been towards the other extreme, and very remarkable results have been obtained with quite small doses of the thermal springs. In cases of very feeble digestion only very small doses should at first be prescribed. A short time before breakfast and dinner is considered the best time for drinking the water, the dose varying from three to twelve ounces according to the case. The Vichy physicians consider the baths an important part of the cure. They are usually taken daily for half an hour at a time at a temperature of 86° to 93° F., the mineral water being mixed with an equal quantity of fresh water. This is said to be an important precaution, the neglect of which may lead to sleeplessness, headache, congestion of the brain, and many febrile and nervous phenomena. The addition of bran to the bath is a method commonly adopted for diminishing its stimulating effect.

The douche, tepid or warm, is more suitable to some cases than the bath, especially to the neurasthenic or nervous dyspeptics, and the irritable gouty and congestive subjects. The cold douche is reserved for torpid anæmia, for certain forms of atonic dyspepsia, and for those cases generally in which it is desired to rouse and stimulate functional activity.

The *douche-massage* as applied at Aix les Bains has been introduced at Vichy and found most serviceable in the treatment of the gouty, the rheumatic, the obese, and certain diabetics. The *ascending* douche has also been largely used, and is highly esteemed at Vichy. The effect of the local application of the douche in cases of gallstone and of engorgement of the liver and spleen is highly spoken of. The cases, then, to which the course of treatment at Vichy is appropriate are those of dyspepsia, gastric and intestinal, when not due to organic, malignant disease, African dysenteries, the sequelæ of malarial fevers, congestion of the liver and gallstones, with the jaundice which frequently accompanies these conditions. Hepatic colic is a malady especially amenable to treatment by the thermal springs of Vichy.

Cases of gastric ulcer (non-hæmorrhagic) are said to do well here when treated with the mineral waters combined with a milk diet. The Vichy course proves particularly valuable in gastro-hepatic dyspepsias, cases in which hepatic torpor and inadequacy plays such an important *rôle*.

Lavage of the stomach with Vichy water is not practised so much now as formerly, as cases of a moderate degree of gastric dilatation recover without recourse to this disagreeable proceeding. Some forms of nervous dyspepsia do well here if the course is combined with hydrotherapy.

Some years ago a violent dispute arose among the doctors of Vichy as to whether *gout* could or could not be advantageously treated there. The dispute grew so warm that it was referred to the Minister of Agriculture and Commerce, who referred it to the Academy of Medicine, and this body, in turn, refused to give any very definite decision on so delicate a question. The conclusions of one of the greatest medical authorities in Vichy and in France on this subject may be thus summarised : Seeing that gout is a particular error or vice of nutrition, and that the maintenance in their integrity of the natural phenomena of nutrition is the chief condition that can preserve from gout, and seeing that one of the most manifest effects of the waters of Vichy, properly administered, is the regulation of the digestive and eliminating functions, and to excite in them a special activity, it follows that the waters of Vichy tend to prevent gout or to correct the gouty constitution by maintaining nutrition intact or by re-establishing it when disturbed. It is in this general way, and not as a specific antidote, that the waters of Vichy are valuable in gout.

While it was imagined that these waters acted as a kind of chemical antidote to gout, they were often administered in excessively large and injurious quantities; but now that a different and more rational view of their *modus operandi* is accepted, the use of small doses, the effects of which are carefully watched, is the order of the day. "Of all the diseases treated at Vichy," writes the eminent authority to whom we have already alluded, "gout is the one whose treatment requires the greatest amount of precaution and watchfulness."

Some cases of gouty eczema do well there, and so do cases of acne rosacea and urticaria when dependent on gastro-hepatic disorder.

With respect to renal calculous affections so constantly treated with so much success at Vichy, it is to be remembered that it is especially in the *uric acid* forms that it proves serviceable, and that in cases of phosphatic and oxalic gravel it should be avoided.

In cases of diabetes the course at Vichy has been frequently found of the greatest advantage; but in these cases, as, indeed, in cases of gout, the Vichy waters must not be regarded in any sense as a specific remedy, but as producing their good effects through a general amelioration of the processes of nutrition and assimilation. It is to the fat and gouty diabetics that these waters do so much good, while they are of no service to the young, thin diabetic, whose case is almost always incurable; nor are they applicable to the pancreatic and nervous forms.

Vichy is also one of the many spas to which obese persons resort for the cure of obesity. Douche massage is applied to these cases, together with the internal use of the water. Hereditary forms of obesity have not been found to benefit at Vichy.

Cases of anæmia, pure and simple, would scarcely come to Vichy for a cure; but cases of cachectic or symptomatic anæmia—*i.e.* anæmia the consequence of other disease, especially of disease of the organs of digestion and assimilation—are no doubt frequently benefited to a great extent by the alkaline iron springs which are met with there.

The high estimation in which the Vichy waters are held in the treatment of the morbid results left behind by malarial disease, is testified to by the fact that a military hospital has been established there with accommodation for 750 soldiers and officers, invalided after service in the French colonies.

The physiological action of the Vichy waters is thus explained by the medical authorities experienced in its application: The warm, gaseous, alkaline water taken fasting, by its local action on the stomach, relieves gastric pains and discomfort. Its digestion is easy and rapid, and it promotes appetite. It relieves and often cures the symptoms of gastric dyspepsia, as weight, flatulence, and a feeling of distension after food. The urine is increased in quantity; its acidity is at first increased and subsequently diminished. About the eighth day a discharge of uric acid and urates has been observed, which with some patients will continue throughout the cure. This points to an acceleration of tissue changes and the promotion of the eliminating function of the kidneys. Towards the twelfth day some disturbance of digestion may occur, such as loss of appetite, furred tongue, constipation, sometimes diarrhœa. Interruption of the course for two or three days, and a few doses of a purgative water, such as Apenta, will usually suffice to remedy this *crise thermale.*

The sum of the physiological effects of the cure at Vichy is to regulate the assimilative functions—acting on the liver, the kidneys, and the intestinal tract, but especially on the liver. Its alkalinity in part explains its action. Exercising a modifying action on the secretions it is in a special degree the remedy for defects of assimilation.

The dietetic *régime* prescribed at Vichy is not a very severe one, nor is it in any way special. A fair and moderate amount of wholesome food and wine is all that is insisted upon. A breakfast at ten o'clock of two or three courses, of which one is usually of cooked fruit and vegetables and frequently carrots—for stewed carrots is a speciality of the breakfasts at Vichy—a little red wine and water, or tea or coffee for a beverage; a dinner at half-past five, which differs in no respect from the dinners met with at the *tables d'hôte* of any good French hotel—these two meals form the *pension* at the hotels. Early hours are the rule there. At six o'clock drinking and bathing commence seriously. Half an hour or an hour of absolute repose after the bath is *de rigueur.* After the ten o'clock breakfast, a lounge in the open air, or a very gentle promenade, or a ride on a donkey passes the time till two or three in the afternoon, when water drinking begins again, and those bathe who do not like the early morning hour.

Only two miles from Vichy is another town, *Cusset,* with important mineral springs. It has this advantage over Vichy, that it is two miles nearer to such picturesque scenery as the neighbourhood offers, and it possesses a spring, the Sainte Marie, much richer in iron than any of those at Vichy. In other respects the waters are of the same composition. The season extends from May 15th to Oct. 1st.

The following table gives the analyses of the three principal springs at Vichy—La Grande Grille,

L'Hôpital, Les Célestins, as well as that of the spring containing the largest amount of iron :—

	La Grande Grille. Grammes.	L'Hôpital. Grammes.	Les Célestins. Grammes.	Mesdames. Grammes.
Bicarbonate of soda ...	4·883	5·029	5·103	4·016
„ potash ...	0·352	0·440	0·315	0·189
„ magnesia	0·303	0·200	0·328	0·425
„ strontia...	0.003	0·005	0·005	0·003
„ lime ...	0·434	0·570	0·462	0·604
„ oxide of iron ...	0·004	0·004	0·004	0·026
Sulphate of soda ...	0·291	0·291	0·291	0·250
Phosphate of soda ...	0·130	0·046	0·091	traces
Arsenate of soda and lithia		traces		
Chloride of sodium ...	0·534	0·518	0·534	0·355
Silicic acid	0·070	0·050	0·060	0·032
	7·914	8·222	8·244	7·811
	Litre.	Litre.	Litre.	Litre.
Free carbonic acid ...	0·908	1·067	1·049	1·908

Vittel is more or less a rival of Contrexéville, possessing springs of the same character, composition, and uses. It is only three miles off, and has the advantage of a more open and agreeable situation. Its elevation above the sea is, like that of Contrexéville, about 1,100 feet, and its climate is temperate but rather cold, and the nights are fresh. Those who object to the "shut-in" situation of Contrexéville will find Vittel more to their taste.

As to the springs at Vittel, thirteen in number, there are only two in general use—the Grande Source, which resembles in all essentials the Pavillon at Contrexéville, but is weaker (it contains 1·65 grammes of solid constituents in a litre against 2·3 grammes in the Pavillon), and the Source Salée, a more active spring with 2·75 grammes of solid constituents to the litre. The former is diuretic, and is given in the same cases—*i.e.* affections of the urinary tract, gravel, etc.—and in the same manner as the Pavillon, but it is said to be more digestible though weaker. The Source Salée is laxative and applicable to cases of stomach and liver affection, biliary colic, and to the cure of habitual constipation. These springs are drunk in large quantities—six to twelve glasses a day—and the same class of cases are sent to Vittel as to Contrexéville. Two subordinate springs are also in use—the Source Marie and the Source des Demoiselles. These are all cold springs of a temperature between 52° and 50° F.

Baths and douches are used in subordination to the drinking cure, and hydrotherapeutic methods are well carried out. But baths and douches are considered to be counter-indicated in cases of gout. What has been said as to the physiological action of Contrexéville waters applies equally to those of Vittel; and the maladies treated there are the same—gout and renal and biliary concretions mainly, diabetes, dyspepsia, and hepatic congestion when dependent on the uric acid diathesis.

Like the cure at Contrexéville, here also the excretion of urea is augmented and that of uric acid, after a temporary increase (eliminative), is diminished, and so is the total acidity of the urine.

Valdieri, in North Italy, Piedmont, has *simple thermal* waters, one of which, the Sorgente San Lorenzo, has a temperature of 156° F. Valdieri lies in the valley of the Gesso, distant five and a-half hours from the railway station of Cuneo, at an altitude of 2,700 feet. Its waters are used for drinking and bathing—a *slimy mud* is collected from the bottom of the springs, composed in part of organic substances, and is used for local or general applications to the surface of the body, like the mud, or *fango*, at other Italian spas. The diseases treated there are chronic rheumatism, rheumatoid arthritis, scrofula, and skin diseases.

Vallacabras, a Spanish *purgative* water, rich in sodium sulphate.

Vals, in Switzerland, Canton Grisons, has *warm calcareous* springs, the temperature not exceeding 77° to 79° F. It is situated in the Valserthal, fourteen miles from Ilanz, at an altitude of 4,100 feet. Its reputation is wholly local, and it is but little frequented.

Val Sinestra, in Canton Grisons, Switzerland, has springs which may be termed *gaseous, ferruginous, and arsenical*. The springs are near Sens, in the Lower Engadine, and about three hours distant from Tarasp-Schuls.

The waters are brought to Schuls chiefly, and they are also *exported*. They contain per litre 0·0017 to 0·0019 of sodium arsenate, 0·03 of bicarbonate of iron, and 1·5 of bicarbonate of lime.

Vegri di Valdagno, in the vicinity of Recoaro, has *sulphate of iron* waters.

Veldes, in Upper Carniola, Austria, on the Lake of Veldes, in the Savethal, at an altitude of 1,560 feet, has an *indifferent thermal* spring of a temperature of 80° F. The situation is a fine one, and it is resorted to in the summer for "sun-baths" and hydrotherapy. The railway station at Lees-Veldes is about three-quarters of an hour's drive.

Vicarello, about sixteen miles from Rome, has *simple thermal* waters. Temperature 113° F. Said to be the Roman Aqua Apollinaris.

Vic le Comte (or **St. Maurice**), France, Puy de Dôme, on the line from Clermont Ferrand to Issoire—station, three miles from the bath—has *thermal* springs, containing sodium bicarbonate and sodium chloride, of the type of the Royat waters. The Source St. Marguerite is the most important, and contains, per litre, nearly 5 grammes, together of sodium bicarbonate and chloride, 0·002 of sodium arsenate, and 0·05 of bicarbonate of iron. Its temperature is 88° F. These waters are exported.

Vic sur Cère, Department Cantal, France, a small bath about twelve miles from Aurillac, at the foot of the mountains of Cantal, in Central France, having *cold gaseous chalybeate arsenical* waters. They are reported to contain, per litre, sodium arsenate 0·008, in addition to sodium bicarbonate 1·8, sodium chloride 1·2, and bicarbonate of iron 0·05, and some salts of lime and magnesium. These waters are chiefly exported.

Vidago, a Portuguese bath, having waters somewhat analagous in composition and therapeutic properties to those of Vichy. The strongest are reported to contain, per litre, sodium bicarbonate 4·6, lithium bicarbonate 0·03, calcium bicarbonate 0·9, and bicarbonate of iron 0·01; also some free carbonic acid gas. The water is bottled for exportation.

Villach, in Carinthia, has *indifferent thermal* springs.

Vinadio, North Italy, Piedmont, has *thermal common salt and sulphur* waters and natural vapour baths (*stufe*), also *fango* or hot mud for outward application. It is twenty-two miles from the railway station of Cuneo.

Viterbo, Province of Rome, has *thermal sulphur* waters.

Voeslau, in Lower Austria, about thirty miles south of Vienna, has *warm, indifferent* springs (75° F.), only used for baths in neurasthenic conditions in women. The grape cure is also carried out there.

Weilbach, a *cold sulphur* bath in Hesse-Nassau, Germany, is situated between Frankfort and Wiesbaden, a short drive from Flörsheim station, at an elevation of 440 feet above the sea. It has two springs, known as the Schwefelquelle and the Natrionlithionquelle. The former is a cold and feebly mineralised spring, but contains sulphuretted hydrogen gas. It is considered to be useful in the treatment of obese persons with a tendency to hypertrophy of the liver and hæmorrhoids. The spray and vapour of this water are inhaled in cases of catarrh of the respiratory organs. It is used also for the preparation of sulphur baths.

The water of the Natrion-lithionquelle is an alkaline common salt water, containing sodium chloride 1·2, sodium carbonate 1·3, and lithium bicarbonate 0·009. It is applied in the treatment of gouty and renal affections and gastro-intestinal catarrh.

The sulphur water is used not only in the cases mentioned, but also in metallic poisoning, and in the treatment of constitutional syphilis.

The season is from the beginning of May to the end of September.

Weissenburg. — A Swiss *weakly mineralised slightly warm calcareous* or *earthy* spring in Canton Bern, a three hours' drive from the railway station of Thun. Weissenburg is situated at an altitude of 2,820 feet in a sheltered and well-wooded valley leading out of the Simmenthal in a north-westerly direction. The *new* bath establishment is a mile and a-quarter from the village.

The bath establishment is surrounded by dense forests of pine and beech trees, so that there is almost entire freedom from dust and from high winds, while there are many shady and agreeable walks. The mean humidity of the atmosphere is rather high in summer, and this may be accounted for by the spray from the neighbouring torrent and its cascades, and the influence of surrounding forests.

The mineral spring has a temperature of about 80° F., and is practically only used for drinking. It is feebly mineralised, its total solids per litre only amounting to 1·39, of which calcium sulphate forms 0·95. It also contains small amounts of carbonate of calcium and magnesium and of sulphates of magnesium, sodium, and potassium. This water is diuretic in its action, and at first tends to constipate, but it is said to act later on as a laxative.

It is usual to commence with very small doses, an ounce or two, which are gradually increased until about twenty ounces are taken daily. If it causes constipation, it is usual to add to the water a little magnesium sulphate. Feeble patients are advised to take the early morning doses of the water in bed. It is said to facilitate expectoration in pulmonary cases.

The speciality of this spa is the treatment of respiratory affections, catarrh of the respiratory passages, chronic bronchitis, asthma, and the early stages of pulmonary tuberculosis. The water drinking has perhaps less curative influence in these latter cases than the soothing and invigorating climate, the regulated, hygienic mode of life, and the calm and restful surroundings with the out-of-door exercise in the pine woods.

The season is from May 15th to Sept. 30th.

Wiesbaden, in Hesse-Nassau, a few miles from Frankfort on the Main, at an elevation of 380 feet, is one of the oldest as well as one of the most popular spas in Germany, and the reputation of its baths reaches back to the time of the Romans. Unlike most of the other spas, it is open all the year round, having a winter season as well as a summer season. So Wiesbaden has grown to be a considerable town, and presents on that account many advantages to the invalid visitor. It has excellent hotels and lodging-houses of all kinds and of all prices. Education is good and not expensive, and the same may be said of its amusements.

Wiesbaden aims at providing nearly everything that all classes of invalids may require, and possesses special resources for all kinds of special maladies. There are excellent establishments for the application of hydrotherapy, with douches, large swimming-baths, etc., and for the application also of electro-therapy. Milk and whey cures are available, cows and goats being fed in a special manner for the purpose; and the grape-cure is introduced in the autumn. This is particularly recommended as an "after-cure," after a course of the waters. Wiesbaden is also well supplied with special medical skill in the shape of oculists, aurists, dentists, etc., so that it forms a sort of invalids' compendium; while it lays claim to virtues as a winter climate which, it must be admitted, can scarcely be granted it as a summer residence. Surrounded on all sides by hills, except to the south, to which it lies completely exposed, it has the disadvantage of being very hot in summer during the daytime: the early mornings and the evenings are, however, cool, for cold currents of air blow down into the valley from the Taunus mountains after the sun goes down.

With regard to the springs at Wiesbaden, their virtues are widely known. Their chief characteristic is their *high temperature*, the Kochbrunnen having a temperature of 150° F.; and their chief constituent is, like so many of the neighbouring spas, *common* salt. Out of 8·20 grammes of solid ingredients in a litre of the water, nearly seven consist of common salt. There is nothing characteristic in the other ingredients, which are for the most part those generally found combined with common salt in other salt springs. There are many other springs, but the only ones used for drinking besides the Kochbrunnen are the Wilhelmsquelle, the Adlerquelle, and the Schützenhofquelle.

In what is known and sold as Wiesbaden *Gichtwasser*, a considerable quantity of sodium bicarbonate is added to the water of the Kochbrunnen. The complaints which are said to be especially benefited by the Wiesbaden springs are those, in the first place, which fall under the category of chronic rheumatism, chronic atonic gout, and neuralgia, old rheumatic and gouty deposits, and thickenings about the joints, as well as muscular rheumatism, and, of neuralgic disorders, sciatica in particular. Cases of paralysis due to chronic inflammation of the coverings of the spinal cord are benefited by the hot baths; so are diseases of the bones, and especially those resulting from gunshot injuries. Chronic ulcers of the skin and some forms of skin diseases, such as eczema, and scrofulous enlargement of glands, are appropriate to treatment at this spa as well as at other salt spas. Cases of protracted syphilitic infection are treated at Wiesbaden in the same manner as at Aix la Chapelle, and those of inflammation of the female pelvic organs as at Kreuznach. It is generally believed that the high temperature of the baths is the chief special influence which is operative in the Wiesbaden cure, but most of the patients are expected to drink the water as well as bathe in it; and, regarded as a drinking spring, other ailments must be added to the list of those already named, chiefly catarrhal conditions of the mucous membranes—*e.g.* chronic gastric catarrh, chronic intestinal catarrh, and chronic laryngeal and bronchial catarrh; all these are said to be amenable to cure, or, at any rate, to great amelioration, by drinking the Wiesbaden waters. *Inhalation* chambers are provided for the treatment of catarrh of the respiratory passages.

The routine of drinking begins at 6 a.m., and from that hour till eight the young women at the Kochbrunnen are busily engaged in supplying the crowd of applicants for glasses of the steaming hot beverage, too hot to be drunk at a draught, so that it has to be slowly sipped or allowed to cool a little before it can be swallowed.

The baths are taken either early in the morning or about an hour after breakfast; patients are required, according to the case, to remain in the bath from twenty minutes to an hour, and a period of complete repose after the bath is earnestly enforced. The water is much too hot to be used as a bath as it issues from the springs, and it is therefore allowed to cool during the night, either in the baths themselves or in reservoirs connected with the bath-houses. The baths are mostly given in certain hotels and bath-houses. These are for the most part in the neighbourhood of the hot springs. It is undoubtedly an immense convenience, especially to those who are crippled by their maladies, to be able to get their baths in the hotels they live in. The baths are taken in the form of full baths and douches. A rain douche of moderately cold water must indeed be an excellent method of refreshing the patient after half an hour in these hot baths.

In connection with the hotel Kaiserhof, a very complete new bath establishment has been erected, the Augusta Victoria Bath, which aims at providing invalids with all the varied resources of "physical therapeutics." It includes mud (*fango*), hot sand, electric, medicated, and Turkish baths, Swedish gymnastics, inhalations, pneumatic chambers, etc.

The period of the cure must not be circumscribed by a hard and fast line. The typical twenty-one baths must often be extended to perhaps twice that number. The environs of Wiesbaden are exceedingly agreeable, and many beautiful walks and drives may be taken through the forests which cover the surrounding hills. A funicular railway recently made up the Nersberg provides easy access to beautiful views and to the fresh air of the Taunus forests.

Wildbad, in the Würtemberg Black Forest, is the type of *indifferent thermal* waters, or, as they are termed in Germany, Wildbäder. It lies in the narrow but beautiful valley of the Enz, at an altitude of 1,400 feet. The river Enz runs through the little town, and there are pleasant walks in the grounds on both sides of the river, as well as in some gardens about a mile from the town. There are also steep zigzag walks up the wooded slopes of the valley. The climate is mildly bracing, and though it may be hot at midday the nights are usually cool.

The temperature of the hot springs, which are numerous, ranges between 92° and 104° F. Most of the springs are alike in being very feebly mineralised, containing minute amounts of sodium salts, chloride, sulphate, and bicarbonate, and a little lime. The springs chiefly used for drinking are the Eberhardsbrunnen and the Königsbrunnen. The waters of other spas are often drunk at Wildbad when an active water is required.

The characteristic bath—the *Wildbad*—given there is an ordinary thermal bath, the water of which bubbles up through a sandy floor, and by means of an overflow pipe is also continually running off, like the French bath *à l'eau courant*. In this way the temperature of the bath is maintained constant.

Other mineral baths are also provided—cold and hot—as well as hot air and vapour baths, douches, electric baths, and Swedish gymnastics, with Zander's appliances.

All the bathing arrangements are commodious and even luxurious.

The diseases suitable for treatment at Wildbad are such as are sent to other simple thermal spas. They are cases of gouty and rheumatoid arthritis in debilitated subjects, and stiff joints, the result of injury; cases of retarded convalescence from acute disease, functional nervous disorders, and even organic nervous affections at an early stage, hysteria, hypochondria in irritable subjects requiring reposeful surroundings, neurasthenia, old hemiplegias or paraplegias, cases of over-work, combined with general debility, and needing rest in a moderately bracing and sedative climate. Pleasant walks and drives of almost any distance can be taken in the surrounding forests. The season is from May 1st to the end of September.

The railway station is the terminus of the

Pforzheim - Wildbad line; the usual route from London being Cologne, Carlsruhe, Pforzheim.

Wildungen, in the principality of Waldeck-Pyrmont, Germany, represents in that country the type of bath of which Contrexéville is the chief representative in France. Its springs are classed amongst the *earthy* or *calcareous* waters. Wildungen is pleasantly situated at an altitude of nearly 1,000 feet, in an open valley, sheltered to some extent from cold winds, and can be reached from Cassel in two hours by the Wildungen-Wabern branch line. The *Bad*, with its hotels and villas, is at the western part of the town, and it has shady woods close at hand, affording every attraction for out-of-door exercise. The three springs most resorted to are the George-Victorquelle, the Helenenquelle, and the Königsquelle. The water of these springs is cold and gaseous, and contains chiefly calcium and magnesium bicarbonate (0·5 to 1·3 grammes per litre), and some bicarbonate of iron (0·018 to 0·036).

The George-Victor is the most feebly mineralised, the Königsquelle contains the most iron, and the Helenenquelle a certain amount of sodium bicarbonate (0·84), and these two springs each contain about 1·0 per litre of sodium chloride, as well as calcium and magnesium bicarbonate in about the same proportion.

Other springs occasionally drunk at Wildungen are the Thalquelle, an earthy, chalybeate water, and the Stahlquelle, a gaseous chalybeate spring rich in carbonic acid and containing 0·07 per litre of bicarbonate of iron. Both these springs are at some distance from the town, but the water of the Stahlquelle and of the Helenenquelle are supplied at the George-Victorquelle.

The bath-house, where patients can also reside, has a spring of its own. The Königsquelle has also a bath-house attached to it.

The *speciality* of Wildungen, as of its French rival, Contrexéville, is the treatment of maladies of the urinary organs, such as calculous patients, renal or vesical, cases of chronic pyelitis and cystitis, cases of prostatic hypertrophy and its sequelæ, cases of uric acid gravel and irritative albuminuria.

Naturally the majority of the patients are men, but women are also treated there when they suffer from gravel, or vesical irritability from other causes.

The waters are usually taken in the morning fasting, often again before the midday meal, and occasionally in the afternoon also. It is a usual practice to warm the water before drinking. Mixing a little hot whey or milk with it renders it more digestible and more agreeable to some patients.

Only a certain section of the patients are ordered to take baths, usually those with renal (uric acid) calculi or gravel, which are given at a temperature varying from 80° to 100° F.

The Helenenquelle, on account of its greater alkalinity, is usually prescribed in cases of great bladder irritability, with acid urine, and it is often prescribed at the commencement of the course, because it is more readily tolerated by the stomach. The George-Victorquelle is thought more suitable when there is much vesical catarrh with alkaline, phosphatic urine. The Stahlquelle is a useful resource in anæmic cases.

The diet in the hotels is regulated to the requirements of the cases treated there; rich and highly seasoned dishes are avoided, beer is prohibited, and sweets and wine or spirits are only allowed in great moderation.

Wildungen has been termed a *surgical* spa, which is a tribute to the surgical skill of its medical men. Surgical methods of treatment are frequently called for and practised, as lithotrity, division or dilatation of urethral structures, etc. It is maintained that the use of these waters often induces a condition favourable to operative methods. Few other patients than those enumerated seek relief from their maladies at Wildungen, yet the alkaline Helenenquelle is well adapted to the treatment of chronic bronchial catarrh and certain forms of dyspepsia, which, moreover, could not fail to be benefited by the tonic air of the forests and the wholesome diet.

Though this spa is open to patients all through the year, the season generally chosen for a cure there is between May 10th and Sept. 25th.

Woodhall Spa, near Horncastle, Lincolnshire, 37 feet above the level of the sea, has acquired a great reputation on account of its so-called *bromo-iodine* spring. Woodhall is situated in an elevated part of Lincolnshire, twenty-three miles due west of the coast. Its subsoil is dry sand with iron stone, and the climate is dry and invigorating. The country around is wooded and agreeable. Woodhall Spa is near enough to the sea to be influenced by the sea breezes. It is in a part of England which has the smallest annual rainfall— not much more than twenty inches.

The hotel accommodation is good, and comfortable lodging-houses near the baths can be found. The water supply is good, being brought from the Wolds, fifteen miles off.

Dr. Frankland, in his analysis of this water (1891), found that it contained per litre 19·5 sodium chloride, 1·27 calcium chloride, 1·114 magnesium chloride, 0·0635 of sodium and potassium bromide together, and 0·0075 of potassium iodide, and no free iodine and no arsenic. The Woodhall Spa water is therefore a moderately strong *common salt* water with small amounts of bromides and iodides. Its temperature is 56° F.

The water when drawn from the well was found by Frankland to be very turbid, and on long standing to deposit reddish matter consisting almost entirely of hydrated peroxide of iron.

A *Mutterlauge*, or "mother lye," is also prepared here by evaporation of the salt water, as at other common salt spas on the Continent, and is used for local compresses and for fortifying the baths.

Although the amount of bromides and iodides may appear small, it must be remembered that in the large bulk of water required to make a full bath the total amount of these compounds would assume a very respectable figure, and as there seems to be little doubt that iodine compounds, at any rate, can be absorbed by the skin, under favourable conditions, it may be concluded that this is the case in connection with treatment at Woodhall.

These waters are applied in various ways at the spa—as full and partial baths, as douches, with or without Aix massage, as uterine and vaginal injections, vapour baths, and as sprays for inhalation and irrigation in chronic nasal, pharyngeal, and laryngeal catarrhs.

The diseases which have been found especially benefited by treatment at Woodhall are the following: rheumatism and gout, chronic rheumatoid arthritis, chronic catarrhal states of the mucous membranes, respiratory and genito-urinary, uterine and vaginal leucorrhœa, functional hepatic disorders, biliousness, scrofulous and syphilitic affections of the skin, bones, and joints, chronic periuterine inflammatory exudations, and fibroid tumours of the uterus.

Woodhall Spa is about four hours from London, and the spa is open all the year round, but the summer and autumn months are the most favourable for the cure.

Warasdin-Teplitz, in Croatia, at an altitude of 920 feet, three hours from the railway station of Csakathurn, has weakly mineralised *thermal sulphur* waters, temperature 136° F., said to be the Aquæ Jasæ of the Romans.

Warmbad, near Wolkenstein, in the Erz Mountains, Saxony—railway station, Flossplatz, on the Chemnitz-Weipert line—lies at an elevation of about 1,500 feet, in a well-wooded branch valley of the Zoschopau, and has *simple thermal* waters (temperature about 80° F.), containing a little sodium chloride and carbonate. They are used for drinking and for baths and douches in cases of nervous affections, rheumatism, gout, gastro-intestinal and female complaints. Season, May 1 to Oct. 1.

Warmbrunn, on the northern slope of the Riesengebirge, in Prussian Silesia, at an elevation of about 1,100 feet, railway station on the Hirschberg-Petersdorf line (it also has electric railway to Hirschberg), is a summer resort, and has several *simple thermal* springs with temperatures varying from 77° to 109° F., containing a little sodium sulphate and carbonate. They are used for drinking and for baths. There is also a swimming bath. A chalybeate spring is likewise used there, the Victoriaquelle. Mud, carbonic acid, and electric baths, hydrotherapy and massage are also available. The season is from May 1 to Oct. 1.

Werl, a small *brine* bath in Westphalia.

Werne, a *thermal brine* bath in Westphalia.

Wildegg, in the valley of the Aar, Switzerland, about two and a-half miles from Schinznach, has a cold spring belonging to the *common salt* group, but containing sodium *iodide* and *bromide*, together amounting to 0·041 per litre, in addition to sodium chloride 10 grammes, magnesium chloride 1·6, and calcium sulphate 1·8. It is made use of at the neighbouring spa of Schinznach in scrofulous diseases, and is exported.

Wimpfen, on the Neckar, has *brine* baths, the brine coming from the Ludwigs-hable salt works. Franzensbad *Moor* baths, pine-needle baths, and hydrotherapy are also available. Railway station on the Heidelberg-Jagstfeld line.

Wipfeld, in Lower Franconia, Bavaria, has *cold calcareous* springs, one of which, the Ludwigsquelle, is strongly *sulphurous*. It contains 1 gramme per litre of calcium sulphate and 24 volumes of H_2S. It has also weak chalybeate springs. The sulphur water is used for drinking and for preparing sulphur mud-baths; gout and rheumatism are the maladies especially treated.

Wittekind, a *common salt* water, near the University town of Halle, in Saxony; also a sanatorium. The water is aërated with carbonic acid for drinking and exportation, and is strengthened with *Mutterlauge*, or bath salt, for bathing. It contains 35 grammes per litre of common salt.

Yverdon, Canton Vaud, Switzerland, on the line between Lausanne and Neuchâtel, has feebly mineralised *warm sulphur* waters containing 3·4 volumes per litre of H_2S. The bath establishment is well equipped for treatment by pulverisation and inhalation, douches, massage, etc.

Zaizon, in Transylvania, at an altitude of 2,600 feet, has a *weak gaseous alkaline common salt* spring, having sodium bicarbonate 1·3 and chloride 0·6 per litre. It has also a weak chalybeate water. It is frequented by women and children chiefly.

as well as of declared "scrofulous" manifestations, not only by sodium chloride waters and "brine" baths, as at La Mouillère, Salins de Jura, Salies de Béarn, Salins Moutiers, Bourbonne les Bains, etc., but also by the stronger sulphur waters such as Luchon, Barèges, etc., or the springs containing both sodium chloride and sulphur, as Uriage, which has been described as "a veritable sulphurous *sea-bath* in the mountains." The saline and arsenical water of La Bourboule is also prescribed in the same cases, and it is maintained that there are cases of scrofulous disease in which sea air proves too exciting, and which do better under the calming but tonic influence of mild mountain air which can be obtained at most of these spas.

If we wish to carry out this method of treatment in England, we have many suitable resorts. The bromo-iodine and sodium chloride spring of Woodhall Spa has a well established reputation for the treatment of these affections. The brine baths of Droitwich and Nantwich, the sodium chloride and sulphur springs of Harrogate, may be applied in the same class of cases. In Germany and Austria there are many baths having a like renown, such as Kreuznach, Aussee (Styria), Hall (Upper Austria), Baden-Baden, Krankenheil-Tölz (Bavaria), and others. Wildegg, in Switzerland, and Salso Maggiore, in Italy, belong to the same group.

It is believed that the drinking of mild sodium chloride water increases albuminoid metabolism, while the brine baths, and other external appliances, exert a stimulating local effect, and those containing iodine and bromine promote absorption of glandular infiltrations.

PULMONARY TUBERCULOSIS.

With regard to *pulmonary tuberculosis*, the climatic and sanatorium treatment of this affection will be considered in the second part of this work, and we shall only, here, refer briefly to those mineral-water resorts that have a time-honoured reputation in the treatment of certain forms of this malady. The success that has attended the "open-air" treatment of phthisis, in suitable and well arranged sanatoria, has greatly diminished the interest that was at one time taken in the treatment of these cases by mineral waters.

The mild sodium chloride waters (Soden) and the alkaline sodium chloride waters (Ems, Gleichenberg in Styria, Obersalzbrunn in Silesia) have been found useful in relieving the catarrhal symptoms associated with chronic, quiescent, torpid forms of phthisis; Ems enjoyed at one time a considerable reputation in this respect, but its somewhat relaxing climate is now generally regarded as unsuited to cases of phthisis.

Weissenburg, near Thun, in Switzerland, with warm weakly mineralised calcareous springs, in a sheltered position in a pine forest, at an elevation of nearly 3,000 feet, owes its reputation, in the treatment of early apyretic forms of phthisis, probably quite as much to its favourable subalpine situation as to its mineral waters.

In France the arsenical springs of La Bourboule and Mt. Dore, and certain of the sulphur springs in the Pyrenees especially, enjoy the reputation of being of value in the treatment of certain forms of pulmonary tuberculosis.

It is most probable that this reputation rests partly on the anti-catarrhal action of these waters, and partly on the favourable hygienic and climatic influence, to which the patients are submitted in those stations, most of which are situated in salubrious mountainous districts, and at moderate elevations. The suggestion put forward at one time that the sulphur components in these springs, especially sulphuretted hydrogen, exercised an anti-bactericidal effect, has not been sustained.

It seems clear that in so chronic and progressive

an affection as pulmonary tuberculosis, a mere course of mineral water, of three to six weeks' duration, could exert but little curative effect, although it might be of service, combined with other measures, in relieving certain symptoms.

We can understand that the tonic arsenical water of La Bourboule, combining also anti-catarrhal effects (from its relationship to the alkaline sodium chloride springs) with bracing mountain air, may have a remedial influence in the cases for which it is deemed appropriate—those, according to the local physicians, are the "pre-tuberculous," or cases in the first stage of the disease, and even more advanced cases when "torpid and of slow evolution."

Those Pyrenean spas which have been especially recommended in the treatment of this disease are all of them situated in mountainous districts, and most of them at an elevation of 2,000 to 3,000 feet: Ax les Thermes (over 2,000), Eaux Bonnes (about 2,300), Cauterets (3,000); Amélie les Bains is not so high (900 feet). Allevard, in the Chambéry district, is also at an elevation of about 1,300 and St. Honoré, near Nevers, nearly 1,000 feet. In all these the indication is for early, torpid, apyretic cases, with a fair amount of constitutional vigour and capacity of resistance to the disease. La Vernet (2,300 feet) trusts more to its sanatorium treatment than to its sulphur springs.

The idea of sending young children with *rickets* for treatment at mineral springs is not a very feasible one. Suitable dietetic and tonic medicinal treatment, in a country or seaside home, seems far more appropriate.

SYPHILIS.

The treatment of constitutional *syphilis* by mineral waters and baths, and the manner in which they act, has been the subject of much controversy. We shall endeavour to summarise briefly the views now generally accepted. The idea that they exert any specific effect is no longer entertained, but their usefulness, in many cases, is not doubted.

It is believed by the physicians at those spas in which syphilitics are especially treated, as Aix la Chapelle, Aix les Bains, Luchon, Barèges, Uriage (combination of sulphur and sodium chloride), etc., that the sulphur water enables the patient to bear much more energetic specific treatment than he otherwise could; and that this is mainly due to the fact that the mineral-water and bath treatment increases metabolic activity and promotes general nutrition. Not only are mercurial inunctions freely used—from two to three drachms of mercurial ointment daily—but hypodermic injections of soluble salts of mercury, with or without iodides, are frequently administered. The association of tonic mountain, or forest, air with the thermal treatment, as at Barèges, Luchon, Uriage, and other resorts, has doubtless an excellent effect in cachectic cases.

This has been remarked upon by the physicians at Luchon, who maintain, and we believe rightly, that this combination is a most valuable auxiliary in the cure of syphilis. At Uriage, also, it has been observed that, in its mountain climate, the mineral-water and bath treatment, combined with mercurial frictions and injections (the patient being able to tolerate much larger doses), has proved of great value in some of the most serious cases of syphilitic infection; as in the pre-ataxic period of tabes, in cerebral syphilis and syphilitic myelitis, and in children the subjects of hereditary syphilis.

In such cases improved nutrition, increase in weight and strength, disappearance of anæmia and cachexia, have been observed.

The diagnostic value of treatment by sulphur baths, in revealing the existence of latent syphilis, is no longer generally admitted.

To sum up, the advantage of sulphur spa treatment in syphilis is that it offers a convenient opportunity for vigorously pursuing specific treatment, and it appears to favour the tolerance of large doses of mercury and to prevent, or counteract, cachectic symptoms.

Some authorities think the arsenical waters of La Bourboule and Levico of use in syphilitic cases, and others point to the utility of sodium chloride waters containing iodine and bromine, in tertiary forms; as Woodhall, Kreuznach, Hall (Upper Austria), Krankenheil-Tölz, etc. Anti-syphilitic treatment is also carried out successfully at Baden-Baden.

CHRONIC METALLIC POISONING.

Cases of *chronic metallic poisoning* (lead, mercury, etc.) are benefited by treatment with sulphur waters and baths—it is believed that the elimination of the poison by the intestines, kidneys, and skin is promoted by mild sulphur waters internally, and warm baths. The latter may be of ordinary water or of the indifferent thermal class, and these are probably as useful as sulphur baths. The warm sodium sulphate waters, such as Carlsbad or Brides, may be of use in cases in which stimulation of the liver is especially indicated.

GLYCOSURIA AND DIABETES.

We have elsewhere discussed the pathology and general and dietetic treatment of glycosuria and diabetes; * we have only in this place to consider the value of mineral waters in the treatment of this disease. We accept the view that all more or less permanent forms of glycosuria are cases of diabetes, and exclude only those cases of the occasional or temporary appearance of sugar in the urine, which occur in certain persons from the excessive consumption of saccharine substances, which appear to have no serious import,

* *See* the Author's "Manual of Medical Treatment," New Edition, vol. ii., p. 531; also "Food in Health and Disease," New Edition, p. 363.

and which may be termed cases of *non-diabetic* or alimentary glycosuria.

It will be convenient, and of some practical importance, especially in connection with the use of mineral waters in this disease, if we recognise three forms of diabetes. First, the *slight* cases—to which the term diabetes is refused by some authorities—such forms often occur in *fat* and *gouty* persons, and the sugar disappears entirely, or almost entirely, from the urine, when carbo-hydrates are excluded from their diet. Such persons are often restored to health by mineral water treatment and a restricted dietary, but are apt to again become glycosuric on the free consumption of carbo-hydrates. Secondly, the cases of *moderate* severity, of which there may be several degrees, in which there is a greater or less diminution in the excretion of sugar, when a rigid diet is enforced; but it does not entirely disappear from the urine, and the general symptoms also, although capable of considerable amelioration by treatment, are not wholly recovered, and become aggravated by any deviation from a strict dietary. There are differences of opinion, as we shall see, with regard to the utility of mineral-water treatment in this group; these cases are, moreover, prone to be attacked by intercurrent maladies, as pneumonia and phthisis, and to pass into the Third or *grave* form. This form is usually rapidly assumed when diabetes attacks *young* persons; in these the glycosuria is maintained, in spite of the strictest dietetic measures, and the patients quickly pass into a cachectic state and generally die of diabetic coma.

There is a general agreement, amongst all authorities, that these *grave* cases are not benefited by mineral-water treatment, and even if we are desirous of trying the effect of mineral waters, it is best to do so at home, and not run the risk attending a journey to a foreign spa; as such patients bear the fatigue of travel very badly, attacks of diabetic coma often supervening on undue exertion.

The French, in considering the applicability of mineral-water treatment to diabetics, divide them into *fat* and *thin* diabetics, or those in which there is diminished and those in which there is increased nitrogenous metabolism. In the latter there is "azoturia" as well as "glycosuria."

It may, then, be accepted as a sound general conclusion that only diabetics of the first group and the more vigorous and chronic cases of the second group should be submitted to mineral-water treatment. But French authorities are disposed to admit a much wider application of mineral water treatment, even to somewhat advanced cases, than German or English physicians. The waters best suited to the treatment of diabetes are undoubtedly the warm *alkaline* waters; the *simple* alkaline waters (Vichy, Neuenahr), the *alkaline* and *mild* sodium chloride waters (Royat), the alkaline sodium sulphate waters (Carlsbad), and the alkaline arsenical waters (La Bourboule).

The three spas most resorted to by diabetics are Carlsbad, Vichy, and Neuenahr. Carlsbad is particularly adapted to the fat and gouty diabetic who is fairly vigorous, with sluggish hepatic functions, constipation, and a tendency to uric acid deposits, and perhaps a little albumen in the urine. The cold waters of Marienbad, with the same composition as those at Carlsbad, have also been found serviceable for obese diabetics with only a small amount of sugar in the urine.

Even thin diabetics, beyond middle age, who retain a fair amount of vigour and in whom the disease is very chronic, and who suffer from gouty symptoms, often gain advantage from Carlsbad. A course of four to five weeks annually is desirable, and in some cases good results follow two courses in the same year, with three or four months' interval.

The same kind of cases also do well at Vichy, but this course is also applicable to a rather more extensive group, comprising those in whom the constitutional symptoms are somewhat more severe, with wasting and azoturia. The excretion of urea is often observed to return to the normal—together with a diminution and, in recent cases, a disappearance of the sugar from the urine; at the same time the nervous irritability and the insomnia are relieved, the dryness of the mouth and throat are removed, and exercise can be taken with less fatigue. The cold alkaline waters of Vals are also useful in the fat and gouty cases.

The warm mildly alkaline and common salt springs of Neuenahr have proved useful to a vast number of diabetics; they may be prescribed for all cases suitable for spa treatment, and especially for those patients who are not vigorous enough to be sent to Carlsbad.

Brides les Bains, in Savoy, is suitable to much the same class of cases as Carlsbad, viz. those with a tendency to hepatic congestion and constipation.

The *alkaline arsenical* waters of La Bourboule, on account of the arsenic they contain, should be preferred in those cases in which the nitrogenous and phosphatic elimination is increased, and there is progressive wasting. These waters are believed to lessen tissue change and organic waste. They are suited to the thin chronic diabetic who is weak and neurotic, and who needs a more tonic treatment than that of Vichy, the climate being more suitable to such cases; but it must not be thought that they can be of service to really cachectic patients. Baths are to be avoided in the cases adapted to La Bourboule.

Contrexéville has been suggested in cases in which glycosuria alternates with attacks of uric acid gravel. It is suited to what the French term "*petits diabétiques*," gouty cases in which the excretion of sugar does not exceed 600 grains per diem; as the sugar lessens, the tendency to uric acid gravel increases.

Royat is regarded as suitable for the more feeble and anæmic diabetics.

In France nearly all the sodium chloride waters are said to be suitable for the treatment of fat diabetics. We may mention the following less well known resorts:—

Bourbonne les Bains (sodium chloride) in gouty cases in which nitrogenous elimination needs stimulation.

Bourbonne l'Archambaut (weak alkaline and common salt) for gouty diabetics with tendency to feebleness.

Châtelguyon (alkaline common salt) for fat diabetics.

Le Boulou, in the Eastern Pyrenees (cold sodium carbonate), said to be efficacious in diabetes "in general."

Santenay (sodium chloride and sulphate) for cases with defective nitrogenous metabolism accompanied with nervous depression.

Obersalzbrunn, in Silesia (sodium bicarbonate), is recommended in the same class of cases as Neuenahr.

In our own country good accounts are given of the treatment of gouty diabetics at Harrogate and Llandrindod.

The combination of warm baths with the drinking cure is of service in promoting a healthy action of the skin, in many cases of the fat and gouty type, but it must be borne in mind that such baths prove injurious to those cases in which there is marked azoturia, as they tend to increase the tissue waste, and aggravate the emaciation, and must therefore be avoided.

In all cases in which a mineral-water cure is found to agree, we shall find a great diminution of the sugar in the urine, or its entire disappearance, a removal of the thirst and dryness of the mouth, an improvement in the general nutrition and ability to assimilate normally a certain amount of carbohydrates, an increase of weight, in the emaciated, and a renewed capacity for muscular exercise. In those who are too fat to take much exercise, Swedish gymnastics and massage may prove useful auxiliaries, in promoting oxidation and a more normal metabolism.

It is probable that much of the benefit derived from treatment at a well-organised spa is referable to a well-ordered diet and regimen, a cheerful life, free from care and anxiety, amidst picturesque and healthy surroundings, with a due amount of out-of-door exercise. Residence in an establishment under medical dietetic supervision is a great advantage. Some recommend, in anæmic cases, that a course of chalybeate water and baths at Schwalbach, Spa, or Pyrmont should succeed the treatment with alkaline waters; an after cure in some restful and moderately bracing place is certainly desirable.

The general use, at home, of gaseous table waters containing sodium bicarbonate and sodium chloride is to be commended in all cases of glycosuria; Vichy and Vals waters are too alkaline to be drunk with food, but may be taken at bed time or on rising in the morning. Giesshübel and Apollinaris are best suited for table and general use.

Apollinaris has much the same composition as Neuenahr water, and when mixed with a little hot water may be regarded as almost identical and quite as useful for home consumption.

GOUT AND THE URIC ACID DIATHESIS.

There is no chronic disease in which recourse is so commonly had to treatment by mineral springs as gout; and nearly every kind of mineral spring has, in its turn, been advocated as a remedy for this disease. The acute arthritic forms of gout are, of course, altogether unsuited to spa treatment, and it is to the various manifestations of *chronic* gout that treatment by mineral waters is applicable. In all such cases we have mainly two things to consider: (*a*) the treatment of the *general* gouty state—the disturbances of normal metabolism, the excessive production of uric acid, and the need for its elimination; (*b*) the treatment of the particular *local affection* or affections attending it, due to the influence of the excess of uric acid on the joints, muscles, viscera, and other structures.

1. Of the various kinds of mineral springs and baths that are available, and that have been advocated, in the treatment of these morbid states, we may mention first the large group of *simple alkaline* waters which occupy a very important place in the treatment of gout. Vichy and Vals are perhaps the most important representatives of the stronger waters of this group.

These springs, especially when warm, are applicable to the treatment of gouty states associated with acid dyspepsia and chronic gastric and intestinal catarrhs; or with biliary and renal gravel and calculi; or with hepatic congestion in feeble persons; or with vesical catarrh and prostatitis associated with excessively acid urine. In the latter condition a course at Vichy is often exceedingly useful.

Other springs of this class are Neuenahr (the only *warm* alkaline spring in Germany), Ober-salzbrunn in Silesia, Fachingen, Bilin, Assmannshausen, especially rich in lithium, and many more of less importance. These waters produce free diuresis and promote renal elimination. They also, by diluting the bile, promote its free discharge and so favour hepatic elimination.

They are all of special value in the treatment of the intercurrent attacks of renal and bladder irritation to which the gouty are prone.

2. The warm *alkaline* and *sodium chloride* springs are applicable to much the same class of cases as the preceding, but they are especially suitable to the treatment of *catarrhs of the respiratory organs* in the gouty. The presence of a small amount of common salt increases the expectorant

properties of these waters, and acts also as a stimulant to digestion in the frequently co-existing dyspeptic states. Ems and Royat belong to this class; Royat is especially useful in *atonic* forms of gout, and has a wide application in the treatment of gouty states in feeble persons.

3. Another group of alkaline waters of great importance in the treatment of the gouty is the aperient *alkaline sodium sulphate* waters; they combine an active aperient and eliminative effect, together with the alkaline action of the simple alkaline springs. Carlsbad and Marienbad, in Bohemia, are the most remarkable and the most highly-reputed representatives of this class, Carlsbad being hot and Marienbad cold.

At these spas the hot mineral mud and vapour baths, together with the application of massage, gymnastics, and electricity, give an additional value to the treatment. Elimination and excretion, which are defective and disturbed in most gouty persons, are powerfully stimulated and promoted by the employment of these mineral waters and baths. The excretory functions of the skin, kidneys, and intestinal canal are brought into greatly increased activity, complete and normal nutritive metabolism is restored, and waste products are eliminated.

This treatment is especially indicated in fairly vigorous patients in whom active eliminative treatment is called for, and in whom the hepatic and intestinal functions are especially sluggish. It is counter-indicated in atonic cases, in cases of advanced arterio-sclerosis, or where cardiac debility is pronounced. Recent gouty deposits in the neighbourhood of joints will often disappear after treatment of this kind.

The cold springs of Marienbad have not so wide a range of application as those of Carlsbad. They are well adapted to the treatment of constipation in the gouty, and to cases complicated with obesity, and where the disturbances of nutrition and excretion are not so serious as in those treated at Carlsbad.

They are suitable to all those gouty cases in which migrainous headaches, dyspepsia, loss of appetite, and other troublesome symptoms are associated with torpor of the intestines.

Tarasp, in the Lower Engadine, is another spring belonging to this group. Its situation at an elevation of 4,000 feet is bracing, and it is especially suited to those cases of gout in which we desire to combine tonic with eliminative influences.

In France, Brides les Bains falls under this class, and has been termed "the French Carlsbad." It may be recommended to those gouty patients who suffer from hepatic and intestinal torpor.

4. The class of *common salt* springs are largely used in the treatment of certain forms of chronic gout. The weaker springs, such as Homburg and Kissingen, are drunk, and also used as baths.

The strong *brine* springs, such as Droitwich, Rheinfelden, Salso Maggiore, and many others, are mainly used for external treatment.

The cold drinking springs, as represented by Homburg and Kissingen, are especially applicable to gouty dyspeptics with tendency to constipation and hepatic congestion. They are often found somewhat tonic in their action; and as they are highly impregnated with free carbonic acid, they are usually easily digested, and, in cases of atonic gout, prove somewhat stimulating, and improve the assimilative functions. Some of the Homburg springs contain an appreciable amount of iron.

In many cases, however, they are not so well tolerated as the alkaline springs. The brine baths, the hot salt springs and the gaseous salt springs (Wiesbaden and Nauheim) are chiefly applicable to the treatment of the chronic joint affections of the gouty—ankyloses, deformities, thickenings and exudations, and neuralgias of the large nerve trunks, etc.

They exercise a stimulating effect on the joints, especially the *gaseous* salt springs; when applied generally or locally they are found to promote the absorption of gouty exudations, and tend, when associated with mechanical treatment, to restore mobility to the stiffened and crippled articulations.

5. The *simple thermal* baths are largely employed in the treatment of chronic articular gout and for the removal of gouty exudations. Bath, Buxton, Wildbad, Gastein, Ragatz, Teplitz, are examples. They are applied to the removal of gouty exudations and in the treatment of peripheral paralyses and neuralgias of gouty origin. Their efficacy is usually augmented by massage, gymnastics, and electricity.

6. The large class of *sulphur* springs are greatly used in the treatment of the chronic articular, and especially of the chronic cutaneous and respiratory, affections of the gouty.

The *cold* sulphur springs (Allevard, Heustrich) are especially useful in the treatment of chronic gouty catarrhs of the pharynx, larynx, trachea, and bronchi. They are drunk usually in small quantity, previously warmed, and are also used as sprays, gargles, and inhalations, as well as in the form of warm baths.

Gouty eczema is especially benefited by the baths at Harrogate and Strathpeffer.

The chronic articular forms of gout are especially benefited by *hot sulphur baths.* They are found useful in the removal of periarticular gouty exudations, in restoring mobility to crippled limbs, and in relieving certain forms of gouty neuralgias, sciatica, lumbago, etc. At Aix les Bains the vigorous and skilful method in which these springs are applied, their thermality, and the warm dry climate, all contribute to the good effects obtained. Baden, near Vienna, enjoys a similar reputation.

The calcareous or *earthy* springs are of great value in the renal and vesical affections of the gouty, uric acid gravel and calculi, vesical catarrh, prostatitis, etc. (Wildungen, in Germany, Contrexéville and Vittel in France). The very feebly mineralised waters of Evian, on the Lake of Geneva, have been found valuable in the same class of cases. It is difficult to understand the precise manner in which these waters act as solvents of uric acid and other urinary concretions, but at these baths, as a rule, very large quantities of the springs are drunk, and a certain amount of mechanical flushing of the urinary passages may probably account for a great part of their action.

At many of these resorts for the gouty, additional remedial influences are brought to bear on the manifestations of this malady in the shape of local or general baths of mineral mud, peat, pine-needle infusions, hot sand, etc.; and, as has already been stated, massage, gymnastics, and light, dry heat, and electrical treatment are obtainable at most.

Another most important remedial agency, which can hardly be over-estimated, is the extremely careful dietetic management which is applied in such resorts as Carlsbad.

We must bear in mind, also, that there is an important condition common to most of these courses of treatment and that is the regular daily consumption of water, a solvent and eliminative agent of great potency.

Amongst our British resorts we have no representatives of the simple alkaline, or the alkaline and sodium chloride springs, but we have at Harrogate strong sulphur waters and chloride of sodium springs, applicable to the treatment of chronic articular gout, gouty neuralgias, and gouty skin affections; as well as of cases of intestinal and hepatic torpor.

Bath and Buxton are examples of thermal springs, useful in the treatment of articular and neuralgic forms of gout. Strathpeffer is useful in the same cases, and has proved very efficacious in the treatment of gouty eczema. Cheltenham and Leamington springs are applicable to much the same kind of gouty manifestations as Homburg or Kissingen, viz. disturbances of hepatic and renal elimination. Woodhall Spa can be utilised for the same class of gouty cases as those that are sent to Kreuznach or Salso Maggiore; and Llandrindod Wells has cold saline, sulphur, and chalybeate springs which admit of being largely utilised in the treatment of gouty affections.

LITHIASIS, OXALURIA, PHOSPHATURIA.

Lithiasis, the deposition of uric acid and urates in the urine, is closely allied to the gouty state, and commonly arises from like causes, viz. too liberal consumption of rich food and alcoholic beverages, too little ingestion of pure water, insufficient exercise, and consequent hepatic inadequacy and tendency to constipation. It is very amenable to treatment by mineral waters, and with the exception of the sulphur waters, most of the waters that are suitable for the gouty are suitable for the subjects of lithiasis and with the same qualifications. Those of robust habit of body, with a tendency to obesity and constipation, should be sent to take the alkaline aperient sodium sulphate waters, such as Carlsbad, Marienbad, Tarasp, or Brides. The warm springs (Carlsbad, Brides) are best suited to those cases attended with hepatic congestion. The simple warm alkaline waters (Vichy, Neuenahr) or the cold gaseous alkaline springs (Vals, Fachingen, Apollinaris), are more suitable to feeble persons or those with a tendency to diarrhœa. The Royat springs, containing some sodium chloride and minute amounts of arsenic and lithium, are especially suited to atonic, feeble patients. The very feebly mineralised water of Evian is largely prescribed for these cases. The sodium chloride waters of Kissingen, Harrogate, Homburg, Châtelguyon, etc., are considered well adapted to thin dyspeptic persons with defective nutrition and appetite. The calcareous waters of Wildungen, in Germany, and of Contrexéville and Vittel, in France, are also employed in the treatment of these cases; and in cases in which there are symptoms pointing to the probable presence of concretions in the kidney they may be preferred, especially in the case of patients who find alkaline waters depressing. These earthy waters are usually prescribed in much larger doses than the alkaline waters. At home much good may be derived from the regular use of the alkaline effervescent table waters, such as Apollinaris, Johannis, Selters, Giesshübel, etc. The utility of these waters in lithiasis depends chiefly on their diuretic influence, and not so much on any solvent effect, but this may not be without some influence, as their alkalinity certainly is in many cases. The flushing of the urinary passages is, however, a very important part of their beneficial effects. Careful regulation of diet is an essential auxiliary to these mineral water cures.

The presence of oxalate of lime crystals in the urine (*oxaluria*) is often found associated with symptoms of dyspepsia and nervous depression. Recourse to suitable mineral waters where the spa is situated in a bracing climate, with quiet but pleasant and cheerful surroundings, often proves effectual in restoring health to such patients. The gaseous alkaline waters, as Giesshübel, the weaker Vals springs, Neuenahr and Apollinaris may be freely drunk, not necessarily at their sources, but in any convenient health resort where the surroundings might be more congenial and appropriate.

Evian is a suitable resort—cheerful and quiet, and with appropriate springs. Pougues les Eaux has been found useful in these cases. Some authorities think the earthy calcareous waters the best, as those at Contrexéville, Vittel, or Wildungen. The slightly alkaline and mildly tonic waters of Bussang, most appropriately situated in the Vosges, may be recommended.

Phosphaturia is apt to occur in the over-worked student or man of business, and is dependent probably on too sedentary a life and insufficient exercise in the open air. It often disappears with "change of air," increased physical exercise, and a cheerful out-of-door life. It is rarely advisable to prescribe a mineral-water course unless other symptoms or conditions are present which render this desirable.

If atonic dyspepsia or a tendency to constipation co-exist, the sodium chloride waters of Kissingen or Homburg may be recommended, and if there is decided anæmia the gaseous iron waters of Schwalbach or St. Moritz, or the mild iron and arsenical water of Bussang. Some advise the calcareous waters of Contrexéville.

OBESITY.

The appropriate mineral-water treatment of *obesity* will depend, to a great extent, on the nature of the conditions which accompany the obesity.

There are the plethoric obese, with abundant muscular activity; there are the pale, feeble, and anæmic obese, with ill-nourished, feeble muscles; there are the young obese and the old obese; there are the gouty obese with feeble fatty hearts and diseased arteries; and there are the diabetic obese. The mineral-water treatment suitable to the two latter groups has already been discussed. The object of treatment in most of these cases is to produce a diminution in adipose tissue without causing any loss in the nitrogenous tissues—a waste of albumen.

In all cases we need the co-operation of dietetic

measures and of suitable exercises, which may take the form of massage or Swedish gymnastics.

It is generally admitted that the best results are obtained from the alkaline sodium sulphate waters, as Carlsbad, Marienbad, Tarasp, Franzensbad, Elster, and others. Good results also follow the use of the "bitter waters," containing magnesium and sodium sulphates, as Apenta, Æsculap, Rubinat, but these are exclusively for home use; waters containing sodium chloride as well as the aperient sulphates, such as Brides les Bains, are also very useful.

The cold sodium chloride waters of Kissingen and Homburg are applicable to many cases.

In France sodium chloride waters are much used in the treatment of obesity; they are believed to stimulate defective metabolism and to promote oxidation. The stronger ones are used only as baths (La Mouillère, Salins de Jura, Salies de Béarn), the weaker springs (Châtelguyon, Santenay) also as drinking cures. It is also maintained, by the Vichy authorities, that the course there is efficacious, if a suitable diet is at the same time adhered to.

Some discrimination is needed in the recommendation of these different cures.

The plethoric obese are best treated by the *cold* alkaline sodium sulphate waters of Marienbad or Tarasp; they are less exciting to the vascular system than the thermal waters of Carlsbad, which are, however, to be preferred in the gouty and diabetic obese.

Marienbad is especially indicated in cases originating in excess of food, and in hereditary cases, also in those cases occurring in women at the climacteric period, and in cases associated with abdominal stasis and hæmorrhoids. Normal metabolism and oxidation are promoted by the free action of the liver, intestines, and kidneys induced by the waters. It must be seen to that free diuresis accompanies the water-drinking, and that vascular pressure is not raised. The course should be of four to eight weeks' duration.

The treatment at Brides les Bains is suited to gouty cases and to lymphatic and anæmic cases with defective oxidation; it is also recommended in cases of abdominal plethora with fatty heart and the earlier stages of arterio-sclerosis. In cases referable to over-feeding, the use of the water is supplemented by douche massage, the induction of free perspiration, and a "Terrain-Kur."

The fat *anæmics* are difficult cases to deal with. Some are best treated with water containing a combination of iron and sodium sulphate, as at Franzensbad (Stahlquelle), Elster (Marienquelle); some by the less energetic cold common salt springs containing iron, as at Homburg and Kissingen; or Tarasp, with its more tonic climate and combined iron and alkaline sodium sulphate spring, may be tried. Such cases are undoubtedly benefited by being much in the open air in a bracing situation.

The various baths employed at these different spas may greatly promote the desired effect in many cases, but they are not to be applied indiscriminately, and it should first be ascertained that the heart is sound and the arteries free from disease.

Vapour baths, warm peat and brine baths, gaseous brine baths, gaseous steel baths, are all of value in appropriate cases. By stimulating the action of the skin and promoting free cutaneous excretion, they further oxidation and healthy metabolism.

Electric light or radiant heat baths are useful for the same purpose.

RHEUMATISM—CHRONIC, ARTICULAR, AND MUSCULAR. RHEUMATIC NEURALGIAS (SCIATICA, LUMBAGO). "RHEUMATOID ARTHRITIS."

We include "rheumatoid arthritis," so called, in this group of maladies, not because we think its relation to rheumatism a close one, but because the term is one generally employed, and because the impression is so widely diffused that it is intimately related with rheumatism and gout. So far as we have been able to observe, its closest pathological affinities are with neither, and we have had reason to think that the term is often wrongly applied to some forms of chronic articular gout and rheumatism, and inferences drawn with regard to its treatment which are not to be relied upon. The French pathologists use largely the word "*arthritisme*," a term of very vague signification, which is made to cover a vast number of morbid conditions that are believed to be associated with an original constitutional tendency to the development of affections of the joints, just as they employ the term "*herpétisme*" to signify a constitutional tendency to cutaneous affections. Patients afflicted with "rheumatoid arthritis" are therefore grouped by French authorities with the rheumatic and gouty, under the vague designation of "*arthritiques*"!

In approaching the consideration of the treatment of rheumatic affections by mineral waters and baths, the first thing to be noted is that nearly every spa, especially if it possesses *thermal* springs, claims to be a remedy for these maladies. It would be difficult to mention a single spa, in Great Britain, which does not include chronic rheumatism amongst the complaints for which it is suitable, and in France the same may be said of fully sixty per cent. of its mineral-water resorts. A similar reflection applies to Germany, Italy, and Switzerland. We may conclude, from these facts, that all *hot* baths, and the auxiliary mechanical and other treatments associated with them, are more or less beneficial to most forms of chronic rheumatism.

It is a question whether patients slowly recovering from attacks of *acute* rheumatism, with or without implication of the cardial valves, should be submitted to mineral-water treatment. The tendency in the present day is to answer this question in the affirmative, and to direct such patients to those common salt baths which are rich in free carbonic acid gas. We shall have to refer to this matter again when dealing with the subject of the treatment of cardiac disease by mineral waters, but we may say now, that we see no good reason for sending these convalescents to foreign spas, so long as well-arranged artificial warm gaseous salt baths, or warm artificially aërated sea-baths, can be obtained in pleasant and healthy resorts in this country. Indeed, it seems to us much better to spare such patients the fatigue and possible risks of foreign travel ; more particularly do we think this view is the correct one in all cases which tend to a protracted subacute course, with occasional slight rises of temperature. It can scarcely be right to remove such a patient to an overcrowded popular German spa. If, however, in such cases there is an entire absence of fever, but certain joints remain stiff and swollen, gentle thermal and mechanical treatment, at one of our own baths, may be useful—such as Buxton, Bath, or Woodhall Spa, or at the seaside, according to circumstances.

In France the spas recommended for these convalescents are the warm weak sodium chloride springs of Bourbon Lancy, Bourbon l'Archambaut and La Motte les Bains, the simple thermal baths of Néris and Plombières, and the hot sulphur baths of Vernet in the Eastern Pyrenees, where the climatic conditions are considered to be very favourable. In Germany the gaseous salt springs of Nauheim and Oeynhausen are most popular.

But it is in those cases of chronic rheumatism which, probably, have but little pathological affinity with the acute disease, that spa treatment is so greatly resorted to.

In chronic articular and muscular rheumatism the following classes of mineral springs are commonly used, sometimes one, sometimes the other, according to individual requirements, place of residence, degree of severity and chronicity, or past experience in particular cases, and often because of the perfection of the methods, thermal and auxiliary, put into practice at the particular resort.

1. *Simple thermal springs* (Bath, Buxton, Wildbad, Gastein, Ragatz, Plombières, Bormio).

2. *Thermal sulphur baths;* if cold, the springs are artificially heated (Harrogate, Strathpeffer, Aix la Chapelle, Aix les Bains, Luchon, Schinznach, Acqui).

3. *Thermal salt or brine baths*—or cold waters heated (Droitwich, Woodhall, Bourbonne les Bains, Wiesbaden, Nauheim, Rheinfelden, Salso Maggiore).

4. *Thermal peat and mud baths* (Strathpeffer, Dax, St. Amand les Eaux, Franzensbad, Elster, Bex, Battaglia).

The object of these baths is to promote absorption of effusions and exudations by stimulating metabolism; to excite and increase the cutaneous functions, and promote elimination by the skin; to influence favourably the circulation by causing dilatation of the capillaries, while the warm temperature of the bath is soothing to the peripheral nerves. It is usual to endeavour to maintain the stimulating action on the skin, by removal, after the bath, to a warm bed, where perspiration is encouraged. The diaphoretic action is further promoted, in the case of the simple thermal baths, by giving the patient some of the hot mineral water to drink.

In nearly all cases the baths and local or general douches are associated with some mechanical treatment, such as massage or Swedish gymnastics. Vapour baths, sand baths, electric light baths, pine-needle baths, and local applications of peat, mineral mud, or "fango," after the manner of poultices, are also employed and prove serviceable in the treatment of these very chronic and often obstinate maladies. Hot compresses, together with friction, have been found useful in relieving the pain referred to particular spots, in lumbago and other forms of muscular pain.

The thermal sulphur and the thermal salt baths are more stimulating than the simple thermal baths, and are usually found more serviceable in obstinate cases of articular rheumatism.

Sciatica and neuralgia of other large nerves is often of a rheumatic or gouty nature, and the mineral-water treatment of such affections is practically identical with that of chronic rheumatism. Apart from those acute cases (neuritis) that require absolute rest, douching and massage, either with the hottest of the simple thermal waters (Bath, Dax, Teplitz), or the thermal sulphur waters (Aix les Bains, Harrogate), or the hot common salt springs (Droitwich, Bourbonne les Bains, Wiesbaden), are most appropriate. Sensitive patients who require baths of rather a lower temperature and more sedative may be directed to Buxton, Ragatz, Wildbad and Gastein.

All those patients require an "after-cure" in as dry and sunny a station as can be conveniently obtained, and to prevent relapses they should, if possible, choose a residence in a dry, sunny district, with a sub-soil of gravel and sand, and good natural drainage. It is good for such patients to be much in the open air, and hence the value of a climate where this kind of life can be followed without risk of chill.

The subject of the treatment of *rheumatoid arthritis* or *osteo-arthritis* by mineral waters is one of some difficulty, and a great difference of opinion exists amongst authorities as to the value of such treatment in these cases. Those who believe this disease to be a microbic infection of the joints, having no direct relationship with rheumatism, maintain, and we think justly, that the proper treatment of those cases is a tonic and supporting one, and that change to a dry and bracing climate, and to cheerful and hygienic surroundings, is of great importance, and most serviceable; while little direct benefit can be expected, or is actually found, to accrue from any *special* action of mineral waters. This has been more particularly observed in chronic cases, in which permanent good results from spa treatment must not be expected. In such cases massage, electricity, baths, douches, and passive movements, perseveringly applied, may prevent further deformity and secure some increase of mobility in the affected joints, especially when aided by general tonic influences, such as good air, plenty of sunshine, and a generous diet. In the acute and painful stage, however, rest is essential, even a splint may be needed; but we must, at the same time, bear in mind that some precautions have to be taken to prevent and counteract the great tendency there is to fixation of joints and consequent deformity in this disease, so that, even in the acute stage, occasional passive movements may be indicated.

In early cases the application of the Dowsing hot-air treatment has been strongly advocated, either locally to the joints affected, or to the whole body, and even in chronic cases good results appear sometimes to follow this method, which is now instituted at many English and Continental spas. It has been suggested that where thermal baths are attended with benefit it is wholly due to the *heat* of the water, and it is to be noted that in France, where bath treatment of these cases is in some repute, it is to the *hotter*—the "hyperthermal"—waters that these cases are sent; the authorities at these spas, however, require that the cases should be in the *early* stage, and do not pretend to cure or permanently benefit the advanced, chronic forms.

At Aix les Bains good results are reported in cases that come under treatment at the early stage, and repeated courses are sometimes found to "arrest the evolution of the disease," but success is uncertain. The *hot* calcareous waters and the cheerful surroundings and favourable climate of Bagnères-de-Bigorre—the hot sulphur springs of Barbotan and Barèges—the latter having also its bracing mountain climate as an auxiliary—the hyperthermal but feebly mineralised springs of Evaux les Bains—the alkaline arsenical waters and mild mountain climate of La

Bourboule—the hot gaseous common salt springs of Bourbonne les Bains—the very hot common salt springs of La Motte—the hot alkaline and mild common salt waters of Bourbon l'Archambaut, containing also minute amounts of arsenic and iodine (this place claims "frequent cures in forms of rapid evolution in young subjects")—and the hot muds of Dax and St. Amand les Eaux—these are the principal spas to which cases of rheumatoid arthritis are sent in France.

In this country recourse may be had to the experience and skill, in the treatment of this affection, of the physicians at Bath, Buxton, Harrogate, Woodhall Spa, Llandrindod, etc.

CHRONIC MALARIAL AFFECTIONS. MALARIAL CACHEXIA. "IMPALUDISM" OF FRENCH WRITERS.

These affections, gastro-intestinal, hepatic, and splenic, associated commonly with an anæmic state, and occasionally with febrile recurrences, the result of residence in tropical climates, are often very favourably influenced and not unfrequently cured by recourse to mineral waters.

It is a distinct advantage if we can find suitable springs, for this purpose, in moderately bracing sub-alpine districts with tonic air and cheerful, picturesque surroundings. It should, however, be borne in mind that many of these patients are highly sensitive to cold, and apt to become chilled if exposed to too low a temperature, and even in a warm resort like Vichy it is found that such patients often do best in the warmest part of the season.

When there is considerable enlargement of the liver and spleen, and much sluggishness of the hepatic functions, with a tendency to constipation, the warm alkaline aperient (sodium sulphate) waters answer best, as Carlsbad or Brides les Bains (aperient sulphates with sodium chloride). The

Tarasp waters are also very useful in such cases as will tolerate its bracing mountain climate. They are, however, cold, which is perhaps a disadvantage. Saint Gervais, with its warm springs of sodium chloride and mixed sulphates and its mild mountain climate, is also a suitable resort. In such resorts the hepatic and splenic enlargements are often much reduced and the blood conditions improved.

The simple warm alkaline waters of Vichy also enjoy in France "a great reputation in the treatment of these affections"—after a prolonged course the gastro-hepatic troubles are usually greatly relieved if not entirely cured. The waters of Vals have a like reputation. Royat is also resorted to for its arsenical, alkaline, and sodium chloride springs, and is found especially suitable to the anæmic forms.

Le Boulou, in the Eastern Pyrenees, with cold sodium carbonate springs, is resorted to by the same class of cases.

Arsenical waters are especially indicated in the febrile and anæmic cases, and good results are obtained from the alkaline arsenical waters of La Bourboule.

The feebly mineralised thermal waters of Plombières have been found serviceable in the treatment of the more delicate patients, and French authors seem inclined to refer their utility to the very small amount of arsenic they contain.

The arsenical waters of Val Sinestra, near Tarasp, can be taken, at the latter place, together with or supplementary to the saline springs.

Some consider the simple thermal waters of value when situated in bracing localities, as at Gastein.

In cases in which anæmia is the predominating symptom, the sulphate of iron waters have been thought to be indicated, such as those at Mitterbad (Tyrol), Parad (Hungary), and Hermannsbad-Muskau (Prussia), and when there is a tendency to febrile recurrences the arsenical iron waters such as Levico, Roncegno, Trebernik and Recoaro.

DISEASES OF THE DIGESTIVE ORGANS.

DYSPEPSIAS.

The same difficulties which we encounter in the *home* treatment of the various forms of disordered digestion, will meet us also when we endeavour to apply mineral - water treatment to their relief.

The obstacles which arise in our endeavour to ascertain the real causes, or to determine, with precision, the true nature of the gastric disorder, impart an element of uncertainty to the results to be expected from the particular course prescribed. The French physicians attempt to establish a marked distinction between what they term dyspepsia from *hyperchlorhydrie, i.e.* an excessive formation of hydrochloric acid in the stomach, and dyspepsia from *hypochlorhydrie,* a defective secretion of that acid. They also recognise a *hypersthénique* and a *hyposthénique* form, but they advocate the same mineral-water treatment in both these last forms. In a semi-official pronouncement as to the applicability of the Vichy springs to the treatment of dyspepsia, it is said, "Painful or *hypersthenic* dyspepsias, simple or complicated with *hyperchlorhydrie* . . *atonic* flatulent or *hyposthenic* dyspepsias . . are usually cured or advantageously modified"* by treatment there. But they commonly distinguish between the waters suitable for cases of "hyperchlorhydrie" and those indicated in cases of "hypochlorhydrie."

We are accustomed, in this country, to recognise chronic gastric catarrh as a dyspeptic state often induced by the abuse of food, alcohol, tobacco, and other irritating agencies. We recognise atonic forms of dyspepsia in the debilitated, as a sequel of acute or chronic illness, in the neurotic (the "nervous dyspepsia," which is the most difficult of all to deal with), in

* Index Medical des principales Stations Thermales et Climatiques de France, Paris, 1903.

the neurasthenic, as the consequence of over-work and worry; and we are familiar with what is perhaps the most common form, the *acid* dyspepsia—the *hyper-chlorhydrie* of the French—often intermittent in occurrence, and provoked, in the predisposed, by slight dietetic errors.

In determining the fitness of a particular spa for the treatment of particular cases of dyspepsia, we shall be assisted chiefly by a consideration of the accompanying conditions, the individual constitution, the probable causation, and the co-existence of other maladies. The comparatively robust, vigorous, gouty dyspeptic will usually require different treatment from that suited to the feeble neurotic dyspeptic.

But in prescribing a course of mineral waters, at a Continental spa, we shall be prescribing conditions, other than the mere water drinking, which are calculated to be beneficial to nearly all dyspeptics. Change of habits of life and of climatic conditions, release from work and home worries, inducements to exercise in the open air, the regulation of diet and the constant medical supervision, the tonic as well as soothing influence of baths and douches—all these influences tend to the restoration of gastric tone and healthy functions.

The following are the different classes of mineral waters that are prescribed for the treatment of dyspeptic states:—

1. The *simple alkaline* waters, such as Vichy, Vals, and Neuenahr. Vals has the advantage of possessing a great number of springs differing in degree of alkalinity, and having, therefore, a wide range of applicability. Neuenahr has very useful warm alkaline springs, but they are very mild, and are suitable to those who do not bear strong alkaline remedies.

The Vichy waters are strong alkaline waters, and some of the springs are warm and others cold. They are adapted to the treatment of many forms of dyspepsia, but especially to cases of excessive gastric acidity and of chronic gastric catarrh. They are of comparatively little use to the neurotic dyspeptic with an insufficient secretion of gastric juice. They are very serviceable in cases of intestinal as well as gastric catarrh, in which constipation and diarrhœa often alternate; but they are not so useful, as certain other springs, for dyspeptics who are the subjects of habitual constipation.

2. The *alkaline weak common salt* waters are suitable to a more limited class of dyspeptics; to those cases of chronic gastric catarrh associated with general debility; and to dyspeptic states in the thin, neurotic, and sensitive, who require very mild and soothing treatment. Ems, Royat, Gleichenberg, are examples of this group of waters, the two former being warm, the latter cold. Dyspeptic symptoms, in the subjects of atonic gout, are likely to be relieved by these waters. Royat is suited to the treatment of gastric atony and dyspeptics with insufficient secretions of gastric juice, the "hypochlorhydric." The presence of a small amount of arsenic in the water gives it a tonic effect, and the situation is not relaxing like that of Ems.

3. The *gaseous common salt* springs, such as Kissingen and Homburg, are largely prescribed in the treatment of certain forms of dyspepsia. Those springs only are suitable which contain but a *moderate* amount of sodium chloride and a large amount of free carbonic acid; the Rakoczyquelle at Kissingen is the type of this class.

The dyspeptic cases suited to these spas are those of chronic gastric catarrh with defective secretion, associated with gastric atony; some cases also of "nervous dyspepsia" improve much at Kissingen, in others the results are disappointing, as is the case with *all* remedies in these very troublesome neurotic cases.

Soden, near Frankfort, Neiderbronn in Alsace, and Châtelguyon in France, are also suitable places of resort for these patients.

4. The *alkaline aperient sodium sulphate* waters Carlsbad, Marienbad, Tarasp, Bertrich are examples; with these may be classed the laxative waters of Brides les Bains, St. Gervais, and Leamington.

To these resorts may be sent the large class of dyspeptics, often gouty, often gross feeders, often alcoholic, who, with catarrhal stomachs, have also congested livers, are constipated, suffer from hæmorrhoids, lithiasis, and generally from defective elimination and hyperacidity.

The warm alkaline waters of Carlsbad are more suitable to the catarrhal cases, and those of Bertrich, which are much milder, to those sensitive, delicate patients who might find the waters of Carlsbad too strong. Marienbad is adapted to the obese and robust, Tarasp to those who require the tonic influence of mountain air. Brides is very useful in cases of habitual constipation, and in those gastro-hepatic troubles induced by residence in hot climates.

Leamington may be recommended to those who desire to avoid the fatigue of travel.

There are a few other mineral-water resorts, which cannot well be included in either of the preceding classes, which, however, are in repute for the treatment of the class of cases we are considering. There is Harrogate, with its Kissingen well, adapted to the treatment of the same class of dyspeptics as the fourth of the preceding groups. There is Evian, with its very feebly mineralised spring, which is recommended in cases of "hyperchlorhydrie," and Pougues, near Nevers, with its gaseous alkaline carbonate of lime water, which is resorted to in cases of gastric atony, and dyspeptic states in the neurotic and neurasthenic with defective gastric secretion. In most of these cases the waters that are *cold* should be *warmed* at the commencement of the course.

The uncertainty as to some of these waters being well tolerated by dyspeptic patients is so great, that Kisch has very wisely suggested "the tentative use, for a few days at home, of the mineral water that is under consideration, in order to determine whether or not it is well borne."*

Home treatment by mineral waters can also be satisfactorily instituted and applied in the milder forms of dyspepsia. The gaseous mildly alkaline table waters, such as Apollinaris, Bilin, or Giesshübel are well suited for this purpose. The first of these, mixed with one-third as much hot water, is an effective substitute for Neuenahr water, and can be taken, in any desirable quantity, half an hour before breakfast or lunch.

Co-existing constipation can be similarly treated by mixing five or six ounces of Apollinaris water with three or four ounces of Apenta or Friedrichshall and drinking this, in two doses, some time before breakfast. Or one or two tumblerfuls of the imported Carlsbad water can be taken at this time.

Many authorities recommend the treatment of cases of *gastric ulcer* at some of these resorts, but we hardly think it desirable, under any circumstances, to send cases of ulcer of the stomach away from home for treatment by mineral waters.

HABITUAL CONSTIPATION.

Habitual constipation is often associated with gastric disorders—especially with gastro-intestinal catarrh, and in treating appropriately the dyspeptic conditions, we have to adopt such measures as will remove the constipation, as we have just seen. Constipation may, however, exist without any notable dyspepsia, and recourse to mineral waters may be had for its relief. The Hungarian "bitter" waters, containing the aperient sulphates of magnesium and sodium and also some chloride of sodium are largely used at home for this purpose; and the spas visited for the treatment of habitual constipation are those which contain springs rich

* Mineral Waters and Their Uses. "Cohen's System of Physiologic Therapeutics," vol. ix., p. 478.

either in these aperient sulphates or in sodium chloride. The gaseous chloride of sodium springs of Homburg and Kissingen are found efficient in some cases, while they entirely fail in others. The alkaline sodium sulphate waters of Marienbad, Franzensbad, and Tarasp are usually found much more effective, but these will wholly fail and even cause constipation in some patients; in such instances we have found the waters of Brides les Bains more uniformly succeed in remedying this condition. In persons advanced in life, and in stout women of sedentary habits, the constipation is often due to muscular torpor of the large intestine; in such cases abdominal massage, combined with a course of laxative waters, proves of great value.

The chloride of sodium and magnesium waters of Châtelguyon are valued in France as a remedy for habitual constipation.

Hæmorrhoids often co-exist with habitual constipation, and are relieved by the same means.

CHRONIC DIARRHŒA AND MUCO-MEMBRANOUS COLITIS.

The employment of mineral waters in the treatment of chronic diarrhœa is naturally only had recourse to in those cases, and they are not rare, in which ordinary medicinal and dietetic treatment has failed.

In those cases of intestinal catarrh, in which frequent mucous discharges have been the result of previous constipation, or dietetic errors, and consequent irritation of the intestinal mucous membrane, the warm alkaline sodium sulphate waters of Carlsbad have often proved of great service, and the same has been observed when the diarrhœa has been traceable to disturbed hepatic functions. But this treatment needs the most careful and skilful supervision, and the mildest possible course, at starting, is usually desirable. In cases where there is a probability that portions of irritating fæcal matter are still retained in the bowels, an initial dose of castor oil is sometimes prescribed.*

The somewhat analogous waters of St. Gervais, in Savoy, have also been employed successfully in cases of painful "enteritis and the dysenteric diarrhœas of hot climates," and the tonic, subalpine climate must be a valuable aid to the recovery of such cases at St. Gervais.

The Vichy course has always been regarded by French authorities as of great service in cases of "gastro-intestinal dyspepsia with alternation of constipation and diarrhœa, and in simple or muco-membranous enteritis." Dujardin Beaumetz maintained that in the case of chronic diarrhœa originating amongst Europeans in tropical countries, the only efficacious treatment consisted in restricting the patients to a diet of milk mixed with Vichy water. Le Boulou, in the Eastern Pyrenees, with waters belonging to the same group as those of Vichy, are resorted to in similar cases.

The very feebly mineralised waters of Evian and Alet have also been found beneficial for the same class of patients. But the soothing influence of the warm baths, of intestinal irrigations, and of a carefully ordered dietary, are probably of far more concern than the drinking of these feebly mineralised waters. This observation is suggested by a consideration of the great success which has attended the treatment of cases of chronic diarrhœa and *muco-membranous colitis* at *Plombières*. This spa has acquired quite a special reputation in this respect, and the *drinking* cure is there regarded as altogether secondary to the influence of the warm baths and the local application of the warm water to the irritated intestine; the *intestinal* douche or "intestinal lavage" forming an important part of the treatment.

* "Carlsbad, its Thermal Springs and Baths, and How to Use Them," by Dr. J. Kraus.

In "lymphatic" and anæmic cases, with general debility of the mucous membranes, Plombières is not suitable, and more tonic waters are to be preferred, viz. those iron waters containing lime salts (Forges-les-Eaux, Schwalbach, St. Moritz), or earthy calcareous waters containing iron (Driburg, Antogast, Wildungen). Waters containing sulphate of iron or sulphate of iron and arsenic (Alexisbad, Levico) have been recommended for the diarrhœa of anæmic and feeble children.

DISEASES OF THE LIVER AND BILE DUCTS.

Mineral waters are found of great service in the treatment of hepatic disorders.

Congestion of the liver, whether due to over-feeding, to alcoholism, to insufficient exercise, or to malarial influences, is especially amenable to mineral-water treatment. The springs which are found most useful in the treatment of this condition are the warm alkaline sodium sulphate springs (Carlsbad, Brides), or the cold ones, in obese, vigorous patients with constipation (Marienbad, Tarasp), or the gaseous common salt waters (Kissingen, Homburg): these last are more suitable to thin and feeble persons. The simple alkaline waters are also very useful, and those of Vichy are frequently prescribed with benefit in the less vigorous malarial, alcoholic, and gouty patients, more particularly if there exists a tendency to diarrhœa rather than to constipation. In anæmic cases the presence of a little iron in the sodium sulphate waters of Elster or Franzensbad renders them more appropriate; and in very sensitive persons the warm alkaline and weak common salt springs of Ems may prove of value.

The same class of waters are applicable to the treatment of the *large fatty liver* of the obese. The purgative "bitter" waters are also suitable for the treatment of these cases, but they can be, and are, usually drunk at home. The waters of Harrogate,

Llandrindod, Leamington, and Cheltenham can be prescribed for the same purpose. Châtelguyon in Auvergne, and St. Gervais in Savoy, are prescribed for the same class of patients.

Early cases of *cirrhosis*, with much hypertrophy in the obese alcoholic, are often very greatly benefited by one or more courses at Carlsbad or Brides or Marienbad, or at one of the other resorts of this class that have been named.

Cases of *gallstones*, biliary sand, or inspissated bile, are treated with advantage at a very great number of mineral-water resorts. One of the indications in these affections being the dilution of the bile so as to promote its free flow along the bile ducts, it is obvious that many mineral springs may rightly claim to have this property. Their free, prolonged, systematic administration is one of the reasons for drinking them at their source rather than at home. The *warm alkaline sodium sulphate* waters (Carlsbad) stand first in repute for this purpose, and the *warm simple alkaline* waters (Vichy, Neuenahr) are of nearly equal importance. The great number of sufferers from gallstones who resort annually to Carlsbad or Vichy bear testimony to the repute in which these springs are held.

The *earthy* or *calcareous* waters, such as Contrexéville, Vittel, and many others, are also advocated for the treatment of these cases when they occur in the gouty; they are usually administered in very large doses. The same may be said of the feebly mineralised waters of Evian. The springs of Ems and Royat (alkaline and weak common salt springs) are also used for the treatment of the slighter cases.

It is generally considered desirable that the course of mineral waters should be repeated annually for a few years to prevent a return of the malady.

A suitable treatment for these cases can be instituted at home (if the patient will consent to the adoption at the same time of an appropriate diet and *régime*) by drinking several glasses daily, at prescribed hours, of a mixture composed of one-third of one of the aperient bitter waters, such as Apenta or Friedrichshall, made hot, and two-thirds of an effervescing alkaline water, such as Bilin, Apollinaris, or one of the weaker Vals springs.

Chronic forms of *jaundice*, when believed to be due to catarrh of the bile ducts, or associated with biliary concretions, require the same kind of mineral-water treatment as that pointed out above for the treatment of gallstones, the warm alkaline springs or the warm alkaline sodium sulphate springs being the most appropriate.

In certain of these chronic forms of jaundice, it will occasionally happen that the disease is due to obstruction of a malignant nature which has not been diagnosed, and such cases may become rapidly worse when sent for treatment to a Continental spa at a distance from home. Such an event often leads to much discontent, and discredit is cast both on the spa and on the medical attendant, and pains should always be taken to avoid, if possible, such an occurrence.

Warm peat poultices have been found serviceable in some forms of hepatic enlargement, of gallstones, and of catarrhal jaundice.

DISEASES OF THE RESPIRATORY ORGANS.

There are certain chronic diseases of the respiratory organs which are specially suited to treatment by mineral waters, and these are catarrhal affections of the upper air passages, such as chronic rhino-pharyngitis, pharyngo-laryngitis, laryngitis, tracheitis, and certain forms of chronic bronchial catarrh. Pulmonary emphysema, when not too advanced, is benefited as a result of the relief afforded to the bronchial catarrh with which it is commonly associated, and also by the co-operation of pneumatic treatment, which can usually be obtained in the localities in especial repute for the treatment of respiratory affections. The forest air and mildly tonic mountain air, at the moderate elevations at which many of these resorts are situated, undoubtedly prove valuable accessories. In asthma, especially bronchial asthma, *i.e.* when the attacks are associated with a tendency to chronic bronchial catarrh, excellent results are frequently obtained by such systematic treatment as is applied, for instance, at Mont Dore.

The mineral springs most commonly resorted to for the treatment of these affections are, in the first place, the *warm alkaline weak common salt* waters, of which Ems may be regarded as the type; secondly, the *warm mild simple common salt* waters, of which Soden is a good example; thirdly, the *warm sulphur* springs, especially the sodium sulphide springs, as exemplified at Eaux Bonnes in the Pyrenees; and the warm *sulphur and common salt* springs such as those of Aix la Chapelle. In a few special cases, as we shall presently see, the *alkaline aperient sodium sulphate* waters (Carlsbad, etc.) are recommended.

The *petrolated* common salt waters of Salso Maggiore have also recently been strongly recommended in the treatment of certain of these maladies.

It is needless to say that in the treatment of these chronic respiratory affections, it is often of much consequence that we should select a spa with suitable climatic surroundings and where the methods applied, especially in connection with *inhalatory* treatment, are of the best and newest.

We shall now pass on to consider the mineral-water treatment of these diseases somewhat more in detail.

Cases of *rhino-pharyngitis*, of *chronic pharyngitis*, and *chronic laryngitis* and *tracheitis* are all amenable to the same forms of mineral-water treatment. The influence of local spraying and douching, which are practised at all the resorts where these affections are treated, and the passing of some considerable time daily in chambers specially arranged for the inhalation of the vapour and spray, at certain of these spas, contribute greatly to the good results obtained.

These measures tend to soften, fluidify, and detach the sticky adherent mucus and mucous crusts that are prone to adhere to the mucous membrane in these chronic maladies; they also soothe the irritated mucous membrane, and some doubtless exert a cleansing, antiseptic action and destroy or diminish bacterial activity.

The *alkaline* chloride of sodium waters most frequently prescribed for these affections are Ems, Gleichenberg, Royat, La Bourboule, and Mont Dore (the three last containing arsenic also); these are especially suitable when the secretion from the mucous membrane is scanty and there is an irritative cough—the *catarrhe sec* of French writers. The waters are drunk warm, as well as applied locally as spray or gargle, and favour expectoration by their solvent action on mucus. The arsenic in the Bourboule and Royat springs has also a tonic effect.

If we also consider a mild moist climate indicated we should choose Ems; where a more bracing influence is desirable we may select Royat, La Bourboule, or Mont Dore.

A great number of *professional* speakers and singers—priests, actors, operatic artists—resort to Mont Dore, Royat, and La Bourboule—the last-named is also specially prescribed by French physicians for "lymphatic" and "herpetic" subjects—by "herpetic" is meant those patients who also have a marked tendency to cutaneous eruptions. Royat and Mont Dore (but particularly Royat) are considered most useful when these affections occur in the gouty.

The *simple mild chloride of sodium* springs, such as Soden, Baden-Baden, Woodhall Spa, Reichenhall, are less useful in these throat maladies than the preceding, and are more frequently used for bronchitic affections.

The *warm sulphur* springs, so serviceable in the treatment of these diseases, are especially abundant in France and particularly in the Pyrenees; Cauterets, Eaux Bonnes, Luchon, Le Vernet are perhaps the best known. Other sulphur spas in France, frequented for the same purpose, are Marlioz, close to Aix les Bains, Challes, Allevard, near Grenoble, St. Honoré, and Enghien, close to Paris. Weilbach, in Hesse-Nassau, and Neundorf, near Hanover, are cold sulphur springs, and these and the warm sulphur and common salt springs of Aix la Chapelle are recommended for the treatment of these affections, but they are not so specially adapted for the purpose as those we have already named.

In Switzerland the cold alkaline sulphur springs of Heustrich, near the Lake of Thun, have a special reputation for the treatment of these throat affections, and in a less degree the warm sulphur springs of Schinznach.

Most elaborate methods have been established at Salso Maggiore for the treatment of the same class of cases, and the mixed vapour and spray of its petrolated salt water has proved of much service to many sufferers from these troublesome chronic throat catarrhs.

CHRONIC BRONCHIAL CATARRH, ETC.

Perhaps the most serviceable waters in this disease are the *alkaline* common salt waters, such as Ems, Gleichenberg, Royat, La Bourboule (arsenical also), Mont Dore, etc. In some cases the mild, moist climate of Ems, in others the dryer climate of Royat, and in others the more bracing mountain air of La Bourboule or Mont Dore will be indicated. The moister climate is advantageous in those cases with scanty secretion and irritative cough.

The local effect of the warm spray of these waters and the influence of the warm alkaline drink are alike beneficial.

The *mild sodium chloride* waters (or the stronger ones diluted) are better suited to cases with profuse secretion, as Soden, Baden-Baden, Reichenhall,

Kissingen, Ischl. Besides the brine spray inhaled, the adjacency of pine woods and the co-existence of pneumatic and inhalatory treatment at some of these resorts are useful aids.

Weissenberg, in Switzerland, not far from Berne, with tepid earthy calcareous springs, has an established reputation in the treatment of these cases of chronic bronchial and laryngeal catarrh, but the mildly bracing mountain air, and the adjacency of pine woods, exercise probably as much, or more influence, than the earthy waters, in the good results obtained.

The *sulphur* and the *sulphur and salt* waters have hardly so great a reputation in the treatment of chronic bronchial catarrh as they have in that of catarrh of the pharynx and larynx; they have, however, their application in the cases of long standing bronchial catarrh of a torpid nature, accompanied with abundant secretion—the *catarrhe humide* of the French. Recourse can be had to such springs as Luchon, Cauterets, Eaux Bonnes, Amélie, St. Honoré, Heustrich, Schinznach, Aix la Chapelle, and the like.

Inhalations of sulphuretted hydrogen are applied at some sulphur spas to allay irritability of the respiratory mucous membrane. Inhalations also of nitrogen, obtained from some of the earthy and calcareous springs (Lippspringe, Inselbad) have been advocated as beneficial in the treatment of chronic bronchial catarrh, but it is difficult to understand how they can produce any curative effect.

The addition of a little hot milk or whey to many of these waters renders them more pleasant to drink, and seems also often to promote their beneficial effects.

In cases of chronic bronchial catarrh occurring in the obese and plethoric, in free livers, and those addicted to alcohol, with a tendency to pulmonary and hepatic engorgement, the *alkaline aperient sodium sulphate* springs (Carlsbad, Marienbad, Tarasp, Brides) or the active sodium chloride waters (Kissingen or

Homburg) may prove the most useful by causing intestinal derivation and unloading of the portal circulation.

The stimulating and invigorating tonic effect on the skin of warm brine baths, followed in young subjects with friction with cold brine, is believed to prevent relapses by diminishing the sensitiveness of the surface to chill.

For home use, both in acute and chronic catarrhal affections of the air passages, the cold gaseous, alkaline sodium chloride waters of Apollinaris, Bilin, Selters, etc., mixed with a little hot milk or whey, are extremely beneficial on account of their solvent action thinning and promoting the expectoration of viscid mucus, and so allaying cough.

Chronic emphysema can only be benefited by mineral waters through their curative influence on co-existing catarrhal states, and to those cases the same indications apply as already set forth. It is, however, a decided advantage, in dealing with such cases, to have the aid of suitable pneumatic treatment, such as is practised at Reichenhall, and the adjacency of pine woods, at moderate elevations, is also a gain.

Asthma.—We have entered so fully into the question of the treatment of asthma at Mont Dore in our account of that spa, that it is not necessary to dilate on that subject now. We may add that the bronchitic cases, associated with pulmonary emphysema, are often treated with advantage at the sulphur springs of Luchon, Cauterets, Eaux Bonnes, and Amélie les Bains. Treatment of catarrhal asthma is also undertaken at Inselbad, close to Paderborn, and good results have been reported.

A suitable "after-cure" is of great importance in all these respiratory catarrhal cases. Places of moderate elevation, with a fairly dry, sunny climate, and in the neighbourhood of pine woods, or places on the sea coast which are protected from cold winds and get much sunshine, are specially indicated. A still atmosphere, with abundant sunshine, is what is needed.

DISEASES OF THE CIRCULATORY SYSTEM.

Until within comparatively recent years it used to be taught that cardiac maladies were counter-indicated at all baths. But in former times all valvular cardiac diseases were looked upon with much greater concern than in the present day, and it was the custom to give a far graver prognosis of some forms of cardiac disease than would now be thought justifiable. With a much truer appreciation of the nature and course of such affections, a much more hopeful view of their therapeutic management has gained ground, so that remedial appliances are now highly valued in cardiac therapeutics which would have been regarded as attended with great risk less than half a century ago.

Not only are cardiac patients sent to drinking cures for the relief of collateral disturbances of health, whether they are dependent or not on the heart affection, but certain baths are now largely resorted to for their *special* influence in relieving morbid conditions referable directly to cardiac defects, functional and organic. Not only so, but such natural baths are now imitated artificially, and largely and successfully applied at or near home.

In the selection, however, of cases for thermal bath treatment, the modern tendency has been to go to the other extreme and to submit nearly all cases of cardiac disease to bath treatment and the mechanical methods associated with it, and serious results have naturally followed such indiscriminate action. Moreover, there has grown up a tendency, in connection with the popularisation of these therapeutic methods, to discover the presence of heart disease where none exists, and many persons, within our own knowledge, have been persuaded to undergo treatment by baths and "resisted movements" for the relief of cardiac affections which had no existence!—neurotic persons readily lending themselves to these minutely detailed and introspective methods.

In considering the usefulness and applicability of mineral springs to the treatment of cardiac affections, it will be convenient to refer, in the first place, to those waters which are not credited with any *special* influence over these maladies, but are prescribed for their beneficial effect in the removal of collateral functional disturbances, apt to be associated with cardiac disease.

In cases of cardiac hypertrophy, in free livers with threatened arterial changes, and in cases of right-sided hypertrophy and dilatation, associated with chronic pulmonary emphysema, in which our object is to relieve blood stasis and promote the regular distribution and circulation of the blood, by unloading the intestinal veins, and so lessening the labour of the heart, we may have recourse to the cold laxative alkaline sodium sulphate waters of Marienbad, Tarasp, or Brides, or the cold sodium chloride waters of Harrogate, Homburg, or Kissingen. The *cold* springs are thought more suitable than *warm* ones, because the warmth of the latter may excite cardiac action and may lead to over-filling of the blood vessels. It is also thought desirable to get rid of any free carbonic acid there may be in the water by stirring briskly or pouring from one glass to another, again for fear of over-stimulating the action of the heart.

The above mentioned waters may be appropriate also in compensated valvular lesions when symptoms of venous stasis in the abdominal viscera seem to show that compensation is in danger—such as gastro-intestinal catarrh, hepatic enlargement, hæmorrhoids, and menstrual abnormalities dependent on abdominal stasis.

When there is much cardiac excitement with heightened blood pressure, and when it is important to subdue quickly co-existing symptoms of portal engorgement, the purgative bitter waters are often of much service for home use, as Apenta, Friedrichshall, Püllna, etc.

In many of these cases where aterio-sclerosis is imminent it is highly important to further hepatic and intestinal elimination as well as to promote renal excretion; for this purpose we may combine the use of *bitter* waters with the use of alkaline common salt waters, as Ems, Neuenahr, Apollinaris. They lessen the work of the heart by promoting diuresis and intestinal activity. They should be freed from gaseous carbonic acid, and in mild cases the alkaline water may be given in much larger quantity than the *bitter* water, one dose daily of the latter being often sufficient.

In certain *cardiac neuroses* the etiological condition may indicate the use of mineral waters. The palpitations associated with anæmia and chlorosis at puberty may be benefited by iron waters, such as those of Spa, Schwalbach, Bocklet, and Pyrmont, while the same symptom coming on at the climacteric period, or dependent on intestinal torpor, may be benefited by the aperient sodium sulphate waters of Marienbad, Brides, or Tarasp.

Hitherto we have referred only to the *drinking* of mineral waters in these cases, but it is to the influence of *thermal baths* in the treatment of cardiac disease that attention has been chiefly directed of late years, and especially to the gaseous thermal brine baths of **Nauheim**, which are exceptionally rich in pure carbonic acid.

Similar springs are found at Oeynhausen and Rehme, and somewhat similar ones at Salins Moutiers in Savoy.

There can be no doubt of the beneficial effect of these thermal gaseous salt springs in certain cases of cardiac disorder. The following are the cases which have been shown by experience to be most benefited by bath treatment at Nauheim:—

1. Cases of dilatation of the heart unaccompanied by hypertrophy and not associated with any cardiac lesion, beyond weakness of the heart muscle, brought about either by excessive physical effort or over-work

(heart-strain); or occurring as the result of toxic action, as in the post-influenzal cases; or following attacks of rheumatic endocarditis in young people. These are the cases that do especially well at Nauheim.

2. Valvular disease, in the early stage and in young people, in which compensation has not been thoroughly established or in which it appears, for some reason, to have become temporarily disturbed.

3. It has been stated by those who have had large opportunities of observing cases of convalescence from attacks of acute rheumatism, that during the prolonged period of rest which should always be enjoined after such illnesses a course of Nauheim baths will, at this period, do more than rest alone to prevent the occurrence of valvular lesions; that while undergoing this treatment murmurs will be observed to disappear. But it must be borne in mind that, in these recent cases, murmurs will also disappear under suitable treatment at home.

Physical examination appears to show that in cases of simple dilation from muscular asthenia, and in dilation the result of valvular lesion, imperfectly compensated, the baths determine a diminution in the size of the heart by restoration of muscular tone, and this result is explained by the following considerations:—The effect of the bath is at first to cause constriction of the cutaneous vessels and a consequent rise of blood pressure, which quickly passes away and is succeeded by flushing of the skin through dilatation of superficial aterioles—this change is referred to the stimulating effect on the skin of the constituents of the water, especially the free carbonic acid and the sodium and calcium chlorides, the latter salt being credited with a highly exciting effect. It is argued that this freer distribution of blood to the skin must lead to a withdrawal of blood from the deeper seated tissues and therefore to an acceleration of the circulation through them; that by the dilatation of the peripheral vessels the strain on the heart is lightened, the over-distension of its cavities is removed, and it is rendered fitter for the work it has to do—as a consequence the heart beat is strengthened and slowed, and the area of cardiac dulness is often notably diminished.* The slowing of the heart beat, notwithstanding the vascular dilatation, has been hypothetically explained by referring it to a reflex stimulation of the cardiac regulator nerves.

4. This treatment is also stated to have been found useful in certain cardiac *neuroses*, especially in cases of pseudo- or vaso-motor angina, due to arterial spasm, and occurring often in gouty subjects from the presence of irritating substances in the blood. The heart is assumed to be sound, but submitted to sudden and severe strain by more or less suddenly increased arterial resistance—in these cases the Nauheim bath acts, as has been seen, by dilating the superficial arterioles and so diminishing excessive blood pressure.

It is, however, very doubtful if this treatment should ever be applied to cases of *true angina;* in such cases it is best to avoid all spa treatment and the fatigue of long journeys, and even in the vaso-motor forms the greatest possible caution is needful, and it is questionable whether other spas are not more suitable to these cases than Nauheim.

At Nauheim and elsewhere, where artificial Nauheim baths are used, it is the custom to apply also what are termed "resistance exercises," which we have described elsewhere.† These are applied either during or after the course of baths. We are not satisfied that these are of any great use—and it has been recorded by those who had experience of the Nauheim treatment, before these movements were introduced, that as good results were obtained then as now.

* We have shown that the effect on the *respiration* has, in many instances, a marked influence in diminishing the area of cardiac dulness on percussion. "Manual of Medical Treatment," new edition, vol. i., p. 398.

† "Manual of Medical Treatment," new edition, vol. i., p. 400.

It must also be borne in mind that *all* baths containing much free carbonic acid—such as the gaseous chalybeate baths—exercise a powerful stimulating effect on the skin: they promote diuresis and general metabolism, and so exert a tonic effect on the heart and tend to relieve cardiac dilatation.

Gentle stimulation of the surface and promotion of the cutaneous circulation by *simple thermal* baths, cautiously applied, has proved of service in cases where the heart has been left weak and irritable after attacks of acute rheumatism attended with myocarditis, endocarditis, or pericarditis.

But the value of the Nauheim treatment has been seriously questioned by such eminent authorities as Huchard, of Paris, who states that he has seen most grievous consequences result from its indiscriminate application. These carbonic acid baths, he maintains, are dangerous in certain cases, and he instances death from apoplexy as occurring not rarely as a consequence of this treatment. He continues, "Even this year* I have seen three patients affected with *arterial cardiopathy* whose condition was considerably aggravated by the Nauheim cure, and who died in Paris, two from morbid conditions due to vasoconstriction and arterial hypertension, and the third from a violent attack of acute œdema of the lung." He refers these serious consequences to the *action hypertensive* of the carbonic acid baths—an effect which has been observed to last for one or two hours or even longer after the bath. He therefore urges that in the condition he terms "présclérose" and in all "arterial cardiopathies" characterised by hypertension, the Nauheim treatment is formally counter-indicated, and he very pertinently points out that this treatment is quite without any anti-toxic or eliminative action. He would reserve its application for cases of valvular disease with persistently low arterial tension.

* "La Médication Hypotensive." *Revue du Therapeutique Medico-Chirurgicale*, 1903.

Huchard, however, advocates thermal baths in the treatment of cardiac affections, and considers that they exercise an important influence on the central organs of the circulation by their thermality causing hyperæmia of the skin and having a vaso-dilator effect on the peripheral circulation; he also thinks it important to select a resort having waters of high or varied temperature, which, when taken internally, exert an anti-uricæmic action, and so lower arterial tension. He considers the springs of Bourbon Lancy especially indicated in these cases of arterial hypertension.

There are many other spas in France which claim to be of use to the cardiac invalid, and especially Aix les Bains, where they specify the following cases as suitable for thermal treatment:—

(1) Endocarditic lesions at their onset, if possible in the month following the acute attack.

(2) Cases of recent origin—a few months to a year—that are subject to frequent recurrences of acute or sub-acute articular rheumatism, and which are therefore constantly threatened with fresh cardiac mischief.

(3) Older cases with good and regular compensation. But no cases with endarteritis, or degeneration of the cardiac muscle, or with visceral complication from failing compensation, or over sixty years of age, should be sent there.

At Aix, in addition to the douche massage for which it is noted, artificial Nauheim baths are prepared, and mechanical exercises, according to the Zander system, are made use of.

This combined method is reported to have yielded excellent results in cases of recent origin.

At Uriage cases of recent endocarditis are said to be favourably modified, especially in children. The same remark applies to La Motte.

At Bagnols, with warm sulphur baths, at an elevation of about 2,500 feet, they treat the same class of cases as at Aix, but they extend the indication to cases of arterio-sclerosis at its commencement, to cases of commencing failure of accommodation, and to cases of fatty heart.

At Aulus, which is situated at about the same elevation as Bagnols, they treat early cases of arterio-sclerosis and the "renal" heart, and also cardiac neuroses and the fatty heart.

At Ax les Thermes they treat arterio-sclerosis, phlebitis, and varicose veins, and the first of these diseases is also treated at Evian. At Bagnoles de l'Orne the various forms of *phlebitis* and diseases of the veins are *specially* treated.

Brides les Bains, with its laxative eliminant water, combined with the adjacent gaseous salt baths of Salins Moutiers, possesses a combination of resources of undoubted value in certain forms of circulatory disorders—the commencement of arterial-hypertension and arterio-sclerosis cases, with threatened failure of compensation, cases of fatty heart in the obese with symptoms of abdominal plethora, enlarged liver and portal engorgement.

It will be seen by the foregoing and by reference to the descriptions in Section B of the spas here alluded to, that mineral waters and baths have come to take a place of some importance in cardiac therapeutics, and that the presence of compensated valvular lesions does not necessarily counter-indicate the prescription of chalybeate warm baths for co-existing anæmic states, or of aperient eliminative waters for hepatic or abdominal venous congestion, or of alkaline diuretic waters in states of uricæmia. We claim also that in cases of *arterio-sclerosis* the eliminant laxative and diuretic springs are of value in that they not only get rid of toxic substances that may be circulating in the blood, but by unloading the intestinal veins they tend to relieve vascular tension and promote a better distribution of the circulating fluid, especially when aided by the stimulating influence of thermal baths on the peripheral circulation. When we have to deal with these cases in the obese and muscularly vigorous patients the alkaline sodium sulphate waters are indicated (Marienbad, Tarasp, Brides), but in the thin and less vigorous the sodium chloride waters of Kissingen or those of Bourbon Lancy may be more appropriate. In all cardiac cases much caution is needed, and it is desirable to have some experience of the patient's capacities of re-action and the degree of compensation which exists, before determining whether or not the case is suitable to thermal treatment. It should also be remembered that some nervous cardiac patients are particularly sensitive to thermal baths, and feel much exhaustion after their use—when this is the case it is advisable not to prescribe them.

RENAL AND URINARY DISORDERS.

Mineral waters prove of great utility in the treatment of many affections which fall under this head. The *earthy calcareous* waters come into especial prominence in the treatment of *urinary concretions* and the morbid conditions of the bladder and urinary passages associated therewith.

Contrexéville, Vittel, Martigny, Wildungen are largely resorted to by sufferers from these maladies. The very feebly mineralised waters of Evian have also a great reputation in the same class of cases.

The class of *simple alkaline* waters, as exemplified by Vichy, Vals, and Neuenahr, retain the popularity they have for many years enjoyed in the treatment of urinary concretions, and although at one time the idea of an "alkaline cachexia" being attributable to the too free use of Vichy waters, advanced by Trousseaux, led to their replacement largely by waters of the earthy calcareous class, this idea is no longer believed to be tenable, and their ancient reputation has been quite regained.

The alkaline and mild sodium chloride waters, like those of Ems and Royat, are preferable in certain cases requiring very mild treatment, while in others the alkaline and sodium sulphate waters of Carlsbad, Marienbad, or Tarasp are to be preferred. In selecting a suitable spring, much must necessarily depend on the constitution of the patient, the cause of the malady, and the co-existence of other morbid states. The occurrence of uric acid gravel and calculi, associated with the gouty constitution, often depends on a disorder of the hepatic functions, and the appropriate treatment must include measures directed to restore healthy action of the liver. For such cases the alkaline sodium sulphate waters (Carlsbad) or the warm simple alkaline waters (Vichy) may be most appropriate, the former when there is a tendency to constipation and hæmorrhoids.

The free use of the alkaline waters, and also of the calcareous springs in case of renal gravel and calculi (uric acid), often leads to the passage of numerous concretions, and this is dependent not on any solvent action of the water, as was at one time supposed, but on its diuretic action and a mechanical *flushing* of the urinary passages. The alkaline waters also tend to reduce the acidity of the urine and maintain it neutral or slightly alkaline, and to prevent the re-formation of concretions. The action of the stronger alkaline waters should be carefully watched, so that the urine may not be rendered too alkaline and the risk of phosphatic precipitation be incurred.

The alkaline waters are also most useful in the treatment of *catarrhal conditions* of the renal pelvis, and of the urinary passages, when caused by uric acid deposits and hyperacidity of the urine, for, as has been pointed out, the "abundant and long continued drinking of those waters" renders the urine neutral or alkaline, lessens the irritation of the acid urine, liquefies the mucus, and influences favourably the diseased mucous membrane.

But when the mucous secretion is profuse and the disease very chronic (chronic pyelitis), the *earthy calcareous* waters may prove more serviceable (Wildungen, Driburg, Contrexéville), and, indeed, they can always be regarded as an alternative to the alkaline waters, and preferable to them in all those cases that do not well tolerate alkaline remedies. The use of Evian water applies to the same cases. It is appropriate to those individuals in whom we desire to effect a simple *flushing* of the urinary tracts and a dilution of the urine.

In cases of great irritability of the vescial mucous membrane, prolonged *simple thermal* baths (Wildbad, Ragatz) combined with the internal use of some mild gaseous alkaline water (Bilin, Apollinaris, Giesshübel) has a sedative and soothing effect.

Neither the alkaline nor the earthy waters should be prescribed in cases of *phosphate* concretions, but springs rich in free carbonic acid, and containing only nominal quantities of sodium bicarbonate and sodium chloride (Selters, Johannis, Bussang) are useful.

In the case of concretions of oxalates we may prescribe the free consumption, for long periods, of the mild gaseous simple alkaline waters (Bilin, Apollinaris, Giesshübel), and in the home treatment of uric acid deposits these or the weaker Vals springs, with occasional aperient doses of a "bitter water," prove of great service.

The imported water of Luhatschowitz, containing bicarbonate and chloride of sodium and much free carbonic acid, has been strongly recommended for home use in these cases.

Prostatic irritation and hypertrophy, when associated with uric acid deposits, is sometimes greatly relieved and reduced by a Vichy course.

Albuminuria.—Although mineral waters prove so useful in the case of renal gravel, calculi, and in catarrhal conditions of the urinary passages, we must not expect much benefit from their use in cases of *albuminuria* dependent on *renal* disease.

In cases of gouty kidney (*interstitial nephritis*) in the early stage, with slight albuminuria, mineral-water treatment, directed to the relief of the gouty state, may be of service, and by correcting the gouty state may cause the albumen to disappear; but any such treatment must be carried out with great care and caution, and we must see that the mineral water ingested is freely excreted by the kidneys, for if this is not the case there is the risk of increasing arterial pressure, which we should do our best to avoid in these cases, as arterio-sclerosis is often present, and almost always impending.

In albuminuria, dependent on digestive disturbance (a condition not so common as some seem to imagine), mineral waters directed to the relief of the dyspeptic condition may be useful.

French physicians seem to have much confidence in the usefulness of mineral waters in albuminuria. Functional albuminuria is reported to be cured at St. Nectaire le Haut, and at Pougues—not only functional forms, but nephritic cases are claimed as appropriate for treatment at those spas. Of other French spas which claim to be indicated in certain forms of albuminuria, we may mention Royat, Evian, Brides, Martigny, and Châtelguyon.

The waters of Contrexéville have been reputed as useful in the nocturnal incontinence of urine in children.

DISEASES OF THE NERVOUS SYSTEM.

There are many diseases of the nervous system which are obviously quite unsuited to treatment by mineral waters and baths, and to these we need not refer; there are others in which bath treatment is permissible, but not very hopeful, and still a few others in which treatment at natural thermal baths proves advantageous.

In most of these cases it is the *bath* treatment—the *external* treatment and not the *internal* use of the mineral waters—that is mainly relied upon, and there can be no doubt that much of the benefit experienced at the spas to which these cases resort is to be attributed to the accessory means there applied—

to the electrical appliances, the mechanical measures, such as massage, re-educating movements, regulated exercises, and proper periods of rest, and the appropriate diet—as well as to the co-operation of a suitable tonic and sedative climate. It is to the whole system of detailed attention and skilful supervision and management, and the perfection of the physical resources at the disposal of the physicians at these resorts, that the good results, not unfrequently obtained, must be referred.

Even in certain chronic cases of structural nervous lesions, where little or no permanent benefit can be looked for, the patient, and the patient's friends, are naturally not content to relinquish all hope of amelioration, and when it is clear that no harm can accrue from bath treatment, it is permissible to allow such cases the satisfaction of some hopeful anticipations, and the feeling that nothing has been left untried. We shall now mention, briefly, the principal nervous affections in which bath treatment has been recommended.

Chronic paralysis and painful contractions following cerebral hæmorrhage.—These cases are not very hopeful ones, and it is generally admitted that bath treatment should not be undertaken until several months have elapsed since the acute attack. The object of treatment is to maintain nutrition and tone in the affected muscles, to allay nervous and circulatory irritability, to relieve painful spasm, and to promote the general health. The indifferent or *simple thermal* springs and the *mild sodium chloride* springs are those mainly resorted to. In France, Néris (*simple thermal*) has a special reputation, so has Bourbon l'Archambaut (*mild warm sodium chloride*). In the latter it is suggested that the original lesion should not be severe, and that the case should not be sent there until *after* the inflammatory stage has disappeared, and *before* atrophy and definite contractions have set in. The somewhat stronger warm sodium chloride springs of Balaruc, close to Cette, on the Mediterranean coast, also enjoys a reputation for the treatment of such cases; it is, however, pointed out that the "cure" must be directed with "extreme prudence" on the part of the medical attendant, and should not be undertaken till long after the hæmorrhagic attack, and when all risk of recurrence is absent.

Cases of the same kind are also treated at Gastein, Ragatz, Wildbad, and Teplitz.

Cases of *cerebral hyperœmia* with "apoplectic tendencies" are not very suitable subjects for spa treatment, but the aperient "bitter waters" or the alkaline sodium sulphate waters have been recommended as "intestinal derivatives"—but these can be taken at home.

Paralysis referable to *spinal* disease, and especially when due to "cold" or rheumatic affection of the spinal meninges, or the sequel of acute disease; paraplegia, recent, and particularly when due to chronic myelitis of rheumatic origin, and spasmodic paraplegia; these are treated at such *simple thermal* baths as Buxton, Bath, Néris, Plombières, Ragatz, Gastein, Schlangenbad, and also at some thermal common salt and gaseous common salt baths, Bourbonne, Balaruc, Nauheim, according as sedative or stimulating effects are desired—also at the feebly mineralised warm springs of La Malou and Bagnères-de-Bigorre.

At Néris it is maintained that the "cure" there is beneficial to cases of *general paralysis* at its onset, and to those of *progressive muscular atrophy* if adopted at the earliest manifestations. But it may be doubted if these diseases are ever greatly benefited by thermal treatment.

Locomotor ataxy or *tabes* is claimed to be amenable to thermal treatment at many Continental spas. La Malou, in France, has a very widespread reputation for the treatment of this affection, which was greatly contributed to by the advocacy of the late Professor Charcot. It is maintained by the local physicians that the painful symptoms —the lightning pains, the visceral crises, the loss of power of the sphincters and the greater part of the trophic disturbances and the general debility—are efficaciously dealt with there, and that the motor inco-ordination is beneficially modified by the thermal treatment combined with the re-education exercises.

It is mainly to the influence of the external application of the waters that the good effects are referred, and the internal use of the waters is quite secondary. Néris also claims that the sedative action of its baths exercises a very beneficial effect on those cases of tabes in which the painful and excitable symptoms predominate.

Bagnères-de-Bigorre has been recommended in cases of incipient tabes.

The *simple thermal* waters of Ragatz, Gastein, and Wildbad have also been found useful. Re-education exercises, to remedy the motor inco-ordination, are practised at most of these spas.

In early cases, but when the painful manifestations have ceased, the warm sodium chloride springs, and even the stimulating gaseous sodium chloride waters, have been found of service at Bourbon l'Archambaut, Bourbonne les Bains, Balaruc, Droitwich, Nauheim, and Oeynhausen.

The warm mud baths of St. Amand have been found useful in relieving the lightning pains of tabes in many instances.

In cases that can be distinctly referred to syphilis, much benefit may be derived from treatment at the *thermal sulphur and salt baths*, as at Aix la Chapelle and Uriage, combined with specific treatment, which can be applied so much more freely at these spas. We may say here that all affections of the nervous system of *syphilitic origin*, like other manifestations of constitutional syphilis, can be advantageously treated at these spas and by the same methods.

Neuritis (and consequent loss of muscular power),

peripheral and multiple, due to alcoholic, metallic, or other intoxication, or to cold (rheumatic) or to injury, may be benefited by suitable thermal treatment. The *simple thermal* baths in cases that require sedative treatment — Buxton, Bath, Néris, Ragatz, Schlangenbad; in those requiring more stimulating treatment we may prescribe *warm sulphur* baths, as Aix les Bains, Aix la Chapelle, and others, or *warm sodium chloride* baths at Droitwich, Bourbonne les Bains, Kissingen, etc. In the cases due to metallic intoxication (lead, mercury, etc.) the warm sulphur or sulphur and sodium chloride baths are especially indicated.

Chronic neuralgias of various origin, whether due to toxic affections, to constitutional states, to anæmic conditions, or to inflammation of the great nerves or their sheaths, are frequently submitted to thermal treatment, and sciatica perhaps more frequently than any other form. Massage, douching, and electricity are employed as auxiliary influences in many instances. Cases of rheumatic, gouty or syphilitic nature are usually sent to *thermal sulphur* baths-Aix les Bains, Aix la Chapelle, St. Sauveur, Acqui— or to the *thermal salt* baths, Bourbonne les Bains, Balaruc, Droitwich, Wiesbaden.

Cases requiring more soothing treatment are directed to *simple thermal* baths, as Bath, Buxton, Gastein, Ragatz, Plombières, Néris, or to the feebly mineralised thermal baths of La Malou or Bagnères-de-Bigorre. The mud baths of Dax have been found serviceable in some cases.

The *anœmic* forms may be treated with the baths and chalybeate waters of Spa, Schwalbach, or Franzensbad.

In some cases of *sciatica* associated with habitual constipation and abdominal stasis the laxative waters (with hot mineral or mud baths) of Carlsbad, Brides, Marienbad, or Kissingen may be most appropriate.

Cases of *infantile paralysis* are not frequently submitted to spa treatment, but it is stated that benefit is derived from the methods applied at Bourbon l'Archambaut, Bourbonne les Bains, and Barèges.

The various *neuroses* and functional nervous disturbances are usually best dealt with at spas situated at moderate elevations in mountainous or forest regions, where a soothing as well as mildly bracing treatment can be applied.

Hysteria and its chronic manifestations, paralysis, contractions, etc., *neurasthenia, insomnia,* some forms of *chorea* and professional spasm, as *writer's cramp,* etc., are often beneficially affected by treatment at St. Gervais, St. Sauveur, Evian, Plombières, Buxton, Gastein, Schlangenbad, Bagnères-de-Bigorre, La Malou, and others.

CUTANEOUS DISEASES.

There are many mineral springs which have a considerable reputation for the treatment of skin diseases, especially the *sulphur* springs, warm and cold, as Luchon, Schinznach, Strathpeffer, Harrogate, and the *sulphur* and *sodium chloride* springs, as Uriage, Aix la Chapelle, Acqui, Herculesbad; also the *arsenical* and *alkaline* springs of La Bourboule and Royat, and the *iron and arsenical* water of Levico; and in a minor degree the *simple thermal* or *thermal earthy* spas, as Bath, Schlangenbad, and particularly Leukerbad. When for the accompanying constitutional state or disorder *alkaline* or *saline* waters are indicated, the French physicians prescribe such spas as Vichy, Royat, and Le Boulou, or Evaux and La Mouillère. In some cases the mud baths of St. Amand are thought useful.

It is, of course, important to consider any coexisting constitutional disease or tendency which may be of etiological importance; for instance in some gouty cases the *alkaline sodium sulphate* waters of Carlsbad may be indicated.

Many skin diseases are associated with the

rheumatic and *gouty* constitutions, and it will be noted that many of the spas which are recommended, in the treatment of skin affections, are precisely those which are found useful in the treatment of chronic rheumatism and gout.

To many others scrofula is believed to have a causal relation, and for these the sodium chloride, and the sulphur and sodium chloride, baths are considered most appropriate.

It is not improbable that in certain forms of skin disease some of these baths, and particularly the sulphur ones, may exert an anti-bacterial influence.

It is naturally the *chronic*, intractable forms of cutaneous disease that are sent to mineral-water resorts.

In some resorts, as at Leukerbad, *prolonged maceration* of the skin, by immersion for many hours at a time, is obviously an important physical agency which has the effect of cleansing the skin of adherent secretions and washing away old epidermal scales, and of exerting a tonic and sedative effect on the cutaneous peripheral nerves.

We shall now mention briefly the spa treatment suitable to the chief and most prevalent forms of skin disease.

Eczema.—This is one of the commonest of skin affections, and one that is most frequently benefited by bath treatment. Uriage may be taken as the type of bath which is most universally applicable to the cure of eczema. The *moist* forms are the most favourably influenced, and the course seems to be equally useful in the lymphatic, the scrofulous, the gouty, and the anæmic. The favourable climatic situation, at a moderate elevation (about 1,400 feet above the sea), with much sunshine, in the mountains of Dauphiné, no doubt is an effectual aid to its mineral springs.

Other *sulphur* baths that enjoy a reputation for the cure of this malady are Strathpeffer (in gouty cases), Harrogate, Schinznach, Luchon (especially the *humid* forms), Enghien (the dry forms and those requiring stimulating treatment), Challes (scrofulous forms), Barèges, St. Gervais, St. Honoré, Ax les Thermes (all forms), Allevard (the impetiginous form), Lenk, in Canton Berne (moist form), Aix la Chapelle, Acqui, etc.

In *scrofulous* forms with tendency to glandular enlargements the following *sodium chloride* waters have been recommended—La Mouillère (Besançon), Salins-du-Jura, Kreuznach; also the arsenical waters of La Bourboule. In *diabetic* forms, Vichy, Royat, Neuenahr, La Bourboule; these are also useful in certain gouty and rheumatic forms. In certain nervous, irritable forms the simple thermal springs prove soothing and beneficial, as Néris, Plombières, Gastein, Schlangenbad, Ragatz; in very chronic forms maceration of the skin by prolonged baths at Leukerbad, or at Bath, may be of great use. Leukerbad is said to be especially useful when the nails are the seat of the disease.

The arsenical and iron water of Levico is prescribed in some anæmic forms. For gouty subjects with hepatic inadequacy the Carlsbad waters often prove of service.

Psoriasis.—This most rebellious of skin affections is often ameliorated, but seldom or never cured, by mineral baths. The skin is often cleansed and freed from scales and crusts, and "whitened" for a time by thermal *sulphur*, with vapour, or *sulphur and sodium chloride* baths (Uriage, Luchon, Aix les Bains, Strathpeffer, Harrogate), or by prolonged maceration in such baths as Leukerbad, or in other simple thermal baths.

The arsenical waters of La Bourboule, Levico, and Roncegno are sometimes prescribed.

Acne.—Uriage (pulverisations), Challes, Allevard, Cauterets, Schinznach, Luchon, Enghien, Barèges, the mud of St. Amand. The accompanying constitutional states may need alkaline waters (Vichy, Royat, Ems), or common salt waters (in scrofulous cases) or chalybeate waters in the anæmic, or the laxative waters of Marienbad, Tarasp, etc., in the hepatic, gouty forms with constipation.

Prurigo and Pruritus.—Harrogate, Strathpeffer, Enghien, Aix les Bains, Luchon, Schinznach, or the sedative springs of Néris, Plombières, Evaux, Ragatz, Gastein, Buxton, the prolonged baths at Leukerbad, the alkaline arsenical baths of La Bourboule, Mont Dore, Royat. The constitutional states must be carefully considered and appropriately treated.

Lichen.—Enghien, St. Gervais, Luchon, La Bourboule, Schlangenbad.

Pityriasis.—Simple thermal waters to allay irritation (Buxton, Plombières, Ragatz, Néris). In very chronic torpid cases the sulphur waters of Aix la Chapelle, Uriage, Enghien, Schinznach, St. Honoré.

Chronic Furunculosis.—Harrogate, Llandrindod, Lenk, Schinznach, Uriage, La Bourboule. The constitutional condition and its appropriate treatment is of chief consideration.

Urticaria.—The constitutional disorder should be the chief object of treatment. The alkaline waters (Vichy, Vals, Royat) may be of use in the gouty or rheumatic. The *simple thermal* sedative baths (Néris, Gastein, Schlangenbad, Buxton) in the neurotic.

DISEASES OF THE FEMALE GENITAL ORGANS.

Chronic disorders of the female sexual organs have been largely dealt with at certain mineral springs: disorders of menstruation—amenorrhœa, dysmenorrhœa, menorrhagia; disturbances of health attending the menopause; catarrhal conditions of the vagina and uterus (vaginal and uterine leucorrhœa); the results of inflammatory affections of the pelvic viscera—metritis, endometritis, perimetritis, parametritis; pelvic cellulitis, inflammatory exudations, fibroid tumours; tendency to abortion; the causes of sterility. All these conditions, when no longer attended by acute inflammatory symptoms, have been beneficially influenced by mineral-water treatment.

Certain spas have obtained a great and special reputation for the treatment of these maladies; Ems, Baden-Baden, Franzensbad, Kreuznach, Woodhall Spa, St. Sauveur, and Luxeuil are all well known in this connection.

We will first refer to disorders of menstruation, and in these, as in all other cases, we must, of course, always pay careful attention to etiological considerations and constitutional tendencies.

Amenorrhœa.—In cases dependent on anæmia the chalybeate baths and waters are indicated—Spa, Schwalbach, St. Moritz, Pyrmont. If associated with constipation and dyspeptic states, or due to passive uterine congestion, the sodium chloride waters (Homburg, Kissingen, Châtelguyon, Baden-Baden, Salins Moutiers), or the gaseous thermal salt waters (Nauheim, Oeynhausen), may be more useful.

If intestinal torpor and tendency to abdominal stasis are very prominent features, the *Moor* baths and the aperient sodium sulphate and iron waters of Franzensbad, Elster, Tarasp, and Marienbad are indicated, as they are also in those cases that occur towards the menopause, often combined with gouty and rheumatic symptoms and a tendency to obesity.

The French school also recommend the sulphur and sodium chloride waters of Uriage, and those of Bourbon l'Archambaut for their stimulating action in lymphatic, torpid constitutions, while for sensitive, nervous cases, requiring sedative treatment, they prescribe such spas as St. Sauveur and Ussat.

In some of these spas local applications in the form of douches of dry carbonic acid gas, peat poultices, and packing the vagina with peat are employed.

It is always an advantage to select an attractive and bracing or soothing climate (according to the individual needs), where the patient can be tempted to be much in the open air.

Dysmenorrhœa.—In *obstinate chronic* cases the *Moor* baths and the ferruginous sodium sulphate waters of Franzensbad and Elster promise the best results.

In *neuralgic* and *ovarian* cases a protracted course of *simple thermal baths* (Plombières, Bagnères-de-Bigorre, Gastein, Wildbad, Ragatz), for their sedative effect, is useful; or if constipation is a prominent feature treatment may be begun at Elster or Franzensbad, and concluded at a simple thermal bath.

The *congestive* form, with enlarged uterus coming on after abortion or uterine gestation, may be treated at sodium chloride springs (Bourbon l'Archambaut, Kissingen, Châtelguyon, Salins Moutiers), or alkaline sodium chloride springs (Ems in particular). In the neurotic and irritable the sedative springs of Ussat, St. Sauveur, Eaux Chaudes, and Luxeuil are serviceable.

It is generally recommended that a prolonged period of bath treatment should be prescribed—eight to ten weeks—during which period the restful life in such pleasantly situated resorts, as most of those mentioned, could not fail to be advantageous.

In the *membranous* form a prolonged course at Ems or Baden-Baden (alkaline sodium chloride), or at one of the simple thermal baths mentioned, is usually prescribed.

Menorrhagia.—In some cases a long course of chalybeate waters proves useful (Spa, Schwalbach, St. Moritz, Pyrmont); in others the waters and baths of Franzensbad, followed by a long after-cure at a moderate elevation.

In France a course at Châtelguyon or Salins Moutiers (sodium chloride) is often prescribed with advantage.

The troublesome symptoms associated with the *menopause*—gastric, hepatic and nervous—are often benefited by a course of mineral-water treatment.

In those case with a tendency to constipation and obesity the sodium sulphate and iron waters of

Marienbad, Franzensbad, and Elster prove very useful. In thin subjects the sodium chloride waters (Homburg, Kissingen, Baden-Baden or Châtelguyon) are more suitable. The sulphur and sodium chloride waters of Uriage, applied according to the methods of hydrotherapy, prove most beneficial in certain cases, in which also the somewhat similar springs of Harrogate and Llandrindod may be prescribed.

In delicate, neurotic subjects the soothing springs of Luxeuil or Eaux Chaudes, or the simple thermal waters of Gastein, Ragatz, Wildbad, or Buxton may be most appropriate.

A prolonged after-cure in an agreeable seaside or mountain resort, of moderate elevation, is essential in these cases.

Leucorrhœa.—Vaginal leucorrhœa is perhaps best treated with the alkaline sodium chloride water of Ems. St. Nectaire le Haut, in Auvergne, has also a reputation to the same effect; its *source intermittente*, which contains much free carbonic acid, is applied as a "natural ascending vaginal douche." If anæmia is a prominent feature the iron waters (Spa, Schwalbach, etc.) are suitable, and if there is habitual constipation the sodium chloride waters (Kissingen, Homburg, Salins Moutiers). In *uterine* leucorrhœa mineral water treatment is not so successful, but co-existing abdominal congestion may be relieved by the sodium chloride waters, or the alkaline sodium sulphate waters of Franzensbad or Elster. If pain and tenderness are prominent features, the simple thermal, or the gaseous sodium chloride, springs may be applied. The *sulphur* and *sodium chloride* waters of Uriage have been found useful in the torpid, lymphatic, and strumous; and the *sulphur* waters of Luchon and Enghien have also proved useful, applied by means of vaginal injection, or with the aid of the wire bath speculum.

Chronic inflammatory affections of the uterus and its annexes and their consequences are frequently submitted to bath treatment—*endometritis*, *metritis*, *perimetritis, parametritis, pelvic cellulitis*, etc.—and a great variety of spas are resorted to for this purpose. Perhaps the most popular are certain *sodium chloride* waters, as Kreuznach, Woodhall Spa, Kissingen, Reichenhall, Ischl, Châtelguyon, Bourbon l'Archambaut, La Mouillère, Salins-du-Jura, Salins de Béarn, La Motte, etc.; or the *alkaline sodium chloride* springs, as Ems, Neuenahr, Royat, St. Nectaire le Haut, combined with long periods of repose.

Drinking cures with the laxative sodium sulphate or sodium chloride waters (Marienbad, Franzensbad, Elster, Kissingen, Homburg, Tarasp) are often useful to relieve hyperæmia and stimulate absorption, by lowering blood pressure in the abdominal vessels and relieving co-existing constipation. *Uriage* has been found useful in chronic debilitated cases with absence of acute symptoms. In chronic painful metritis, and cases requiring soothing treatment, the more sedative springs should be advised, as Ussat, Eaux Chaudes, St. Sauveur, Luxeuil, and Plombières. In anæmic forms an after-course of iron waters may prove beneficial.

Uterine fibroids.—It must not be expected that mineral waters will cause the disappearance of these tumours, although very confident statements have occasionally been made to this effect; but no doubt great benefit and relief to symptoms have been found to attend treatment at certain spas, especially the strong thermal sodium chloride springs at Kreuznach, Ischl, Woodhall Spa, Salins-du-Jura, Salins de Béarn (occasional *cures* are claimed at this spa), La Mouillère (Besançon), Salins Moutiers, La Motte les Bains, etc. Good effects have also been claimed from treatment at Luxeuil.

Tendency to miscarriages.—In anæmic cases chalybeate waters, with long periods of rest, may prove useful. In suspected syphilitic cases the usual specific treatment at sulphur baths may be prescribed. In neurotic cases the sedative baths and climate of Eaux Chaudes and St. Sauveur have been advised. A prolonged after-cure in a soothing and bracing resort is always essential.

Sterility.—Many and diverse spas have been credited with the cure of sterility—the *iron* waters of Schwalbach, Pyrmont, Spa, St. Moritz—the *sodium chloride* springs of Homburg, Kissingen, Baden-Baden—the *alkaline sodium chloride* springs of Ems—the *sulphur* baths of St. Sauveur—the *simple thermal* springs of Gastein, Ragatz, Luxeuil and others. Ems has a very great reputation in this respect. Mineral waters can only act by causing the disappearance of material or functional defects. Chronic leucorrhœa and acidity of the vaginal secretions may be removed: by the application of vaginal douches the circulation and nutrition of the uterus may be improved; iron tonics and a bracing climate may improve the general health and tone. But doubtless one of the most influential circumstances is the long separation of husband and wife and the consequent tonic effect on both.

Part II.

CLIMATE AND CLIMATIC RESORTS.

CHAPTER I.

CLIMATE AND CLIMATES.

WHAT do we mean by climate? What is the kind of information we require when we ask the question—what kind of climate has any particular place? We generally mean by a question of this kind that we desire to know how the natural conditions and surroundings of a particular place affect the life and well-being of its human inhabitants. That, practically, is what we want to know when we make inquiries about climate; with the geographical distribution of plants and animals, or with any other considerations connected with climate, we are only now concerned in so far as they affect the well-being of mankind.

It is evident that the climate of a place must depend, first and chiefly, on the conditions and character of its atmosphere—its aërial cloak*—which may be hot or cold, moist or dry, still or agitated, pure or foul, uniform or variable, etc.; and, second, on the nature of its surface, which may be land or water, low or elevated, level or broken, barren or cultivated, sand, clay, rock, marsh, wood, meadow, country, or town, etc., and these conditions also act through their influence on the atmosphere.

* "The term *climate*, in its broadest sense, implies all the changes in the atmosphere which sensibly affect one's physical condition."—*Humboldt.*

The characters and quality of the atmosphere differ considerably in different places on the surface of the globe. The atmosphere over Manchester differs from the atmosphere over a Yorkshire moor or a Swiss mountain; the atmosphere over the table-lands of Central Asia differs from the atmosphere over the Indian Ocean; the atmosphere over the plains of Lombardy differs from the atmosphere in the Upper Inn Valley; and although these differences are not so considerable as to actually interfere with the maintenance of human life, they may be sufficient to materially influence the health and well-being of men, at certain times and under certain circumstances.

The chief conditions of the atmosphere that affect the climate of a place are these: 1, its temperature; 2, its movements (winds); 3, the amount of aqueous vapour and its precipitation as rain or snow; 4, its electrical conditions; 5, its purity; 6, its density or pressure; and 7, its composition.

And these conditions depend mainly on the following influences:

1st, and chief, distance from the equator;

2nd, adjacency to, or remoteness from, seas or other large tracts of water;

3rd, elevation above the sea;

4th, the prevailing winds; and

5th, strictly local influences, such as configuration and inclination of surface, relation to mountain chains, nature of soil and vegetation, absence or presence of plantations, cultivation, aspect, drainage, population, manufactures, etc.

The most important factor in the determination of climate is undoubtedly **temperature**, and the temperature of a place is, with certain qualifications which will immediately be stated, dependent on its distance from the equator.

Those countries are hottest upon which the sun's rays fall vertically, or almost vertically, and the warmest climates are therefore those of the intertropical regions. The further we go from the equator the more and more obliquely the sun's rays fall on the surface, and for that reason the same amount of solar-rays are spread over an increasing extent of surface, while they also have to traverse a greater mass of air. The nearer we approach the poles, the less the amount of heat received from the solar rays, and these climates therefore are the coldest.

The influence of distance from the equator is well shown in some European countries in the difference of time in the flowering or ripening of widely-distributed plants. At Naples (N. lat. 40° 5′) the elm comes into leaf at the beginning of February, at Paris (N. lat. 48° 5′) not until late in March, and in the centre of England (N. lat. 52° 5′) not until the middle of April. In the South of Italy ripe cherries may be gathered about the beginning of May, in northern France and central Germany at the end of June, but not in England usually till three or four weeks later.

Were it not, then, for counteracting influences we might say that, universally over the surface of the globe, *temperature is regulated by latitude*. But this statement is by no means of universal application; indeed, places which are on the same parallel of latitude rarely enjoy exactly the same temperature, and in some instances there are wide divergences.

If, for example, we compare London and Labrador, which coincide in latitude, we find that while in both the summers are mild, in England the winters are not very cold, while in Labrador they are excessively so.

By means of numerous thermometric observations taken at various parts of the world, at different times and seasons, it has been possible to construct maps upon which lines are drawn through all places having the same temperature at the same season, or the same average annual temperature, and these *isothermal lines* as they are called show the general distribution of temperature over the globe.

Isothermal lines, or lines of equal temperature, are

named after the degrees of temperature they express, *e.g.* "the isotherm of 60°" means the line drawn through all the places on the map which have the average annual temperature of 60°.

Now it is found that these isothermal lines, drawn round the globe, instead of following the parallels of latitude, bend up and down, and these bendings are determined by the place of continents and oceans. They are noticed to be least irregular over the wide expanse of ocean in the southern hemisphere, while they show the greatest deflections across North America, the Atlantic, Europe, and Asia. It is thus seen that temperature is more uniform and more directly dependent on latitude in the oceanic parts of the globe than in the continental, or where the oceanic and continental come together as they do in the basin of the Atlantic.

If we take the isotherm of 50° (mean annual temperature), viz. that passing through London, it continues in nearly a straight line westward toward the coast of Wales; it then bends south-westward, and crosses to the west coast of Ireland. If we trace it to the opposite side of the Atlantic, we shall find that in crossing the ocean it bends much further south, and reaches the coast of America, near New York, so that the mean annual temperature of London and New York is the same, though New York is as far south of London as Madrid.

On reference to a map of isothermal lines, it will be seen that these divergencies of belts of equal heat from the same parallels of latitude are determined by the manner in which the great areas of land and sea are grouped.

"Land gets sooner heated by the sun's rays than the sea, and also gives off its heat again sooner. The sea, though it does not get so hot as the land does, retains its heat longer, and is enabled by virtue of its liquidity and motion to diffuse it. Hence the influence of the sea tends to mitigate both the heat and the cold of the land. Its warm currents heat the air resting on them, and so give rise to warm winds which blow upon the land, while its colder waters in like manner temper the air, which reaches the land in cooling breezes, or it may be in cold, damp winds and fogs. Thus, in the basin of the North Atlantic, a warm ocean current, called the *Gulf Stream*, issues from the Gulf of Mexico, and, augmented by the surface-drift of warm water which is driven onward by the prevalent south-west winds, flows across the Atlantic to the shores of Britain, and even of Spitzbergen. It brings with it the supplies of heat which make the climate of the west of Europe so much less cold than it would naturally be. On the other hand, an icy stream of water coming out of Davis Strait brings a chill to the coasts of Labrador and Newfoundland. The ocean, therefore, by its cold currents is depressing the temperature in America along the same latitudes, where in Europe, by its warm currents, it is raising it."*

Again, the influence of a large tract of land situated in high latitudes lowers the temperature below what it would be if the same regions were occupied by sea, because it allows of the accumulation of vast masses of snow and ice; and a similar tract of land in low latitudes, by exposing a broad, motionless, and quickly-heated surface to the tropical rays of the sun, gives rise to a far higher temperature than would be observed over a tract of ocean in the same region.

But we must not conclude that two places which have the same average *yearly* temperature have the same climate. Take, for instance, Dublin and Munich, which have nearly the same annual means of temperature, viz. 48° to 49° F.; but the winters at Munich are 9° colder than in Dublin, and the summer about 6° warmer.

In order, then, to compare the climate of different places on the surface of the globe, it is necessary not only to know the mean annual temperature, but also

* Geikie's "Physical Geography," p. 61.

how the temperature is distributed through the different seasons, and maps are prepared for this purpose, with isothermal lines showing the distribution of temperature for each month or season.

"Range maps" have also been constructed, enabling us to contrast different localities with regard to the extent of variation, or range, of temperature which they experience in the year, which is a very important factor in the determination of climate.

These "range maps" show that:

(*a*) The range increases from the equator towards the poles, and from the coast towards the interior of a continent: (*b*) the regions of extreme range in the northern hemisphere coincide approximately with the districts of lowest temperature in winter: (*c*) the range is greater in the northern than in the southern hemisphere: (*d*) in the middle and higher latitudes of both hemispheres, with the exception of Greenland and Patagonia, the western coasts have a less range than the eastern: and (*e*) that in the interior of the continents the range in mountainous districts diminishes with the height above the sea.

On inspection of such a map, the influence of the sea in moderating extremes of climate is unmistakable, "but even more decidedly do the agencies of prevailing winds and prevailing currents show their effects. Where the prevailing winds are westerly, the so-called anti-trades, and where the ocean currents are flowing from the equator into higher latitudes, the cold of winter is mitigated, and the curves of equal range bent polewards. On the other hand, on the eastern coast of America, and even more so on that of Asia, the prevailing winds are northerly and cold, so that the temperature in winter falls very low, while the summer is comparatively warm, and the contrast between the opposite seasons is very marked."*

We thus see how temperature is regulated, and the effect of distance from the equator modified by the *distribution of sea and land.*

* Scott's "Meteorology," p. 342.

The temperature of the air is also regulated, and the effect of distance from the equator modified, by the *elevation of a region*, by its height above the sea. It is a matter of common observation that in ascending mountains the air gets cooler the higher we go.

It may be taken as a somewhat rough average that the decrease of temperature with elevation is about 1° Fahrenheit for every 300 feet of ascent; so that *height above the sea* is an important element in climate. There is an apparent exception to this observed in very cold, calm weather, when, in a valley, the cold, heavier air sinks to the lowest level, and the warmer and lighter air rises on the hill sides, so that a residence on a slight eminence, or on the side of a hill, secures immunity from the greatest severity of the frosts. Evergreens suffer less in such situations than in low-lying bottoms.

Before we consider the important influence of the movements of the atmosphere, *i.e.* of the prevailing currents of wind on climate, it will be desirable to consider shortly the influence of **atmospheric pressure** or density, and of **atmospheric humidity**, as it is on them that the movements of the air are dependent.

The use of the barometer to foretell changes of weather is founded, as everybody knows, on the fact that variations in atmospheric pressure give rise to winds and storms, and all those movements of the air upon which weather depends.

But if we ask, in the next place, what causes these variations of atmospheric pressure, we shall be told that they are greatly affected, first by temperature, and secondly by aqueous vapour.

We can readily understand how temperature acts. Air when heated expands, when cooled it contracts; therefore cold air is heavier than warm air, and warm air ascends while cold air descends.

The ascent of warm air must necessarily diminish atmospheric pressure. When a broad tract of the earth's surface, such for instance as the centre of Asia, is greatly heated by the sun's rays, the hot air in contact with the ground rises and flows over into the surrounding regions. Hence the atmospheric pressure is lowered there during the hot months of the year.

The influence of the presence of water-vapour on the pressure of air is due to the circumstance that water-vapour is very much lighter and has less pressure than air; so that air saturated with vapour of water is lighter than dry air, and the difference in weight increases with the temperature, because the warmer the air, the more water-vapour can be dissolved in it. For instance, a cubic foot of perfectly dry air at 32° F. weighs a grain and a-quarter more than a cubic foot of air saturated with vapour at the same temperature, whereas a cubic foot of perfectly dry air at 80° F. weighs six and a-half grains more than air saturated with moisture at the same temperature.

The amount of aqueous vapour in the air is constantly varying; the addition of a large volume of vapour to the atmosphere lowers its pressure and causes the mercury to fall; the removal of this vapour, by its condensation into rain for instance, restores the pressure, and the mercury rises.

How these changes in the volume of vapour in any part of the atmosphere are brought about is still unknown.

Every surface of water exposed to the air gives off vapour into the atmosphere so long as this remains unsaturated; when the air reaches its point of saturation, evaporation ceases, and the higher the temperature of the air, the greater its capacity, as we have seen, of absorbing moisture. Wind greatly favours evaporation, for it blows away the vapour from the surface of the water as it is formed, and brings other and dryer air to absorb and carry off the fresh supplies.

It is clear, then, that more vapour of water must be added to the air during the warmer day than during the colder night, and during the summer than in winter, during a brisk wind than in still weather, and in far greater amount in warm tropical regions than in temperate or cold ones.

The water which passes into the air in the form of this invisible vapour is condensed, and reappears in such visible forms as dew, rain, snow, clouds, and mists.

The presence of this water-vapour in the atmosphere has a very important influence on the temperature of the surface of the earth. It surrounds the earth with a kind of cloak, sometimes invisible, sometimes in the visible form of cloud, and by lessening the diathermancy of the air it serves to protect it from the too great intensity of the solar rays during the day, and from the too rapid loss of heat by radiation into cold space during the night, when the influence of the sun is removed. "If it could be removed for a little from around us, we should be burnt up by day and frozen hard at night."

It is well known that when water passes into the state of vapour it absorbs a considerable amount of heat which is rendered *latent* or imperceptible, and that when the vapour is again condensed into water, the latent heat is again given out and becomes sensible. Every pound of water which is condensed from vapour liberates heat enough to melt five pounds of cast iron. When, then, in nature, the vapour of the air is converted into water on a large scale, the temperature of the air is thereby considerably raised. Rainfall is dependent on the amount of aqueous vapour which passes into the air, and its subsequent condensation; it is therefore usually greatest in tropical regions, where the amount of evaporation is greatest, and it diminishes in amount as the temperature falls towards the poles. This rule is, however, subject to important exceptions, dependent on the distribution of sea and land, and on the great aërial currents.

As condensation is more active over land than over sea, the rainfall also is greater over land than sea, and over the northern hemisphere, much of which is land, than over the southern hemisphere, most of which is water. Most of the vapour of the atmosphere being furnished by the ocean, it follows that the condensation of vapour into rain upon the land is greatest at the coast-line, so that the sea-board of a country may be rainy while its interior is comparatively dry. Rainfall is much influenced by the form of the surface; as mountains act as condensers, they are therefore much wetter than plains. "Places which lie in the path of any of the regular air-currents are wet when they cool the current, and dry when they warm it. Hence winds blowing towards the equator, since they come into warmer latitudes, are not usually wet winds; but when they blow towards the poles they reach colder latitudes, and are chilled and therefore rainy.

"Some of these laws are well illustrated in the British Islands, where the rains are chiefly brought by the south-westerly winds, which have come across the Atlantic. The coast-line facing that ocean is more rainy than the east side looking to the narrow North Sea. In the former part of the country, away from the hills, the amount of rain which falls in a year would, if collected together, have a depth of from 30 to 45 inches. On the east side, however, the average annual rainfall does not exceed 20 to 28 inches. Where the western coast happens to be mountainous, an excess of rain falls; hence the wetness of the climate along the north-west coast of Scotland and in the lake district of England, where the annual rainfall ranges from 80 to 150, and sometimes even more than 200 inches."*

Owing to the enormous evaporation which goes on between the tropics, a constant stream of vapour is rising into the upper regions of the atmosphere, and, becoming chilled there, falls in the form of heavy and frequent rains.

If a high mass of land, in these rainy regions, lies in the path of the warm, moist air-currents, the rain-

* Geikie's "Physical Geography," p. 77.

fall is still greater; thus, in India, on the Khasi range of hills, the annual rainfall reaches the enormous amount of 500 to 600 inches.

On the other hand, a tract of country lying behind a high mass of land upon which moist winds blow may be almost rainless.

When it happens, as it does in some countries, that in one part of the year the wind blows in one direction, and in another part of the year in the opposite, we shall find that these periodical winds are usually accompanied with rain when they blow from warm to colder regions, and with dry weather when they blow from a cold to a warmer region; therefore in these countries rainy seasons alternate with dry ones.

Great irregularity of rainfall is characteristic of North-Western Europe, but as a rule there is more rain at the end of autumn and in winter than in summer.

So far as the health of human beings is concerned, the cleansing effect of rain on the air is important, for a downfall of rain washes the air and carries away suspended and other impurities which, in dry weather, are blown about and diffused by the aërial currents.

The influence of prevailing winds on climate has already been mentioned, and it has been shown that the **movements of the air** are produced by differences of pressure. The following is the law which governs the direction of these movements: *Air always flows in spirally from areas of high pressure into areas of low pressure.* It is clear that this must be the case, as low pressure indicates a deficiency, and high pressure a surplus of atmosphere. The column of air is heavier in the latter case than in the former, consequently, obeying the universal law of gravitation, the heavier column must necessarily flow out at the base to supply the deficiency in the lighter one.

A familiar and instructive illustration of the influence of temperature in producing currents of air can be observed on the sea coast of any country, where the days are warm and the nights cool. The surface of the land during the day, under the influence of the sun's rays, becomes much warmer than that of the sea, and thus heat is communicated to the air resting on it, which becomes hotter than that resting on the sea. The hotter air on the land expands, its pressure is diminished, and being lighter it ascends, while the cooler air from the sea streams in towards the land to take its place; thus a light breeze, blowing from the sea on to the land, is developed, which increases in force as the day advances. This is the familiar *sea breeze!* As the sun disappears it dies away, for as soon as the sun is set the land parts with the heat it has absorbed during the day by radiation into space, and it does so much more readily than the sea does; thus the air over the land becomes cooler, and therefore denser than that over the sea, and this denser air moves towards the sea to take the place of the ascending lighter current now flowing upwards from its surface; and thus a *land breeze* arises. This increases in force, as the difference in temperature between the air over the land and that over the sea increases by continued radiation from the former; it again dies away towards morning, when the sun's heat again becomes felt on the land, and the temperature of the air over land and sea becomes equalised.

A somewhat similar illustration may be observed in mountainous districts; during the day the air on the mountain sides, heated by the sun's rays, ascends, and a breeze blows up the mountains from the valley; while at night the cold, heavy air on the mountains flows down as a cool breeze into the valleys.

The large masses of land in the northern hemisphere interfere considerably with the regular distribution of the aërial currents as they are observed over the broad unbroken expanse of ocean presented by the southern hemisphere. "In January the high and cold table-lands of Central Asia become the centre of a vast area over which the pressure of the air is high. Consequently, from that elevated region the winds issue on all sides. In China and Japan it appears as a north-west wind. In Hindostan it comes from the north-east. In the Mediterranean it blows from the east and south-east. But in July matters are reversed, for then the centre of Asia, heated by the hot summer sun, becomes part of a vast region of low pressure, which includes the north-eastern half of Africa and the east of Europe. Into that enormous basin the air pours from every side. Along the coasts of Siberia and Scandinavia it comes from the north. From China, round the south of the Continent to the Red Sea, it comes from the Indian Ocean, that is, from south-east, south, and south-west. Across Europe it flows from the westward. Hence, according to the position of any place with reference to the larger masses of sea and land, the direction of its winds may be estimated." *

Monsoons is the Arabic name (meaning any part or season of the year) given to the summer and winter winds on the shores of the Indian Ocean. We have seen that the air is drawn in towards the centre of Asia in summer, and flows out from the centre in winter; so in India the winter wind is the north-east Monsoon, which corresponds to the north-east Trades of the North Atlantic and North Pacific Oceans; whereas the summer wind is the south-west Monsoon, which is a complete reversal of the natural course of the Trade Wind, owing to the enormous indraught caused by the low summer pressure over Asia. On the Chinese coast the winter wind is a north-west Monsoon, and the summer wind a south-east Monsoon. Something similar occurs in North America, for in the Southern States the winter wind comes from the north-east, the summer wind from the south-west.

There are certain well-known *local winds* which blow in certain countries, and which have received local names, of which the following are the chief.

* Geikie's "Physical Geography," chap. xi., "The Movements of the Air."

If these winds come from a tract over which the pressure is high and the temperature low, to a region where the pressure is lower and the temperature higher, they come as cold blasts condensing the humidity in the air of the warmer region into torrents of rain. But if the area of low pressure surrounds hot desert regions, like Africa and Arabia, it draws out towards it the hot air lying over these burning sands; such a wind is that known in Italy as the *Sirocco*—a hot, moist wind, causing extreme languor to men and animals. In Spain it is known as the *Solemo*, and it sometimes brings with it to this country, across the Mediterranean, fine hot dust from the African deserts. This wind from the desert is known in Africa and Arabia as the *Simoom*, and it sometimes blows with such violence as to whirl up clouds of sand, in which whole caravans have been buried. A similar hot wind is encountered on some parts of the West Coast of Africa (Guinea), in December, January, and February, blowing from the interior out to sea; this is the *Harmattan*. In Egypt there is a similar wind called *Khamsin* (fifty), a hot and very dry wind laden with fine sand; it is the prevailing wind for about fifty days in spring. The *Föhn* is a warm and dry wind frequently met with in the north-eastern cantons of Switzerland, and is generally very much dreaded on account of the physical and mental depression it produces. It "blows down from the crest of the Alps with great violence from a south-easterly, southerly, or, less frequently, from a south-westerly direction." Some difference of opinion exists as to its source and origin. The view that it comes from the desert of Sahara and gets laden with moisture by its contact with the surface of the Mediterranean, and that this moisture becomes precipitated in its passage over the Alps, so that it is felt in Switzerland as a warm and dry wind, is disputed by Professor Hann, who argues that it "must come down from aloft, from the summits of the Alps, to replace that which has been removed from the valleys," and that "its high temperature is explained by the law . . . that a mass of air, descending to levels where the pressure is greater, warms at the rate of 1° C. for every 100 metres."*

The numerous names and other significations given to local winds on the Mediterranean coasts will be referred to in the chapter on the Riviera.

Winds often serve a useful purpose in distributing temperature and moisture. A wind blowing from a warm or mild region raises the temperature of the district to which it comes. The prevailing west and south-west winds of Great Britain, for example, are warmed by their passage over the Gulf Stream, and keep our climate much milder than, from its latitude, it would otherwise be. But when a wind blows from a colder to a milder region it produces a depression of temperature ; thus it is that the winds that blow from the vast cold expanse of elevated land in central Asia westward into Europe, make the weather in winter and spring colder and drier there than when west winds blow.

Winds also distribute the moisture of the atmosphere, and if it were not for them the condensed vapour of the air would be discharged upon the same area from which it had been evaporated; but the winds convey vapours from the sea, and these become condensed on the land, so that, speaking generally, the wetness or dryness of any place will depend on the direction from which its prevalent winds come. If they come over a wide and warm expanse of sea they will bring moisture, if they come from the interior of the continent they will be dry, and hot or cold according to the temperature of the regions from which they come.

The preceding considerations show how climate, *generally*, is influenced: 1, by distance from the

* For the facts and arguments in support of this view, *see* "Handbook of Climatology," by Professor Hann, translated by Ward, chap. xix. Macmillan: New York, 1903.

equator; 2, by nearness to or distance from the sea; 3, by elevation above the sea; 4, by the prevailing winds; 5, by atmospheric humidity and its influence on the intensity of solar radiation; and 6, by less general local conditions; and that in estimating the climate of any particular place we have to take into consideration the *temperature*, not only its annual mean and annual range, but its seasonal and even its daily variations, and not only the air temperature in the shade, but also the intensity of solar radiation; the *rainfall* and not only its annual amount, but the manner of its precipitation, whether in short and sudden torrents, or prolonged over considerable periods, and its distribution in the different seasons and months; the average atmospheric humidity, amount of cloud and mist; the *elevation* above the sea; the direction of the *prevailing winds*, during the different seasons of the year; and, finally, *local conditions* such as the presence or absence of protecting hills, forests and mountain chains, the shape and position of the ground, its relation to adjacent masses of water, sea, lake or river, the nature of its soil, whether porous and absorbent or the reverse, cultivation, vegetation, population, etc. etc.

It will also be seen from the foregoing that the elementary division of climates into *insular or oceanic* and *continental* is well founded. Owing to the fact that water absorbs heat more slowly, and parts with it more slowly than land does, the ocean and other large masses of water act as store-houses of heat which they absorb slowly during the hot seasons, and give out again slowly during cold seasons to the air lying on their surface; it follows, therefore, that the climates of the sea and sea-coasts are much moister and more equable than those of the interior of continents, and that in proportion as places are distant from the sea, their climates become more extreme. An insular and oceanic climate is one where the difference between summer and winter temperature is reduced to a minimum, and where there is a copious supply of moisture from the large water surface. A continental climate is one where the summer is hot, the winter cold, and where the rainfall is comparatively slight. This difference is well brought out by the fact that such evergreens as the Portugal laurel, aucuba, and laurustinus grow luxuriantly even in the north of Scotland (57° 5′ N. lat.), while they cannot withstand the severe cold of the winter at Lyons (45° 41′ N. lat.).

Little more need be said on these points. With regard to that important element of climate, the *prevailing winds*, we have seen that winds which come from a cold region are cold, and those from a warm region warm. Sea winds are usually moist, those from the land generally dry. Sea breezes are not subject to the same extremes of temperature as those from the land. They serve to cool the heat of summer and diminish the cold of winter; whereas winds from the interior of a continent are usually hot and enervating in summer, bitterly cold and dry in winter. We have also seen that winds which come from lower into higher latitudes, or from warmer to colder regions, deposit their moisture in the form of rain and are therefore wet winds, while those which come from higher to lower latitudes, or from cold to warm regions, are dry winds.

Of *local* influences, one of the most important is the nature of the soil. Where the ground is wet and marshy the mean temperature is lowered, for the water absorbs and conveys downwards the heat which would otherwise be retained on the surface and warm the soil; when such ground is properly drained the mean annual temperature is found to rise. This rise of temperature from efficient drainage has been known, in our own country, to raise the annual average as much as 1·5 to 3° F., which is as great a change as if the ground had actually been transported 100 to 150 miles further south.

A sandy desert presents the greatest extremes of climate, for while the dry surface readily absorbs the sun's heat so as to rise even to 200° F. during the day, it cools rapidly by radiation, and during a clear night may grow ice-cold.

The presence or absence of vegetation is also an important local element of climate. When the surface is covered with vegetation the heating effect of the sun's rays on the soil is necessarily diminished, at the same time that the radiation of heat, during the night, from the surface into space is hindered, so that the soil is neither heated nor cooled as much as it would be if it were bare; and as leaves never become so hot as the soil, the presence of vegetation is an equaliser of temperature. The influence of a large forest on the local climate is, therefore, to moderate both the heat of day and the cold of night.

The adjacency of lakes and other large inland surfaces of water also exercises a similar equalising effect. As the temperature of the water on the surface becomes lowered by the cold of winter, this cold surface water descends to the bottom, and the deeper, warmer water rises to the surface; as this becomes cooled in its turn, it sinks and allows another portion of warmer water to take its place. The temperature of the air lying over the water is thus raised above that lying on the adjacent land, and the colder, heavier air over the surrounding land flows down on to the surface of the water, displacing the warmer air and becoming itself warmed in turn. Thus it is that deep lakes, which do not freeze over in winter, serve as reservoirs of warmth to keep the temperature of the surrounding ground higher than that of places only a short distance away. The reverse happens during summer, when the water cools the air on its surface and so lessens the heat of the locality.

We have seen how the neighbourhood of hills and mountains may act on local climates, either by serving as a screen or protection from prevailing winds, or by cooling the upper air and precipitating rain, or in causing local currents of air moving alternately up and down valleys, or in generating cold gusts of wind which rush down from the hills on to the plains.

There are also local influences affecting the *composition* of the air, which have an undoubted influence on the well-being of men. It is well known that the air on the sea-coast and in the open country is purer and richer in oxygen than it is in the densely crowded districts of populous cities; whether its salubrity is associated with the presence of *ozone*, as used to be generally admitted, is now regarded as debatable. Professor Hann observes "it cannot be doubted that the presence of ozone in air shows that this air has active oxidising properties, whether this fact is to be ascribed to the more active form of oxygen which is called ozone, or to the presence of peroxide of hydrogen. When ozone is present in considerable quantity in the atmosphere, it is a sign that the air is free from organic impurities and products of decay."*

The presence or absence of floating organic particles in the air has, no doubt, a great influence on its salubrity. Dr. Angus Smith has calculated that in Manchester the air that a man breathes in ten hours contains 37,000,000 spores! Whereas, the air over the sea and in high mountain regions is usually remarkably free from these organic impurities.

Various attempts have been made to classify climates, with more or less want of success; for, in most instances, what has been gained in precision has been lost in accuracy.

We may, however, as we have said, accept as well grounded the fundamental division into:

A.—Sea or insular climates.

B.—Inland or continental climates.

The suggested subdivision of climates into (a) humid climates and (b) dry climates, rather indicates approximately the characters of the climate of

* "Handbook of Climatology," p. 80. New York, 1903.

different places, than affords a basis for accurate classification, and the following division is partly comprised in the foregoing: (*a*) climate of plains; (*b*) climate of altitudes.

No less imperfect is the classification founded on the annual distribution of temperature into 1, hot; 2, cold; and 3, temperate climates, although it has a certain practical value, when qualified by a knowledge of the seasonal and diurnal variations of temperature.

A.—*Sea or insular climates* are represented by the climate of the open sea, of small and moderate-sized islands, and of sea coasts. These have much in common, although they, of course, vary according to latitude and to those other determining conditions of climate which we have considered.

They agree in possessing the following characters:

1. Their atmosphere is usually freer from organic and inorganic impurities than that of inland plains.

2. Owing to the constant evaporation from the surface of the sea their atmosphere is comparatively moister than that of inland regions, and the amount of atmospheric humidity is less variable.

3. Their temperature is more equable than that of inland climates, there is less difference between summer and winter and day and night temperatures.

B.—*Inland or continental climates* differ from sea and coast climates in being less equable and more exposed to extremes, to great heat in summer and severe cold in winter. The east coast of continents usually shares in these extremes.

The difficulty attending the further subdivision of climates is at once seen when we consider that the suggested classifications of climates into (a) humid and (b) dry climates very nearly coincides with the preceding, *humid* climates being usually sea or insular or coast climates, and dry climates being ordinarily continental or inland climates. There are of course exceptions determined by local conditions. Then, again, in the division into (*a*) climate of plains and (*b*) climate of altitudes, it is obvious that the first of these will coincide with sea or coast climates if the plains are adjacent to the sea, and with continental climates if situated inland.

In the next chapter the characters of sea and mountain climates will be more fully discussed.

CHAPTER II.

SEA OR MOUNTAIN?

THE CHARACTERS AND RESTORATIVE ACTION OF SEA AND MOUNTAIN AIR.

WE must, in the first place, realise that there is much in common in the properties of sea and mountain air. The presence of ozone, or some active oxidising agent, in *sea* air in greater proportion than in the air of inland plains is well established. This is a property which it shares with mountain air. Its greater abundance on the sea-coast depends, in all probability, on the influence of sunlight, which is one of the most important sources of ozone. It purifies the air, especially by determining the oxidation of decomposing organic substances. The excess of this active oxidising agent in sea air is, therefore, one of its most important properties, as it is also one of the most important properties of mountain air.

Another hygienic property which sea air shares with mountain air is the absence in it of organic dust. This applies with especial force to the air of the open sea, or on small islands, or to points of land standing well out into the sea. As the sea presents an ever-moving fluid surface, no impurities in the shape of organic dust can rest upon it, so as to be again blown about, in mischievous activity, with every fresh breeze.

Equableness of temperature is another characteristic of sea air, and one to which it owes much of its beneficial influence in many cases. In this respect it is contrasted with the air of elevated regions, in which the diurnal variations of temperature are often very considerable. The temperature of the sea-coast is warmer in winter and cooler in summer than that of inland districts. This admits of easy explanation. In the first place the rapid cooling of the surface of the land by radiation into space, after the sun has gone down, is checked by the amount of moisture in the air. The aqueous vapour which is abundant in sea air absorbs the heat given off from the soil during nocturnal radiation, and acts as a kind of screen to retard the loss of heat in this way. Hence great variations between the day and night temperatures are rarely observed at the seaside.

"Wherever the air is dry" (Tyndall) "we are liable to daily extremes of temperature. By day, in such places, the sun's heat reaches the earth unimpeded, and renders the maximum high; by night, on the other hand, the earth's heat escapes unhindered into space, and renders the minimum low. Hence the difference between the maximum and minimum is greatest where the air is driest."

During the heat of the day the air over the sea is always cooler than that over the land; for the surface of the land gets rapidly heated and communicates its heat to the superjacent strata of air; but when the sun's rays fall on water they are not, as in the case of land, arrested at the surface, but penetrate to a considerable depth, so that water is heated much more slowly by the sun's rays, as well as cooled more slowly by nocturnal radiation than the land. Moreover, the evaporation which is always going on at the surface of the sea, and going on rapidly where the sun's rays are powerful, carries away some of the heat of the surface-water, and helps to keep the air in contact with it cool.

We have already referred (Chap. I.) to the refreshing currents of air produced by the inequality in the heating and cooling of the atmosphere on the land and over the sea.

On account of their equableness of temperature, oceanic climates—the most equable of all climates—are said to afford almost absolute immunity from colds.* It is only on board ship that such a climate in its perfection can be found. A very near approach to it, however, may be obtained on small islands situated at some distance from land.

The chief characteristics of sea air—an equable temperature and a high degree of humidity—are soothing rather than bracing properties, and if it were not for the currents of air induced on the sea-coasts, as has been explained, they might be found actually relaxing, and this is no doubt the case in warm and cloudy weather on our own south-western shores. In these respects, therefore, sea air offers a great contrast to mountain air. The same is the case with regard to its density. The absolute density of sea air is, of course, greater than that of the air at any higher level, and it must therefore contain, bulk for bulk, more oxygen; and it follows that in breathing sea air we take more oxygen into the lungs in a given time than in the air we breathe at places above the level of the sea; that is, supposing in both cases we breathe with equal frequency and equal amplitude. But it does not necessarily follow, because an absolutely larger quantity of oxygen exists in a given volume of sea air than in the same volume of mountain air, that more oxygen, on that account, is taken into the blood at the seaside than on higher ground. In the first place, the oxygen may be, for aught we know, in a more active form in mountain than in sea air; its chemical energy may be greater, and therefore the nutritive changes dependent on respiration may be accelerated, though the air be thinner, and poorer in its absolute quantity of oxygen; or, in the second place, the respiratory act may be so much increased in frequency on the mountains, that although less oxygen is taken into the lungs at each breath, yet by deeper and more frequent inspirations much more may be received into the organism in a given time.

* It has also been observed that, after a sea voyage, on landing, there is much greater proneness to take cold, and extra precautions are necessary to guard against it.

Another important point to be attended to is the great and frequent variations of barometric pressure met with on the sea and on sea-coasts. Now it has been shown by careful experiment that all rapid variations in atmospheric pressure increase the activity of the circulatory and respiratory organs, and that the perfection of organic life depends on these alternations of excitement and repose.

It has also been shown that the barometric variations at the seaside, besides being greater in amount than inland, occur with far more regularity, a circumstance which is regarded as tending to promote the accommodation of the organism to these conditions.

These, then, are the most important properties of sea air: 1, Excess of what has been known as "ozone"; 2, excess of aqueous vapour and consequently greater equability of temperature; 3, great purity and absence of organic particles; 4, maximum density and great but regular variations of barometric pressure. Of minor importance are the presence of saline particles suspended in the air, which, of course, vary greatly in amount, according as the sea is calm or agitated, and probably exercise a mildly stimulating effect on the respiratory mucous membrane. The small amount of iodine and bromine diffused in sea air may not be without a real influence on some organisms.

In the next place let us examine the characteristic properties of *mountain* air. And here, at the very outset, we come upon a very remarkable contrast. There was no need to define what we meant by sea air, although its effects may be greatly modified by circumstances of locality. But are we always sure what we mean when we use the term mountain air? In Scotland and Wales we speak of mountain air at a few hundred feet above the sea, considerably below the level of the towns of Lucerne or Geneva. In Germany we hear of mountain air at 1,200 and 1,500 feet above the sea, and in the Engadine at 6,000 feet, in

Mexico at 12,000! Now if we think only of one quality of mountain air, viz. its rarefaction, it is quite clear that we must be using the same term to express very different things. But if we are thinking only of the *general* bracing effects and hygienic qualities of mountain air, we may find these, no doubt, at very various elevations, and we may even find them in great perfection at comparatively low levels. An open plateau in a temperate climate at an elevation of 2,000 or 3,000 feet above the sea will certainly possess a more bracing air than a close valley, in a hot climate, at twice that height.

If we confine our attention to the continent of Europe we may take the Upper Engadine (5,000 to 6,000 feet) as the extreme limit of a permanently inhabited mountain district. For all practical purposes of comparison we may take an elevation of 6,000 feet as the limit in one direction of a habitable European mountain climate, and in the other direction such elevations as Glion, above Montreux, 2,900 feet; and Seelisberg, 2,400 feet, on the Lake of Lucerne. Places at a lower elevation than these, although they may have many advantages as health resorts, can scarcely be admitted into the category of mountain climates. Of localities such as these, then, ranging between 2,000 and 6,000 feet above the sea level, we have, within tolerably easy access, a great number to choose from; while there are a few, for exceptional needs and for short periods of residence (in the summer season), between 6,000 and 8,000 feet.

There seems good reason to believe that at higher elevations than these the air reaches a degree of rarefaction which is inconsistent with the maintenance of vigorous health.

Diminution of atmospheric pressure is, then, one of the chief properties of mountain air. It has been calculated that at an elevation of 2,500 feet we lose about one-eighth of the atmospheric pressure, at 5,000 a sixth, at 7,500 feet a fourth, and at 16,000 a half.

Another important property of mountain air is its lower temperature. It is well known that the temperature of the air diminishes in proportion to the altitude. From observations made in the Alps of Switzerland the medium loss of temperature was found to be 1·8° F. for every 520 feet of elevation during summer, and for every 910 feet in winter. Whence it follows that the tops of mountains are relatively warmer in winter than in summer. It has, however, been pointed out that there are extraordinary modifications, amounting frequently to subversions of the law, of the decrease of temperature with the height, owing to the circumstance that "the effects of radiation will be felt in different degrees and intensities in different places. As the air in contact with declivities of hills and rising grounds becomes cooled by contact with the cooled surface, it acquires greater density, and consequently flows down the slopes and accumulates on the low-lying ground at their base. It follows, therefore, that places on rising ground are never exposed to the full intensity of frosts at night; and the higher they are situated relatively to the immediately surrounding district the less they are exposed, since their relative elevation provides a ready escape downwards for the cold air almost as speedily as it is produced." Hence a southern slope at a considerably greater elevation may have a higher night temperature than a neighbouring valley. "On the other hand, valleys surrounded by hills and high grounds not only retain their own cold of radiation, but also serve as reservoirs for the cold heavy air which pours down upon them from the neighbouring heights." And at the numerous meteorological stations in Switzerland it is observed that "in calm weather in winter, when the ground becomes colder than the air above it, systems of descending currents of air set in over the whole face of the country. The direction and force of these descending currents follow the irregularities of the surface, and, like currents of water, they tend to converge and unite in the valleys and gorges, down which they flow like rivers in their beds. Since the place of these air-currents must be taken by others, it follows that on such occasions the temperature of the tops of mountains and high grounds is relatively high, because the counter currents come from a greater height and are therefore warmer." So the "gradual narrowing of a valley tends to a more rapid lowering of the temperature, for the obvious reason that the valley thereby resembles a basin almost closed, being thus a receptacle for the cold air-currents which descend from all sides. The bitterly cold furious gusts of wind which are often encountered in mountainous regions during night are simply this out-rush of cold air from such basins."*

Considerations such as these are of importance in determining the hygienic character of any particular mountain health resort.

The question of the humidity or dryness of mountain air is one not easy to resolve. The air on the summits of high mountains is no doubt dryer than the air at lower levels. But at intermediate levels, considerations other than those of altitude alone determine the relative humidity or dryness of the atmosphere; so that each mountain station must, to a great extent, be judged of by itself with regard to this very important point. Perhaps, as a general rule, one may say that the higher the locality the less rain falls; but, on the other hand, we have to face the startling fact that twice as much rain and snow fall at the St. Bernard and St. Gothard stations as at Geneva! Much will, however, necessarily depend on the configuration of the ground, as well as its aspect. A mountain ridge facing the direction from which moist winds habitually blow will condense their moisture and precipitate it in the form of rain or snow on its sides, or on the valleys or plains at its

* Article "Climate," "Encyclopædia Britannica." New edition

base; while more remote summits of the same mountain chain and the higher mountain valleys on the other side of the chain may be thus protected and screened from heavy and prolonged rainfalls.

Thus the moist Atlantic winds blowing against the western ranges of Scotland and Cumberland determine the great rainfall in these regions; and the town of Santa Fé de Bogota in the Andes, at an elevation of 8,600 feet, is visited with almost incessant rain, owing to its situation at the foot of a mountain on the sides of which the warm trade-winds of the South Pacific Ocean become cooled, and condense their moisture.

The presence or absence of vegetation will also exercise a determining influence as to the relative humidity of the atmosphere. We must, therefore, bear in mind that certain topographical conditions will frequently induce, in stations of considerable altitude, a moister atmosphere than is found on the neighbouring plains. But if we consider the effect of altitude alone, it is easy to understand how the air of elevated regions must be, *cæteris paribus*, dryer than that of lower situations.

In the first place, the lower the atmospheric pressure the more rapid is the process of evaporation, and hence the boiling-point of water is 28·3° F. less on the top of Mont Blanc than at the sea level.

Secondly, the energy of the sun's rays, and therefore their drying effect on the atmosphere, is greater the less the thickness and density of the layer of air they have to traverse. The slope of the soil, the absence of vegetation at great heights, and the greater intensity of the aërial currents all tend to promote dryness of the atmosphere.

Mountain air differs, then, from sea air in three main particulars: 1, In its diminished density; 2, in its lower temperature; 3, in containing less humidity. The temperature is not only lower than that of sea air, it is also less equable. Owing to the clearness of the air, the absence of moisture, and the energy of the sun's rays, very great differences between the day and night temperature are constantly found at great elevations. There is but little aqueous vapour in the air to prevent nocturnal radiation into stellar space from the surface of the soil, greatly heated during the day by the solar rays; thus there is usually a rapid fall of temperature when the sun goes down. In summer a difference of 40 to 50° F. between the day and night temperatures will sometimes be registered. There is often also a very great difference between the sun and shade temperatures during the day.

Mountain air resembles sea-air in containing an excess of ozone, in its freedom from organic and other impurities, in being cooler in summer than the air of inland plains, and in the fact that its monthly and annual variations of temperature are less than on inland plains.

The study of mountain climates has hitherto taken the form, chiefly, of an investigation into the physiological effects of diminished atmospheric pressure on the human organism. Since different individuals are very variously endowed with the power of accommodating themselves to altered external conditions, it is not to be wondered at that some discrepancies are to be found in the statements of different observers as to the effects upon themselves and others of alterations of atmospheric pressure.

Jourdanet maintains that persons who are not accustomed to a rarefied atmosphere begin to suffer inconvenience when they attain an elevation of between 6,000 and 7,000 feet. Most of those who have reported their experiences of mountain ascents in Europe have not experienced any noticeable inconvenience until they reached nearly 10,000 feet. Soldiers going to Himalayan stations at 7,500 feet complain at first of shortness of breath, and have a quicker and more feeble pulse; but these effects are temporary. Of the serious effects of exposure to the highly rarefied air of very considerable elevations we have most valuable evidence in the records of

Glaisher's balloon ascents. Acceleration of the pulse was one of the first effects noted. At 16,000 feet it had risen from 76 to 100. Between 18,000 and 19,000 feet both Glaisher and his companion suffered from violent palpitations, with difficulty of breathing; then their lips and hands became of a deep blue colour. As they continued to ascend their respiration became more laborious. On another occasion, at 27,000 feet, Glaisher became unconscious. The attack came on with indistinctness of vision, inability to move arms or legs, though he could move his neck; then he lost his sight completely, though he could still hear his companion speak, but he could not answer him. Then he became wholly unconscious. He also describes a feeling of nausea, like sea-sickness, coming on at great elevations.

The following are the various symptoms of "Mountain Sickness" that have been recorded by many different observers as occurring during the ascent of lofty peaks or on elevated plains. Great loss of muscular power, palpitations, quick and laborious respiration, bleeding from the nose or gums, drowsiness, severe headache, nausea and vomiting, great thirst, mental depression, enfeebled senses, and impaired memory. The superficial veins become distended, the face pale and bluish. These symptoms were aggravated by exertion and mitigated by rest. Another significant symptom, reported on good authority, both in mountain and balloon ascents, is *increasing coldness of the body* beyond what would be accounted for by the lower temperature of these elevations.

It seems certain, then, both from the evidence of these actual observations, and from the experimental researches of the late M. Bert in the laboratory of the Collége de France, that when the rarefaction of the air reaches a certain degree, the due oxygenation of the blood is interfered with, and we get symptoms developed which point to oxygen-starvation, and to obstruction in the circulation through the lungs. In M. Bert's experiments it appeared that slight degrees of diminution of atmospheric pressure did not lessen the affinity of the aërial oxygen for the blood corpuscles; but when that diminution approached, or reached, one quarter of the whole atmospheric pressure, perceptible disturbances ensued.

M. Jourdanet * believed that the oxygenation of the blood is not injuriously affected by residence at an elevation below 6,500 feet, but that above this elevation the respiratory functions become disturbed, and the due oxygenation of the blood is interfered with. Lombard also states that the monks of St. Bernard, after several years' residence there, present various signs of anæmia, and that these are occasionally so grave as to necessitate a removal to the plains.

Not less important than its rarefaction is the *dryness* of mountain air. Dryness of the air has an important influence on the activity of the bodily functions. Herbert Spencer has pointed out that "other circumstances being alike, there will be more bodily activity in the people of hot and dry localities than in the people of hot and humid ones," and that in tracing the progress of different races of mankind "we get strong reasons for inferring a relation between constitutional vigour and the presence of an air which by its warmth and *dryness* facilitates the vital actions."

Mountain air is not only dryer than sea air and the air of inland plains, but, as we have seen, it is also colder. Now this lowering of temperature tends, to a certain degree, to compensate for the deficiency of oxygen dependent on its elevation. For instance, in a given volume of air at 1,400 feet above the sea, at a temperature of 32° F., there is as much oxygen as in the same volume of air at the sea level at 60° F. So that such virtues as are

* "Influence de la Pression de l'Air sur la vie de l'Homme."

lessened in mountain air by its elevation are, in part, restored by its coldness.

Having now considered the properties of sea and mountain air, having noted in what particulars they agree and in what important points they differ, we are prepared to approach the consideration of the following highly practical questions: Who should go to the mountains? who should go to the sea? and who should go to neither? There is no greater mistake made than that very general one of sending *all convalescents* to the seaside, except the still greater one of actually embarking them on a sea voyage! It arises from the very natural desire to hasten convalescence after acute disease. But these unwise attempts to hasten convalescence are the very frequent cause of serious relapses. In the general debility which follows a fever, or an acute inflammation, all the organs share—the organs of nutrition, the secretory, the circulatory, the eliminatory organs, are all feeble and unable to do much work without exhaustion. If an attempt is made to over-stimulate them, if an appetite is induced before digestive power has been regained, a feverish state is frequently re-excited, and the very effort that has been made to hasten recovery retards it.

Sea and mountain air are alike too stimulating and exciting for many such cases. They arouse to premature activity when the organism can best strengthen itself by absolute repose. Pure, unexciting country air, in a locality where the patient can be much in the open air while thoroughly protected from cold winds—that is the safest and best place for the invalid to slowly, but steadily, regain health after severe acute disease. Sea or mountain air may, however, be beneficial later on, when a stronger tonic influence is needed.

Speaking generally, those who seek health in high mountain districts should be capable of a certain amount of muscular activity. Those who suffer from great muscular debility as well as general exhaustion, and who need absolute or almost absolute repose, are unsuited for mountain climates. These climates are too changeful, and too exciting; and such persons, when they find themselves in cold, rarefied, exciting mountain air, are apt to become chilled, depressed, and dyspeptic. Much repose at an agreeable seaside resort, with a residence at a little distance from the sea, is more suitable to such persons.

There are others, however, who, with vigorous frames and much actual or latent power of muscular activity, become mentally exhausted by the strain of incessant mental labour, anxious cares, or absorbing occupations. Mental irritability usually accompanies this exhaustion, great depression of spirits, with unrest of mind and body. These are the typical cases for the mountains, which both stimulate to and afford opportunity for muscular exertion, the bracing atmosphere rousing the physical energies and re-awakening the sense of powers unimpaired and unexhausted, while the soothing effect of the quiet and stillness of high mountain regions brings rest and renovation to the over-worn mind.

For convalescents after surgical operation, where the processes of tissue-change require hastening without necessitating any activity in the patient himself, the seaside is best.

Sea air is better suited than mountain air to persons who cannot bear great and sudden changes of temperature, as is the case with most of those who suffer from grave chronic maladies.

A certain morbid sensitiveness to cold, or rather to "taking cold," is often greatly lessened by a residence in the bracing rarefied air of elevated localities, and the same good effects are also to be obtained from exposure to a bracing sea air, especially if accompanied by sea-bathing.

Speaking within very wide limits, mountain air is less suitable to persons advanced in years than sea air. The very stimulus to muscular exertion which mountain air produces is to persons much past middle life often a pitfall and a snare. *Qui va doucement, va loin,* is especially applicable to this period of life, and the state of feverish activity which is sometimes induced in aged persons in the mountains is not by any means for their good.

We must not forget to consider that the effects of sea air vary very much with locality. The very bracing effects which German physicians observe in the isle of Norderney would not be found in the often warm, moist air of some parts of our own south-western coast. The former locality is, no doubt, much under the influence of the cold, dry, continental east winds. The watering places on our east coast enjoy a much more bracing and less humid atmosphere than those on our west and south-west coasts, and those on the north coast of France and Belgium have a dryer air than either.

In the following chapters we shall pass in review the sea-coast and mountain resorts which are of chief interest to invalids.

CHAPTER III.

SEASIDE RESORTS IN THE UNITED KINGDOM.

I.—England and Wales.

IT will be convenient to describe our own seaside resorts in the following order; passing westward from the mouth of the Thames, round the Land's End to the north-west coast of Cornwall and north coast of Devon; then the Welsh coast and the north-west resorts of England and, leaving Scotland for the present, return by the north-east and east coasts again to the mouth of the Thames.

Herne Bay is the nearest seaside resort to London on the Kentish coast. It is sixty-three miles from London and eight from Canterbury, and is reached in rather less than two hours by the South Eastern and Chatham Railway. It is situated on a fine bay on the estuary of the Thames, with a beach of shingle, and like the neighbouring resorts, Westgate and Margate, it has a north-eastern aspect, and is open to the breezes from the North Sea, and its climate, like that of those places, is tonic and stimulating. There is a good promenade, a mile long, where are the baths, and it has an iron pier. The surrounding country is flat, and there is little protection from prevailing winds. Its rainfall is said to be below and its amount of sunshine above the average. Fog is rare.

Birchington-on-Sea, which has recently come into notice as a seaside resort, is sixty-nine miles from London and only three and a-half from Margate. It is situated on elevated ground and is bounded on the sea-coast by bluff cliffs. It has a sandy beach. The village, about three-quarters of a mile in length, lies on the old London and Canterbury road. It is a quiet resort, well suited to those who are seeking rest and retirement. Its climate is dry, windy, cold and breezy. There is a fair amount of sunshine, a relatively small rainfall, and but little fog.

Westgate-on-Sea has grown rapidly into popularity as a health resort. It is one and a-half miles from Margate, of which parish it once formed a part. It is in an open situation facing north without much protection from winds. It enjoys a good deal of sunshine, and the soil dries rapidly after rain. Good roads have been made and sea walls built round the curves of St. Mildred's and Westgate Bays, forming two promenades over a mile in length, from which by steps the sands or cliffs are easily accessible. Gardens also have been made on the cliffs, where there is a marine drive two miles in length. The air is bracing and pure, and the water supply is pure, abundant, and continuous. The sea bathing is good and safe, on a sandy bottom.

Westgate is a salubrious and convenient seaside resort for families with children who require good bracing sea air and pleasant, quiet sea bathing.

Margate is one of the most bracing of our seaside resorts, within two hours' railway journey of London, and within about five hours by river steamer. It must not be forgotten, in estimating the special qualities of the climate of Margate, that its aspect is north or north-east. In this respect it differs entirely from the neighbouring coast town of Ramsgate, which is so placed in an indentation of the coast-line as to look south-east. From this difference of aspect it not unfrequently happens that the local weather differs considerably in these two places, only a few miles apart, for a storm may be raging at Margate which is scarcely felt at Ramsgate. It happens also from this northerly or north-easterly aspect of Margate that during the prevalence of the north-easterly winds of spring it is one of the very few conveniently accessible seaside resorts where, during that season, pure *sea* air can be obtained. For the prevailing north-east winds blow directly over the North Sea and the northern portion of the British Channel on to Margate and the line of coast of which it forms a part, whereas during the same season the prevailing winds at the resorts on the southern coast are land-winds, and blow off the land out to sea, driving off, as it were, the sea air—hence probably the great value which Margate air is known to possess in scrofulous affections.

It has a chalk subsoil, and the ground quickly becomes dry after rain. The water supply is abundant and pure.

The best residential part of the town is at Cliftonville; it lies much higher than the rest of the town.

Margate is too windy for ordinary cases of chest disease, except in the summer months, but it is especially beneficial to cases of scrofulous disease in children and to those of convalescence after surgical operations. This fact has led to the establishment there of that excellent institution, "The Royal Sea-Bathing Infirmary, or Royal National Hospital for Scrofula."

The air of Margate is excellent for promoting the progress of slowly healing wounds and ulcers, and it is valuable in cases of debility from inherited feebleness of constitution.

Its autumn climate is often very fine.

Margate is celebrated for its sands, which are very extensive owing to the shallowness of the water. They are therefore the delight of children. Its relative humidity varies between 80 and 90, the mean being 82. The average annual rainfall is about 23 inches, and the number of rainy days about 170. The average winter temperature (October to March) is reported to be 42·1° F., and in January, the coldest month, 38·9° F.

Broadstairs is a quiet little seaside town, especially the resort of young children, who can bathe and amuse themselves all day long on its sheltered sands. It is built on the cliffs about half-way between Ramsgate and Margate, and looks almost due east.

The climatic characteristics of the place are the same as at the other resorts in the Isle of Thanet. The subsoil is chalk. The greater part of the district is from 120 feet to 150 feet above the level of the sea. Some of the residential parts enjoy much protection from winds, except from the south-east.

Ramsgate (and St. Lawrence, its north-western surburb), unlike Margate, has a south-eastern aspect. It is somewhat warmer than Margate, and is more protected from northerly and north-easterly winds. Its air is, however, bracing and tonic, and, like Margate, it has fine sands for bathing. Its climate has been described as "relatively warm, relatively equable, and moderately dry—sky moderately free from cloud—rainfall and number of rainy days smaller than those of the great majority of stations in England."* The drainage and water supply are good.

The harbour and town lie between two cliffs, the east and west, where most of the visitors reside. Ramsgate may be reached by rail in two hours from London. There are steamers also from London Bridge in six hours. The five preceding resorts are in the Isle of Thanet and partake of the characters of its climate, which are mainly due to its chalky soil and its exposure to winds. Owing to the flatness of the country it gets a great amount of sunshine.

St. Margaret's Bay, situated between Deal and Dover, is a small and quiet seaside retreat that has much to recommend it, but so long as it remains three miles from a railway station (Martin Mill) its development is likely to be slow. A portion of the residential part is built on the shingly beach and a portion on the chalk cliff, which rises to a great

* "Climates and Baths of Great Britain." Published for the *Med. Chirurgical Society*. Macmillan & Co.

height above the sea, and the two portions are connected by a very steep path. The lower portion enjoys considerable protection from the cliffs behind it. The climate is "dry and bracing, and is particularly adapted for all kinds of pulmonary disease and cases of nervous exhaustion. The effect of the air in cases of phthisis, attended by debility, etc., is remarkable."*

Dover has many merits as a health resort. Its climate is, for the most part, dry, tonic, and invigorating. It is not, however, to be recommended at all seasons of the year. It is very cold in January, very windy in March, and very hot in July. It is usually pleasant in May and June, and again from August to the end of October. The winter is often mild up to January. Dover is a good deal exposed to sea fogs. The cases that are said to do well at Dover are those of early phthisis; of bronchial catarrh in young people, with sensitive nervous systems and languid circulations; of nervous dyspepsia, of chronic diarrhœa from residence in tropical climates; of insomnia; of scrofulous disease in children. Most of the houses at Dover are built with a southern or south-eastern aspect, and are exposed to the direct influence of the sea breezes blowing from the Straits. It is protected by the chalk hills behind it, to some extent, from winds coming from the north, the north-east, and the north-west. Its subsoil is chalk, but most of the houses are built upon the beach, *i.e.* on shingle, flint, and sand overlying the chalk. The soil is, therefore, porous, and rain rapidly drains off the surface. The water supply is good and pure.

Folkestone, with its excellent service of trains, and situated so conveniently on the great highway of Continental traffic, possessing, moreover, attractions in itself of no mean order, has naturally become one of the most popular of health resorts.

* "Climates and Baths of Great Britain." Macmillan & Co.

The town is built on a lofty, porous cliff of greensand, and seen from the sea, or from the cliffs to the east of the harbour, it has a most picturesque appearance. The "Lees," on the west cliff, form a fine extensive promenade, high above the sea, commanding a vast sea-view up and down the Channel; on the high ground Folkestone is rather exposed, especially to south-westerly winds, but the chalk hills at the back protect it somewhat from the northerly land winds. The houses built on the lower part on a level with the harbour enjoy much protection from the high cliff which is directly behind them. A hydraulic lift connects this part and the pier with the Lees. The open chalk downs behind the town, and the many attractive country roads, afford abundant resources for horse and carriage exercise. The water supply is good, pure, and abundant, and the drainage has been most carefully provided for. The annual rainfall is said to scarcely exceed twenty-five inches, which is very small for a town on this coast.

The climate is considered suitable to many forms of chest disease, to cases of early phthisis, to cases of chronic catarrhal tendencies in the over sensitive and scrofulous, to some forms of asthma. It is also highly useful in cases of depressed nervous tone, with irritability, sleeplessness, loss of appetite, and hypochondriacal tendencies, also in cases of protracted convalescence after attacks of acute disease.

One drawback, from the point of view of sea-bathing, is the rather rough shingly beach; but baths of all kinds, including a large tepid sea-water swimming-bath, can be obtained at the Bath Establishment. On the east cliff is built the St. Andrew's Convalescent Home for poor patients.

Sandgate is about a mile west of Folkestone; it stretches for some distance along the coast, with a fine sandy beach in front, furnishing great facilities for bathing, and a range of hills behind, affording protection from the north.

Shorncliffe Camp lies on a plateau above, and on the north side of Sandgate. There are pleasant walks and drives towards Folkestone, or Hythe, or Shorncliffe, and the promenade in front of the sea forms an agreeable and sunny lounge. Sandgate has the same character of climate as the lower part of Folkestone, but it is quieter and less expensive, and the sea-bathing is decidely better. There is a sea-wall and parade between Sandgate and Hythe, which is two or three miles further west, and has the same climate and character as a health resort as Sandgate.

Hythe is now much resorted to for its excellent golf links and its well-managed hotel on the sea front with a fine garden.

Littlestone-on-Sea, between Dungeness and Dymchurch, is also frequented for its golf links.

Hastings and **St. Leonards**, sixty-two miles from London, have a complete southern aspect, and they are protected to the north and north-east by high cliffs, and hills at the back; but there is little or no protection at St. Leonards from winds blowing due east; these enfilade the promenade along the shore with considerable force.

These adjoining towns appear to have a remarkably equable temperature, both in winter and summer, and on that account they are considered suitable to cases of pulmonary disease. The air is warmer along the shore than on the hills behind the town, where it is said to be cool during the warmest summer months. Pulmonary invalids are recommended to choose the former, and convalescent patients, suffering from debility and want of tone, the latter situation.

The soil is porous and sandy, and the rain that falls is rapidly absorbed, so that the air is free from the humidity which might arise from evaporation of water retained on the surface. Hastings enjoys great immunity from land fogs, but sea-fogs are not uncommon in the spring. Its relative proportion of sunshine is large. The system of drainage, and of disposal of sewage, is excellent. The mean annual temperature is 49·4, for the winter quarter 39·6, the spring 45·9, and the summer 59·9. The mean daily range is 10·4. The mean relative humidity is 83·8. There is a mean annual rainfall of 30 inches and 183 rainy days.

Hastings is resorted to in the winter on account of its relatively mild climate by persons who are subject to chronic bronchitis and to catarrhal throat affections, and by cases of chronic stationary phthisis and by feeble and sensitive invalids generally, in search of winter sunshine.

Hastings has a very fine pier with a large covered pavilion. St. Leonards also has a pier. On the esplanade are very convenient glass-covered shelters. There are numerous places of beauty and interest to be visited in the neighbourhood. There is an extensive public park—St. Andrew's Park—in a sheltered valley at the back of the town.

Bexhill-on-Sea lies between St. Leonards and Eastbourne, about six miles from the former place. It is somewhat less sheltered from the north and north-east than Hastings, but it has a full southern exposure. The beach, composed of shingle and sand, affords good sea bathing. Its drainage and water supply are good. Bexhill has made much progress in the last few years.

Eastbourne is a highly popular and attractive health resort. The roads and streets have been skilfully planned and laid out, on a uniform system, so as to secure abundance of space and free ventilation, and trees are planted throughout the streets of the town. Moreover, the streets and other residential parts of the town are not all huddled together, close to the shore, as in some resorts, but spread out over a considerable tract of land, stretching towards the magnificent downs behind the town, for some distance from the seashore. So that a choice of residence is provided either close to the sea or some distance from it.

Eastbourne is situated on the coast of Sussex, between St. Leonards and Brighton, at a distance of sixty-five miles from London; its train service is good, and the fast trains accomplish the journey in little more than an hour and a-half.

The old town of Eastbourne is a mile inland; the new town, which has naturally been built towards the sea, has a south-eastern aspect. There is a level frontage to the sea, with three parallel promenades at different elevations, extending from the pier westward for nearly three miles till it ends in the steeply rising ground reaching to the magnificent promontory of Beachy Head. There is an extensive sandy beach, affording admirable sea-bathing. Between the sea front and the downs are very fine golf links.

The sanitary arrangements are as complete as they can well be made. The salubrity of the town has led to the establishment of a great number of high-class schools there for both sexes. The death-rate is low.

During the summer, phthisical patients often do extremely well at Eastbourne, especially if they begin their stay by living away from the sea. The dryness of the air is in certain fine seasons very notable, and is said to be due to the fact that the upper parts of Eastbourne lie on chalk and the lower on alluvial soil of a very porous nature.

Cases of torpid scrofula, of slow convalescence from surgical operations or injuries, cases of anæmia and general want of tone, cases of depressed function, nervous or digestive, are all suited to this place. In houses built to the west of the town, and with rising ground between them and the east, the winter temperature is not unpleasantly low, and they get more than the average amount of sunshine. But those parts of the town which are unprotected from the east suffer much from the prevailing winds in spring. January and Febuary are the coldest months, with a mean average temperature of 39·7. July and August are the hottest months, with a mean average temperature of 60·2. The mean annual daily range is 10·1. Mean annual rainfall, 30·6 inches. Mean annual relative humidity, 83·0.

Seaford is nine miles west of Eastbourne, the range of chalk cliffs and downs, of which Beachy Head forms the culminating point, lying between them. It is three miles from the port of Newhaven.

The air is pure and bracing, and there are fine downs (with golf links) stretching up to Beachy Head, which is six miles distant. The climate has much in common with that of Eastbourne, except that the great mass of cliff which intervenes between the two places affords a great protection from the east; it is, however, fully exposed to the south-west, and has but little protection from the north. The beach is shingle.

Brighton is too familiar a resort to need detailed description. No seaside place is so accessible to those who live in London. Its strong sea-air, coming from a wide open sea-board, is most invigorating to many, but for others it is too irritating; and it is important to recognise a form of dyspepsia with torpidity of liver which becomes developed in certain constitutions at Brighton—as well as in some other seaside places—and does not disappear so long as the patient remains there. Brighton is also not at its best when the north-east spring winds prevail, for then the wind is off the land, and the smoke, etc., from the town is blown down over the esplanade, and, instead of pure sea-air, we breathe not very pure land-air. South-south-west and westerly winds bring the best air to the shores of Brighton.

But the climate of Brighton differs considerably in different parts of the town. The houses in the King's Road, for example, are much more under the influence of the sea than those high up, near Montpellier Square; and the high east cliff (Kemp Town) is more bracing and has altogether finer air than the low western side, which is, however, more sheltered, and far more frequented and popular.

Under the east cliff, and extending along its whole length, a fine summer promenade has been made, which is completely sheltered from the north and north-west, but the east and north-east winds are felt there keenly ; this is the so-called "Madeira Walk."

The soil of Brighton is exclusively chalk. In the spring the winds are variable, in summer they come most frequently from the west, in autumn and winter from the south-west. It has a good and abundant water supply.

The sea-bathing is good, the water is clear, and the bottom is sandy. There are numerous private bathing establishments, where hot and cold sea-water baths can be obtained ; as well as Turkish baths and *massage*. The South Downs, which stretch along the back of the town, are a great and valuable resource for healthful exercise.

Brighton is especially serviceable in cases of retarded convalescence, especially after surgical operations, and also after some acute febrile maladies. It is useful in cases of anæmia, and general loss of tone induced by over-work, by chronic illnesses, or by other depressing agencies. It is of value in giving vigour to delicate young people, especially when of scrofulous constitution, during the most trying periods of rapid growth and development. Its bracing sea-air and sea-baths are also beneficial, in diminishing that sensitiveness of skin and mucous membranes upon which the prevalent tendencies to catarrhal and rheumatic affections depend. The autumn up to the end of November is the best and healthiest season at Brighton.

The mean annual temperature is 49·4. January is the coldest month, 39·3. August the hottest, 61·2. The mean annual daily range is 12·0. The mean annual rainfall is 30·4 inches, and the number of rainy days 163. The relative humidity, 78. Brighton has rather less sunshine than Hastings and Eastbourne.

Worthing is about twelve miles to the west of Brighton, and fifty-two miles from London. It is a much more quiet resort than its popular neighbour, and enjoys much the same climatic character. It has been said, however, that while the climate of Brighton is keen and bracing, that of Worthing is soft, mild and equable, and the character of the vegetation, and the testimony of the inhabitants seem to support this statement, but the meteorological data do not.

The town is clean and well laid out, and the drainage is good. It is a very suitable station for sea-bathing, as the sands are firm and good. There is an esplanade facing the sea about a mile long, composed chiefly of lodging-houses; there is also a good pier. *West Worthing* is built at a little distance from the sea, to the west of Worthing, and is an attractive residential neighbourhood, consisting chiefly of villa residences with their gardens. Worthing is surrounded by agreeable country, with some charming rural scenery, a few miles from the shore, amongst the South Down hills.

Littlehampton, on the Sussex coast, is sixty-two miles by rail from London, ten from Worthing, four from Arundel, and eleven from Chichester. It is resorted to on account of its bracing air, its comparative retirement, its excellent sea bathing, firm and clean sands, and its adjacency to the fine scenery around Arundel. When the tide is low the sands are left firm and dry, affording delight to young children. The town is situated at the mouth of the river Arun, and as this river flows across the sea front it stops all possibility of going westward except by ferry—a most uncomfortable feature of the place. The water supply and drainage are good.

Littlehampton is a suitable resort for families and children requiring sea change in the summer months, but it is otherwise without attractions, and is at times very bleak and cold.

Bognor, on the Sussex coast, is about sixty-three miles from London, twenty miles west of Brighton, and twenty-five east of Portsmouth. It is a quiet resort, and having a firm, clean, level, sandy beach, is well adapted for sea-bathing. The air is pure and mild. The elevated downs lying behind it afford a protection from the north winds. There is a fine pier. Bognor is a very suitable resort for delicate children and convalescents.

Hayling Island has only recently come into repute as a seaside resort, and for those who like to get away from the beaten track, it has much to recommend it. It is reached by a short branch of the London, Brighton, and South Coast Railway from Havant, the journey from London taking a little less than three hours, or it can be approached from Southsea by crossing the ferry at Fort Cumberland, from which it is distant about half-a-mile. Numerous good villas and a commodious hotel have recently been built there. Pure air, fresh breezes from the open sea, excellent sands and good bathing, exceedingly well suited to children, good golf links, and the absence of a fashionable crowd—these are the attractions of Hayling Island.

Southsea has many attractions. It is within two hours by rail of London, and within half-an-hour of the Isle of Wight. It looks due south, has a fine common facing the sea, two piers, and, from its adjacency to a great military and naval arsenal, constant social activity and interests, and frequent military and naval displays. The beach is shingle, and is not so pleasant as sand for bathing from; the extensive Common lies between it and the town.

As a winter residence Southsea has been highly commended. A six years' resident testifies: "We have much less rain than inland, and the ground, except in one low-lying part, rapidly dries when a fall does occur, the soil being gravel and shingle. In the winter house-rent is very moderate." The death-rate is low. One of the medical authorities of the place states that "more people come now in winter who have delicate chests, and they do well here if they live on the Common. Speaking roughly, our average temperature is, in winter, 5 or 6° F. higher, and in summer 5 or 6° F. lower, than at Kew." Southsea enjoys considerable protection from the north from the Portsdown hills behind it. There is a good system of drainage and a good supply of water.

Southsea brings us to the neighbourhood of the **Isle of Wight.** This island is about twenty-three miles in length from east to west, and about thirteen miles wide at its widest part, from north to south. A range of high chalk downs stretches right across the island, near the middle, from Bembridge Down, not far from the extreme eastern part of the island, to the extreme western part. There are other chalk downs at the southern end of the island.

Its chief places are Newport, Ryde, West and East Cowes, St. Helens, Sandown, Shanklin, Ventnor, Yarmouth, Alum Bay, and Freshwater. Newport, the capital, is situated in the centre of the island, and does not, therefore, concern us in this place.

Cowes, chiefly associated with yachting meetings, is divided by the river Medina into East and West Cowes. Of these, West Cowes is the more resorted to by visitors, and is the more fashionable ; its houses are less crowded together. During the yachting season, and especially in the regatta week, Cowes is crowded with visitors, but it really possesses little interest as a health resort. Its aspect is due north.

Ryde is a pleasure resort rather than a health resort, and is the most fashionable place in the island. Its long pier is a well-known and popular lounge, and military bands play there during the season. It is a great centre for yachting and boating, and for excursions into the interior and around the island.

The town occupies the face of a hill which slopes mainly in a north-easterly direction, but partly also in a north-westerly direction. It lies on the steep north-easterly slope, and is much exposed to the north-east winds. The most elevated part of the town is 155 feet above the sea. The highest part of the whole district, at its boundary, is 193 feet. The subsoil at the lower and northerly parts is clay, with here and there gravel and sand, and a little stone. At the higher parts the subsoil is brick-earth, with gravel and some sand. Owing to its north-easterly exposure, and its open and comparatively unprotected situation, Ryde is only adapted for a summer resort, and for this purpose it is cool, cheerful, and attractive.

St. Helens is the name of a district stretching for about three miles to the east of Ryde. The slope and summit of the hill at its western extremity are largely built over, and there are two villages along the shore.—*Spring Vale,* about a mile, and *Sea View* about three miles, east of Ryde. Sea View is a very quiet little bathing-place much resorted to by families with children. It has a steamboat pier.

Sandown is about fifteen minutes by rail from Ryde. It is built on the shore of a fine open bay, which affords great facilities for bathing and boating. The town is delightfully placed on the slopes of a low hill, and these stretch with a gradual fall towards the sea at the south-east. To the north-east a sea-wall protects the low marsh land from incursions of the sea. The streets, which are many feet above the sea-level, are wide and well laid out, and the houses have gardens attached to them. The subsoil of a great part of the town is clay, but the westerly and upper third is built on sand. The town is well drained. Public walks and pleasure grounds have been laid out at great expense.

The surrounding country is attractive, and excursions to various parts of the island can readily be made from it.

Sandown is a pleasant, quiet, picturesque, sea-bathing resort, much frequented in the summer by families with young children, but is too exposed and windy for invalids in winter.

Shanklin is about three miles by road and five minutes by rail from Sandown, and is situated in a valley stretching inland from the shore of the bay of Sandown. Like Sandown, it has a firm sandy beach. The air is fresh and pure, and bracing on the higher ground. Shanklin Chine is a beautiful rocky glen covered with luxuriant verdure. The walk from Shanklin to Bonchurch is considered one of the most beautiful in the island, passing, as it does, through the romantic Chine of Luccombe. There is also a fine walk across the high downs to Ventnor.

The houses at Shanklin are built on the sloping sides of a hill which, at its highest part, is 200 feet above the sea. It has for the most part a sandy subsoil.

Shanklin is a resort of great beauty and attractiveness; its sea-bathing is excellent, and the excursions which can be made from it, both by sea and land, are most varied and delightful. It has a chalybeate spring and a thermal bath establishment.

Ventnor is situated at the most charming part of the southern side of the island, and is built in a series of terraces on the wooded rocky slopes of the beautiful and celebrated Undercliff. It is sheltered from the north and north-east winds by a steep range of limestone rocks, and the downs to the north rise to a height of 400 to 800 feet above the sea. It is greatly sheltered also from the north-west, west, and south-west winds, but is open to the south and south-east. Owing to its protected situation, it has become a popular resort for pulmonary invalids; on this account it has been selected as the site of the National Hospital for Consumption. There is a large open piece of ground between the Hospital and the sea, where patients can sit or take exercise in the open air. Very good results are, as might be expected, obtained there.

Besides the winter season, which begins in November, Ventnor has also a summer season from June to September. It has good sea-bathing in deep, clear water, with sandy bottom. There is an esplanade by the sea and a fine pier.

Ventnor has different climatic characters in its different parts, some houses being close to the water and others stretching up the face of the cliff in terraces reaching to 500 feet above the sea, while some are more exposed to the sun's rays, and for a longer time, than others; and some, again, are nearer the shelter of the rocks, while others are in more open and airy situations.

The climate of Ventnor partakes of that of the whole Undercliff, the name given to the curious landslip which forms a kind of terrace six miles in length on the south-eastern coast of the island, stretching from near Bonchurch to Black Gang Chine. This district enjoys protection from the north, north-east, north-west, and west. The character and luxuriance of its vegetation bear striking testimony to its mild winter climate. The rain that falls is rapidly absorbed by the chalk and sandstone rocks, so that the ground, which is almost wholly rocky, is generally dry. There is plenty of space for out-of-door exercise, and the warmth of the sun is reinforced by reflection from the cliffs, and in some parts by reflection from the sea. The mean temperature at Ventnor during the coldest winter months (January and February) is 41·8, the mean relative humidity 87, the mean sunshine 129 hours for the two months; 4·6 inches of rain and 29 rainy days in these two months. Average rainfall for the whole year, 27·53 inches, with 164 rainy days.

The climate, then, is mild and equable, but at the same time fairly dry and tonic, and is adapted to cases of early phthisis and to those who have reason to fear they may become phthisical, to chronic catarrhal throat affections, to scrofulous and anæmic and debilitated persons, and to convalescents from acute diseases.

Ventnor, being built on a series of terraces stretching up the steep cliff, has the drawback that there are no level walks except on the beach. Bonchurch, its eastern suburb, is better off in this respect, and is preferred by many as a residence on this account and for its better protection from the east.

Yarmouth, on the north-west coast of the island, and **Freshwater** and **Alum** and **Totland Bays** on the western, come under the influence of the Atlantic, and in the three latter, especially, fine breezy sea air, and the adjacency of high downs, can be enjoyed, in comparative quiet and seclusion, during the hot months of summer.

Milford-on-Sea, on the south coast of Hampshire, is situated between Lymington and Bournemouth, fourteen miles to the east of the latter place. Its nearest station is New Milton, on the direct Bournemouth line. It lies just opposite the Needles, and is close to the borders of the New Forest. It has golf links finely situated, and is well placed for pure sea air and for walks and drives amidst beautiful scenery. It is rather exposed to prevailing winds, and is a summer rather than a winter resort.

Bournemouth is well known as a winter resort for persons with delicate chests and others, and it is also a suitable place for summer visitors. Indeed, there is no reason why a place of *winter* resort at the seaside should necessarily be unfit for *summer* resort, as is popularly supposed, for the possession of an equable climate, which renders such a place warmer than inland districts in winter, often also renders it cooler than those places in summer.

As a winter resort Bournemouth has many advantages. The houses chiefly occupied by visitors are situated on the higher ground to the east and west of the sheltered depression occupied by the older part of the town. Many of the villas are built in the midst of the pine trees, which here cover a considerable tract of the sandy soil. These pine forests not only afford a certain protection from winds, but they also exert a salutary influence on the atmosphere, and embalm the air with their aromatic exhalations. The soil, composed of sand and sandstone, is dry and absorbent, so that the rain falling on the surface rapidly drains away, and the atmosphere is left dryer than it would be were the water retained longer on the surface of the ground by a less readily permeable soil.

There is fair shelter from the north and north-east, and, to a less extent, from the east winds; but the surrounding hills are low, and the protection they afford must be at times very imperfect. Bournemouth is, however, much exposed to the west, south-west, and south winds. There is more shelter from cold winds on the eastern than on the western cliff. Compared with Torquay it is somewhat less sheltered, but is dryer and more bracing. It has a moderate rainfall, and a medium degree of atmospheric humidity.

Taking the two coldest winter months (January and February), the mean temperature is 39·7, and the mean relative humidity 87. The mean annual rainfall is 27·26 inches, and the number of rainy days 158·3. The drainage and water supply are good.

The adjacency of many interesting and picturesque places of resort ought to add to its popularity as a summer resort.

"The smooth hard sands, and the almost uniform height of the tide, permit the bathing to be peculiarly safe and agreeable."

Boscombe is merely an extension eastward of Bournemouth.

Southbourne-on-Sea is three and a-half miles east of Bournemouth. It is built on a plateau surmounting a sandy cliff, and is less sheltered than Bournemouth, but more bracing. It is a good summer and autumn resort, quiet and invigorating.

Swanage is the chief place in the "Isle of Purbeck," and is reached in about four hours by fast train from London. It can also be approached by steamers from Poole, Bournemouth, or Weymouth. Its situation is charming. It lies quite open to the east or south-east, and is pleasantly cool in summer.

It commands extensive and varied views of the coast of Hampshire and the Isle of Wight, which is only fifteen miles off. It has smooth and fine sands, with excellent bathing. There is a pier from which the steamboats land and take up passengers.

To the north the cliffs are precipitous, and rise to a height of nearly 600 feet above the sea. The surrounding country is very interesting, and a variety of agreeable excursions can be made into it; especially to Corfe Castle, St. Aldhelm's Head, Lulworth Castle, etc.

Swanage is particularly appropriate as a seaside resort to persons requiring quiet and soothing surroundings in a cool and somewhat sedative atmosphere, and opportunities for exercise in the open air amidst pleasing rural scenery.

Weymouth, distant three and a-quarter hours by rail from London, is a popular resort on the Dorsetshire coast, which here runs out towards the south, and bending a little eastward forms a wide, open bay, which looks to the east. A projection of the shore divides this bay into two parts, Weymouth Bay and Portland Roads. The new part of the town is built along the curving shore of the bay, and commands a fine view of the coast to the east as far as St. Aldhelm's Head. There is an esplanade and a pier of stone and wood, and these afford good promenades by the sea.

The reputation of Weymouth as an invigorating seaside resort dates from the end of the eighteenth century. Its chief attractions are its wide open bay and its smooth, level sandy shore, affording great facilities for sea-bathing.

Lyme Regis, on the Dorsetshire coast, is five miles and a-half from Axminster station, which is about four hours from Waterloo by fast train. It is most picturesquely situated, being built on the slopes of a hollow on a wild, rocky coast. Miss Austen said of it: "He must be a very strange stranger who does not see charms enough in the immediate vicinity of

Lyme to make him wish to know it better." It is sheltered from the north and east winds, so that its winter climate is mild, while the sea-breezes make it cool and fresh in summer. There is good bathing on pleasant sands. The place is quiet, and the surrounding scenery is charming.

Sidmouth is the first seaside resort of any consequence we come to on the south coast of Devon. Its reputation as a winter resort has been growing rapidly of late years. It is between four and five hours from London by rail (S.W.R.). It is situated at the mouth of a valley running at nearly right angles to the coast, and enclosed especially on the north and east by lofty hills terminating seawards in the sheer precipices of Salcombe and High Peak, about 500 feet above the sea. The coast view from the beach is admirable, owing to its situation in the centre of the Great Bay, which is bounded to the east by the Isle of Portland, and to the west by Start Point. "The characteristic features of the sea view are the blood-red cliffs, which rise to a height of about five hundred feet above the beach." The air is mild and at times moist and relaxing. The amount of *winter* sunshine is said to be greater than at south coast resorts generally. Numerous interesting excursions can be made amongst the neighbouring hills and valleys.

It is a very suitable resort for cases of chronic bronchitis, catarrhal asthma, cardiac debility, and convalescents from acute disease. The Nauheim system of baths for cardiac weakness is applied there. Good accommodation can be obtained a little distance from the sea as well as on the beach.

Exmouth, between ten and eleven miles (railway) from Exeter, is a popular watering-place on the Devon coast. **Budleigh Salterton**, five miles from Exmouth, is much more sheltered, and has a warmer climate, as it is placed in a narrow valley, and is well protected from cold winds.

Dawlish is about midway between Exmouth and Teignmouth. It is a pleasant and popular resort, with many attractions to recommend it. It is in a sheltered valley on a sunny coast, with neat, well-built houses, some facing the sea, others built round public gardens; and it has very picturesque rural scenery surrounding it. It has a bright and cheerful aspect, which is not a little enlivened by the railway running across the mouth of the valley close to the sea.

There is a fine esplanade by the side of the line of railway. There is safe and pleasant bathing on beautiful and extensive sands. The climate is, perhaps, as mild as that of Torquay and as equable, and living is quieter and less expensive. The cliffs of the bay are of bright red sandstone, and some of them assume fantastic forms.

Dawlish can certainly be commended as a charmingly quiet, and yet bright and cheerful, resort, with a mild climate, cooler in the hottest part of summer than most of the seaside resorts near London, and with a sedative, and at times somewhat humid, relaxing atmosphere. It is well suited to delicate invalids and children who do not tolerate a too bracing seaside climate. The drainage and water supply are good.

Teignmouth is a pleasant town on the south coast of Devon, only three miles from Dawlish, and fifteen from Exeter. It is situated on the estuary of the river Teign, Shaldon being on the opposite side. Like Dawlish and Exmouth, it faces a minor depression in the west of that large bay, which is bounded on the east by the Bill of Portland, and on the west by the Start Point; adjacent to this depression in the coast, and west of it, is the much deeper indentation known as Torbay.

Teignmouth looks south and south-east, and is protected to the north by somewhat distant hills.

The surrounding scenery, like that adjacent to most of this coast, is exceedingly picturesque and varied; the rich red soil is most productive.

The climate of this district is characterised by milder winters and cooler summers, and by greater equability of temperature, than is found inland or further east.

The following are some meteorological facts, founded on an average of ten years' observations, applying to the coldest and hottest months in the year, and which afford a very fair criterion of the climatic elements which are found on this part of the south coast.

January—Mean temperature	... ...	41·8° F. per cent.
Humidity, 9 a.m.	... ...	88·0
Mean total rain in inches	...	3·40
,, number of wet days	...	16·0
July—Mean temperature ...	...	61·8° F. per cent.
Humidity	... ...	76·0
Mean total of rain in inches	...	2·33
,, number of wet days	...	13·0

March is the dryest month, with a mean of twelve wet days and a rainfall of 1·98 inches; the next dryest is May, also with twelve wet days, and a rainfall of 2·3 inches. The wettest month is October, with eighteen wet days, and a rainfall of 4·77 inches.

There are 180 wet days, distributed pretty equally over the whole year, and 37 inches of rainfall annually.

The defects of this climate are very evident from these data, viz., a high degree of atmospheric humidity—a large proportion of wet days—often a cloudy sky, which, together with its equability of temperature, form a rather relaxing climate, modified somewhat by the tonic effect of the sea-air.

Torquay is one of the most popular and fashionable winter resorts in England. It enjoys a magnificent situation, facing one of the finest bays on any part of our coast. It is encircled by hills, which shelter it from the north and north-west, and, to some extent, from the north-east. North-east winds are, however, sometimes felt there severely.

Villas stretch up these hills at various elevations above the sea up to 450 feet.

The air of Torquay is said to be dryer than at any other place on this coast; but different parts of the town differ greatly, the nearer the sea the more sedative and relaxing the air, the higher up the hills the more bracing it becomes.

The luxuriant growth of sub-tropical plants testifies to the general mildness of the climate. Its climate is no doubt very equable, more so even than that of Teignmouth, but, like neighbouring resorts on this coast, there is frequently a great deal of humidity in the air. The rainfall is considerable, and the number of rainy days very great. If, for instance, we compare the rainfall and the number of rainy days at Torquay and at Bournemouth, we find that at Torquay the rainfall is 35 inches, at Bournemouth it is 27·6; while the rainy days at Torquay are 187, and at Bournemouth 153. The mean temperature in the two coldest months (January and Febuary) is 41·4 and the mean relative humidity 86·6.

It is claimed for Torquay that it is much cooler in summer than the seaside resorts further east. Bathing, boating, yachting, and sea fishing can be pursued with great advantage at Torquay, and beautiful excursions into the surrounding picturesque country, extending even to the wild hills of Dartmoor, can easily be made.

The water supply is very good, and so is the drainage.

The town appears to be exceedingly healthy, and the death-rate is low. The cases which appear to do well at Torquay are those of chronic bronchitis in old people, some forms of chronic phthisis, with tendencies to catarrhal attacks, some irritable throat affections; also young and delicate children during the trying periods of rapid growth and development, and some elderly people, who find themselves more comfortable in a moderately mild and soft climate rather than in a dry and bracing one.

Torquay can now be reached in four and a-half to five hours from London, by express trains.

Salcombe, about eighteen miles west of Dartmouth, and nine miles west of Start Point, lies on a protected inlet in the southernmost part of the coast of Devon. It is not well known, although by its position it is so sheltered as to be one of the warmest coast towns in Britain.

Falmouth, on the south coast of Cornwall, is beautifully situated on the shore of one of the finest harbours in England. The town itself is not very attractive, but from the ramparts there are grand views of the adjacent coast, and a great variety of interesting excursions about this picturesque coast can be easily made. Although so far from London—eight hours by express train—its reputation as a seaside resort is rapidly growing, especially as a residence for bronchial invalids during winter and spring, on account of its mild climate.

Many houses and handsome detached villas have been built on the heights above the old main street of the town.

The village of Flushing on the opposite side of the harbour looks west, and is more sheltered. The mean temperature in the two coldest winter months (January and February) is 42·9, more than 3° warmer than Bournemouth, and the relative humidity is 84·5. But it has a large annual rainfall, 44 inches, and 212 rainy days. The mean daily range of temperature is 8·5.

Penzance is the westernmost of seaside resorts on our coasts. It is 321 miles from London, but there is one fast train in the day which is timed to accomplish the journey between Paddington and Penzance in a little over eight hours.

The town is built on the west side of Mounts Bay, so that it has a south-east aspect. It commands a fine view across the bay, and the long, low line of coast to the Lizard. It is sheltered by a lofty plateau on the west and north, but is fully exposed to winds from other quarters. Notwithstanding this exposure to the winds, its temperature is remarkably equable, like that of the *Scilly Islands*, forty-two miles further west. These possess "the most equable temperature in the British Islands, if not in all Europe." St. Mary's, Scilly, is warmer than Penzance, the mean winter temperature for four years was 47·9°; the mean maximum, 50·5°; the mean minimum, 44·5°; the mean daily range, 6°; the mean monthly range, 18·7°; the mean relative humidity, 89°; number of rainy days, 107; rain in inches, 17·13; winds from north and east, 56 days; from south and west, 90 days. The mean temperature in the two coldest months of winter (January and February) is 45·3°, while at Penzance it is 43°.

Penzance is 5° warmer than London in winter; 1° warmer in spring; 2° warmer in autumn; and 2° cooler in summer. It has rather a large annual rainfall, 43 inches, and a large number of wet days.

There are many interesting excursions to be made from it both by land and sea.

For persons whom a mild, equable, somewhat humid climate agrees with, Penzance, like Falmouth, is well suited. The place is sedative, and the prevalence of winds from the sea must confer upon it a certain tonic element.

Turning round the Land's End to the north coast of Cornwall, we come to St. Ives, Newquay, and Bude. These, with Tintagel and Boscastle, all have a more or less northern exposure, and, although well adapted for summer and autumn visitors, are unsuited as winter resorts for invalids. We now reach the north coast of Devon; the first of the picturesque resorts on this coast which we come to is Clovelly. This charmingly romantic fishing village can scarcely be called a health resort, and must not detain us now.

We soon, however, reach **Westward Ho**. This is a comparatively new resort twelve miles east of Clovelly. The coast immediately around it is flat and not very interesting, but very beautiful scenery is not far distant. It is a quiet retreat, with fine bracing air, and a long reach of tolerably firm sands. Its golf links are said to be "only surpassed by those of St. Andrews and Musselburgh."

Ilfracombe, on the north coast of Devon, offers great attractions to the lovers of the picturesque, situated as it is in a part of England unrivalled, perhaps, for the beauty of its scenery. It has a very fine swimming-bath, filled at every tide.

It is chiefly a summer resort, but its winter climate has also been recommended for invalids who can bear a certain amount of bracing wind, as its winter temperature compares favourably with other well-known winter resorts; in the coldest month (January) its mean maximum temperature was 47·2° (Ventnor 45·7°) and its mean minimum 39·4 (Ventnor 37·4), so that it is warmer than Ventnor and nearly as warm as Falmouth, for which resort the corresponding temperatures are 47·3° and 39·8°. It is reputed, however, to suffer much from boisterous winds from the east and west.

The promenades and excursions are numerous and attractive.

Ilfracombe is six hours by express train from London.

Lynton and **Lynmouth**, only seventeen miles by coach-road from Ilfracombe, are amidst the most exquisite scenery of the North Devon coast. Lynton is built on hilly ground, at an elevation of 430 feet above the sea, while Lynmouth lies on the sea-shore, at the mouth of the Lyn.

Lynton has the disadvantage of being separated from the sea by one of the steepest of hills, which is traversed by zig-zag paths; but the grand prospects that it offers, of which perhaps the loveliest is that of the gorges through which the East and the West Lyn flow, more than compensate for this drawback, and the provision of a water-balance railway up the cliff is a great convenience to those who object to the hill. There is no flat sandy beach, and the place for bathing is rocky and limited in extent. Owing to its hilly character, this country is not altogether suitable for invalids or weakly persons. The one way to see the locality is on foot; those who cannot walk will miss some of the most charming features. The drainage arrangements and the water supply are alike excellent. There is one train daily from Waterloo viâ Barnstaple, in about seven hours.

Weston-super-Mare and the adjacent resorts, Minehead and Clevedon, on the shore of the Bristol Channel, have the disadvantage of large muddy sand-fields at low water, and their climate is rather relaxing than bracing. Weston is, however, greatly frequented for sea air and sea bathing by the inhabitants of some of the large towns in the west of England, Bristol, Bath, etc., as well as by people from the Midlands. The season lasts from July to October.

Passing now to the opposite Welsh coast, **Penarth**, close to Cardiff, and the **Mumbles**, near Swansea, are well situated and pleasant summer coast resorts.

Tenby is the most important and the most popular seaside resort on the south coast of Wales. It has a decided sea climate, mild, and fairly dry, and is about seven hours by fast train from London. The town stands upon the western side of Carmarthen Bay, on the south-west coast of Pembrokeshire. It is built upon the point and north-eastern margin of a rocky peninsula, composed of mountain limestone, rising to nearly 100 feet above the sea, with fine land and sea views. The sands, which are not surpassed at any watering-place in the kingdom, are most extensive. The bathing is therefore very good and free from danger. Sea fishing can be had all the year round.

Tenby has its summer and its winter season. As a winter resort Tenby is becoming more and more popular as a residence for invalids suffering from pulmonary and cardiac affections. The mildness of the climate, the absence of frost, and the sheltered situation, render it very suitable for such cases. It has about 1,700 hours of bright sunshine in the year.

Aberystwith, on Cardigan Bay, is one of the chief resorts on the west coast of Wales. It is sheltered by hills from the north and east, but it is exposed to the west, south-west, and north-west. Its climate is somewhat mild and humid, and the rainfall is large, 46 inches in the year. But it is said to prove both soothing and invigorating to those whose nervous systems have become irritable and enfeebled by over-work. It has a mild and equable temperature in winter. The beach is shingle, and is considered very safe for bathing. The drainage is good, and the water supply is abundant and pure.

A few miles to the north of Aberystwith, on an arm of the bay, is **Aberdovey**, a small seaside resort of recent growth, with a southern aspect and mild climate.

Another neighbouring and popular resort on this coast is **Towyn**, with very firm safe sands for bathing.

Barmouth is, like Aberystwith, on the shores of Cardigan Bay, but some little distance further north. It has much the same climate, the same protection from the north and east, and the same exposure to the west. Owing to the nearness to Barmouth of some of the finest of the mountain scenery of Wales, it is a favourite summer resort, but it has the disadvantage of large muddy sand-fields at low water. Its winter climate is very equable. It is said to be dry and mild, and suitable as a winter residence for pulmonary invalids who are not over-sensitive to cold winds. The soil is sandy, and the rainfall is soon absorbed.

The town is situated on a rocky eminence, facing southwards, and the houses are mostly built in terraces one over the other on the slope of this hill. The bathing is very good. The beach is sandy, with no shingle. The best time to visit Barmouth is in the early summer. In August the heat is apt to be oppressive, and there is an unpleasant glare from the sands.

Criccieth and **Pwllheli** are in sheltered positions

on the north coast of Cardigan Bay, and are pleasant summer resorts.

Beaumaris, on the Menai Straits, fully exposed to the east, has fine bracing air and beautiful sea and mountain scenery; the prospect is further enlivened by the frequent passage of shipping.

Bangor, **Penmaenmawr**, and **Conway**, adjacent resorts facing north, are much resorted to in summer.

Llandudno, on the north coast of Wales, occupies an exceptional position, and enjoys an exceptional climate, owing to the protection it receives, chiefly from the Great Ormes Head, rising to an elevation of 678 feet above the sea, which shelters it from the west, north-west, and north. It is also protected by a lower range connected with the Little Ormes Head, to the south and east.

The town lies in a valley formed by these two elevations, and this valley opens at both ends to the sea—to Llandudno or Ormes Bay on the north, and Conway Bay on the south-west.

As a summer resort Llandudno is highly and justly popular on account of the freshness of its atmosphere, its two beautiful bays, and the admirable facilities for bathing enjoyed there in almost all weathers.

The Ormes Head Marine Drive is one of the great attractions of the place. From end to end this is about five miles in length. Its air—a combination of sea and mountain air—is pure and exhilarating, the views are varied and attractive.

Llandudno has also been recommended as a winter resort, especially for invalids who can support a certain amount of windy weather. Its annual rainfall—31·14 inches—is somewhat below the average rainfall of England and Wales, which is 35 inches. The mean humidity of the air in winter is 82%, so that it has a drier winter atmosphere than some of our south-west coast resorts; this is partly due to the porousness of its subsoil, which is mostly gravel and sand.

Colwyn Bay, a few miles east of Llandudno, is also a popular resort, and affords excellent sea bathing and many picturesque excursions inland.

Rhyl is only twenty-four miles west of Liverpool, and six and a-half miles east of Llandudno. It has little that is attractive beyond its pure sea air and firm and extensive sands.

New Brighton, at the mouth of the Mersey, and close to Birkenhead, with a north-west aspect, looking partly out to sea, and partly over the opposite Lancashire coast, is one of the most accessible seaside resorts for the inhabitants of Liverpool, by whom it is much frequented.

Southport, on the Lancashire coast, is a popular seaside resort for some of the large towns of the north of England, as it is only eighteen miles by rail from Liverpool, and thirty-seven from Manchester.

Southport has a fine Marine Promenade, raised well above the level of the sands, a most exhilarating and inviting place for exercise.

The pier is one of the longest in England. The water goes out a great distance, but leaves behind it broad and firm sands.

Southport has an Art Gallery, a Free Library, Winter and Botanical Gardens, a Public Park, and a Convalescent Hospital and Sea-Bathing Infirmary.

The climate of Southport seems well suited to the various classes of invalids who require the tonic and alterative influence of bracing sea air.

Blackpool, on the Lancashire coast facing the Irish Sea, has become a very popular resort in the north of England. It lies about midway between the mouth of the Ribble and Morecambe Bay. It is only sixteen miles from Preston, and is also quickly reached from Manchester and Liverpool.

Blackpool lies fully open to the westerly winds which prevail on this coast. It has a fine sea-port, bracing air, and miles of good sands for bathing.

It is said that the easterly winds of spring are felt to be less trying there than further south.

The promenade and carriage drive runs for a length of nearly four miles, and from it and the two piers a series of remarkably fine views can be obtained. The drainage and water supply are satisfactory.

The rainfall is moderate, and averages 32 inches per annum.

From the middle of July to the middle of September Blackpool is crowded with visitors.

Morecambe and **Grange**, both on the coast of Morecambe Bay, have considerable attractions as seaside resorts for those who inhabit the great manufacturing towns in this part of the north of England. Morecambe commands fine views of the Bay and the Lake hills. It has a good pier, from which extensive views of the Lake mountains can be obtained in clear weather.

Grange is popular as a seaside resort on account of the beauty of the adjacent scenery and the protection it obtains from the lofty crags around it, which renders its climate a mild one and suitable for winter residence.

St. Bees and **Silloth**, further north, are quiet, pleasant sea-coast resorts in Cumberland.

Crossing to the eastern coast of England, the most northern of the watering-places on the Yorkshire coast is **Redcar**, which faces a fine open sea, and has extensive sands ; but it is too near the manufacturing town of Middlesbrough to make it an attractive resort to visitors from the south.

Saltburn-on-the-Sea, only a few miles from Redcar, enjoys a fine position on the coast between it and Whitby. Two picturesque wooded glens run down to the sea. There are beautiful sands for bathing, and the fine, bold, lofty cliffs afford admirable promenades and fine sea views. Saltburn is very picturesquely situated, the town is well built, and offers very considerable attractions as a bracing, healthy, seaside resort. It has brine baths, the brine being obtained from wells at Middlesbrough.

Whitby is situated about midway between Saltburn and Scarborough, and is reached in about seven hours from London by Great Northern Railway. It depends for its prosperity greatly on its fisheries. It is also famous for the manufacture of jet ornaments, the material of which is found in the neighbouring cliffs.

Whitby is a pleasant, bracing, summer resort. The sea view is enlivened by the frequent passage of large ships close to the piers, of which there are two—east and west. Boating is a favourite amusement. There is good sea fishing, and there is also good salmon and trout fishing in the river Esk. The sea bathing is very good; the sands generally are firm and smooth.

The water supply is excellent—pure and abundant. The beautiful grey ruins of St. Hilda's Abbey form an interesting feature on the cliff.

There are many pleasant villages and woods within a short distance of Whitby. Robin Hood's Bay, a village of considerable antiquity, lies to the south.

August to November is considered the best season for Whitby. July is sometimes rainy, and the spring months are to be avoided. Its fine weather comes late in the season.

Scarborough, the most popular of northern seaside resorts, is situated in the N. Riding of Yorkshire, at a distance of five hours and a-quarter from London (G.N.R.).

The greater part of the town is built upon a site elevated more than 100 feet above the level of the sea, surmounting a range of precipitous cliffs. The Castle Hill on the north-east of the town rises to an altitude of 285 feet, it juts out into the sea, and serves to divide the town into two parts, the North Bay and the South Bay. It is on the borders of the latter that most of the attractions of Scarborough are situated.

Oliver's Mount, more to the south, is, at its summit, 500 feet above the sea.

Scarborough is healthfully situated, and as it is well looked after, from a sanitary point of view, by the local authorities, it has high claims to favourable consideration as a tonic and exhilarating seaside resort. For the health-seeker, pure and simple, it is perhaps a little too fashionable, too gay, and at times a little noisy.

Its mean temperature for January is 38° F. and for July 59·3. The mean annual rainfall is 28 inches.

The water supply is good, and comes from springs nearly four miles from the town, and the sewage arrangements are very satisfactory. There are fine sands for bathing, and there are chalybeate and saline springs at the Spa.

The walks and drives in the neighbourhood are numerous and attractive.

Filey, eight miles from Scarborough, has the same fine bracing climate as the larger town, without its noise and excitement. It stands on an elevated position above the sea, has excellent bathing, and many interesting walks in its neighbourhood. The death-rate is reported to be very low, and to those who desire a healthy and quiet but bracing seaside resort without the gaiety of a fashionable populous town, Filey will prove more attractive than Scarborough.

Separated from Filey Bay by the bold promontory of Flamborough Head is **Bridlington Quay**, with fine cliffs and good sands, only three miles from Filey.

Hunstanton, on the southern side of the mouth of "The Wash," is a popular seaside resort for the adjacent towns of the Eastern Counties. It stands near a fine cliff, a mile long, and sixty feet high at its highest point. It commands an extensive sea view, and there is a firm sandy beach for sea bathing. It is a quiet resort, and shares in the dry bracing climate of this coast.

Cromer, in a fine, bracing situation, on the north-east coast of Norfolk, now reached by express train from London in about three hours, has, of recent years, become very popular and fashionable, chiefly on account of the high estimate which has been formed of its salubrity by the medical profession. For those who are seeking a bracing summer seaside resort it certainly possesses great attractions. It is surrounded by fine country, affording admirable drives to places of interest at varying distances; it has high cliffs on each side, reaching to some 200 feet above the beach; and on the gorse-covered Lighthouse Hills to the east of the town there are very fine golf links, with a club-house and two finely-situated adjacent hotels. There are extensive firm sands for bathing, and a fine pier, at the end of which a large enclosure, with glass-panelled shelters, capable of accommodating a large number of persons, has been erected. The shelters are so arranged as to afford protection from the wind from whatever quarter it may blow. Shelters are also provided on the fine parades adjoining the pier.

As to the climate, it is essentially a bracing one. Cromer is said to enjoy fine weather in the late *spring*, and May and June are often very agreeable months. In the *summer* it is cooled by breezes from the North Sea, and is rarely oppressively hot as are some of the southern resorts. *Autumn* is a fine season, with much sunshine, little rain, and exceptionally few fogs. In *winter* it is said to be warmer than a few miles inland. In 1902 the rainfall for the second half of the year was only 9·5 inches, and of these 2·9 fell in August, the wettest month of the year. During the same six months there were 782 hours of sunshine. The mean maximum temperature for the summer three months was 64° F., and the mean minimum 50° F. It is said to be one of the dryest and healthiest places in England. Its death-rate is low, only 8·4 per 1,000 for 1902, and an average of 11·5 for the last eight years. The town is well drained and well supplied with water. There is an excellent isolation hospital three miles from the town, to which infectious cases can be sent. Cromer is often very full during the summer season, and proportionately costly; it has therefore been recommended that visitors who are able to do so, and who have to study economy, should come early in the year, before the summer season sets in, or later, after it is over.

Sheringham, only four miles to the west of Cromer, has similar attractions and a like climate. It has fine high cliffs and beautifully situated golf links (18 holes). It is quieter than Cromer, and less expensive in the height of the season.

Mundesley, which is situated a few miles on the other side of Cromer, has a sanatorium for the treatment of consumptive patients, built in a protected situation, looking south, and with high ground between it and the sea, affording a protection from the more prevalent winds.

Great Yarmouth, on the coast of Norfolk, facing nearly due east, is 121 miles from London, rather more than three hours by fast train. There is also regular steamboat communication with London during the summer season. It is one of the great seats of the herring fishery. It has extensive sands for bathing, and the sea air is fresh and bracing. It is, however, at certain seasons of the year much exposed to violent winds, which blow the sand from the surface into the air, and make out-of-door exercise unpleasant.

There are a great number of cheap lodging-houses, which are filled during the summer months by visitors chiefly from the poorer districts of London.

Gorleston-on-Sea, close to Yarmouth, but rather quieter, has the same climatic characters.

Lowestoft, about ten miles from Great Yarmouth, on the Norfolk coast, is a very popular seaside resort. Like Yarmouth, it looks nearly due east, and has good bracing sea air; it is, however, quieter than Yarmouth, and is resorted to by a better class of visitors.

It has a fine harbour, a good pier, and a good beach, partly sand, partly shingle, with excellent bathing. It has a public park with fine views of the sea. Its adjacency to the Norfolk Broads makes the neighbourhood attractive to yachting men and anglers.

It has excellent accommodation for visitors.

Southwold and **Aldeburgh**, quiet summer resorts, are situated between Lowestoft and Felixstowe.

Felixstowe, upon the Suffolk coast, about twelve miles from Ipswich, has a southerly aspect, and its merits as a health resort have made it deservedly popular. The air is bracing and dry, its cliffs being sixty feet above the sea level. There are some well-sheltered spots, which are suitable to chest cases even in the winter months. The weather in most seasons is generally delightful until the end of February. The colder months of the year are March, April, and perhaps May ; the prevalent east winds are then, as elsewhere, trying, although the high crag cliffs much shelter the houses along the under-cliff. The water is very pure, though hard, and contains some iron derived from the iron pyrites in the red crag. The bathing is safe, and excellent in every respect. A Convalescent Home, on a large scale, has been established there. The medical men of the surrounding neighbourhood think highly of Felixstowe as a health resort.

Felixstowe is within two and a-half hours from London, by rail. The warrens at Felixstowe are used as golf links. One of the largest golf clubs in England has established itself there.

Harwich, well known as an important port for the steamers of the Great Eastern Company, and as an ancient fishing town, is also a great resort during the sea-bathing season for excursionists from London, who come in great numbers by steamboat and by rail. **Dovercourt**, which is a kind of suburb of Harwich, has better sea bathing. It has fine firm sands, and is altogether a pleasant place to reside in.

Walton-on-the-Naze and **Clacton-on-Sea**, near one another, on the Essex coast, have become very popular of late years as good bracing seaside resorts, providing facilities for bathing on a sandy shore, and conveniently accessible by steamboat or by rail from the East End of London. They are usually cheaper than the more fashionable resorts on the south coast.

Southend, on the north bank of the estuary of the Thames, finishes our survey of the watering-places on our English coast. It has the merit of being readily accessible, and is a convenient resort for the inhabitants of the crowded districts at the east of London. Though at the mouth of the river, its adjacency to the eastern coast obtains for its climate a certain bracing character, and it has extensive sands for bathing and for recreation.

Classification of English and Welsh Seaside Resorts.

From the point of view of climate the foregoing seaside resorts on the English coast admit of a somewhat rough classification, according to their situation. Those on the west coast are warmer and moister than those on the east coast, owing to their contact with a warmer sea, and owing to the prevalence of comparatively warmer and moister winds. In winter, when this difference of temperature is chiefly manifested, there may be an increase of from 3° to 6° F. of warmth on the west coast over that on the east. But from January to May this gradually decreases, and as summer advances, owing to the sun heat and the prevalence of warm winds from the continent on the east coast, the conditions of temperature may be reversed.

It has also been noticed, especially in the resorts on the Norfolk and Suffolk coasts, that in autumn, often up to November or December, owing to the comparative absence of easterly winds, and the slighter influence of westerly and south-westerly gales over the eastern counties, the weather is warmer and dryer and sunnier than at any other part of the year, or than the weather on the west and south-west coasts.

The east coast towns are much dryer than those on the west or south-west coasts, the easterly winds to which the former are exposed being continental and dry winds, and blowing over a comparatively narrow expanse of sea.

It follows that the climate of the seaside resorts on the east coast are, generally speaking, dryer and more bracing than those on the west and south coasts, and less suited for residence in winter, and especially in spring, during the prevalence of easterly and north-easterly winds; whereas their superior dryness and sometimes even greater warmth make them valuable in summer and autumn.

Of course, the further north we go on the east coast, the colder and more bracing the climate of the sea coast becomes, except in localities which enjoy some exceptional amount of shelter, or, from indentations of the coast-line, some unusual aspect.

A great drawback to the resorts on the west and south-west coasts is their large rainfall, which is spread over a great number of rainy days, and the associated humidity and dulness of their atmosphere. Such conditions are the opposite of bracing, and these places may be said to possess a sedative and somewhat relaxing climate, modified, no doubt, in certain places by strictly local conditions of shelter from prevailing winds, nature of soil, etc.

On the west coast, as on the east coast, latitude makes itself felt in lowering temperature as we proceed north, but less so, owing to the warmth of the Atlantic currents.

The resorts on the south coast have been grouped into three main sub-divisions, according as they approach its eastern or western extremity.

Those situated furthest east—from Westgate to St. Leonards—are considered to partake somewhat of the character of the east coast resorts; to be dryer and more bracing than those further west, while they are warmer in winter than those east of them.

Those furthest west—from Weymouth to the Land's End—are especially moist and warm (in winter), more equable both in winter and summer, and for these reasons more sedative and relaxing.

A third or intermediate group, extending from Eastbourne to Weymouth, and including the Isle of Wight, are fairly warm and dry, less relaxing and moist than those further west, less bracing than those further east.

This classification is by no means free from defects, as strictly local conditions constantly come into play, greatly determining the bracing or relaxing influence of particular places.

II.—Ireland and Scotland.

Of popular seaside resorts in Ireland and Scotland, the following, beginning with *Ireland*, are the chief:

Queenstown, in the Cove of Cork, the most popular winter resort in Ireland, has a southern aspect. It is built in terraces on the side of a hill rising from the sea, completely open to the south, and well protected from the north and east. Its climate is remarkably mild and equable, if somewhat humid and relaxing.

Its mean annual temperature is 51·9° F.
„ winter „ 44·2 „
„ spring „ 50·17 „
Its annual rainfall is 34 inches.

It would seem to be somewhat warmer than Hastings, Bournemouth, or Ventnor, and to have about the same temperature as Torquay. It has a good sandy beach for sea bathing.

Tramore, with its bay, is also on the south coast, not far from Waterford, and is frequented as a summer bathing resort, but has not acquired a reputation as a winter residence.

Glengarriff, on Bantry Bay, has also a southern aspect, and enjoys considerable protection from cold winds by mountains which protect it on the north, east, and west. It has a mild and equable climate, like that of Queenstown, but slightly warmer, and is surrounded by beautiful scenery. The coast around is very interesting and romantic. Thackeray wrote of it as "a country the magnificence of which no pen can give an idea." It merits to be better known and more frequented as a winter resort for persons with delicate chests. Its mean winter temperature is 45° F. The luxuriant vegetation testifies to the mildness of its winter climate.

There are many beautiful spots on the south-west coast of Ireland with a comparatively mild winter temperature, but the rainfall is large and the atmosphere extremely humid, so that they are not attractive or suitable as winter resorts. At Valencia the mean annual rainfall is as much as 55·8 inches, and it has been stated that in certain places as much as 90 inches have been recorded in the year!

Other picturesque resorts on this coast to which the above observations apply are **Parknasilla**, on the northern shore of the Bay of Kenmare, with a combination of mountain, woodland, and sea views. **Waterville**, **Dingle**, **Tralee**, **Ballybunnion** at the mouth of the Shannon, **Kilrush** on its estuary, **Kilkee**, Co. Clare—the two last have good sands for sea bathing and a healthy climate, but they are necessarily much exposed to Atlantic gales and not rarely enveloped in fog and mist.

Milltown-Malbay lies north of Kilkee, and is resorted to in the summer for bathing and fishing. Still further north on the shores of Clew Bay are the summer resorts of **Westport**, **Newport**, and **Mallirany**. To the north of Clew Bay is **Achill**.

Bundoran, on the Bay of Donegal, is one of the most popular summer resorts on the north-west coast, as is **Buncrana**, on Lough Swilly, on the north coast.

Portrush has been called the "Brighton" of Ireland, its proximity to Giant's Causeway making it a very frequented resort. It is situated near the extreme north of Co. Antrim, and has very grand coast scenery. It has a fine sandy beach, but the sea is rather rough and the air keen and bracing. It has rather a large annual rainfall, about 47 inches, but the soil, being porous, dries rapidly after rain. It is cold during the winter, from its exposed situation. The accommodation for visitors is good.

Port Stewart, three miles from Portrush, has similar climatic characters.

Bangor is a very popular summer resort, being only ten miles from Belfast on the Co. Down side of the Lough. It has a history extending back to earlier than the ninth century, when the Danes destroyed an abbey there. Situated on the southern shore of Belfast Lough, it enjoys very fine and bracing air.

Hollywood is practically a suburb of Belfast, from which it is distant only five miles.

Donaghadee, a small seaside resort in Co. Down, twenty-two miles by rail from Belfast, and only twenty-one miles from the nearest port in Scotland (Port Patrick). It has a fine harbour and a lighthouse. It is sheltered from the south and west winds but open to the east and north-east, which gives it a bracing summer climate. There are good public promenades and gardens. There are excellent public baths and good bays for sea bathing adjacent to the town.

Rostrevor, a beautiful summer resort on Carlingford Bay, at the southern extremity of Co. Down. It is protected from the north and east by the Mourne mountains, and lies open to the south. It is a delightful quiet retreat, the valleys covered with verdure and enclosed by rugged mountain summits. Its protection from the north-east makes it a most agreeable resort in spring. Good accommodation is provided for visitors in the hotels and lodging-houses.

Rail from Dublin or Belfast to Warrenpoint, a distance of two miles (tramcar). Many pleasing excursions can be made in the neighbourhood. The drainage and water supply are good. As the subsoil is sandy the surface dries quickly after rain. There is in the neighbourhood a sanatorium for the open-air treatment of consumption.

Newcastle, in Dundrum Bay, Co. Down, is about twenty miles from Rostrevor, and, like it, is a favourite summer resort. It is beautifully situated at the foot of the highest of the Mourne mountains, and has a fine sandy beach. There are numerous attractive walks and drives in the country around, with a combination of sea and mountain air. There is a recently erected bathing establishment. The accommodation for visitors is good.

Malahide, on the east coast, is near Dublin, and **Howth** is still nearer, both a little to the north of the capital. They are popular summer resorts.

Kingstown is really a suburb of Dublin, being but a few miles distant, and on the southern shore of the beautiful Bay of Dublin. This district has the smallest rainfall in Ireland, but is much exposed to east winds in spring.

Bray, on the coast of Wicklow, is only fourteen miles from Dublin, and is very picturesquely situated with the Wicklow mountains behind it. Bray Head reaches to 650 feet above the sea. Bray is an extremely popular summer resort owing to its nearness to the capital and its great physical attractions. **Greystones,** a little further south, is a much quieter resort.

Scotland has so many attractions in its mountains, lochs, and rivers that its seaside resorts sink into minor significance, and are not numerous.

Rothesay, on the west coast, the capital of the Island of Bute, at the mouth of the Firth of Clyde, is popular both as a winter and as a summer resort. The climate is moist and mild, the scenery very fine, and the bathing good. The island, which is only eighteen miles in length, and four or five in breadth, is almost surrounded by the lofty hills of the opposite coast. Its climate is characterised by great equability; the temperature rarely falls below freezing point, and rarely rises above 70° F.; for the winter three months it is 39·3° F.; the mean annual rainfall is 40 inches. The difference in temperature between Glasgow and Rothesay is sometimes as much as 10 or 15°.

The **Isle of Arran**, in the Firth of Clyde, is resorted to by great numbers in the summer for its sea bathing and fine scenery.

There is very little accurate information to be obtained as to other resorts on this coast, but there are probably many with almost similar advantages of mildness and equability to those of Rothesay. One of these—

Ardrossan, on the coast of Ayrshire, is certainly popular. It is frequented chiefly for its sea bathing. It has cool, humid, and equable summers, and mild winters, with rather much rain, however. The amount of humidity and cloudiness of this district in winter makes it unsuitable to most invalids.

Other small resorts on the same coast are Wemyss Bay, Millport, Largs, Tunellan, Dunoon, etc.

Oban, on the coast of Argyllshire, is a very popular summer resort, and serves often as the starting point for tours in the Western Highlands. Much yachting and boating takes place there. It has a moist climate, and a large annual rainfall (52 inches). Its mean January temperature is 39·8°, and for July and August 57·3° F.

The following are the chief seaside resorts on the east coast:

North Berwick, twenty-two miles from Edinburgh, at the mouth of the Firth of Forth, is a pleasant seaside resort in summer, and is much frequented by visitors from Edinburgh and adjacent towns for sea bathing on its excellent sands. It also has extensive Links, for golf players, between the sea and the town. It has a fine sea view, enlivened by the constant passage of ships. Its climate is tonic and invigorating.

Largo, in the bay of that name, **Crail, Elie** with **Earlsferry**, are seaside resorts on the Fifeshire coast.

St. Andrews, on the coast of Fifeshire, forty-four miles by rail from Edinburgh, is situated on the small bay of St. Andrews. From its position on the bay it is exposed to the north-east winds, which are the prevailing winds in spring. For fairly strong persons, however, the climate is bracing and healthy. The city stands on a high cliff or rock, forming a peninsula jutting into the North Sea between the bay on one side, and the Burn of Kinness, or Nether Burn, a small stream skirting the town, on the southern and eastern sides. To the north-west of the town stretch the celebrated Links—uneven downs formed by the sea. These are nearly two miles in extent, and there are similar downs south-east of the town. St. Andrews is the headquarters of the old Scottish game of golf, and for the sake of this game, as well as for fine bracing sea air, it is much resorted to in the fine months of summer. There are many antiquities and objects of interest in this ancient town, and there are the ruins of an old castle on a cliff on the bay, the foundation of which dates back to the thirteenth century.

Broughty Ferry, situated at the mouth of the Firth of Tay, may be regarded as a seaside suburb of Dundee, and is greatly frequented in the summer.

Stonehaven, on the coast of Kincardineshire, sixteen miles south of Aberdeen, is very picturesquely situated near the mouth and on both sides of the river Carron, and is popular as a bathing-place. It is a pleasant, cheerful, summer resort, with fine bracing sea air.

Aberdeen.—There are magnificent sands at Aberdeen for sea bathing, on the coast just to the north of the port, but they are a little distance from the city. A large bathing establishment has been built near the sea. The north-east coast of Scotland gets a fair amount of sunshine, and has a comparatively small rainfall.

Dornoch, the chief town of Sutherlandshire, has golf links and good sea-bathing.

Cruden Bay, thirty miles from Aberdeen, has recently become popular as a bracing seaside resort with excellent golf links, and good bathing from a firm sandy beach two miles in length. It is six and a-half hours from Edinburgh. Good hotel accommodation.

Nairn is the county town of Nairnshire, and is situated on the left bank of the river Nairn, near its confluence with the Moray Firth, about eighteen miles north-east of Inverness. It is much frequented for sea bathing on account of its good sands and its accessibility. It has also been recommended as a winter resort, as its climate has been stated to be much warmer owing to local conditions (having the Highlands to its windward) than might have been expected from its latitude. The mean temperature for January is 37·1° F., for July 57·3° F.; and the mean annual temperature is 46·2° F. Its rainfall is relatively small, the annual mean being 24·53 inches. Owing to the porousness of the subsoil it dries rapidly after rain.

Having now passed in review the chief seaside resorts on our own coasts, we propose in the next chapter to describe briefly the chief resorts of this kind which are frequented on the Continent.

CHAPTER IV.

CONTINENTAL SEASIDE RESORTS.

It will be convenient to consider, first, the neighbouring resorts on the other side of the English Channel, together with those on the North Sea coast, beginning with the French resorts.

Passing from east to west, the first we encounter is **Dunkirk**, an old Flemish town of 33,000 inhabitants, situated in the midst of barren downs. It is an important fortress and garrison town, as well as a commercial port.

As a sea-bathing place, Dunkirk is chiefly frequented by visitors from the country round about. It has a large number of English residents, life there being cheap and pleasant.

There is a railway from Calais to Dunkirk. There is also communication with London by steamboat, every few days.

Calais is not attractive as a sea-bathing station; the beach is shingle, and the resources for visitors are very limited.

Boulogne-sur-Mer is one of the most popular French watering-places. The old town stands on a hill on the right bank of the river Liane, and is connected with the new town, lower down and nearer the port, by the Grande Rue, a handsome thoroughfare, with good shops. The great attraction of Boulogne is its fine sandy beach for bathing.

The climate is fairly dry and bracing. Dryer and sunnier than on the opposite English coast.

Berck-sur-Mer, a few miles west of Boulogne, is noted for its sanatoria for scrofulous children. The city of Paris has established a vast sanatorium there capable of accommodating 700 to 800 children. There is a great extent of fine sands, and the air is decidedly bracing.

Le Crotoy is close to Berek, and on the right bank of the Somme, opposite Saint Valéry. It is resorted to greatly by Parisians on account of the excellent sea bathing on its fine sandy beach.

It has a large Etablissement des Bains, with an extensive terrace facing the sea, and on the other side a large garden.

It has much the same climate as Boulogne, but it is much quieter.

Saint Valéry-sur-Somme, at the mouth of the Somme, and on its left bank, is connected by rail with Abbeville, from which place it is distant about forty minutes.

It is a clean, neat, agreeable town, with many ancient monuments of interest. William the Conqueror is said to have sailed from this port when he invaded England.

The bathing here is not so good as at Le Crotoy, as the water is generally sandy, except at high tide.

The next well-known resort on this coast is **Le Tréport**. It is about two hours from Longpré, a station between Amiens and Abbeville. It is at the mouth of the river Bresle, and consists of an old town half-way up the cliff, and a new town extending to the beach, where the Etablissement des Bains, and many elegant villas and *chalets* have been erected.

Bathing (at high tide on shingle, at low tide on sand) is carried on in three different reserved spaces; that on the right being for ladies only, the next for families, and that on the left for men only.

Close by is a hydropathic and warm sea-bath establishment.

The population is exclusively composed of fishermen.

Dieppe is the most popular of seaside resorts on this coast, and justly so. It is reached in about four hours from Newhaven. It is picturesquely situated between two ranges of hills, forming on both sides high white cliffs, visible from a considerable distance. The harbour divides the town into two parts, Dieppe proper on the west, and a suburb (Le Pollet) on the east, where the fishermen and sailors live.

Dieppe, during the bathing season, is full of life and gaiety. The beach is more than two-thirds of a mile in length. The Casino and Etablissement des Bains are united in the same building. A theatre has been added to the Casino; it is an elegant house, with room for 800 people.

Behind the Casino is a fine, carefully laid-out and well-kept garden, a special portion of which has been set apart for children. It also contains a gymnasium and a hydropathic establishment.

There is an establishment, in the Rue de l'Hôtel de Ville, where warm seabaths can be taken. It is open all the year round, and comprises reading, billiard rooms, and a fine concert room.

Excursions into the beautiful country around Dieppe are numerous and interesting.

Veules is a very picturesque little seaside resort on the line from Paris to Fécamp. It is rapidly becoming popular, on account of its good beach for bathing and its charming situation. It is on the river Veule, in the valley of which there are lovely walks.

Saint Valéry en Caux, a little further west on this coast, and about two and a-half hours by rail from Rouen, is situated at the end of a small bay between two high cliffs. It is a place resorted to greatly during the season by families desirous of a quiet and inexpensive life and good sea bathing, which its firm, sandy beach affords.

Fécamp is an active sea-port, with one of the safest harbours on this coast. It is a town of 12,000 inhabitants, two and a-half hours from Rouen by express train. It is built in a picturesque, winding, narrow valley, and has a simple, quiet, and peaceful aspect.

The beach is of shingle, and a little distance from the town. There is a very grand Etablissement des

Bains de Mer, "one of the finest buildings of the kind ever constructed." It contains a very good hotel, theatre, concert-hall, and reading and recreation rooms.

Warm seabaths are a speciality at Fécamp, where the custom is to line the bath with a thick layer of seaweed. This has the effect of imparting to the water the peculiar properties of the weed, so rich in bromine and iodine. The mean temperature of the air in the hottest summer month (August) is 63·6° F.

Good hotels and pretty villa residences are found on the cliffs behind the Casino.

A cliff, 300 feet high, rises to the north of Fécamp, with a chapel seven centuries old on its summit. It is visited by a number of pilgrims on the 25th of March. There are some curious grottoes in the cliff.

Yport, four miles west of Fécamp, is another of those small picturesque fishing villages on this coast which have of late years become converted into fashionable seaside resorts. The beach (all sand), sheltered by two high cliffs, is somewhat small, and bathing can only take place at low tide. There are very few stations on the coast more pleasantly situated than this one, as on no other point are trees to be found so near the sea. The forest of Hogues slopes down almost to the very edge of the cliffs.

Not far from Yport is the pretty sand beach of **Les Petites Dalles,** generally resorted to by families.

Between Fécamp and Havre is **Etretat,** situated between two cliffs, 270 feet high, and renowned for the beauty and picturesqueness of its landscapes. It is one of the most frequented sea-bathing places on the Channel coast.

It is unlike any of the other watering-places; its aspect is striking and original in the highest degree. The ground, lower than the water at high tide, is protected by a barrier of fragments of rocks which has often been destroyed by the waves. An old custom, derived from this peculiar position, still prevails. On Ascension Day the local clergy, in a curious ceremony, including the benediction of the waves, bid the sea not to come beyond its limits, and to respect the little village.

Etretat has been a favourite resort for artists and literary men.

The Casino is erected on the highest and most central point of the beach. From the terrace the view of the country around is magnificent.

The environs of Etretat are most charming, and abound in beautiful walks.

Le Havre, the chief port on the north of France, has also bathing stations in that part of the bay which extends from the North Jetty to **Ste. Adresse**; the most important are the well-known Etablissement Frascati and that of *Ste. Adresse* at the foot of the hills. The beach is pebbly, and bathers require shoes.

Honfleur, on the left bank of the Seine, opposite Le Havre, can scarcely be called a health resort; its beach is muddy, and the sea bathing is not therefore attractive to visitors; it has, however, many points of interest for the tourist. Steamers go from Newhaven to Honfleur twice a week.

Villerville, six miles from Honfleur by a picturesque and shady road skirting the sea, is a small bathing-place, with a fine sandy beach and a bracing climate.

Trouville and **Deauville** form practically but one town; they are five and a-half hours by express train from Paris. Small steamboats also ply between Trouville, Le Havre and Honfleur.

Trouville is one of the most fashionable and most pleasant watering-places on this coast.

The situation of the town is particularly fine. It stands at the mouth and on the right bank of the river Touques, at the foot of a pleasant hill studded with pretty villas and gardens.

The Casino of Trouville is composed of several detached pavilions, in front of which is a wide terrace, communicating with the beach by a flight of steps. The interior decoration of the Casino, and particularly of the "grand salon," is of great beauty and richness.

The bathing season extends from June 1st to the middle of October. The beach, a very fine sandy one, is divided into three separate parts—the first on the left being reserved for ladies, the second for ladies and gentlemen, and the third for gentlemen only. Trouville is also provided with a very good hydropathic establishment.

A fine stone bridge connects *Deauville* with *Trouville*.

The country around is very picturesque and well wooded, and there are a number of interesting places to be visited.

Five miles west of Trouville and Deauville is **Villers-sur-Mer,** which is now connected with the main line of railway from Paris to Caen. It is much quieter than its fashionable neighbours, and it is less expensive. It is therefore a popular resort for families, who come in great numbers in the summer months to enjoy its cool sea breezes and to bathe on its excellent sands. It is most charmingly situated at the opening of a wide valley, and has most agreeable and picturesque surroundings.

A few miles further west we come to **Houlgate** and **Beuzeval**, connected together by a street bordered with pretty houses. Houlgate, with its beautiful villas, splendid hotels, and admirably appointed Casino, is an aristocratic and fashionable bathing-place. The sands, sloping gently towards the sea, are lined with rows of bathing-machines or cabins; and large *umbrellas*, firmly set in the ground, afford excellent shelter against the overpowering rays of the sun. Bathing at Houlgate is very convenient, and there is, besides, a very complete hydropathic establishment, where baths and douches of all descriptions can be taken at all times.

Beuzeval, on the other side of the small stream which separates it from Houlgate, is essentially a quiet place, a family bathing station, where all the visitors know each other. Its proximity to Houlgate enables the residents, who feel so inclined, to share in all the amusements going on there, without experiencing the disadvantages inherent to fashionable watering-places.

Still further west, close to the little town of Dives, and on the left bank of the river of that name, at its mouth, is

Cabourg, with a fine sandy beach four or five miles in length, where bathing can be indulged in at any state of the tide. A pleasant, smaller and quieter bathing-place, **Home-Varaville,** is only two and a-half miles from Cabourg; and many prefer it on account of its greater quiet and retirement.

A number of small watering-places succeed one another on the coast of Calvados, west of the mouth of the river Orne. The first of these is **Lion-sur-Mer,** a little distance from the sea, with a small bathing establishment. Next comes **Luc-sur-Mer,** about two miles from the former. It is frequented in summer by bathers, chiefly from Caen. Here the celebrated belt of rocks—the rocks of Calvados—commences. Next we have **Langrune-sur-Mer,** with a small bathing establishment; then, about a mile further west, **Saint Aubin-sur-Mer,** where, as most of the houses are on the beach, visitors can take their sea-bath from their own door—a plan both convenient and economical. Three miles further still is **Courseulles,** a small port at the mouth of the Seulles, with productive oyster beds and a small bath establishment.

These and others adjacent are all pleasant, quiet seaside resorts where good sea bathing and pure sea air can be obtained, and where living is simple and inexpensive.

S. Vaast la Hogue is a small seaport with a fine bay looking east, on the Normandy coast. Previous to the rise of Cherbourg it was the chief port of the Cotentin. It has good sea bathing, and fine coast views can be obtained from the country around.

Barfleur, on the same coast and with the same aspect as the preceding, is only seven miles from it. It is about a mile from the extreme point of the Cap de Gatteville, where there is a fine lighthouse 271 feet above the sea.

Fifteen miles west of Barfleur is **Cherbourg**, the principal naval port of France; it is situated in the centre of a bay at the north extremity of the peninsula of the *Cotentin*. It is nearly opposite Portsmouth, from which it is distant seventy miles. There is good and safe bathing on the sands to the end of the *avantport* and *jetée*, where there is a bathing establishment, with a casino for balls, concerts, etc. In front the Casino has a garden and fine terrace, with a beautiful view over the harbour and pier.

At Cap de la Hague the coast line turns again sharp to the south, and at nearly the end of this indentation of the coast line we find the seaport of **Granville**, situated at the foot of a rocky promontory, projecting into the British Channel. It is about twenty-five miles from Cherbourg by land. It is a busy trading town, and many ships are built there.

The baths lie close under the cliff, and can only be approached through a breach in the rocks. There is a fine expanse of smooth, broad sands, quite shut out from the town. Instead of using machines the bathers are enclosed in canvas cases, carried like sedan-chairs.

About two miles from Granville is **St. Pair**, a pretty little bathing place, on a creek or bay, with excellent sands, and much frequented in the summer.

Avranches, a few miles from the coast, but with a fine view over the sea and opposite Mont St. Michel, is a favourite resort, and has many English residents.

Cancale is three hours by sea from Granville, across the bay of St. Michel. It is celebrated for its rocks and its oysters, and is beautifully situated on the east of the fine bay of Cancale, at an elevation from which a grand panorama is commanded. To the south of the town is the port named *La Houle;* this is inhabited almost exclusively by the oyster fishers. The view from this port comprises not only the whole of the bay, but also, in the distance, Mont St. Michel and Mont Dol.

St. Malo is about six miles from Cancale. There are steamers twice a week to and from Jersey, in about three hours. The town is built on a peninsula, connected by a causeway with the mainland. The situation is very picturesque, and the town and its neighbourhood present many objects of interest to the visitors. It is much frequented for its sea baths, as well as for the beauty and interest of its surroundings. The beach, which is covered with fine sands, descends gently to the sea. From the terraces of the Casino fine views are obtained.

It is a most attractive, healthy, and pleasant seaside resort in summer.

Dinard is on the opposite side of the estuary of the Rance to St. Malo, and a steam-ferry plies hourly between them. The sea bathing here is good, and some prefer it as a residence to St. Malo.

It is only about fourteen miles—steamers make the journey by river—to the most romantically situated town of Dinan, amidst the most beautiful scenery in Brittany. Numbers of English families are settled there.

The Channel Islands (49° 10′—49° 42′ N. lat.), belonging to Great Britain, lie at a short distance off this part of the Norman coast. Jersey is only fourteen miles distant. They are usually, however, approached from Southampton (133 miles) or Weymouth (95 miles). Those who do not dread a long and boisterous Channel passage may find at Jersey (St. Helier's) or Guernsey (St. Peter's Port) a milder and more equable winter climate than anywhere on the English coast, while in the fine weather of summer the air is somewhat cooler, and these islands offer many attractions to visitors.

The climate of these islands is a decidedly marine

one—moist and equable—but much exposed to winds. Vegetation is very luxuriant, and bears witness to a genial and moist climate. The mean temperature for the winter season is 43° F. The islands get more sunshine than the sunniest of our coast resorts. Their mean relative humidity is high, from 82 to 89 per cent.; the mean annual rainfall, 32 to 34 in., with 170 to 180 rainy days. The winds are usually from the south-west or west, but in the spring north and north-east winds make themselves unpleasantly felt. The climate is said to favour growth in the young and promote longevity in the aged; to be useful for scrofulous children, for cases of torpid phthisis in adults, and for aged persons with bronchial catarrh, who find themselves more comfortable in a mild, moist climate than in a dry one; but in winter the rough Channel passage is a serious drawback!

Paimpol, Tréguier, Roscoff, are three small towns on the coast of Brittany, situated in the midst of romantic land and coast scenery and associations, near the mouth of the Channel, too much out of the "beaten track" ever to become popular resorts. The climate of Roscoff is exceptionally equable, as it is much under the influence of winds from the sea, in consequence of which the soil is of extraordinary fertility, and early fruits and vegetables are sent from Roscoff in abundance to Paris and to the English and Dutch ports.

It must be remembered that the whole Department of Finistère is much exposed to storms from the Atlantic, which bring a large rainfall, and at times a good deal of mist and fog.

Before passing round to the west or Atlantic coast of France, we must complete our review of seaside resorts on the coasts nearer and *opposite* to our own, viz., those to the north of the Straits of Dover, on the coasts of Belgium and Holland. These somewhat resemble in their climate the resorts on our own east coast. They are generally dryer and more bracing than those further west, and have a less equable climate; they are quite out of the reach and influence of the warmer Atlantic winds and currents, and the continental winds which blow from the east and north-east are colder in winter and spring, and warmer in summer and autumn, than they are further west.

Between Dunkirk and Ostend, and but a short distance from the latter, is **Nieuport Bains**, with a fine sandy beach and excellent sea bathing. It is rising in importance as a seaside resort, and deserves a visit from those who think Ostend too fashionable and expensive. Other still small but pleasant resorts are **Middle Kerke** and **Maria Kerke**.

Ostend is one of the most popular seaside resorts in Europe, commending itself to persons of nearly all nationalities who require good sea bathing in fine bracing air. The mean temperature in July is 64·8° F. as compared with 60·5° F. at Brighton. The sands of Ostend are very extensive, and every facility for sea bathing is afforded there. Being so popular and fashionable, it is consequently a very expensive resort, and only suited to persons who can afford to be somewhat indifferent to the cost of accommodation.

There are abundant amusements provided, and its undoubted character as a resort of pleasure distinctly detracts from its value as a health resort.

Blankenberghe, near Bruges, about eleven miles to the east of Ostend, on the Belgian coast, has a finer seaside promenade than Ostend, and even more extensive sands; and it had, at one time, the advantage of affording a quieter life and more simplicity than its fashionable neighbour, but it has now become very nearly as gay and costly as Ostend.

Heyst, only five, and **Knocke**, seven miles further east, afford quite as good sea bathing as either of the preceding resorts, while the life at them is much more quiet and simple. The summer climate at these Belgian resorts is rather more bracing and dryer than on our own south coast.

Scheveningen, three miles from The Hague, on the

coast of Holland, has many attractions. The hotel accommodation is good. The sea view is very fine, and the extensive sands are beautifully white and clean and afford the most admirable sea bathing. "The gently-sloping beach makes it a paradise for children." The air has been described as "fine and elastic, with a softness in it which makes it delicious." The mean midday temperature in July is 69·8° F.

It is certainly an advantage at Scheveningen that the most interesting places of this interesting country, the picture galleries, the antiquities, and the many objects of interest, are within easy reach. The Hague, with its deer-park and promenades, its picturesque buildings, its galleries, its canals, is within two or three miles. It is only twenty minutes from The Hague to Delft; it is a short hour from Scheveningen to Haarlem, and twenty minutes from Haarlem to Amsterdam.

Zandvoort, north of Scheveningen, and distant twenty minutes by rail from Haarlem, is a smaller, recently developed seaside resort. Close to Haarlem is a beautiful spot **Bloemendaal**, with a new resort **Duin-en-Dal**, separated from the coast by high dunes or sand hills.

There are many, more or less popular, seaside resorts on the German coasts of the North Sea, with good sea bathing and fine, bracing, tonic sea air.

Some of these are small islands in the North Sea near the mainland, as Borkum, Nordemey, Baltrum, and Wangeroog; Heligoland, ceded by England to Germany, forty-six miles from the mouth of the Elbe; and some are on the adjacent coast, as Cuxhaven, at the mouth of the Elbe, Busum, Dangast, Wilhelmshaven, and others.

Westerland, in Sylt, one of the Schleswig Islands, is a favourite resort of North Germans.

Heligoland is much frequented, and is connected by regular steam communication with Hamburg and

Bremen. It consists of a sand-stone rock, a portion of which, the foreland, is level, and another portion elevated, the latter being reached by an ascent of nearly 200 steps.

Heligoland, being a small island, has the advantage of presenting an entirely insular or sea climate, almost as completely so as in a ship anchored out at sea. From whatever quarter the wind may blow it must come over sea. Much the same applies to the island of Norderney. This island is very accessible, being only about half an hour from the mainland. It has an establishment for warm seabaths and a large marine sanatorium for poor, feeble, and scrofulous children. The mean temperature in July is 60·2° F.

There are several seaside resorts on the German coast of the Baltic, which do not possess much interest, except for those who live within easy reach of them. As sea bathing places they have this peculiarity, that the water contains very little salt. At some the water contains less than one-third the amount of salt contained in the Atlantic. The presence of brine springs in many of these resorts allows of the preparation of "Sool" baths, which may take the place of sea baths. The chief of these are:

Travemünde, which is conveniently near to Lübeck, and has beautiful shady walks.

Heiligen Damm, close to Doberan, in Mecklenburg-Schwerin.

Warnemünde, the port of Rostock; it has fine white sands, but lacks shade.

Sassnitz, with fine forests close at hand, is finely situated on the island of Ruegen, where there are many other resorts.

Heringsdorf and **Swinemünde**, on the island of Usedom, are conveniently near Stettin.

Heringsdorf is very fashionable, and is said to be the "Ostend of the Baltic."

Misdroy and **Berg-Dievenon** are also not far from Stettin.

Kolberg and **Ragenwalde** lie further east.

Zoppot and **Westerplatte** are popular resorts close to Danzig.

Kranz, near Königsberg, is the most easterly of German Baltic resorts.

The mean July temperature at Swinemünde is 63·3° F., and this may be taken as typical of the region. The climate is less bracing and less windy than that of the North Sea coast. The Baltic is a non-tidal sea, and is liable to be frozen in the winter.

These are excellent cool summer resorts, most of them in the neighbourhood of beautiful forests, but with little that can be called truly "marine" in their climate.

Returning now to the west or Atlantic coast of Brittany and France, we find there several summer sea bathing stations. The first we come to after passing Brest is **Douarnenez**, usually reached from Quimper, from which it is distant fourteen or fifteen miles. It is pleasantly situated on a fine bay of the same name. Its chief industry is catching and preserving sardines. The beauty of its bay attracts a certain number of bathers in the season, but the baths are situated in the hamlet of Riz, more than a mile from the town.

Some twelve miles from Douarnenez is **Audierne**, on an extensive bay, which is much exposed to the fury of the Atlantic gales. Its shores are of fine sand, with a few small scattered rocks, and afford good bathing in calm weather. The spot has the most sublime grandeur, not surpassed by any scene of the kind in France, and bearing comparison with the sea-cliffs on the west coast of Ireland and the precipices of a Norwegian fjord. The sea around is almost always tempest-tossed, and the shore of the Baie des Trépassés, so called from the number of dead bodies washed upon it, is perpetually covered with wrecks.

Some few miles further south, in a rather deep indentation of the coast, is **Concarneau**, a town the inhabitants of which are devoted to the sardine fishery; but its chief point of interest is the possession of a great aquarium and marine laboratory for the study of marine natural history, which is open to all comers who are interested in this branch of natural science. The situation is a fine one.

Le Croisic, situated on a point of this coast just before we reach the mouth of the Loire, is a popular resort in summer for sea bathing and for its fine sea air. It has the usual Etablissement des Bains, and several lodging-houses.

There are two beaches from which baths are taken, one close to the Etablissement, and another about half a mile distant. The rocks of the adjacent shore are worn into most curious and fantastic shapes, and are well worth visiting.

Many interesting excursions can be made from Le Croisic.

Pornic, near the mouth of the Loire, on the opposite side to Croisic, and on the shore of the Bay of Biscay, is prettily situated, and has some interesting objects in the neighbourhood. Steps cut in the rock connect the upper with the lower part of the town. It is much resorted to as a sea bathing place by the inhabitants of the adjacent city of Nantes.

Les Sables d'Olonne and **La Tremblade** are also frequented summer resorts on this coast. A little further south is

Royan, situated at the mouth of the Gironde, where it pours its waters into the Atlantic. It is a small seaport town twenty-seven miles from Rochefort. It has a bathing establishment, and is much resorted to in the summer for sea baths. The surrounding country is flat and uninteresting.

Arcachon is a popular summer resort for sea bathing, especially for the inhabitants of Bordeaux and the neighbourhood, from which it is distant about thirty-five miles. It is situated on the south shore of a large land-locked basin or inlet from the Bay of Biscay. This is the Bassin d'Arcachon, which communicates with the open sea by a channel about two miles wide that runs for some miles in a southerly direction before it opens westward into the bay. This protected basin with its shelving beach affords a convenient place for sea bathing, especially for families, as some of the houses facing it have gardens running down to the beach, and protection from the Atlantic rollers makes bathing much safer than at Biarritz.

The merits of Arcachon as a winter resort will be dealt with in a subsequent chapter, as also those of **Biarritz**. It is only necessary to say now that Biarritz is a very popular bathing station, and is thronged with Spanish visitors during the hot months of summer. It is too hot to be attractive to those who live further north.

It is not necessary to do more than mention the sea bathing resorts on the coast of the Spanish peninsula, for they are only of local interest, and although they may appear as comparatively cool retreats to those who live in the adjacent inland towns, they are far too hot in summer to be healthful or attractive to other European visitors. The coolest of these resorts are those on the Spanish coast of the Bay of Biscay, as they are the furthest north and have a northern aspect. The chief of these are San Sebastian, Santander, and Corunna. On the coast of Portugal there are Oporto and Lisbon; on the Mediterranean coast of Spain, Cartagena, Alicante, Valencia, and Barcelona.

Sea bathing can be had at nearly all the coast towns of the French and Italian Riviera. Via Reggia, between Spezia and Leghorn, is said to be better adapted than many of them for this purpose owing to the adjacency of large pine-woods affording shade and shelter from the sun's heat.

Bathing on the Lido is very popular during the summer months with vast numbers of the inhabitants of the inland towns in central, eastern, and south-eastern Europe, who come to Venice and other ports on the Adriatic for this purpose.

Trieste also has a fine sandy beach, and is greatly frequented for sea baths during June, July, and August.

This completes our survey of fairly accessible seaside resorts at home and abroad. Many minor resorts of merely local interest have not been mentioned, but none have been passed over that can claim any great attractiveness or usefulness to visitors from other countries. Many southern health resorts especially adapted to winter residence will be considered in the chapter on Winter Quarters, and also in that on the Western Riviera.

CHAPTER V.

MOUNTAIN CLIMATIC RESORTS.

ST. MORITZ AND THE ENGADINE—DAVOS PLATZ, AND THE MOUNTAIN-AIR CURE FOR CONSUMPTION.

It is fit that we should commence our survey of mountain climates and mountain resorts with the familiar resorts of the Upper Engadine and Davos; for not only are they of great practical importance to us from their therapeutic value and their accessibility, but also because they were the first resorts to call forth that great interest in the curative and restorative action of mountain air which is now so universal.

St. Moritz.

The medical interest of English physicians in **St. Moritz** was at first chiefly centred in its chalybeate springs, and it was, perhaps, hardly realised then how great a share in the good results obtained from the course of mineral waters and baths was, in reality, due to the invigorating effects of the pure and tonic mountain air.

Germans, Swiss, and Italians had long known of the virtues of its waters or of its mountain air, or of both together, and annually came in considerable numbers to go through the regulation cure; but a book by Mrs. Freshfield, entitled "A Summer Tour in the Grisons, and in the Italian Valleys of the Bernina," which was published in 1862, was one of the first publications which drew the attention of English tourists to the, at that time, unfrequented upper valley of the Inn.

Somewhat later H. Weber called attention to the good results obtained in the treatment of phthisis at these altitudes.

St. Moritz is the highest village in the Upper

Engadine, and the projecting ridge of rock upon which it is built is on this account termed the Engadiner Kulm. The highest part, where the Kulm Hotel stands, is placed at an altitude of 6,100 feet above the level of the sea, the general bed of the valley being about 300 feet lower. Green meadows slope from the village to the north-west shore of the beautiful little lake, the St. Moritzer See, which stretches across the valley to the wooded foot of the Piz Rosatsch, a huge mountain mass, which rises steeply on the opposite shore of the lake, its base covered with larch and pine trees, and its summit overhung by a great glacier mass.

Behind St. Moritz, to the north-west, rises the Piz Nair, a mountain very easily ascended; and continuous with this, towards Samaden, rise the neighbouring summits of Piz Padella and Piz Ot. In the opposite direction, towards Campfer, is seen the triangular pyramidal summit of the Piz Munteratsch, a mountain which rises on the eastern side of the Julier Pass.

The village of St. Moritz is built in an irregular, scrambling way, along the hillside, with narrow streets and a terribly rough and jolty pavement. The springs and Kurhaus are about a mile from the village; an electric tram connects them.

One of the chief characteristics of the climate of the Upper Engadine is very sudden and great diurnal variations of temperature. The thermometric variations, in the same day, are often so very considerable that, in summer, a temperature below freezing-point will be registered, and on the same day a temperature of from 40° to 50° above freezing-point; while a westerly wind in the winter will sometimes cause the thermometer to mount from – 13° F. to + 42° F.! —a range of 55°. These sudden changes are admitted by the resident physicians to induce, even in the acclimatised, attacks of inflammation of the lungs, of pleurisy, of chronic rheumatism, and of catarrhal fever, if they are not carefully guarded against.

The early morning is generally cold and damp, as there is a heavy dew-fall; but the damp fogs which are common in the lower Swiss valleys are almost unknown at this great elevation. The midday is often very hot, as the sun's rays act very powerfully, owing to the perfect clearness of the sky, and the diathermacy of the air. The evenings again are cold; but on some few nights in the height of summer, when the south wind comes over the mountain-passes from the plains of Italy, the air becomes positively warm.

Speaking generally, there is in the Engadine a short and temperate summer, and a long and very cold winter. Formerly, owing no doubt to the occurrence from time to time of excessively cold seasons, very exaggerated ideas were current as to the cold of the Upper Engadine in summer, and many persons brought back with them accounts of the rigour of its summer climate which a longer experience could not fail to have modified. We have known invalids who have passed some portion of nearly every day in July and August reclining on a couch in the open air. Of course in order to do this it was necessary to wrap up warmly.

From a series of meteorological observations, continued over many years, at Bevers, near Samaden, by M. Krättli, the following facts have been taken:

The mean annual temperature of the Upper Engadine is 36·5° F. The mean for the three summer months of June, July, and August, 50·8° F.; for the three winter months of December, January, and February, 17·5° F.; for the three months of spring, March, April, and May, 35·4° F.; for the three months of autumn, September, October, and November, 37·8° F. The two extremes of temperature observed by M. Krättli were −25·8° F., or 57·8° F. of frost in February, and 79·7° F. in July.

In November and December there are occasionally thick fogs, but the three first months of the year are generally calm and clear.

For five months in the year the snow covers the ground to the depth of two or three feet, and the lakes are covered with ice several feet in thickness; snow, as we have said, occasionally falls in summer. We have seen the valley covered with a foot of snow in August!

The extreme dryness of the air renders the cold in winter less insupportable than it otherwise would be. The normal barometric pressure is considerably diminished, owing to the greater rarity of the air at this elevation: it ranges between twenty-four and twenty-five inches.

St. Moritz is certainly more favourably situated than most of the other villages of the Upper Engadine; it is sheltered on the north and north-west by the Julier chain of mountains, and on the east by a wooded elevation which projects as a spur from the mountains at the back, and so forms the eastern boundary of the St. Moritzer See. The declivity upon which it is built has also a southern aspect*; but the drawback to nearly the whole of the Engadine is the great height and nearness of the mountains bounding it to the south, so that they intercept a great deal of the sun's light and heat during some hours of the day.

Of the salubrity, then, of the climate of St. Moritz in summer and in fine weather, there can be no difference of opinion. The air is perfectly pure, clear, dry, and bracing. There is an absence of that oppressive heat, even in the hottest weather, which makes the lower valleys almost unendurable; for wherever there is shade in the Engadine there is also coolness. The freshness of the air, moreover, induces an increased capacity for muscular exertion, and the author of "The Regular Swiss Round" (the late Rev. Harry Jones) mentions that he has known some

* Owing to the favourable position of the Kulm Hotel its winter temperature is many degrees higher than at the low-lying Kurhaus.

people come there "who have been so indisposed as to feel scarcely able to make the journey from London to Paris, and after a time have been able to make a twelve hours' excursion on the glacier."

This statement goes more to the root of the matter than the writer of it probably thought at the time he penned it, for this kind of climate is especially useful to those who have been *strong*, but by some accident or other, such as over-work, or illness, or trouble, have become weak : to those who possess a latent power of reaction. It is less advantageous to the essentially weak person, to whom "twelve hours on a glacier" always has been, is, and ever will be, an utter impossibility.

Owing to the want of this power of reaction the Engadine does not suit persons advanced in years, unless they retain considerable bodily vigour.

St. Moritz as a winter resort will be referred to later on. Its mineral springs and their uses have been described in Part I.

Other Resorts in the Upper Engadine.

What is most characteristic of the Upper Engadine is its great extent as well as its great elevation. Nowhere else in Europe is there a valley of the same elevation, and of the same magnitude, and with the same number of permanently inhabited villages.

There are nearly thirty miles of broad valley and good level carriage road, traversed daily in various directions by postal *diligences*, and now penetrated by a railway, at an average elevation equal to that of the Rigi Kulm ; while some of its villages are situated at an elevation of over 6,000 feet above the sea. The direction of the valley is from south-west, where it commences at the low pass of the Maloja, to north-east, where it terminates in the bridge Punt Auta ; its natural boundary is, however, some three or four miles east of this.

Just beyond St. Moritz a ridge crosses the valley leaving only a narrow gap through which the foaming waters of the Inn force their way; this forms a sort of natural division of the Upper Engadine into two portions, which differ considerably in aspect and character. The upper half, viz. that between the Maloja and St. Moritz, is narrower, its mountain boundaries on each side are grander and wilder, and much loftier, and their summits are covered with extensive glaciers and snow-fields; while the floor of the valley is occupied by a series of small but beautiful lakes linked together by the stream of the Inn, which flows through them. The lower half, that which extends from the ridge above mentioned to the termination of the Upper Engadine, has a very different appearance. Here there are no lakes, the floor of the valley is much wider, and is occupied by broad stretches of meadow-land, through which the Inn quietly and tamely flows along. The mountains on each side are of lower elevation, they all rise in gentle slopes from the floor of the valley, and present no bold or striking features of form or outline.

In the upper half of the valley, viz. between the Maloja Pass and the Baths of St. Moritz, there are, besides the well-known Maloja Kursaal, three well-known villages which are resorted to by visitors to this district in the summer months; these are Sils, Silva Plana, and Campfer. In the lower half of the valley, Cresta, Celerina, Samaden, and Pontresina are the only villages which can be said to have any vogue as resorts for strangers. The village of Zuz, has, however, developed into a *Luftkurort*, and must therefore be reckoned amongst the health resorts of the Upper Engadine.

Sils.—This is one of the most characteristic and picturesque villages in the Upper Engadine; or rather there are two villages of that name. One, in a bleak windy situation on the north side of the valley, is called Sils Baseglia, and the larger and better-built village is termed Sils Maria—this is on the south side of the valley, in a protected situation, at the commencement of the ravine which leads into the beautiful Fex valley.

Sils Maria certainly commands some of the finest views in the Upper Engadine. The Silser See, close to which it is built, is the first and finest of the lakes encountered in this upper part of the valley, and, indeed, is the largest lake in the Alps at this elevation, being three miles in length, and a mile in breadth at its broadest part. The village of Sils Maria is 5,880 feet above the sea; it is clean and well built, and possesses two very good hotels. It is especially well adapted to those who desire to lead a very quiet life, as it is far away from the more frequented spots, such as St. Moritz, Samaden, and Pontresina; and as it is well protected from the prevailing winds, it serves as a good summer station for cases of early phthisis and other invalids.

Numerous pleasing walks and excursions into the adjacent Fex valley, and to many picturesque spots along the wooded hills which adorn the southern shore of the lake, are quite within the powers of invalids.

Silva Plana is a village of considerable size, about three miles from Sils and five from St. Moritz. It is very pleasantly situated at the foot of the Julier Pass, in the centre of the lake scenery of the upper part of the valley, having the Silva Plana lake on one side of it and the Campfer lake on the other.

Many families pass the whole summer very pleasantly and comfortably there, and so avoid the crowd of visitors at St. Moritz and at Pontresina. Silva Plana is most conveniently situated for making many of the popular mountain excursions in this district.

Campfer is the next village we come to, and is about midway between Silva Plana and St. Moritz. Its immediate surroundings are exceedingly picturesque, and it possesses excellent hotel accommodation, the "Julier" hotel being a favourite with

English visitors. It is a convenient abode for those visitors to the Baths of St. Moritz who desire a quiet residence; it is as near the Kurhaus and the baths as the village of St. Moritz itself. The walk through the woods on the right bank of the river, between Campfer and the Kurhaus, is infinitely preferable for pedestrians to the hot, steep, and dusty road which leads from the latter to the village of St. Moritz. The wooded and grassy mountain slopes around the village afford facilities for quiet rambles which are not to be found in the more frequented parts of the valley, while for exploring the attractive lake region of the upper part of the valley, it is far more conveniently situated than St. Moritz, Samaden, or Pontresina.

Campfer has an elevation of 5,950 feet above the sea, and from the position of the surrounding mountain-ridges it enjoys considerable protection from the prevailing winds; its warm and sunny situation, and the many easily accessible walks around, rendering it a very suitable summer station for invalids.

Passing now to the lower half of the Upper Engadine beyond St. Moritz, the first village we arrive at is **Cresta**, and a few minutes farther on we reach the village of **Celerina**, to which parish the adjacent village of Cresta belongs. Celerina is situated about midway between St. Moritz and Samaden, where, at present, is the terminus of the Engadine Railway; but between St. Moritz and Celerina we have to descend in steep zigzags the high ridge which here stretches across the valley and forms a natural protection to St. Moritz from the north-east. Beyond Celerina the valley continues at an almost unbroken level to its termination. These two villages, Cresta and Celerina, look particularly neat, with their limewashed walls, green shutters, handsome old doorways, and windows filled with flowers. Celerina is 5,600 feet above the sea, rather more than 400 feet lower than St. Moritz Kulm.

Samaden, the capital of the Engadine, rather

more than three miles from St. Moritz, is situated just at the spot where the Upper Engadine begins to be almost ugly. It has a certain prestige as the capital of the valley, and as the largest and most central village in it. It has long served also as a kind of reservoir for the reception of the stream of visitors waiting for accommodation at Pontresina and St. Moritz, being about equi-distant from both.

There is one fine view from Samaden, and that is the view of the snow-clad summits of the Bernina group, which is well seen from the terrace of the *salle-à-manger* of the Bernina Hotel.

There are many pleasant and invigorating walks along the meadows which cover the lower slopes of the mountains, on the north side of the valley, between Samaden and Celerina; and on a warm summer day, when the high road is exceedingly hot, dusty, and fatiguing, the cool air on these grassy slopes, where there are good paths, 300 or 400 feet above the level of the valley, is often very refreshing and grateful. The mountain-paths along these alps, between Celerina and Samaden, form one of the pleasantest walks in the Upper Engadine; the bracing character of the air there being particularly noticeable. There are also pleasant walks through the pine-woods, on the same side of the valley, but in the other direction, viz. towards Bevers.

But the most popular and interesting excursion from Samaden is that to the Bevers valley, at the entrance to which the village of **Bevers** is situated. This valley is one of the most picturesque and beautiful of the whole of this region. Samaden is nearly 5,700 feet above the sea.

Pontresina, the most frequented of Engadine villages, lies about three miles from Samaden, along the road which turns to the south-west and goes to the Bernina Pass. Its situation is exceedingly picturesque, and it possesses several excellent hotels. It is about 5,900 feet above the sea. It is, moreover, the most convenient station for exploring the high mountains, the valleys, and the glaciers of this portion of the Upper Engadine. It is close to the foot of Piz Languard, the Rigi of the Engadine, and it is about an hour nearer the glaciers of the Morteratsch and the Roseg than either St. Moritz or Samaden. It has been said to have a milder climate than St. Moritz. From its situation, in a wide open space, at the junction of two lateral valleys with the main one, it is much exposed to the direct rays of the sun for many hours during the day; and around and near the village the sun-heat is sometimes great. But for the same reasons it is to be expected that the nocturnal cold would be greater than at St. Moritz, and it is so situated as to receive directly the cold gusts of air blowing down the Roseg valley.

To those who are vigorous enough to devote themselves daily to mountain and glacier excursions, Pontresina is undoubtedly the best resort in the Upper Engadine, but it is not so well adapted for the quieter life of an invalid as some of the other resorts we have mentioned. It is certainly a convenience, to those who need the extremely bracing and tonic influence of glacier air, to be tolerably near, as one is at Pontresina, to so large and accessible a glacier as that of the Morteratsch.

Most visitors to Pontresina make at least one excursion to the hospice on the summit of the Bernina Pass, a drive of about two hours; and this hospice has been occasionally resorted to as an *air cure* by those who have felt that they needed an extraordinary and exceptional amount of bracing! It is more than 1,500 feet higher than St. Moritz Kulm, and the air is there wonderfully keen and cold, especially after sunset. For quite exceptional cases and exceptional constitutions, the extremely rigorous bracing climate of the Bernina may, for a time, be suitable; but it is of extremely limited applicability as a health resort, even to those exceptional cases.

The only other village in the Upper Engadine that can be spoken of as a health resort is the village of

Zuz, about eight miles below Samaden. It has about the same elevation as Samaden, 5,680 feet, and is raised somewhat above the floor of the valley at this part. The scenery around is pleasing.

Tarasp-Bad, is the only place of any great interest in the **Lower Engadine**. Its claims as a mineral-water resort have been dealt with in Part I.

Many of the visitors to Tarasp prefer to live either at Schuls, the principal place in the Lower Engadine and about a mile from the Tarasp Springs, or at the Hôtel Waldhaus, **Vulpera,** situated in a fine position, several hundred feet above the Kurhaus on the right side of this valley.

As to the climate of Tarasp and Vulpera. This district, situated at an elevation of between 4,000 and 4,500 feet above the level of the sea, possesses all the invigorating characteristics of an Alpine climate, while it has the advantage of being much less severe and rigorous than that of the Upper Engadine. There are here fewer sudden changes of temperature, and an unexpected fall of snow in the summer months, by no means an uncommon occurrence at St. Moritz, is at Tarasp quite an exceptional event. The milder character of the climate is indicated by the much greater luxuriance of vegetation ; rye and flax are extensively cultivated in this district, and fruit-orchards flourish near Schuls, while the local flora is exceedingly rich and diversified.

As well as being milder, the air is less dry and rarefied than in the Upper Engadine.

The mean atmospheric temperature in the months of July and August ranges from 56° to 60° F. The maximum and minimum temperatures noted in the same months were 82° and 37·5° F. It will thus be seen that the climate of the Tarasp district especially commends itself to those cases in which it is thought desirable to try the influence of mountain air, without incurring the risk of exposure to the sudden changes of temperature, the highly rarefied air, and often the continuous cold of the Upper Engadine.

Also, on leaving the Upper Engadine, Vulpera offers an admirable intermediate point where patients may break the suddenness of their descent into the lower lying resorts of Italy, Switzerland, and the Tyrol.

Davos Platz, and the Mountain-Air Cure for Consumption.

Davos is situated in a mountain valley in the Grisons, which runs parallel with the Upper Engadine, at a distance of about twenty miles north of it. It is about 5,070 (Davos Dorf Sanatorium) feet above the level of the sea. But it is not its particular elevation alone which gives to Davos its special suitability as a mountain resort. We must seek in other local conditions for the characteristic qualities of the climate of Davos. So far as purity and rarefaction of the air are concerned, it is in almost precisely the same position as the adjacent Engadine valley. It is probably only in the greater stillness of its atmosphere, and in protection from the prevailing local winds, that Davos presents any special advantages in winter over such resorts as St. Moritz, Pontresina, or Samaden. Dr. Frankland (*Proceedings of the Royal Society*, vol. xxii., p. 317) writes :—

The summer climate of Davos is very similar to that of Pontresina and St. Moritz in the neighbouring high valley of the Engadine—cool and rather windy; but as soon as the Prättigau and surrounding mountains become thickly and, for the winter, permanently covered with snow, which usually happens in November, a new set of conditions comes into play, and the winter climate becomes exceedingly remarkable. The sky is, as a rule, cloudless, or nearly so; and as the solar rays, though very powerful, are incompetent to melt the snow, they have very little effect upon the temperature either of the valley or its enclosing mountains, consequently there are no currents of heated air, and as the valley is *well sheltered from more general atmospheric movements, an almost uniform calm prevails until the snow melts in spring.*

And the late Mr. J. A. Symonds, speaking from long personal experience, said of the winter climate of Davos :—

> The position of great rocky masses to north and south is such that the most disagreeable winds, whether the keen north wind or the relaxing south, known by the dreaded name of *föhn*, are fairly excluded. Comparative stillness is a great merit of Davos; the best nights and days of winter present a cloudless sky, clear frost, and *absolutely unstirred atmosphere.* March is apt to be disturbed and stormy, and during the summer months there is a valley-wind, which rises regularly every morning and blows for several hours.

The direction of the valley is from north-east to south-west. It is only about half a mile broad, and protecting mountains rise on each side to the height of from 2,000 to 5,000 feet above the level of the valley. About three-quarters of a mile above Davos Platz, to the north, is Davos Dorfli, a sunnier spot than Davos Platz, but perhaps not so well protected from wind. Still farther north is the Davoser See, or the Lake of Davos, which affords good skating in winter until it becomes too thickly covered with snow.

At the south-west extremity the valley is also well protected and closed in by high mountains, and there are no extensive glaciers and snow-fields in the immediate vicinity of Davos as at Pontresina.

The winter snowfall in the Davos valley, as well as in the Engadine, usually begins early in November. An early and heavy snowfall of three or four feet is considered to promise a good winter. The snow continues to fall through November and a part of December. In the roadways it gets beaten down to a depth of three or four feet. In good seasons, fine settled weather, with absence of snowfall, sets in before the end of December. The atmosphere becomes still and calm, the air intensely cold and dry, and absolutely clear. At night the brilliant starlight, or the cold silvery moonlight streaming over the snow-mantled valley, gives it an aspect of singular beauty. The temperature at night often falls very low, frequently some degrees below zero. The days are cloudless, with an intensely blue sky, and an amount of heat from solar radiation which enables invalids to pass many hours sitting in the open air; and the brilliancy of the sunshine in mid-winter makes umbrellas and sunshades necessary for protection. The instant, however, the sun is withdrawn the intense coldness of the air makes itself felt, and a fall of 50° or 60° F. is common immediately after sunset. Of course all delicate invalids should be indoors before this hour. Owing, however, to the great dryness of the atmosphere, and the absence of wind, the extreme cold at night is by no means so much felt as might be expected. "There are no patients," says one of the local physicians, "who cannot, if they are so inclined, sleep with safety with an open window during the winter." Patients are advised to be in the open air from sunrise to sunset.

Unfortunately, weather at Davos is fickle sometimes, as it is elsewhere, and a remarkably fine winter may be preceded or followed by a remarkably bad one, and a really bad winter will often prove disastrous to many invalids.

The relaxing south wind, the *föhn*, will sometimes prevail to a great extent, in consequence of which the snow is thawed at times in mid-winter, and colds, which are rarely caught at Davos, are then common. In really *good* winters, however, "wonderful recoveries" are numerous. There is then almost an entire absence of wind, the air is remarkably dry and bracing, and for months there may be almost uninterrupted sunshine and clear unclouded skies.

Owing to the absence of aqueous vapour in the clear dry air of this elevated region, the intensity of solar radiation on perfectly clear days is remarkable; and, according to Frankland, at Davos Dorfli, on the 21st December, 1873, at 2.50 p.m., the "mercurial thermometer with a blackened bulb *in vacuo*" recorded 113° F., and on the same day at Greenwich the maximum reading, obtained by the same method, was 71·5°, giving a difference in favour of Davos of 41·5° F. But a maximum of solar radiation amounting to 153° F. was obtained on the 31st January, 1881, while on the same day the maximum temperature of the air in the shade was 42·5°, and the minimum 18° F. So that the difference between sun and shade temperature is enormous. The lowest temperature recorded during the winters 1879-80 and 1880-81 was 16·7° F. below zero on 9th December, 1879. The mean daily minimum for the same month was 5·5° F., and the mean daily maximum 23·13°. The maximum sun temperature 138° F. *This was during a month of the finest Davos winter weather;* the amount of aqueous vapour in the air being exceedingly small, and the readings of the hygrometer very low.

The mean winter temperature at Davos varies between 20° and 30° F.

Davos has flourished greatly and deservedly as a winter resort for consumptives, while as a summer resort its manifold attractions have not met with the esteem they merit. We have found it in summer a most agreeable residence, and preferable to many other mountain stations for its quiet restfulness.

On the other hand, while St. Moritz has not become the great winter resort for the phthisical that Davos has, its summer renown has progressed uninterruptedly.

St. Moritz has been tried and found to answer exceedingly well as a winter resort in a certain number and class of cases. No doubt it is not so well suited as Davos to the feebler class of pulmonary invalids, who are also the victims of more advanced disease. But to many of the stronger patients, and to those in whom the disease is in its earliest stage, or very limited in extent, or to those who are suffering only from general loss of tone, St. Moritz may prove as useful, or even more so than Davos. Moreover, at the Kulm and other hotels at St. Moritz, patients will find winter sanatoria, furnished with all the conveniences which invalids require, and no effort is spared to make the winter life of an invalid cheerful and comfortable. The Kulm hotel possesses an excellent covered terrace for sitting out, and a skating-rink is also close at hand.

St. Moritz is within easy reach of Davos, so that a patient who finds the climate of the Upper Engadine unsuitable can easily remove to the Davos valley. On the shortest day in the Engadine the sun rises at 10.45 a.m. and sets at 3 p.m., and there is a sudden chill when the sun goes down.

We must now enter into a little detail as to the treatment of consumptive patients in these high mountain valleys.

At one period cases of phthisis in too advanced a stage were not unfrequently sent to winter at Davos or St. Moritz. This was not altogether the fault of medical men, but because patients with advanced disease insisted on trying a cure of which so much was being said. The following extract from a letter from a medical man who was also a patient at Davos at that time calls attention to this :—

> Among the twenty-five to thirty-five guests at the Hôtel —— there were several deaths, some of them people who certainly came much too far gone, but one or two in which it seemed that the peculiar air brought on an increase of disease.

After giving the particulars of a case in which a severe and fatal illness appeared to have been induced by "the exceptional excitement, etc. of the climate," he adds :—

> Other deaths in the house were very sudden, and I knew of some cases of sudden attacks of hæmorrhage. In one or two cases where there was no disease, but weakness and want of stamina, people seemed to have gained considerably when they left. I am sure for dyspepsia the climate is a wonderful remedy.

It would be disingenuous not to admit the fact that other experiences of winters at Davos have been by no means unchequered by calamities, and some fatal occurrences there have been very sad and unexpected. The better results now obtained are certainly to a great extent due to a more careful selection of cases, to the existence of suitable sanatoria and to the acceptance of the teaching that the altitude cure for consumption has its limitations.

The success which has been obtained in recent years, in the treatment of consumptives in sanatoria at various elevations, and in many countries, emphasises the well-known fact that immunity from consumption does not follow any particular level of elevation. It was originally thought that the altitude of immunity from phthisis varied in various latitudes, descending in proportion as we passed from the equator to the poles. In the tropics it was necessary to ascend to an elevation of between 8,500 and 9,000 feet. In the Peruvian Andes patients were sent to mountain valleys reaching an altitude of nearly 10,000 feet. In Mexico to valleys 6,500 and 7,000 feet above the sea-level. On the other hand, in the Pyrenees, we were assured that at elevations varying from 1,760 feet (Bagnères-de-Bigorre) to 4,580 feet (Gavarnie) phthisis was equally rare.

In Switzerland some localities not more than 3,000 feet above the sea appeared to be as free from phthisis as others of twice that elevation. In the Black Forest and in the Harz mountains of Germany, it was stated that consumption was extremely rare at the comparatively moderate height of 1,400 to 2,500 feet; while Brehmer asserted that in the neighbourhood of Görbersdorf, in Silesia (1,700 feet), he had never seen phthisis among the inhabitants.

These statements pointed clearly to the conclusion that the freedom which any particular locality appeared to enjoy from this disease was independent of mere elevation, and due in part to other conditions, and this contention has received remarkable confirmation by the success that has attended the "open air cure," when carried out at suitable sanatoria at home and abroad.

We know that the air of large, densely-populated cities and towns is filled with impurities, both organic and inorganic, and doubtless in many localities this floating dust is largely composed of filthy putrescent organic matter, or infective particles, capable under certain circumstances of exciting or conveying disease. It is amongst those who have to live in the worst parts of this unwholesome town atmosphere that phthisis is most rife and fatal; and therefore to the absence of these impurities in the air of elevated regions, as well as in that of the open sea, we may reasonably attribute their beneficial influence in preventing or arresting tubercular disease.

M. Miquel's observations at the Observatoire de Montsouris show how comparatively free the air is from organic impurities over extensive tracts of water, as well as at great elevations; in his examinations as to the presence of bacteria in the air he found *none* at elevations of two to four thousand metres; he found on the surface of a small lake like that of Thun, in 10 cubic metres 8·0 bacteria only; on the shores of the lake (near the Hôtel Bellevue) 25·0, and in the Rue de Rivoli, Paris, 55,000·0!

Most of the localities which enjoy an immunity from tubercular disease of the lungs are characterised by a pure and dry atmosphere, a dry subsoil, and a scanty population.

And it has been shown that in certain favoured localities in our own country, where these conditions of dryness of subsoil, thinness of population, and purity and dryness of the atmosphere co-exist, there also the occurrence of cases of phthisis is very rare.

If consumption be a disease engendered by city life, by overcrowding, by breathing a damp contaminated atmosphere, we should expect it to disappear in localities where all these conditions are reversed.

It may be interesting to enquire briefly into the nature of the evidence which was originally relied upon in support of the view that elevated districts were those best suited to phthisical patients.

Before we were in possession of all the evidence that has been derived from the results of the past thirty years' experience at Davos and elsewhere, the strongest and the most unequivocal was that derived from the experience of medical practitioners resident in the large towns at the base of the Peruvian Andes, and in similar tropical stations.

In these localities consumption is very rife, and it had long been the established mode of treatment there to remove the patients so afflicted, as early as possible, to one or other of those sheltered valleys at great elevations which the slopes of the Andes afford in abundance. Dr. Archibald Smith, of Lima, was one of the first to call the attention of the medical profession to this method of treatment. He stated that in the Peruvian Andes immunity from phthisis was commonly observed at an elevation of between 7,500 and 8,500 feet. No plan of treatment could be more rational than to remove the consumptive patient from the hot, damp, unwholesome atmosphere of the densely-populated town in which he had been attacked, to the pure, clear, dry, invigorating air of the adjacent mountain valleys. It is very well known that, in temperate climates, some moderately elevated regions enjoy a greater immunity from tubercular disease than others of perhaps twice their altitude. Local conditions, therefore, other than the single one of mere elevation determine the suitability of each particular district. Protection from strong winds appears to be one of these conditions. One important fact appeared to come out of the inquiry so far as it had at that time advanced, viz. that a moderate elevation of 1,500 to 3,000 feet was as useful in some parts of the world as an altitude of from 7,000 to 10,000 feet in others.

After wintering at these altitudes, one of the difficulties always has been what to do when the transitional season of spring sets in, and the snow begins to melt. "When the snows melts," a patient writes from St. Moritz, "winds of icy coldness blow on the snow, surpassing English east winds in their fierce bitterness, making existence barely tolerable in March and April." Some, however, boldly face the inconvenience and remain where they have wintered, and, so far as we can learn, without taking any particular harm. But some springs are much more trying and disagreeable than others, and, no doubt, there is a craving for a little change when spring, with its unpleasant weather, reaches the snow-covered valley. To return to England at once seems scarcely advisable, knowing what our own spring weather is like. To seek some other intermediate mountain station, of lower elevation, for a few weeks before descending to the sea-level would perhaps be the best thing to do, if such suitable stations were easily found. But there are difficulties in doing this. Many of the summer resorts between 2,500 and 3,500 feet above the sea are not open and available at this season, and in those that are available the accommodation is perhaps not such as invalids require. Moreover, even if a suitable intermediate station is found, it will occasionally happen that pulmonary invalids find themselves worse for the change, and begin to think they have been ill-directed in their choice; whereas they should bear in mind that the spring is a difficult season everywhere, especially for those who suffer as they do.

Thusis, 2,448 feet above the sea, is convenient and accessible from the Engadine, but little is known about its spring climate, and, from its situation, it would, we fear, be draughty in spring. Fair accommodation can be obtained there, and it has the advantage of being on the way homeward.

Seewis, nearly 3,000 feet above the sea, a village in the Prättigau, quite close to Landquart, is exceedingly conveniently situated, in a picturesque position, with a good sunny aspect, and, we are assured by those who have spent a whole winter there, has good but limited accommodation.

Glion, above Montreux on the Lake of Geneva, about 2,300 feet above the sea, is a pleasant, sunny station with very good accommodation and most picturesque and cheerful surroundings; but it is rather out of the way for those who are returning to England from Davos or the Engadine.

Heiden, 2,660 feet above the sea, near Rorschach, on the Lake of Constance, is also conveniently accessible and in a pleasant situation, but it would probably be found dull and unprepared for spring visitors.

The Dolder Hotel, close to Zürich, is finely situated, and conveniently placed on the homeward route.

In conclusion, two questions must be briefly dealt with: First, what class of invalids may fairly expect to derive benefit from resorting to these high mountain valleys? and, secondly, what are the curative agencies at work there?

It is of the first importance to remember that these mountain climates are by no means adapted to the treatment of many well-defined forms of consumption; that cases have to be selected with great care and discrimination; and that regard must be had as much to the constitution and temperament of the individual as to the extent of local disease. Hereditary predisposition, other circumstances being favourable, offers no counter-indication to the suitability of these stations. But their remedial power is especially manifested in persons who have become accidentally the subjects of chronic lung disease, and who were the possessors of an originally sound constitution, and have obvious reserve stores of physical vigour. It is the universal experience of physicians that the phthisical constitution is the most difficult of all to control; consumptive patients are for ever committing indiscretions which are perilous to themselves, and in the last degree exasperating to their doctors. Cautions against over-excitement and over-exertion are therefore specially needed in climates such as we have been considering. Hence the value of treatment in sanatoria. The following summary of cases suitable to these high mountain health resorts is founded on a long practical experience in one of them, collated with that of the author.

1. Where there is an obvious and well-ascertained predisposition to consumption, and when perhaps a slight hæmorrhage has occurred without the manifestation of any definite local disease, as a *preventive* measure a residence for two or three seasons in a high mountain station is to be recommended.

2. In catarrhal forms of consumption, in the early stage, without much constitutional disturbance, or rise of temperature, the best results may be looked for. But cases with much fever from the commencement, and of nervous and excitable temperament, must not be sent to high altitudes.

3. Chronic inflammatory induration and infiltration of limited portions of the lung, often the result of acute congestion and inflammation, are especially suitable; not so, however, if a considerable extent of lung is the seat of tuberculous disease, or if, owing to the extent of lung involved and consequent changes in the sound lung, there is much dyspnœa.

4. Cases of chronic bronchial catarrh in young people; that is to say, those cases of tendency to repeated attacks of "cold on the chest," often left behind in children after whooping-cough, measles, and other maladies. But this does *not* apply to the chronic winter coughs of persons more or less advanced in life, or to cases where there is much *permanent* shortness of breath. The young patients of this class should begin the mountain-air cure before the end of the *summer* season, and continue it through the succeeding winter, so as to become gradually adapted to the change of climate.

5. The results, in the shape of thickenings and adhesions, of former attacks of pleurisy, to which, too often, the development of serious subsequent lung disease can be traced. The pulmonary gymnastics

excited by treatment in high altitudes prove of great value in those cases.

6. Many cases of purely nervous asthma in young subjects have been cured in these resorts.

7. Apart from cases of pulmonary disease, many other ailments, such as general loss of power, not dependent on organic disease, cases of nervous exhaustion, over-work, retarded convalescence in otherwise vigorous constitutions, certain forms of dyspepsia and hypochondriasis, and other less strictly definable maladies of a neurasthenic or anæmic form, not seldom find restoration to health and strength from prolonged residence in the pure bracing air of these Alpine stations.

Next, what are the curative agencies at work in these resorts? This question is by no means an easy one to answer decisively. When we reflect that cases of consumption are arrested in their course and apparently cured, as they certainly have been, in such a climate, for instance, as that of Arcachon, on the coast of the Atlantic, and in the many "open air" sanatoria in our own country, and also in such an apparently utterly different climate as that of Davos, we are led to the conclusion that we must seek for some *special relation* between the individual to be cured and the particular climate that will suit him. And it is sometimes only by actual trial that such relation can be discovered.

Purity and stillness of atmosphere are two important, and probably the most important, conditions at work. Elevation in itself, as has already been said, may also be of some importance, but it cannot be an essential; it brings with it other conditions, however, such as dryness and purity of air, which are of great consequence. The Tartar steppes, where the Russian physicians send their consumptive patients, and where, we are told, they are cured, are sometimes below and not above the sea-level. It is not the low temperature alone that is the cause of immunity from phthisis in these mountain valleys, for in some of the coldest parts of Russia the mortality from phthisis is more than 20 per cent. of all deaths; but the cold, in these places, is probably associated amongst the poorer peasantry with overcrowding and other insanitary conditions of life, to which the mortality from phthisis is doubtless due. Cold, when associated with dry, calm, pure air, gives tone to the organism and stimulates appetite.

It used to be thought that an equable temperature was of great importance in the treatment of consumption; and within certain limits, and if associated with certain other qualities, equability of temperature is an advantage in a climate; but, unless dryness of the air is associated with it, equability of temperature is not of so much value. Indeed, a too equable temperature may lead to loss of tonic property, and so diminish nutritive activity. We find, for example, that in Ceylon, which has a remarkably equable climate, consumption is exceedingly common. On the other hand, at Quito, in Ecuador, which is 10,000 feet above the sea, its immunity from phthisical disease is considered to be greatly due to its equable temperature; the mean temperature for the year being 60° F., and "in a large room, with doors and windows open day and night, the temperature varied between 57° and 60° only!" But it is obvious that the climate of Quito possesses not only equability, but the other conditions dependent on great elevation.

It has been suggested, and with much reason, that the immunity from phthisis observed in certain places, and at certain elevations, may perhaps be due to the fact that the inhabitants are all agricultural or pastoral, and live out-of-door lives, and also to the relative scantiness of population.

But, as we pointed out some years ago, the chief curative agency at work in these elevated districts is probably the *aseptic* quality of the air. It has been shown that there is an almost entire absence in these localities of those *organic impurities* which play such an important part in the production of disease. To this fact may be added the stimulating and tonic properties of the cold pure air, promoting the desire for muscular activity, as well as increasing the power for the same, by inducing increased activity in the functions of nutrition. Another valuable condition is the rarefaction of the air, which necessitates greater activity of the respiratory organs. The respirations are necessarily more frequent and more profound; the air breathed is relatively richer in active oxygen than the air of the plains; a more complete aëration of the blood is secured; all the portions of the lungs which are capable of admitting air are called into full play and activity; the air-cells are more completely dilated; the functions of all the healthy portions of the lungs are roused and thoroughly engaged in the work of respiration. There is, in short, hyper-ventilation of the lungs. We find that the chest expands considerably during residence in these resorts, and portions of lung ordinarily little used in breathing (and these are the parts specially liable to be attacked in phthisis) become actively engaged, and so a compensatory activity in the sound parts makes up for the inactivity in parts which have become spoiled by disease. The increased activity of the circulating functions, the more complete penetration of all the tissues of the lung by the more active blood currents, promote repair and recovery from the damage inflicted by disease. The low temperature of the air inhaled also has a tendency to diminish fever. The energetic action of the solar rays, the intensity of the insolation, is also a most important factor. These may not be all the influences at work in the restoration to health of the pulmonary invalids who pass their winters in these snow-covered regions, but we doubt not that they are the chief.

Davos has some excellent **sanatoria** for the reception and treatment of consumptive patients, in addition to a vast number of good hotels and *pensions*. Dr. Turban's sanatorium has a wide reputation, and at Davos Dorf there are Dr. Dannegger's and others. Then there are the German and Swiss sanatoria for assisted patients belonging to the working classes, conducted on the same system as that proposed for adoption in the projected Queen Alexandra Sanatorium. There is also the Schatz-Alp Private Sanatorium in an admirable situation—perhaps the finest in Europe, 1,000 feet above the Davos Valley, where it must get more sunshine, especially in the short winter days, than is possible in the valley.

The report of the German Sanatorium states, as a result of a year's experience, that of 143 patients who left the institution during the year, 83·2 per cent. had improved and 54·6 per cent. were able to resume full work, results which appear particularly good when it is borne in mind that only 30 per cent. of these cases were in the first stage.

Comparing results obtained at these high *altitude* stations with those resulting from treatment in low-lying sanatoria, Prof. Erb remarks: "I cannot quite understand how people in some places appear to think and say that similar results have been obtained in the mountains of medium height, in the low countries, on the Rhine and in the lowlands of North Germany; and that the treatment of consumption depends much less upon the climate than upon the special hygienic and dietary conditions. It seems to me indubitable that, on most people, the high mountain climate has a particularly invigorating and strengthening effect, and that it is just a *change* of climate that is needed to obtain a powerful and climatic effect; even though the high mountains need not always be called into requisition. Why should we withhold from consumptives, who need it most particularly, this advantage of a change of climate and especially of a high mountain climate, and leave and treat them in their own home, and in the climate to which they have been accustomed so long?"*

* Clinical Lecture on "Winter Cures in the High Mountains," Leipsic, 1900.

CHAPTER VI.

OTHER MOUNTAIN HEALTH RESORTS: FOR WINTER AND SUMMER CURES.

A MOUNTAINOUS country like Switzerland naturally presents many other stations suitable for the mountain-air cure, both in winter and summer, as well as the Engadine and Davos. There are some in the immediate neighbourhood of Davos—as **Clavadel**, at an elevation of 5,400 feet, in the Sertig Valley. It lies on a sunny slope and has a Kurhaus with a residential physician (Dr. Frey). It is well suited to patients who wish to be in a quieter resort than Davos, and the climatic conditions are practically the same.

Wiesen, 4,770 feet above the sea, only eleven miles from Davos Platz, in the same valley (the Landwasser), is often resorted to in spring, after wintering at Davos, and sometimes also as a preparation for the winter season at that place. It is in a dry and sunny situation, on sloping ground, about 1,000 feet above the river, and is surrounded by very pleasing mountain scenery. It is somewhat better sheltered from cold north winds than Davos. It gets sunshine in the shortest days from 10 a.m. to 3 p.m., which is more than is possible at Davos, as Wiesen is more open towards the south.

Of course the same society and amusements cannot be obtained there, but some may not think this altogether a disadvantage. A patient, a medical man, who stayed there, described it as "more sheltered than any other high Alpine health resort."

Arosa, with a sanatorium for consumptives 6,090 feet above the sea, is a small hamlet at the head of a valley which opens to the west, opposite Langweis, the last village in the Schanfigg Thal, the valley which leads from Coire to the Strela Pass, the most direct way for walkers from that town to the Davos valley. It is about five hours from Coire by carriage road.

In the summer it is a pleasant walk of about five hours from Arosa, over the Strela Pass, to the Davos valley. Arosa has of late years developed considerably as a winter resort—an alternative to its neighbour Davos on the other side of the mountains.

Many visitors of all nationalities now spend the winter there. It is much more sheltered by high mountains than Davos; the surface of the ground is broken and irregular and the scenery more picturesque and less monotonous.

Owing to this shelter it enjoys more protection from winds, and the dreaded *Föhn* is much less troublesome than at Davos and Wiesen. Its mean relative humidity is lower than that of Davos, being only 60·3° in January. It is, however, rather colder owing to its greater elevation (about 800 feet), and for the same reason the snow melts later, which is thought to be an advantage, as it enables patients to remain there till later in the spring. The variations or the range of temperature is less. This also is an advantage. Arosa also has rather less cloudiness.

Arosa is reported to get twenty-eight and a-half more hours of actual sunshine in the three winter months than Davos Platz; it also has a longer period of possible winter sunshine than either Davos or St. Moritz, but this is more than neutralised by its faulty distribution, for the sun rises earlier in the day and sets earlier, so that during six or seven weeks in winter the sun sets before 3 p.m.!

The mean temperature for the three winter months, December, January, and Feburary, is 22·4°, 24·1°, and 27·7° F.

Arosa is a much quieter place than either Davos

or St. Moritz, although it has altered greatly recently in the increased number of winter visitors. It has now many good hotels, *pensions*, and villas, an English toboggan club (!), and six resident physicians. As a summer resort Arosa has many attractions ; it is a spot of great natural beauty, with many mountain walks of various distances.

Leysin (4,783 feet) is at a rather lower elevation than those winter mountain resorts we have just noticed. It is also in western or French-speaking Switzerland, while they are in eastern Switzerland.

This mountain resort, beautifully situated in the Vaudois Alps, is mainly devoted to the sanatorium treatment of phthisis. The sanatoria are built on a plateau, 600 feet above the village of Leysin, protected from the cold north and north-east winds by mountains covered with pine forests, and with a full southern aspect looking across the Rhone valley and facing the Dent du Midi and the majestic mountain peaks which surround Mont Blanc. It would be difficult to find a place more admirably adapted to the purpose for which it has been chosen, viz. the "open air" sanatorium treatment of tuberculosis. There are three large sanatoria : 1st, the Sanatorium Grand Hôtel, the dearest ; 2nd, the Sanatorium Mont Blanc, with prices rather less ; and 3rd, the Sanatorium Chamassain, with quite moderate prices (8 to 13 francs a day, inclusive terms). There are also two charitable institutions—the Popular Sanatorium and a small sanatorium for children.

It is wisely insisted upon that winter patients should "come in September, or, at the latest, October, and not in November only, as many do to their disadvantage ; they should arrive before the cold weather comes on in order to become acclimatised by degrees." The mean *winter* temperature at Leysin is 28·76° F., while that at Davos is 19·6° ; the annual range or variation is also reported to be less at Leysin than at Davos. "The absolute minimum has been −4·9° F. (January 7, 1895) ; at Davos, on the same day, it was – 14·8°; the absolute maximum is substantially the same, 80·6° F."

The average variation from day to day is not great, viz. about 3·8° F. in winter and 3·6° in spring. The mean relative humidity is small, being 61 per cent. in winter, while at Aigle, in the valley, it is 77 per cent. It has more sunshine in winter than Davos or Arosa, owing to the distance of the opposite mountains; in December (the darkest month) it may reach seven and a-half hours in the day. The mean amount of sunshine for the winter quarter is 50 per cent. of the *possible* sunshine. Fog is rare, occurring usually in the summer. As to wind, it is claimed for Leysin that it is "one of the best-sheltered stations in the Alps."

Leysin is very accessible, being reached by electric railway in an hour from Aigle station in the Rhone Valley. There are good paths through the pine woods, and skating and ski-ing are popular in the winter. English patients have not been numerous, hitherto, at Leysin, perhaps because of the absence of an English doctor, probably also because English patients do not like the restrictions of sanatorium life; but to the real invalid they are distinctly advantageous.

Montana (5,010 feet) is at no great distance from Leysin. It is situated high up on the mountain range which forms the northern boundary of the Rhone Valley, and therefore has a full south aspect. It is reached by carriage road in about two hours from Sierre, and nearly faces the grand peak of the Weisshorn and the opening of the Val d'Anniviers. The country around the hotel has been rightly described as a kind of natural park, with beautiful spacious green lawns and grand pine trees, and a number of small shallow lakes which give the impression of humidity. We think it better suited for a quiet, moderately bracing summer retreat than a winter residence.

There are certain other resorts in Switzerland of less altitude, but which are also frequented in winter by invalids, which we must briefly notice. Three of these are in the same district as Leysin, in the Alps of Vaudois, viz. Mont de Caux, Les Avants, and Glion.

Of these, **Les Avants** (3,212 feet) has been established for some years, and has acquired a well-merited reputation as a winter resort. It is in a beautiful situation open to and facing the south—looking over the upper part of the Lake of Geneva and on to the Dent du Midi. It is almost 2,000 feet above the lake and has the disadvantage of all such elevations, in the immediate vicinity of lakes, that mists will occasionally hang over it for hours in the early part of the day. But apart from this it has much to recommend it.

Its situation is very advantageous both on account of its accessibility and its protected character, and also because of its beautiful and varied walks on the wooded mountain sides.

It lies at the foot of the Col de Jaman, and is enclosed by mountains on all sides except to the south-west. It has much sunshine and a somewhat milder winter climate than the higher mountain resorts; the snow melts earlier, and may have disappeared at the beginning of March, so that the spring is a much more agreeable season than at some of the higher resorts, for the sloping inclination of the ground allows of the free draining away of the water from the melting snow.

The accommodation there is very good, and the place is very accessible, being connected with Montreux by a funicular railway, the transit occupying about three-quarters of an hour. Les Avants is also very popular as a summer resort, when it is often crowded with visitors.

Caux or **Mont de Caux** (nearly 4,000 feet) is very near Les Avants—less than an hour's walk—but it stands in a more open situation, the hotels being built on a small plateau which projects from the mountains behind it towards the Lake of Geneva; it therefore enjoys much less protection from prevailing winds, and although it is a winter as well as a summer resort, the managers of its palatial hotels (Grand Hotel and Caux Palace Hotel) announce that it "cannot be recommended to persons attacked by serious maladies, and, contrary to what is done at other alpine stations, those suffering from TUBERCULOSIS OR PHTHISIS WILL IN NO CASE BE RECEIVED." The cases they claim as suitable are, "weak and anæmic persons, convalescents, and those suffering from nervous disorders and heart affection."

The magnificent new Palace Hotel is fitted up with *hydrotherapeutic, medical, and electric baths.* While constructing this new hotel a *terrace* was also made nearly three-quarters of a mile in extent "commanding one of the finest views in the world," and suitable for the *sun cure*, and as a promenade and bicycle track. This terrace is lit up by electric lamps.

Caux is situated directly above Territet and Glion, and between the latter place and the Col de Jaman and the Rochers de Naye, where there is a mountain hotel, open in the summer, at an elevation of nearly 6,500 feet.

Both Caux and Les Avants have the advantage over resorts situated in inhabited valleys, traversed by carriage roads, in that they enjoy complete freedom from dust in summer.

Caux, like Les Avants, is a most popular summer resort, and is often very crowded in July, August, and September. A cog-wheel railway ascends from Territet, on the lake, to the Rochers de Naye, with stations at Glion, Caux, and Jaman.

Glion is only 2,400 feet above the sea, and although open both winter and summer it may be asscciated more closely with Montreux, and has none of the special characters of an altitude resort. It is especially useful as a transition resort in spring and autumn.

Quitting the Canton de Vaud, a few other mountain resorts of no great elevation, which are open for the reception of *winter* visitors, must be mentioned.

The most elevated of these is **Andermatt**, on the old St. Gothard road and also on the Oberalp route, about 4,700 feet above the sea. Although it has been open as a winter resort for some years it has never attained any great reputation, and it must be admitted it is not so well placed as, and has not any advantages which would lead to its selection in preference to, the other winter resorts we have referred to. It has, however, the convenience of being close to a station on an international line of railway (Göschenen). This circumstance, and its situation in the immediate neighbourhood of some of the grandest Swiss scenery, have made Andermatt a very suitable bracing summer resort, and it may be recommended to those who do not wish to go so far as the Engadine, or who prefer the scenery of Lucerne and the Oberland. It is also most convenient for those who propose to continue their journey into Italy.

Adelboden (4,660 feet) is both a winter and a summer resort, but " all the hotels and *pensions* have agreed collectively to *take no cases* of *tuberculosis*." It has a large skating rink, which is found very attractive in winter. The nearest railway station is Frutigen, from which it is a three hours' drive. It is near the Wildstrubel.

St. Beatenberg (3,750 feet) has a Kurhaus open for the reception of *winter* as well as summer guests. It lies on a sort of long natural terrace on the north side of the Lake of Thun, well protected by the mountains behind it from the north and east, and open to the south and south-west. It commands a fine view over the highest peaks of the Oberland, looks over the Lake of Thun, and faces the opening of the Simmenthal. It can be reached in about three hours by carriage from Interlaken or by funicular railway in fifteen minutes from Beatenbucht on the Lake of Thun.

Its climatic characters are not those of a high

mountain station and it must not be regarded as competing in any way with these. It differs from them in being mild and equable and having more cloud and more agitation of the air in winter. When the sky is clear the insolation in winter is intense. Its air is soothing, as well as tonic, and the possession of a nearly horizontal promenade, about three miles in length, offers a great boon to feeble persons who cannot climb, but who require much gentle exercise in the open air.

In winter it may be utilised as a resort for rest and convalescence, and as it has an early spring—the snow melting rapidly in the places exposed to the sun—it may be convenient as an intermediate station between high altitudes and the plains. As a resort in summer it is valuable in cases of chronic catarrh of the respirative mucous membrane, in those of predisposition to phthisis, or in its early stage without the presence of fever, and in slow convalescence from pleurisy and pulmonary affections generally. In winter its action is more tonic, and it may be resorted to by young patients of tuberculous or scrofulous families, or by those suffering from anæmic or neurotic conditions. It is also suitable to some forms of cardiac diseases—the air being mildly tonic and not exciting. It is a very popular summer resort.

Gossensass (3,600 feet), on the southern side of the Brenner Pass, with a station on the railway, about two hours from Innsbruck, has recently advanced claims to be considered a suitable winter resort for the same purposes and the same class of cases as Davos, with what amount of success we are not yet aware. It certainly appears to have some attractions as a summer subalpine resort for those who happen to be in the neighbourhood of Innsbruck or who are coming from Italy in that direction—the accommodation is good, the charges are moderate, and the surroundings attractive.

There are many distant mountain sanatoria and winter and summer resorts out of Europe. We shall reserve the consideration of such of these as are of chief interest until we have concluded our survey of the most popular and useful *summer* mountain resorts to accessible districts in Europe.

Summer Resorts.

If there are but few European mountain stations suitable for conversion into winter sanatoria, there are a very great number adapted for resort in summer. In the remainder of this chapter we shall endeavour to mention most of these and to describe briefly the chief of them.

It may be convenient to group these roughly into those having an elevation of over 6,000 feet, and possessing therefore a highly bracing climate; those with an elevation of between 5,000 and 6,000 feet, and having a decidedly bracing climate; those between 3,000 and 5,000 feet, and having a moderately bracing climate; and finally those below 3,000 feet, which still possess in some respects the character of mountain climates, but whose bracing quality depends much upon latitude, aspect, and surroundings, which is indeed more or less the case with all these resorts, as has been already explained.

The elevated *winter* resorts in the Engadine and elsewhere in Switzerland have been already described. Of *summer* resorts the hotel on the **Riffelberg**, the Riffelhaus, now connected with Zermatt by a mountain railway, is one of the highest in Europe, being 8,427 feet above the sea. The accommodation is fairly good, but the hotel is apt to be overcrowded in fine weather.

A more suitable place for the ailing in mind and body is the **Riffel-Alp**, about 1,000 feet lower. This hotel is in a magnificent position and is greatly resorted to by clergymen, schoolmasters, and professional men who need refreshment and rest from their labours. It is generally found too high for persons with feeble circulation and weak hearts and who are subject to attacks of congestion of the liver.

The hotels on the Gornergrat (10,250 feet) and at the Schwarzsee (8,490 feet) are too high for any invalids.

The hospice on the **Bernina Pass** (7,650 feet), about three hours from Pontresina, is one of the highest spots in Europe where any one has made a prolonged residence solely for the sake of health.* The food and accommodation there are both very fair, and there is a good carriage road which passes by the hospice, providing fairly level walks for those who do not wish to climb. The air is extremely dry and bracing, but the nights, as the writer can testify, are even in summer sometimes excessively cold, and one's very bed feels as if it had been "iced."

The Hôtel Weisshorn, above Vissoye, in Val d'Anniviers (7,690 feet), is in an exposed situation with very little shelter.

On the **Eggischhorn**, the Hôtel de la Jungfrau, 7,362 feet above the sea, offers good accommodation to those who desire to pass a few weeks in fine bracing air, close to one of the largest glaciers—the Aletsch—in the Alps. It is approached from Viesch, in the Rhone Valley, by a safe and not very steep bridle-track, in about three hours. Within ten minutes of the hotel is one of the finest panoramic views in the Alps—of the great peaks around Zermatt. It is also the best starting point for excursions on the Aletsch glacier, and for the ascent of some of the higher peaks of the Oberland.

The hotel on the **Bell-Alp**, on the opposite side of the Aletsch glacier to the Eggischhorn, is 7,153 feet above the sea. It is usually approached from Brieg, the terminus of the Rhone Valley Railway, by a mule-path, in four or five hours. The path is steep in points, and the ascent fatiguing to only moderate

* See "Safe Studies," by the Hon. Lionel Tollemache. Article on "The Upper Engadine."

walkers. Its nearness to a railway station makes it, perhaps, the most accessible high mountain resort in Switzerland, and it is a favourite resort of the English. The drawback, so far as invalids are concerned, is the difficulty of finding level walks. Excursions on the glacier involve a very steep descent in going and a very fatiguing ascent on returning. The ascent of the Sparrenhorn, a pyramidal summit (9,889 feet) rising just behind the hotel, is a walk of two and a-half hours, and from the summit there is a magnificent near view of the great Aletschhorn, and a glorious panorama of the peaks to the south of the Rhone valley.

There is a hotel at a rather lower elevation, the **Rieder Furka** (6,820 feet), and another on the **Rieder Alp**, 6,388 feet above the sea; the latter can be reached in two and a-half hours from the hotel on the Eggischhorn. It can be ascended from Morel, in the Rhone valley, in three hours. It is better adapted for invalids who wish to make a protracted stay in a high mountain resort than its higher neighbours.

There are two hotels on **Mount Pilatus**, but neither quite suited to invalids. The highest, the Hôtel Bellevue, 6,790 feet above the sea, is situated on the ridge between the two highest peaks, and is only eight minutes' walk from the summit. The other, the Hôtel Kleinsenhorn, 5,935 feet, is built on the saddle connecting two of the other peaks—the Oberhaupt and the Kleinsenhorn.

There is a very obvious objection to all resorts in isolated situations on or near mountain peaks, that in bad or misty weather there are no facilities for taking exercise such as can be had in great mountain valleys like the Engadine or at Davos.

There is a fair inn on the **Great Scheideck** (6,434 feet), reached in three hours from Grindelwald.

The Hôtel Jungfrau on the **Wengern Alp** has good accommodation (6,184 feet).

The hotel on the **Engstlen Alp** (6,033 feet) offers a pleasant resting-place amidst beautiful surroundings and the grandest mountain scenery. It is on the road from Meiringen to Engelberg by the Joch Pass, and is about five hours from the former place.

Arolla (6,572 feet), with a fair hotel (Hôtel du Mont Collen), is about three and a-half hours from Evolena by a bridle-path, and is situated at the top of the Val d'Hérens in a fine position opposite the grand pyramid of Mont Collen. It is surrounded by a wood of "Swiss" stone-pines, here called "arolla."

It is a fine bracing locality, fairly accessible, about eight or nine hours from Sion railway station, and well suited to those who wish for exercise in mountain air with quiet surroundings.

Chandolin (6,340 feet) is in a fine situation above St. Luc in the Val d'Anniviers.

On the southern side of the Alps, near **Airolo**, on the St. Gothard Railway, the Hôtel Piora (6,000 feet), in the valley of that name, offers a charming mountain retreat. It is built on a hill, in a sheltered position to the left of a sequestered lake—Lake Riton—in the vicinity of pine woods, and with fine views close at hand. It is about three hours' walk from Airolo.

Sulden (6,050 feet), a pleasant mountain resort with good accommodation in the Suldenthal, in the Ortler district, a valley branching off from the Stelvio road near Trafoi.

Many mountain inns not suitable for a prolonged stay we have not mentioned.

There are many resorts to choose from, amongst the next group, at an elevation of between 5,000 and 6,000 feet.

Perhaps the best known of these are the several resorts on the **Rigi**, which vary in elevation from the Hôtel du Rigi Kulm, about 5,800 feet, to the Hôtel du Rigi Kaltbad, 4,728 feet. At intermediate elevations are the Rigi Scheideck, 5,400 feet, the Rigi Staffel, 5,200 feet, and the Rigi First, 4,750 feet. These resorts are so well known that they do not need to be described. The Scheideck is perhaps the most suitable for invalids.

The **Rhone Glacier Hotel**, at an elevation of 5,750 feet above the sea, is nearly as high as that of the Rigi Kulm. It is well managed, and affords excellent accommodation for visitors, with the opportunity of breathing fine glacier air. Standing at the junction of the Grimsel and Furka Passes, it is apt to be overcrowded in the height of summer, and is, perhaps, too much resorted to by the passing tourist to be altogether suitable for the prolonged residence of invalids.

Santa Catarina (5,700 feet), in Val Furva, seven miles from Bormio. possesses, like St. Moritz, a fairly strong gaseous iron spring. Its situation is exceedingly beautiful, surrounded as it is by a semicircle of grandly shaped snow mountains. Situated on the southern side of the Alps and enclosed on nearly all sides by lofty mountains, its climate is less bracing than many resorts of less altitude,

The village of **Mürren**, 5,348 feet above the sea, is connected with Lauterbrunnen by funicular and electric railways.

It is very finely situated, opposite the precipitous western face of the Jungfrau, and is surrounded by very grand mountain scenery. It has good accommodation for a prolonged stay, and is very popular as a bracing resort in summer, owing to the protection it gets from high mountains close to it.

It is not so dry and bracing as might be expected from its elevation ; but it is well adapted for such as find a somewhat mild mountain air best suited to them.

On the south side of the Bernardino Pass, about thirty-six miles from Thusis, we find the village and baths of **San Barnardino**, at a height of 5,334 feet above the sea. It possesses a chalybeate spring, which is taken internally and used for baths. The place is much frequented by Italians during July and August. The hotel accommodation is fair, and the surrounding scenery is attractive.

Zinal (5,500 feet), in the Val d'Anniviers, is a favourite summer resort, reached in six hours from Sierre.

Zermatt, 5,315 feet above the sea, is well known to all mountaineers. It is in the midst of some of the finest mountain scenery in Europe; but it is more suitable for the active and hardy tourist than for the valetudinarian, unless he be a muscular one only needing rest of mind, in fine invigorating air and amidst grand scenery. It is readily accessible by a branch line from the Rhone Valley Railway.

Gressonay-la-Trinité (5,370 feet), and **Gressonay St. Jean**, nearly 1,000 feet lower, on the Italian side of Monte Rosa, are beautifully situated, and are favourite summer resorts of the Italians.

Ceresole Reale (5,290 feet), with chalybeate springs, is described in Part I.

In the **Adamello** district of the Italian Tyrol, near Pinzolo, at an elevation of about 5,000 feet, in a beautiful situation, is the Hôtel of **La Madonna di Campiglio**, close to the pilgrimage church of the same name. It is much resorted to in summer, and there are fine views and attractive excursions around.

Trafoi (5,080 feet), on the Stelvio road, has good accommodation.

The Karrersee (5,580 feet), in a most picturesque situation in the Dolomites of the Fassa, five hours from Botzen, has excellent accommodation, and is near shady woods.

There are a very great many resorts which have to be included in the next group, viz. those between 3,000 and 5,000 feet above the sea.

Macugnaga (4,354 feet), in the Val d'Anzasca, one of the most beautiful of the southern valleys of the Monte Rosa chain, affords excellent accommodation amidst the finest scenery. Lying on the south side of this great Alpine chain, it enjoys a milder climate than places of the same elevation on the north of it, and is well suited to those invalids who require a mildly bracing climate with, however, decidedly tonic properties.

Some of the highest of this group are found in the Dolomites. These are rather hot in mid-summer, and are better suited for the earlier or later part of the season. They can scarcely be recommended to invalids from England ; but for those who are already in Italy, and who do not wish to travel north, they may serve as useful summer quarters. The accommodation, of course, varies, but is very good in many.

Schluderbach (4,730 feet), **Höhlenstein** (4,615 feet), and, considerably lower, **Cortina** (3,970 feet), in the Ampezzothal, are all on the high road from Belluno, through the Val d'Ampezzo, to Toblach, in the Pusterthal.

In a beautiful situation, looking into thé **Primiero** valley, is the Hôtel **San Martino di Castrozza** (4,800 feet), in a sheltered position, with shady woods in the heart of the Dolomites.

The **Lago Mesurina** (5,760 feet), near Schluderbach and Monte Cristallo, has a good modern hotel.

Toblach (4,080 feet), **Wildbad Innichen** (4,370 feet), **Niederdorf** (3,800 feet), are all in the Pusterthal. In the beautiful Pragserthal are Alt-Prags, New Prags, and the Pragser-Wildsee, between 4,320 and 4,910 feet.

Heiligenblut, in Carinthia (4,600 feet), is an interesting and attractive resort. **Weissenstein**, with an old Schloss restored and converted into a hotel and *pension* (3,410 feet), with mineral baths, and near Windisch-Matrei, is suitable for a prolonged stay.

On the Brenner line, besides Gossensass, already mentioned, there are **Brennerbad** (4,390 feet), **Gries** (3,810 feet), and **Steinach** (3,430 feet) ; **Ladis** (3,880 feet), and **Obladis** (4,530 feet), near Landeck, in the Inn valley. The latter has been described as "one of the best sanitary establishments in the Tyrol."

Lengenfeld (3,820 feet), with sulphur waters in the beautiful Oetzthal.

Gastein (3,430 feet), described in Part I.

The Semmering Hotel (3,280 feet), near the **Semmering** Station, a favourite resort of Austrians.

Hospenthal, near Andermatt, on the St. Gothard road, between 4,700 and 4,800 feet, bracing and extremely accessible, offers very great facilities for interesting excursions in all directions.

The Hôtel Alpenclub (4,790 feet), in the beautiful **Maderaner-Thal**, is in an admirable situation for a quiet health resort. It can only be approached by bridle-path; it has fine pine woods close to it, affording both shade and shelter.

Pralognan (4,670 feet), in Savoy, is beautifully situated, and within a three hours' drive of Brides-les-Bains (*see* Part I., p. 116). It is open only in the summer, and is much out of the beaten track. It is well suited for an after-cure for those who have been taking the cure at Brides or Salins Moutiers.

The **Baths of Leuk**, at the foot of the Gemmi (4,600 feet), described in Part I., p. 234, afford excellent hotel accommodation in a situation easy of access.

Morgins (4,628 feet) is situated in the Val d'Illiez, and is approached by a good carriage road from Monthez, in the Rhone valley, near St. Maurice. It is not far from Champéry, but it is more than 1,000 feet higher. It is well protected from wind, and is freer from mist and fog than the somewhat lower elevations, and its air is decidedly bracing. It has a chalybeate spring, referred to in Part I., p. 268. It is too much enclosed to be bright and cheerful, and there is no distant view of snow mountains. It may be as well to notice **Champéry** (3,450 feet), in connection with Morgins, as it is also in the Val d'Illiez, and is reached from Monthez in three and a-half hours. It is the highest village in this valley (Morgins being in a side valley which opens to the west), and has a beautiful and cheerful situation. There are fine points of view in the neighbourhood, especially of the Dent du Midi. There are several good hotels and *pensions*, and these are much frequented by English people.

Champéry can be recommended as a bright, cheerful, and accessible mountain resort; but the climate is not very bracing, and mists occasionally settle there for a few hours at a time, especially in wet seasons.

Evolena, 4,521 feet above the sea, is approached from Sion in the Rhone valley by carriage road through the Val d'Hérens (six hours). It has a good hotel (H. de la Dent Blanche) and is picturesquely placed in a broad, grassy valley, surrounded by pine-clad hills, beyond which are snow-fields and glaciers. There are several glacier and mountain excursions to be made from Evolena.

Adelboden (4,450 feet), already mentioned amongst winter resorts.

Comballaz (4,416 feet), three miles from Sepey and fifteen miles from Aigle, in the Rhone valley, is an easily accessible mountain resort, and has good accommodation for visitors making a long stay. Beautiful excursions can be made in the neighbourhood.

Not far from Comballaz (about six miles) is **Ormond Dessus,** five hours from Aigle by *diligence*. It lies lower than Comballaz (3,832 feet). It has a good hotel and *pension* (Des Diablerets), and affords the most convenient head-quarters for exploring this interesting neighbourhood.

In a fine situation, about three hours' walk from Brunnen, on the Lake of Lucerne, is the **Stoos Hotel and Kurhaus** (4,342). The accommodation is fairly good, the air clear and bracing, the surroundings extremely beautiful. About an hour nearer Brunnen is the well-known Kurhaus Axenstein (2,330 feet), and a little lower the Hotel Axenfels. These command one of the finest views of the Lake of Lucerne.

Weissenstein (4,213 feet), in the Swiss Jura, is a very accessible mountain resort, being a three hours' drive from Soleure station. There is a large Kurhaus there, surrounded by woods and pastures. It is generally full in the summer. It has a very bracing climate, owing to its open situation.

"No spot commands a better view of the whole Alpine chain from Tyrol to Mont Blanc."

Villars sur Ollon (4,166 feet) is approached from Aigle. There is a *diligence* daily, which takes three to four hours to perform the journey. It commands fine views of the Rhone valley and the surrounding mountains, and has pleasant park-like grounds around, which offer many agreeable excursions. It is built on a plateau open to the south and protected by wooded hills from the north. It is somewhat exposed to mists in wet seasons, but is a most agreeable and bracing resort in fine ones.

A little below Villars there is good hotel accommodation at **Chesière** (3,970 feet), which commands a beautiful view.

The **Schröcken** (4,134 feet) is in a wild and grand situation in the Vorarlberg, between Bregenz and Arlberg. Numerous interesting excursions can be made into the mountains which surround it.

Courmayeur (3,986 feet), on the southern side of Mont Blanc, at the head of the Val d'Aosta, may be approached from Chamounix by mule-track, a journey which usually takes three days, and forms part of the "tour du Mont Blanc." It can also be reached by a good carriage road across the Little St. Bernard from Bourg St. Maurice in the valley of the Isère. From the south it would be reached easily viâ Aosta. It affords excellent hotel accommodation, it is surrounded by the grandest scenery, and its climate is mild, equable, and fairly dry. It is protected from the north by the Mont Blanc range. It is sometimes very warm in the height of summer, but the mornings and evenings are cool, and the dryness of the air renders the mid-day heat less oppressive. It is much frequented by Italians for its mineral waters and its mountain air.

Patients with chronic bronchial catarrh often find the summer climate of Courmayeur extremely agreeable and useful to them.

The hotel on **Monte Generoso** (3,970 feet), situated between the Lakes of Lugano and Como and approached by mountain railway from Capo-Lago, a port on the Lake of Lugano and a station on the St. Gothard line, is a pleasant summer resort and useful as an after-cure for those who have been taking baths in the vicinity or in Italy.

Alagna (Hotel Monte Rosa, 3,953 feet) is a mountain resort in the Val Sesia, one of the southern valleys of Monte Rosa, much frequented by the Italians, in a beautiful situation, eight hours from Macugnaga, over the Turlo Pass. It is easily reached from the south from Varallo.

Bad Gurnigel (3,783 feet), with important mineral springs, is fully described in Part I., p. 196.

St. Beatenberg (3,750 feet), above the Lake of Thun, is described amongst winter resorts, p. 587.

The **Schlucht**, with a hotel (French) on the summit (3,775 feet) and another (German), the Hotel Altenberg (3,300 feet), on the Alsatian side of the frontier, is a pass in the Vosges, between the French valley of Gérardmer and the Alsatian valley of Münster. It has very picturesque surroundings, and commands fine views of the Vosges mountains, and may be frequented as an after-cure by patients from Contrexéville and other spas in the vicinity.

The **Waldhaus-Flims** (3,620 feet), about one and a-half miles from Flims in the Vorder Rhein Thal, is beautifully situated in the midst of pine and beech woods, the walks through which are numerous and interesting. There is a small lake a few hundred feet below the Kurhaus where boating and bathing can be indulged in. It is well adapted as an after-cure for patients who have gone through a serious course of mineral waters. Some sixteen miles higher up the valley is **Dissentis** (3,773 feet). It has the disadvantage of being on the high road.

The village of **Gryon** (3,632 feet), seven miles from Bex, in the Rhone valley, is accessible by carriage road. It is situated on a sunny slope with fine views,

Chateau d'Oex (3,498 feet), accessible from Bulle by *diligence* in four and a-half hours—eighteen miles. It has several good hotels and *pensions*, and is a pleasant and popular summer resort, in a green open valley. It is moderately bracing. It is only seven miles from Chateau d'Oex to **Saanen** (Gesseney), 3,556 feet above the sea, with moderate accommodation, in the centre of the Gruyère cheese manufacture.

The baths of **Lenk** (3,630 feet) are described in Part I., p. 233.

Chaumont (3,845 feet), in the Jura Mountains, is reached in a drive of two hours from Neuchâtel. A forest of fir trees stretches down to the shores of the lake. There are nice level walks around the hotel, and good accommodation. It is protected towards the north, but is somewhat exposed to the east and west. The weather is sometimes cold and foggy, and the north-east wind occasionally makes itself felt unpleasantly.

Soglio (3,569 feet) is in a fine situation in the Val Bregaglia, above **Promontogno,** which is nearly 1,000 lower (2,681 feet). It should serve as a good transition resort between the Upper Engadine and the Italian lakes.

Chamounix (3,445 feet) is too much overrun by tourists to render it an eligible resort for invalids. Its climate is tolerably bracing, and in December and January many visitors go there for tobogganing, sleighing, and winter sports.

Grindelwald, in the Oberland (3,468 feet), lies in a healthy and sheltered situation, but has the drawback of being constantly overcrowded during the summer season. It gets a good deal of the *Föhn* wind in spring and autumn. It is much frequented in winter for skating and other winter sports.

St. Cergnes (3,460 feet), at the foot of the Dôle, the highest summit of this part of the Jura chain, is about six miles from Nyon, on the Lake of Geneva. Its accessibility and its picturesque situation have rendered it a very popular mountain resort in summer, especially for the Genevese. It is also the spot from which the Dôle is ascended, the ascent taking about three hours.

St. Cergnes is built at the bottom of a gorge exposed to the east, and is surrounded with pine woods. Its climate is "essentially tonic, but too irritating for persons impressionable to cold winds."

Höchenschwand (3,326), in the Black Forest, is one of the highest villages in the Duchy of Baden; it has good accommodation, a cool, refreshing climate in summer, and commands a magnificent view of the Alps. It is twelve or thirteen miles from Albbruck station on the Bâle-Waldshut railway.

Engelberg (3,315 feet) has much to recommend it as a mountain health resort, having a mild but, at the same time, somewhat bracing climate, adapted especially to nervous invalids who cannot support the exciting air of higher regions for any length of time. It is very accessible, being connected by a mountain railway with Stanstadt on the Lake of Lucerne (forty minutes from Lucerne by steamboat).

The hotel accommodation is excellent. Engelberg lies in a bright green valley almost completely surrounded by high mountains, and therefore much protected from winds. The valley is six miles long and about a mile broad. It is often resorted to by patients who have wintered in the south, and who require a mildly bracing climate for the summer months.

Les Avants (3,212 feet) is described with winter resorts, p. 585.

Klosters (4,190 feet the highest point) and **Bad Fideris** (3,580 feet), the latter referred to also in Part I., are easily accessible summer resorts in the Prättigau valley with stations on the railway between Landquart and Davos.

Seewis, about 3,000 feet above the sea, is in the same valley as the preceding, but nearer Landquart. This resort ought to be very serviceable for residence during the snow-melting time, in spring and early summer, for those who have passed the winter at Davos or in the Engadine. For the former it is very accessible.

The village has a complete southern exposure, and commands an extensive view over the lower half of the Prättigau. It is built on the southern slopes of the Vilan, which descend very steeply into the valley below Seewis, thus affording most perfect surface drainage during snow-melting or after heavy falls of rain. Pleasant walks through meadow and forests stretch up the mountain and around the village on all sides.

It is protected from the north and east by the Scesaplana, a mountain 10,000 feet high, and it has a mild and equable climate exceedingly free from wind.

There are a vast number of other health resorts at about 3,000 feet or lower in Switzerland, in the Tyrol, in Germany, especially in the Black Forest, and elsewhere, but although many of these are admirably bracing resorts, they scarcely present the special qualities of mountain climates, or only in a very modified degree.

The following list presents a choice of such resorts:

Gais, in Canton Appenzell, a pretty village, devoted in summer to the milk cure, and having an elevation of 3,060 feet.

Schönfels and **Felsenegg**, above *Zug*. 3,000 feet.

Achensee, a beautiful lake in North Tyrol, about sixty miles from Munich, with an hotel (Achensee-hof) much frequented in summer. About 3,000 feet.

Schluchsee, in the Black Forest, nine miles from St. Blasien; prettily situated in the midst of a pine forest, and popular as a summer resort. It has a bath establishment for warm baths. Elevation, 2,958 feet.

Magglingen, on the slope of a mountain, above Bienne and its lake. 2,900 feet.

Uetliberg Hotel, above *Zurich*. 2,860 feet.

Burgenstock, with a fine view over the lake, on the Lake of

Lucerne, with funicular railway; good hotel and shady walks. 2,850 feet.

Seelisberg, a well-known and popular resort above the Lake of Lucerne. 2,770 feet.

Frohburg, near Olten. 2,770 feet.

Vorder-Todtmoos, in the Black Forest, about ten miles from St. Blasien, in a picturesque situation. It has a pilgrimage church much resorted to. 2,693 feet.

Weissbad, three-quarters of an hour from Appenzell. 2,680 feet.

Obertsdorf, nine miles from Southofen station, and about fourteen from Immenstadt, in the Bavarian Alps; a favourite summer resort. 2,666 feet.

Heiden, above Rorschach, on the Lake of Constance. Milk cure in summer. 2,645 feet.

Vorauen, at the foot of the Glärnisch, and about eight miles from Glarus, on a beautiful little lake, the Klönsee, and amidst fine scenery. 2,640 feet.

Walchensee, a small village near the shore of the extremely picturesque lake of that name in the Bavarian Tyrol. It may be approached from Munich or Innsbruck. 2,630 feet.

Schliersee, on the lake of that name in the Bavarian Alps, between Innsbruck and Munich, and thirty-eight miles by rail from the latter; a beautiful spot, frequented in summer. 2,588 feet.

Waidring, four and a-half miles from the St. Johann station, on the Salzburg-Tyrol railway, and on the high road between Worgl and Reichenhall; much frequented in summer. 2,562 feet.

Appenzell. Milk cure in summer. 2,550 feet.

St. Blasien, in the Black Forest, sixteen miles from Albbruck and twenty from Waldshut stations; a popular summer resort in a protected situation, surrounded by pine-clad hills; open also in winter; fine views. 2,532 feet.

Zell-am-See, on the railway between Salzburg and Worgl, a beautiful retired situation on the shore of the Zellersee. 2,469 feet.

Thusis, three hours from Chur, at the entrance to the Via Mala. 2,450 feet.

Monnetier, on the Salève, near Geneva. 2,336 feet.

Schönbrunn, a hydropathic establishment near Zug. 2,300 feet.

Triberg lies in the heart of the Black Forest; it has a station on the railway between Offenburg and Constance. There is a fine waterfall close at hand. It is a pleasant and popular summer resort. 2,245 feet.

Charnex, beautifully situated above Clarens. 2,231 feet.

Gérardmer, a popular and pleasant resort in the French Vosges, with a pretty lake and a hydropathic establishment, much resorted to by the people of Nancy and neighbouring towns, and as an after-cure by patients from adjacent spas. 2,200 feet.

Hohwald, in the Vosges, nine miles by carriage-road from Barr railway station, in a sheltered and picturesque situation; much frequented in summer. 2,198 feet.

The **Geissbach Hotel**, above the Lake of Brienz, and near the celebrated falls, with good accommodation, but overcrowded with tourists. 2,166 feet.

Kochel, on the Kochelsee, in the Bavarian Alps. 1,963 feet.

Starnberg, on the lake of that name (also called Würmsee); about seventeen miles from Munich by rail; crowded in summer. 1,945 feet.

Cheimsee Hotel, fifty-six miles from Munich and sixteen from Rosenheim, on the line of railway between Munich and Salzburg. 1,745 feet.

Divonne, three and a-half miles from Coppet, on the Lake of Geneva, a well-known hydropathic establishment. 1,543 feet.

Distant Mountain Resorts.

Out of Europe there are several elevated resorts for the treatment of consumption and other maladies which, though distant, are becoming well known, and are resorted to occasionally by European invalids. In the Peruvian Andes, near the city of **Lima**, there are some elevated resorts which have afforded some of the best results that have ever been obtained from the climatic treatment of phthisis. It must be remembered that in regions near the equator, even elevations of 7,000 or 8,000 feet have a temperature in winter as high as our own summer temperature, and higher elevations than these have often to be resorted to.

The **Valley of the Jauja river**, in the Peruvian Andes, reaches an elevation of from 8,000 to 10,500 feet. The towns of **Turma, Jauja,** and **Huancayo** are the chief resorts for consumptive patients from Lima. At Huancayo (or at Jauja, which is cooler) the sky is said to be always clear and sunny, the atmosphere always pure and bracing, and the temperature very equable, the annual range not exceeding 10 or 12° F. Invalids are enabled to take much out-door exercise and to be constantly in the open air.

Other resorts in the Andes or the Cordilleras which have been found well suited to the treatment of consumption, actual or threatening, are the following:

Santa Fé de Bogota, the capital of the United States of Colombia, lies on a plateau at an elevation of 8,665 feet, and is in much local repute; as also is **Quito**, the capital of Ecuador, at about the same elevation.

Cuzco, the ancient capital of Peru, is higher, 11,400 feet; and **La Paz**, in Bolivia, still higher, 12,200 feet.

But none of these resorts is so suitable for European invalids as many others that are more accessible.

Consumptive patients in Brazil are usually sent to the high resorts in the Cordilleras. Other mountains of the Argentine Republic offer many suitable sites for sanatoria for pulmonary invalids.

These mountain districts extend, at higher or lower elevations, from the province of Cordoba to the valley of Rimac.

The mountains of Cordoba are preferable for consumptive patients to the Andine heights of Bolivia, as they contain a greater variety of objects to divert the attention and amuse.

The ancient city of **Mexico** lies on an extensive plateau from 6,000 to 8,000 feet above the sea level, surrounded by mountains, and having a temperate and agreeable climate, well suited to the treatment of pulmonary tuberculosis. The same may be said of the city of **Puebla**, seventy-six miles east-south-east of Mexico, which is also situated on a high plateau, 7,215 feet above the sea.

The Rocky Mountains, in Colorado, United States, possess several elevated stations which are used as sanatoria for consumptive patients. **Denver** is the best known of these to Europeans. It is situated at an elevation of 5,280 feet, and has a cool, dry, and stimulating climate. The rainfall there is small, the annual mean being 14½ inches, and Denver also has many clear days, 42 per cent. as compared with 27 in New York, allowing therefore of much out-door exercise. Its mean annual temperature is 47° F. September and October are the best months for commencing residence there; the patient then gets gradually acclimatised to the cold in winter, which is at times very severe. The days are warm and bright, but the nights are very cold, and indeed are cool all the year round. There is not much snow, and that falls mostly in early spring. There is a good deal of disagreeable wind during the spring months. From the middle of September to the middle of April there is scarcely any rain. Changes of temperature are often sudden and extreme, and precautions have to be taken against chill. The city of Denver stands about fifteen miles east of the foot of the mountains. One of the drawbacks to Denver as a sanatorium for invalids is the fact that it is a populous city, with the amusements and excitement inseparable from such a place. It possesses good hotels and lodging-houses, and there are many sanatoria for consumptive patients. The lower part of the city has a damp soil. To those who need not only a cure, but an occupation or a career, Denver may furnish one.

There is also an excellent sanatorium at **Boulder,** in the heart of the Rocky Mountains, at an elevation of 5,500 feet, twenty-five miles north-west of Denver. It is the seat of the Colorado State University.

Seventy-five miles south of Denver is **Colorado Springs,** a city with 21,000 inhabitants. It is situated on a plateau five miles from the foothills of the Rocky Mountains and six from the base of Pike's Peak, at an elevation of 6,000 feet above the sea. So that while Denver is about the altitude of Davos, Colorado Springs is about the altitude of St. Moritz Kulm. Its situation is a very sheltered one, and the town being built over a large area, there is plenty of ground around most of the dwelling-houses. The streets are wide and lined with shady trees. The ground has a very gentle slope from north to south. There is a top soil of two feet resting on seventy feet of sand and gravel, which is very porous, so that there is a perfect natural drainage. A supply of pure water is obtained from the mountain-side six miles off. The air is dry, the relative humidity in winter being 50 per cent. The mean annual rainfall is 15½ inches. There are high winds in March and April. There are two good sanatoria there, and camping out in tents is practicable during a considerable part of the year. There are several good boarding-houses and comfortable villa residences. Farm produce is good and of moderate price, but luxuries are dear. There are plenty of horses and carriages to be hired, and the rides and drives around are numerous and interesting. There is no lack of pleasant society, or of churches, schools, and places of entertainment. But there is no saloon or public bar in the town, the sale of liquor being prohibited.

There are some other less frequented altitude resorts in the Rocky Mountains. The following may be mentioned: **Cañon City** at an elevation of 5,360 feet, situated south of Pike's Peak. It has hot mineral springs used in the treatment of rheumatism. It is warmer and dryer than Denver or Colorado Springs.

Glenwood (5,600 feet), 160 miles west of Denver, is an excellent winter resort on account of its sheltered position. It lies in a protected valley on the western slope of the Rocky Mountains. It is much less windy and dusty than the resorts on the eastern slope. Glenwood has many thermal springs.

Estes Park (7,300 feet), **Manitou Park, San Lui Park,** and many others are as yet undeveloped as resorts for invalids.

In these Rocky Mountain resorts there is great variation between sun and shade and day and night temperature; but they have very many clear days and great dryness of atmosphere. The most agreeable seasons are autumn and early winter; the spring is windy and changeable, and the summer rather too hot; but during the hot summer months invalids camp out or go to higher resorts.

Comparing these with the Swiss altitude resorts, it has been pointed out that the latter are more enclosed and less open, with a colder and rather moister climate, but with less wind and dust. Owing to the very few days in winter during which snow lies on the ground at Colorado Springs the visitors escape the disagreeable snow-melting period in the spring which is so trying in the Swiss resorts.

There is more possible and more actual sunshine in winter at Denver and Colorado Springs than at Davos or St. Moritz. On the other hand, Colorado Springs has occasionally very disagreeable dust storms, accompanied by a very dry and electric state of the atmosphere.

For those who like a sea voyage and who do not fear a long and somewhat rough land journey, the South African highlands present many attractions with their very dry and bracing climate, hot summers, and cold winters. But it is difficult to write about South African resorts at present, and until the country gets more settled. We may, however, say that **Bloemfontein**, 4,700 feet above the sea, has a considerable reputation as a sanatorium for persons with delicate chests. Its climate has proved very valuable in arresting phthisis. It is very dry, having a mountain range between it and the Indian Ocean to the east, and having an extensive plateau of dry, open country to the north and west. Its summers are very hot, its winters very cold, but the dryness of the air enables invalids to bear these extremes of temperature without suffering any injury.

There are many other elevated resorts in South Africa, in the Orange River Colony, and in the Transvaal, but it is clear that they can only be suited at present to a very limited class of invalids, and, in the present somewhat unsettled condition of these countries, it is better to await developments.

CHAPTER VII.

WINTER QUARTERS.

A Review of some Winter Health Resorts.

In searching for a winter health resort, what do we desire to avoid, and what do we desire to find? There are three things which we desire to avoid, especially when they are found combined, as in our own winter climate, and these three things are damp, cold, and variability. It is the combination of these three conditions which makes the winter climate of England so unsuitable to many persons. It is responsible for the catarrhal conditions which are so common, and which often lead to greater disturbances of health. To it is due the prevalence of chronic rheumatism, and of many forms of neuralgia, and not unfrequently its chilling influence determines in delicate persons the occurrence of serious inflammation of internal organs. The combination of climatic conditions necessarily associated with a clouded and sunless sky produces also a depressing effect on the mind and spirits. The more sensitive the organisation, the more acutely will these unfavourable conditions be felt.

What we seek, then, in a winter climate is the opposite of these conditions, viz. dryness, warmth, and equability. But it is always difficult to get all we want; besides, as a matter of fact, while some invalids require a combination of warmth and moisture, others need warmth and dryness, while others do better in a combination of cold and dry air; but no one wants a combination of cold and damp, and all desire sun-heat, a clear sky, and as much of it as possible; and we shall find, as a rule, that *the value of a winter climate depends on the number of clear and sunny days, or the number of days and hours during which an invalid*

U

can take exercise or be in the open air. The mere absolute amount of rainfall seems of small importance, provided the nature and inclination of the soil are such that the water drains off rapidly from the ground, and that there are long or frequent intervals of clear, sunny skies. Indeed, occasional heavy rains often have a salubrious effect in cooling and cleansing the atmosphere. It seems also clear that diurnal variability of temperature, even within wide limits, does not render a climate unhealthy even to invalids, if it is also a dry climate and the invalid learns to protect himself from the danger of sudden chill. Nor does humidity, when accompanied with moderate warmth, seem to be necessarily unwholesome, especially in marine climates. In all these matters individual peculiarities have to be taken into account. There are many other details which cannot be considered here. With regard to the expense attending a change of winter quarters, we are content to quote the words of Dr. Samuel Johnson: "Sir, your health is worth more than it can cost."

Within the limits at our disposal an exhaustive survey of the whole series of winter health resorts would be impossible. It will be expedient, therefore, to confine our attention to those which are tolerably accessible. We have, in other chapters, entered fully into the question of the utility and scope of high mountain health resorts in winter.

We will now give our attention, in the first place, to **Egypt**, which has, since the British occupation, become a very popular winter resort, its climate resembling in some respects the climate of high mountain valleys. It is dry and exhilarating, and it presents a wide range between day and night temperatures, depending upon the powerful heating effects of the sun's rays during the day, and the great and rapid radiation, after sunset, of the heat absorbed during the day, into clear cloudless space. The climate of Upper Egypt is, however, on the whole a more reliable climate than that of any high mountain valley, and less subject to variations. The objections to Egypt are its distance, and the expense attending the journey; and, moreover, whichever route you select, it is impossible to avoid a sea voyage of at least three days.

There is only one period of the year when Egypt is visited as a health resort, and that is from the middle of November to the beginning of April, when it is considered to have the "finest climate in the world." There are several routes from England to Egypt. The shortest is that through Italy to Brindisi. From Brindisi to *Port Saïd* is a three days' voyage by steamer. In this way the journey to Egypt is accomplished in five or six days. The longest but least fatiguing for those who do not mind a sea voyage, is that by P. and O. boat from London to Port Saïd, which takes twelve or thirteen days. There is a third route viâ Marseilles, at which port all the large P. and O. steamers call. This is, perhaps, the most popular and convenient route. It is important to leave Egypt before the heat becomes too great—*i.e.* not later than the middle of April—and as the transition from the climate of Egypt to that of England should not be abrupt it is undesirable to return to England before the end of May. The interval may be conveniently spent in a variety of places of interest, in Syria, Italy, Greece, or some of the islands of the Mediterranean. If it is thought best to remain later in Egypt, Ramleh, near Alexandria, in Lower Egypt, is the most suitable place at this period of the season.

The chief characteristic of the climate of Egypt is its dryness.

"In the richly wooded districts of the equatorial regions of Africa, where the numerous affluents of the Nile take their rise, almost continuous rains prevail; but in the deserts of Nubia and Upper Egypt, through which the great river flows in its course to the sea, sometimes years pass without a single shower. The absence of rain and absence of vegetation are obviously related to one another. The Mediterranean coast and the Delta are less dry than the upper parts of the country, and Cairo occupies an intermediate position."—(*Flower.*)

We have the authority of the same writer for the statement that in an exceptionally wet season there were only eleven days out of one hundred and fifty in which rain fell, and on some of these it was scarcely more than a few drops. The days, as a general rule, are much like one another, fine, clear, bright, and sunny. Another characteristic of the winter climate of Egypt is the warmth or heat of the day (70° to 75° F. in the shade, and very much higher in the sun), as contrasted with the coldness, freshness, and heavy dews of the nights. In the night the thermometer often falls to 40° F. or lower, seldom quite to freezing-point, so that there is a very considerable range between the day and night temperature, as there also is between sun and shade temperature. It has been justly observed that this is an advantage to many constitutions—that a sultry night following a hot day often induces languor and depression, and that the freshness of the Egyptian night and early morning is invigorating and bracing, and enables one better to bear the fatigues and heat of the day. Persons with delicate chests must be careful to protect themselves by appropriate clothing, and by retiring before nightfall, to avoid the sudden change from the day to the night temperature, which they might otherwise find trying or injurious. The air of the desert—that is, all the country above the level of the autumnal overflow of the Nile—is universally admitted to be most invigorating; a refreshing breeze, in winter at least, generally tempers even the heat and glare of the mid-day sun, and in the morning and evening it is decidedly cool. Nowhere, on land, is air so pure, as nowhere else is there such complete absence of all decomposing organic matters in the soil; it has been well compared with the air of the open sea.

The thing of chief importance for the invalid in

Egypt is to breathe as much of the desert air as possible. It has been objected to **Cairo*** that the hotels and all the modern houses are built on low ground, which, until reclaimed, used to be subject to the overflow; and that the whole of the ancient city, with its crowded population and filthy streets, is between them and the desert; that the prevailing winds, being from the north, blow directly across the Delta. "This, and the great amount of not very clean dust which fills the air of a great city full of people and animals, form the principal drawbacks to Cairo as a residence for invalids." But it is not necessary for the invalid to live in Cairo, for the hotel at the Pyramids (*Mena House*) is within half an hour by electric tram of the city, and affords excellent accommodation in purer, fresher, and dryer air than at Cairo. Mena House is one of the best hotels in Egypt, and is open from Nov. 1st to May 15th. It is built at the foot of the Pyramids, and has golf links close by and a large swimming bath, facilities for quail shooting, and other attractions. Or the invalid can find suitable quarters at **Helouan les Bains**. Of its sulphur baths we have already given an account in Part I. (p. 203); it is therefore only necessary to add a few words with regard to its climate as compared with that of Cairo. Helouan is about sixteen miles to the south of Cairo, and about three miles from the Nile and 144 feet above it. It is built on a desert plateau at the foot of the Tura Hills. It has good hotels and a great number of villas, and frequent trains connect it with Cairo, the journey taking about half an hour. It has good golf

* It is interesting to note what Professor Peterson, of New York, says of Cairo. "In winter one may spend some very miserable, cold, damp days in Cairo. I experienced about Christmas time last year four most uncomfortable rainy and cold days in succession in Cairo." The same writer observes: "The desert is sometimes piercing cold at night. Water in a shallow dish will occasionally freeze on exposure to a desert night wind."

links, and is well provided with distractions. It is surrounded by desert, and its air is therefore very free from organic or other impurities. On an average it has nearly eight hours of daily sunshine during the winter months, and its atmosphere seems to be a little warmer, as well as dryer and freer from dust than that of Cairo. Its relative humidity in winter varies between thirty and sixty per cent.; in Cairo it is 63·2.

Many invalids will doubtless prefer to go on, by rail or Nile steamer, to Upper Egypt, and pass the winter at Luxor or Assouan. Others will take the costly Nile voyage in a dahabeeah, and a few may determine to camp out in the desert.

Luxor, 450 miles from Cairo, is reached by Nile steamer in five and a-half days, or by rail (express sleeping cars) in sixteen to seventeen hours. The latter is best for most invalids, especially if they arrive late in the season. Luxor has an admirable climate from November to the middle of March, when it gets too hot. It is warmer, dryer, and sunnier, and has less wind, than Cairo and its suburbs. It is practically rainless—one or two brief showers being all that has been observed in the winter months.

Invalids can be in the open desert air for a great number of hours daily, and its effects are most tonic and stimulating.

The prevailing wind is from the north. The drawbacks to Luxor are that, being close to some of the most interesting monuments of Egypt, its hotels are, in the height of the season, overcrowded, and the place is overrun by swarms of tourists. Invalids should arrive early in the season, before the end of November, so as to make sure of good accommodation, which should be engaged beforehand.

Assouan is 130 miles south of Luxor, and close to the first cataract. It is connected by rail with Luxor. The town stands high above the river. It is drier and warmer than Luxor, but is said to be more windy. Overcrowding in the height of the season was at one time complained of, but hotel accommodation has been, of late years, greatly increased. Assouan has all the characters of the Egyptian climate in a very marked degree, viz. warmth, dryness, almost uninterrupted sunshine, and purity of air from the desert. Its mean minimum temperature in winter, occurring just before sunrise, has been found to be 6° or 7° F. higher than at Luxor or Cairo, a fact of importance to certain invalids.

"The relative humidity is so low that dew never falls, and the annual rainfall is hardly measurable." Risk of chill at nightfall to the invalid is said to be much less than at other Egyptian resorts.

Of the Nile voyage, made in a dahabeeah, little need be said here in the way of description.

"It is a perfect rest from nearly all the little cares and troubles of the world; the weather is almost always fine, so that nearly the whole day may be spent on deck, and the variety and exercise of a walk on shore can generally be got at some time or other in the twenty-four hours; the life on board a dahabeeah is generally a healthy one. It is essentially an out-of-doors, country life. The air, though perhaps not equal to that of the higher parts of the desert, is pure and bracing; for, owing to the narrowness of the strip of fertile land on the sides of the river, the air is practically that of the desert. On the first subsidence of the water, after the autumnal overflow, the banks are muddy and damp, so it is well not to take to the water until December, by which time they are well dried by the sun, though January, February, and March are the best months. The higher the river is ascended, so the salubrity increases. The nights are generally clear, bright, and cool, and warm clothing is essential."—(*Flower.*)

As to camping out in the Nubian desert under tents, Sir Hermann Weber testifies that in his experience it has given results "in several advanced cases of consumption altogether superior to any obtained from any health resort, or from any other treatment."

Egypt as a winter resort has, then, the following advantages: 1. It is almost rainless, especially in upper Egypt; at Cairo the rainfall is a little over one inch annually. There are heavy dews at night along the Nile and in the desert near the Nile. 2. It has a generally dry and clear atmosphere; attended, it is true, with great changes of temperature in the twenty-four hours, a circumstance which proves invigorating rather than otherwise, if the invalid is careful to protect himself from the sudden fall of temperature at sunset, as well as through the cold nights. 3. Extreme cold, as marked by the thermometer, is excessively rare. The mean winter temperature at Cairo is about 58° F., that of the coldest month (January) is 53·6° F., and it rarely falls below freezing-point. 4. Its climate allows of constant exercise in the open air, and exposure, therefore, to the tonic effect of fresh air and sunlight. The climate of the desert has been found to be dryer and to have a much smaller daily range than that of adjacent towns.

Invalids doing the Nile voyage should be careful not to expose themselves, on coming down the river, to the cold north wind when it blows strongly, as it does sometimes for days together, and as there is a great fall of temperature at sunset they should always retire to the saloon a little before sun-down.

The climate of Egypt then is tonic and stimulating, and is useful in a great variety of chronic ailments, the chief of which are the following: In cases of early phthisis or in those cases of torpid phthisis which have a tendency, even in this country, to run a protracted course; it is of great value in chronic gout and rheumatism, and in those vascular and renal changes which gout induces; catarrhal conditions find relief and cure there, so that cases of chronic bronchial, laryngeal, and pharyngeal catarrh get well in Egypt, as do also some cases of asthma. Certain forms of anæmia, persons suffering from exhaustion of the nervous system from too great excitement, worry, or undue application to business or study, are precisely the cases for the Nile voyage. The same may be said of those numerous cases of intractable dyspepsia associated with over-work or worry. Cases of Bright's disease, when not too far advanced, are often greatly benefited by the warm, dry air of Upper Egypt.

The climate of Egypt is not limited simply to the cure of *early* phthisis, but advanced chronic cases often do well there, though it is considered inexpedient that they should venture on the Nile voyage or go beyond the neighbourhood of Cairo. Cases of febrile phthisis with a tendency to rapid progress in irritable or highly nervous constitutions must not, however, be sent to so exciting a climate. The same remarks apply to cases with a tendency to hæmorrhage.

As the journey to Egypt is long and costly, it is desirable that invalids should not undertake it without realising clearly the nature of its climate; we therefore wish to recapitulate and enforce certain drawbacks to be encountered, and certain precautions to be taken.

Although a *warm* climate, it is one in which invalids may feel uncomfortably cold, and there is always danger of chill at sunset. Sensitive persons will tell you they "never felt so cold anywhere as in Egypt," which is owing to frequent cold high winds and the great difference between sun and shade, and day and night, temperature; this is especially the case round Cairo, and on the Nile, and in the months of December and January. The cold *felt* is quite out of proportion to the temperature registered by the thermometer. Coming down the Nile, facing the north wind, the cold, after sunset, is intense. It follows that invalids need more warm clothing there than at home, and should bring their furs; they should be indoors before sunset, and should not go out till two hours after sunrise; they should avoid over-fatigue in sight-seeing. The *steamboat* voyage

U *

on the Nile is unsuited to invalids; it is attended with too much wind and too much exposure to unavoidable changes of temperature. Invalids whose destination is Upper Egypt should get there fairly early in the season, and not remain at Cairo after the middle of December, indeed, it is better to leave Cairo and the Pyramids until the return journey—after the middle of February; between these periods it may be cold, windy, and in some seasons even rainy there, while before December it is apt to be damp, on account of the recent inundation of the plains of Lower Egypt. Then there are always *mosquitoes* in Cairo, while they are absent in the desert—but in March and April the *flies* are a torment all over the country.

Then there is the hot *Khamseen* wind, which blows in the spring and is depressing to most people, and is laden with fine dust that proves very irritating to the lungs. This wind begins in February and blows for a day or two at a time till the middle of April.

The diseases that are apt to be induced by chill are diarrhœa, dysentery, and pneumonia, and if great care is not taken in consuming only perfectly pure water, to these may be added typhoid! As to the cases that should not be sent to Egypt, it ought not to be necessary to say that no cases of advanced organic disease should be sent there; cases of tabes do not do well there, nor do hypochondriacal neurotics, nor persons troubled with habitual insomnia not due to worry or over-work.

Beyrout and **Haifa**, on the coast of **Syria**, have been recommended as winter resorts; especially the slopes of Lebanon *above* Beyrout, which afford an excellent climatic resort for those who have wintered in Egypt and who do not wish to return at once to Europe. Brumana and Alai have been mentioned as suitable places in the neighbourhood of Beyrout. "The valleys of Lebanon offer attractions unsurpassed by mountain scenery in any part of the world. Haifa is quieter than Beyrout and less civilised. There is a German colony there. The adjacent monastery of Carmel is an attraction."

Haifa is about ten miles from Acre, and twenty-two from Nazareth. As a winter resort it combines comfort with economy. "It is impossible to conceive a more agreeable climate during the winter months than it offers. The climate of Carmel is exceptionally bracing and healthy; while the beauty of its situation, commanding a lovely view of the Bay of Acre and the encircling hills of Palestine, over-topped by the snow-clad Hermon, is remarkable. An Austrian Lloyd's steamer touches there once a fortnight, either from Beyrout or Alexandria."*

The tonic and stimulating climates of Davos and Upper Egypt on the one hand, and the soft soothing climate of Madeira on the other, may be regarded as at the two extremes of winter health resorts for European invalids. **Madeira** has been overrated and underrated. It is apt to suffer from those violent oscillations of medical opinion to which all health resorts are liable. It suffered, when it was believed that all consumptives should winter in the high mountains; and when it was shown that many consumptives did remarkably well at Teneriffe, Madeira shared in a measure the popularity of Orotava. Now, we are informed, it has suffered greatly through the popularity of open-air sanatoria at home!

Situated between 32° and 54° N. lat., in the Atlantic Ocean, about 500 miles from the west coast of Africa, it is a typical representative of a warm and humid marine climate. The beauty and diversity of its landscapes and the richness of their colouring give this island a special charm for artistic natures.

Writing of Madeira, the late Dr. Lambron, of Luchon, calls it "la première résidence hivernale du monde,"† and the late Dr. Andrew Combe wrote:

* *Blackwood's Magazine.* † "Choix d'une résidence d'hiver."

"*If I must go abroad*, I shall most likely return to Madeira, on the simple ground that, if I must forego the pleasures of home, it is better to resort at once to the *most* advantageous climate," etc. It is now, we believe, sufficiently well understood that the climate of Madeira is only suited to a limited and carefully selected class of cases; but for the proper cases it is a climate of the greatest utility. If we bear this fact in mind, we shall be able to reconcile the wide discrepancies which we find in authoritative and evidently unprejudiced statements about this island. Madeira is the type of what is termed an oceanic climate, *i.e.* a climate essentially soft and equable. It is also moist and sedative, and, no doubt, to persons with considerable constitutional vigour it seems relaxing and depressing. But to certain persons in a state of great debility, with much feebleness in the organs of circulation; in cases of irritative, chronic bronchitis with scanty secretion, and complicated with emphysema; in some cases of advanced consumption, and particularly those complicated with repeated attacks of bronchitis, even cases that have seemed quite hopeless, a prolonged residence in the climate of Madeira has been attended often with most remarkable amelioration. The feeble flickering lamp burns longer there than in a more stimulating and tonic air, and now and then it seems to gather renewed power and burns up again with some of its old lustre. The sedative atmosphere allays cough in cases of irritable respiratory mucous membrane, but it often causes loss of appetite and bilious disturbance in persons predisposed to such disorders. It would seem to be more useful in cases of chronic laryngeal and bronchial catarrh, and emphysema, than in phthisis. It is also suitable to persons of feeble circulation, who cannot bear bracing treatment, and who enjoy a sea climate.

Funchal, the capital of the island, is the principal resort (there are also some hill stations available); it is built in the form of an amphitheatre, and looks very beautiful from the sea. It is surrounded by luxuriant vegetation, and tropical fruits ripen there all the year round. It is protected by mountains, which rise to nearly 6,000 feet, from winds from the north, north-east, and north-west. One drawback, however, is the difficulty of getting level walks.

The climate of Funchal is extraordinarily equable. The mean annual temperature is about 65° F. The night temperature scarcely ever descends below 48° F., and the day temperature scarcely ever rises above 86° F. The mean winter temperature is 61°, the mean spring temperature 62°, the mean summer temperature 69°, the mean autumn temperature 67°, and the mean difference between the day and night temperature is only 9° F. The temperature of the sea varies between 63° and 75° F. As might be expected, there is considerable humidity of atmosphere, the mean humidity being from 70° to 74° F.; but this varies greatly with the changes in the air currents. There are on an average fifty rainy days in the winter six months, eighty-five in the whole year. Funchal is occasionally visited by violent storms of wind, but as it is protected by mountains from the prevailing wind, the north-east, the atmosphere is generally calm from 7 to 9 a.m.; then breezes blow in from the sea till 8 or 9 p.m.; and the land wind sets in late at night. The air, though humid, is not felt by many to be unpleasantly so, while it is pure and free from dust.

The climate, then, though very equable, is not felt to be relaxing except by a few persons, and it must be remembered that there are great differences of climate to be found in different parts of the island. There are villas to be procured at various altitudes adapted for winter or summer quarters, so that there is no necessity for the invalid to leave the island during the hot summer season. The hotel keepers are always willing to make arrangements to provide invalids with such summer quarters.

The autumnal rains set in at Funchal in October, and last till the end of the year. The rain is not continuous, but, like our heavy April showers, with intervening sunshine. Usually some heavy gales are felt about the beginning of the year from south-south-west. Then continuous fine weather sets in in February, and winter is over. It is usual to sleep with open windows at Funchal, for there is an entire absence of that chill at sunset so commonly experienced in the south of France, and there is no dew-fall.

Besides the maladies I have already named, the climate is said to be particularly suitable to cases of chronic dysentery and malarial fever. Visitors usually live in hotels. There are villas also for families. There is an English club and a good library; good horses are also to be obtained. Steamers leave London and Southampton for Madeira weekly. There is a tendency to suffer from diarrhœa on first arriving in the island.

The **Azores**, a group of islands (38° 30′ N. lat.) in the Atlantic Ocean, 800 miles from the coast of Portugal, possess a climate resembling that of Madeira. There is even greater humidity of atmosphere, however, for "paper hangings will not adhere to the wall, and the veneering of furniture strips off." The principal island, St. Michael, has two chief places of resort, Ponta Delgada and Villa Franca. In the island of Fayal there is also Horta as a place of resort. These islands have frequently been visited by earthquakes. St. Michael possesses numerous hot springs which are renowned for the treatment of cases of chronic rheumatism, skin diseases, and syphilis. Accommodation is very limited.

The **Canary Islands** (28° 15′ N. lat.), possess a warmer and dryer climate than Madeira or the Azores. These islands, under the name of "The Fortunate Islands," have been renowned since ancient times for their beauty and salubrity, but the main interest of invalids will naturally be directed to those places in them that have been chosen and frequented in recent times as health resorts. Of these the chief are Las Palmas in Grand Canary, and Orotava in Teneriffe, and in the latter island also the port of Santa Cruz, and some elevated resorts, as Laguna, Guimar, Tacaronta, and Vilaflor. La Palma, one of the most westernly of the islands, is occasionally visited for its beautiful scenery, and has a fair hotel at its port—Santa Cruz—but it is not a resort for invalids.

Las Palmas, three and a-half miles from the port of Grand Canary, is the nearest of these resorts to the African coast, being only 120 miles from the desert of Sahara and about fifty miles from Teneriffe. The island is very mountainous, rising in its centre to an elevation of 6,000 feet, so that mountain as well as coast climate can be found there for summer residence. Hotel accommodation can be obtained at an elevation of 1,300 feet.

Las Palmas has a dry, almost African climate, and it is sufficiently distant from the mountainous centre of the island to be unaffected by the clouds which collect over the central summits, so that it has habitually a clear sky and much sunshine; the mean temperature in the coldest month of the year (January) is 61° F., as compared with 49·5° at Mentone. The average daily range of temperature for the winter months is about 10° F. which is very moderate. The mean relative humidity for the winter months is about 67 per cent., and dew is rare. The average yearly rainfall is under ten inches, and two-thirds of this falls at night. "Day after day during the winter a bright, bracing air is experienced, with a blue sky, blue sea, white trade wind clouds, and many hours of sunshine" (Milland). The east coast of Grand Canary, where Las Palmas is situated, is cooler and dryer than Teneriffe, as it gets almost constantly the dry and tonic breezes of the north-east trade wind. Las Palmas has a fine, sandy beach four miles long, affording excellent bathing. Here between the town and the port is the English quarter with two good hotels in their own grounds, the Santa Catalina and the Métropole.

It has been reported to us that in very dry and windy weather the wind blows up much fine dust in this situation, which proves very irritating to some chest patients.

Above and behind the hotels, in an open, breezy situation are the golf links. Inland, as the ground rises, the rainfall increases considerably, as is testified by the vegetation. Occasionally when a south-west wind is blowing from the tropics, the air becomes warm, damp, and relaxing. The south-easterly wind blowing from the African desert is also a disagreeable one. Known as the Levante, it causes the air to be hot, dry, and irritating, with considerable difference between day and night temperature, needing care to avoid chill. The winter climate of Las Palmas is breezy and fairly dry at times, perhaps rather too exciting for a certain class of invalids.

Visitors to *Teneriffe* land at the port of Santa Cruz, fifty-two miles from Las Palmas and 256 from Madeira. Santa Cruz is on the south side of the island, while Orotava is on the north. To reach the latter a six or seven hours' drive over the mountains is necessary, passing through Laguna at an elevation of about 2,000 feet; here in winter it is sometimes cold, windy, and wet, and the invalid must be protected with warm wraps.

Orotava is situated in a valley facing the Atlantic with a mountain protection behind it and on both sides, so that it has a very sheltered position. Its surroundings are very beautiful, and Humboldt spoke of it as "one of the most charming spots in the world." Its mean monthly temperature for the coldest month in the year (January) is 61·2° F., and it varies little for the next three months, that for April being 64° F., while that for the hottest month (August) is only 73·3° F., while the mean daily range is 13·8°; it has, therefore, a very equable temperature.

The sea temperature in January is 65·7° F. The mean annual rainfall is about 16 inches, there is rarely any dew, and fogs are almost unknown. There are about sixty rainy days in the year, and in half of these the rain falls at night.

December and January are the wettest months, but in the summer, *i.e.* from April to October there is rarely any rainfall. The prevailing winds in winter are off the sea and from the north; they are light, refreshing breezes. In summer cool N.E. trade winds exercise a cooling influence. There is always a "parasol of clouds" surrounding "the Peak" which intercepts a certain amount of sunshine and moderates the summer heat. There is an average of about five hours' sunshine daily during the three winter months, December to February. Seasons, of course, vary at Teneriffe as well as elsewhere, and occasionally a very wet April may be experienced. We have heard of "drenching rain daily for a week," and nearly three weeks without sunshine. On an average, Orotava appears to be 1·5° F. warmer than Las Palmas, and 3° warmer than Madeira. Although Las Palmas is actually warmer than Madeira, it feels cooler on account of the refreshing north-east trade wind, and its temperature is not quite so equable. A literary friend, not an invalid, a very needful distinction in weighing evidence as to climate, writes of Orotava as "an enervating Eden, a climate which diffuses over one a deliciously dreamy languor." In the month of January he experienced "a positively prostrating warmth." He preferred Las Palmas, as he found it more bracing—"the Canarian climate, the Canarian air," he thought "beyond comparison and beyond description." No doubt the more vigorous invalids who prefer a climate with a decidedly bracing element in it should choose Las Palmas.

Comparing the climate of the Canaries with that of Madeira, we find the latter is moister, with a greater rainfall and more wet days; but we are advised, as a set-off against this, that at Madeira the food is better, the accommodation more varied, and the dust absent!

A few words must be added as to the less frequented resorts in Teneriffe. **Santa Cruz** is the port of arrival, and a sanatorium has been established there, and competent observers have reported of it as the best climate in the island for the months of January, February, and March.

"It has a southern aspect, the clouds which gather round the high mountains do not intercept so much of the sunshine as at Orotava," and it has more protection from cool north and east winds. Its mean daily temperature is higher, and its rainfall less.

Laguna, five and a-half miles from Santa Cruz, with an elevation of 1,840 feet and beautiful surroundings, is utilised as a cool and refreshing retreat in summer, and might suit some cases in winter.

Guimar, at an elevation of 1,200 feet, has a sanatorium for the open-air treatment of tuberculosis, under the experienced medical supervision of Dr. Salmond. A limited number of patients are received and treated on the Nordrach system. Guimar is very favourably situated, being on the south side of the island, twenty miles from Santa Cruz and three miles from the sea by a rather rapid descent. It is reported to be dryer, with less rain and more hours of sunshine, than any other resort in Teneriffe, while it is entirely sheltered from northerly winds by a range of mountains 6,000 feet high.

Tacaronta, 1,700 feet above the sea, is twelve miles from Laguna, between it and Orotava.

Vilaflor, at an elevation of 4,335 feet, is the highest village in the Canaries, and has been indicated as an excellent summer resort, but it is difficult of access, and we have not heard of any satisfactory accommodation there for invalids.

The journey to Teneriffe or Las Palmas takes from four and a-half to eight or nine days, according to the line of steamers selected. There is a considerable choice, the faster boats being more expensive than the slower ones.

Mogador, on the coast of **Morocco**, in nearly the same latitude as Madeira, but a little more to the south (31° 30′ N. lat.), has been highly praised by French authorities as a winter resort for consumptives on account of its warm and very equable climate. It is protected from the hot desert winds by the Atlas range of mountains. The prevailing winds are from the north-east, and these blow over the Atlantic, but a low rocky island lies opposite the town and shelters it from all winds but the west-south-west. The mean winter temperature is about the same as that of Madeira, 61° F. The mean daily range of temperature has been stated to be only 5° F., which is exceedingly small. The relative humidity is fairly high, 78 per cent., but the rainy days are few, an annual mean of about 45 days.

There is only a difference of about 10° F. between the summer and winter mean temperature. There is usually but little cloud, the sky being nearly always clear.

The town is reported as very clean and in good sanitary condition, but the surroundings are not picturesque. Consumption is said to be almost unknown amongst the inhabitants, and the climate has exercised a remarkable curative effect on consumptives who have resorted to it. These exceptional climatic conditions have been attributed mainly to the influence of the north-east trade wind, which prevails there a great part of the year. There are not half-a-dozen days in the year that may not be spent agreeably out of doors. The air is charged with minute particles of salt from the breaking of the Atlantic waves on the reefs near the town. Europeans can find accommodation at the Palm Tree House Hotel, on the hill behind the town.

Tangier is the only town in Morocco that is likely

to prove an attractive winter resort to English invalids, as it is only thirty-five miles from Gibraltar—three hours by steamer. Situated in 35° 42′ N. lat., close to the coast both of the Atlantic and the Mediterranean, it has a very moist, warm, and equable climate. Its mean winter temperature has been stated to be from 57° to 62° F. All its winds are moist winds, coming either over the Atlantic or the Mediterranean, and we are told that nothing dries there spontaneously by mere exposure to the air. The annual rainfall is from 30 to 32 inches, but it has few rainy days, not more than 35 to 40 in a year. Although an interesting and picturesque spot, the climate is too moist and windy for many invalids; but when the temperature ranges above 70° F. the air is not unwholesome, even when nearly saturated with vapour, though it lacks the crisp, tonic effect of dryer air. Sea bathing can be had all the year round. The most serious drawbacks, however, to living in Tangier, are the absence of drainage, the dirt, the bad smells, and the want of roads. The unsettled state of the country is also a disturbing factor. Fairly good accommodation is to be obtained at the hotels there. Those invalids who are not deterred by these drawbacks will find there a warm, moist, fairly sunny winter resort, a place where, owing to the moderate heat of summer, they can remain all the year round. It is suitable to certain cases of early phthisis and to those of bronchial catarrh and asthma, especially when there is scanty secretion. Early cases of chronic Bright's disease often do well there—and convalescents from acute diseases who long for an entire change of *entourage* might find life there both interesting and beneficial.

Algiers may be recommended to many who are in search of winter quarters, and who do not dread a sea passage of twenty-six to twenty-eight hours. The great interest of the town itself, and the variety of interesting excursions in the neighbourhood, are attractions for many of those who have to spend each recurring winter out of their own country. The Transatlantic steamers leave Marseilles on four days in the week at 1 p.m., and the whole journey from London to Algiers may be accomplished in fifty-two hours. Algiers has its admirers and its detractors, which may be taken to prove that it has its bad seasons and its good seasons. Much rain falls during the winter months, and many invalids have complained of having encountered very wet seasons; authorities differ as to which are the wettest months. All, however, seem agreed that March and April are the best months. The winter temperature of Algiers is, on a general average, about 10° F. higher than that of the Riviera. The mean temperature for the coldest month (January) is 54° F. The difference between the day and night temperature is not so marked as on the Western Riviera; but as soon as the sun sets the air becomes highly charged with moisture, and heavy dews fall. The thermometer very rarely descends to the freezing point; one observer found it only do so twice in twelve years. There are winters in Algiers when the rain falls in great quantity, "nearly daily, and often all day," in the months of November, December, January, and February. On an average there are forty to fifty rainy days during the winter season. The mean annual rainfall is 32 inches.

The prevailing wind is the north-west, a cold wind, blowing across the Mediterranean. The Sirocco blows but seldom, perhaps for three or four hours during four or six days in a month; but it is excessively disagreeable while it lasts, for, coming across the great desert of Sahara, it is laden with a fine penetrating dust, and feels hot and burning like a blast from an oven. The climate of Algiers, less exciting and milder and more equable than that of the Riviera, is not humid and relaxing like Madeira; it seems, therefore, capable of exercising a tonic, soothing, and bracing influence in many cases of chest disease, as well as in other chronic maladies. The combination of tonic and sedative climatic influences is peculiarly suitable to cases of protracted convalescence after attacks of pleurisy and pneumonia, and to cases of early phthisis in somewhat feeble, lymphatic constitutions, or in cases where the existence of nervous excitability would counter-indicate a residence on the Riviera.

Persons, however, subject to bilious disturbance, complain that after a little time the climate of Algiers makes them very uncomfortable, and that they are compelled to leave it. Some forms of chronic Bright's disease and certain cases of chronic heart disease do well in Algiers. The climate also suits cases of chronic bronchitis and laryngeal catarrh in the gouty with scanty secretion.

An oft-repeated objection to Algiers is the unhealthy and foul-smelling state of the picturesque old part of the town; and the hotels in the town have not been considered as very safe dwelling-places. But these objections to the town of Algiers do not apply to the suburb of Mustapha Supérieur, which consists of villa residences surrounded by their own gardens and beautifully situated on the slopes of the hills to the south-west of the town. In the selection of a villa it is important that the house and garden should be exposed as much as possible to the sun all the day; for in the shade and in wet weather the atmosphere is often very damp and chilly. It is also very important to inquire carefully into the drainage and water supply.

It should be remembered that you do not get "desert air" in Algiers, for, as Mr. Otter pointed out in "Winters Abroad," "the soil is, in fact, deep, rich, and damp, and there is no desert within 100 miles. It is strange," he adds, "how much even slightly bad weather is felt in Algiers; the cold wind seemed more trying, and the rain colder and wetter, and to leave a damper feeling in the air, than in any other country which I ever visited."

There is usually pleasant English society in

Algiers, and there are beautiful walks, rides, and drives into the surrounding country.

Excellent hotels exist at Mustapha Supérieur, and every foot one rises on the hill of Mustapha one gains in climate. There is, perhaps, more wind on the top of the hill, but there is more sun also, and no damp. The upper level also has an incalculable advantage: once there, the visitor can walk for miles amidst lovely scenery, on level ground, whereas, lower down there is nothing but ascent and descent on high-roads.

It has been recommended, in cases of early or threatening consumption, to spend two winters and the intervening summer in Algeria without returning to Europe; for it has often been observed that the good obtained by wintering there is counteracted by the fatigue and chill inseparable from a visit to England in summer. The summer can be passed in the highest part of the hill at Mustapha, where it has often been noted that the thermometer has not exceeded 80° F. for more than ten days the whole summer.

Hammam R'Irha, with thermal springs and a bath establishment which have been described in Part I. (p. 198), is situated in a depression of the Lesser Atlas range, at an elevation of 2,000 feet above the level of the sea. It is about sixty miles west-south-west of Algiers. There is first a journey by rail of three and a-half hours to Bon Medfa, and then a drive of eight miles to the baths. Hammam R'Irha can also be reached from Oran in nine hours. The place is surrounded and protected on nearly all sides by mountains, and there is an extensive pine wood about a mile and half to the north-west, and ash, oak, olive, and eucalyptus trees flourish on the hills around. Roses, violets, and geraniums bloom throughout the winter. There is, however, a defect in the mountain protection to the place in the shape of a cleft which lets in the stormiest wind in Algiers—the north-west—which blows at times very fiercely.

The hotel accommodation is good, and there are pleasant excursions and walks in the country around. Records of its winter temperature make this place about 5° F. colder than Algiers, and it has many rainy days. It is a suitable climate station in the spring when Algiers gets too warm, and it is resorted to also in summer for its coolness and freshness.

The air is no doubt pure and bracing, and is said to resemble the mountain air of Scotland in the summer months, only it is dryer. In winter frost and snow are not unknown.

It is a suitable resort in winter also for those who are recovering from protracted illness, and for those who, having broken down from worry, anxiety, or over-work, require a quiet place of rest where the air is mild, yet pure and exhilarating. It certainly does not appear to be a suitable winter residence for delicate invalids.

Hammam Meskoutine is another Algerian thermal station which, like Hammam R'Irha, can be resorted to in winter by those who are seeking for treatment by hot baths when the European spas are closed. It is not so accessible, nor has it been as yet so fully developed as a health resort, as Hammam R'Irha. It is a long and tedious railway journey of twenty-six hours from Algiers, as it lies in the centre of a triangle formed by the cities of Philippeville, Constantine, and Bone. It is best reached, from Europe, viâ Philippeville, Bone, or Tunis.

From Tunis it can be reached in eleven hours by rail, and from Bone in three or four hours, and in either case there is a rather tedious sea-voyage. The invalid must be very vigorous, or very restless, who can contemplate such a journey for the purpose of getting hot baths. Once there, the climate and the baths are likely to prove very useful in cases of chronic rheumatism, muscular and articular, in tabes and constitutional syphilis, in sciatica and other neuralgias, chronic bronchitis and emphysema, and some skin affections. It is not thought useful, but the contrary, in phthisis, heart disease, gout and congestive conditions.

It has a warm winter climate, the thermometer rarely falling below 50° F.; but March is often a stormy month. There are several springs, one—the Grande Cascade—is very hot, 205° F., nearly that of boiling water, and has a strong odour of sulphuretted hydrogen, which it loses as it cools.

There is another spring not quite so hot which contains a little iron, and is used when cool for drinking. It also contains a good deal of sulphate and bicarbonate of lime, and is regarded as similar in effect to the Contrexéville water.

It is a quiet, restful place, with interesting and picturesque surroundings.

Biskra.—This Algerian winter resort consists of several villages, in an oasis of the Saharan desert, on the south side of the Lesser Atlas mountains, at an elevation of about 400 feet. It lies in 34° 55′ N. lat., nearly two degrees south of Algiers, and about ten degrees south of Nice.

Its climate is practically that of the desert, very dry and sunny, but not so equable as Algiers. The rainfall is very small, about 6½ inches in the year, but it has the great drawback of being very windy and draughty, and the wind storms bring clouds of dust. It is also fatiguing for the invalid to get at, as it is a twenty-two hours' railway journey from Algiers; it is best, however, to break the journey at El Guerrah (3,000 feet above the sea) and sleep there, and so avoid the fatigue of night travelling. There is an alternative route by sea to Bona or Tunis which shortens considerably the railway journey. There is an overcrowded Arab settlement at Biskra with the usual insanitary surroundings, which tend to diminish the purity of the desert air. The winter temperature at Biskra is said rarely to exceed 80° F. or to fall below 60° F. There is a thermal sulphur bath about four miles from Biskra which is largely resorted to by the Arabs, and is used in the treatment of those maladies for which hot sulphur springs are usually employed, viz. pharyngeal, laryngeal, and bronchial catarrh, chronic syphilitic, rheumatic, and cutaneous affections. With *suitable sanatoria*, Biskra ought to prove a valuable climatic winter resort for pulmonary invalids who are vigorous enough and well enough to bear the fatigue of the long and tedious journey, but this, together with the absence of an English doctor and chemist and the doubtful food and draughty dwellings, renders it unfit at present for delicate, feeble English invalids. Chronic rheumatic cases should do well at the baths, and cases of syphilitic cachexia. Those suffering from over-work and brain fag may find the dry, bracing, clear desert air, the very beautiful and interesting scenery around, and the entire change of *entourage* refreshing and restorative.

The winter resorts on the Western Riviera are of such great importance to dwellers in Northern Europe, from their accessibility and natural attractiveness that we prefer to devote the whole of the next chapter to their consideration. Speaking generally, the climate of the Western Riviera is tonic, stimulating, and exciting, specially useful in cases where the vital energy is drooping and wants flogging into renewed activity. It often proves injurious to persons of a nervous and irritable temperament, and to cases which have a tendency to febrile excitement. It is on this account often ill borne by many hysterical persons and hypochondriacs.

We pass on now to consider the resorts on the **Riviera di Levante**—the Riviera to the east of Genoa. These are not so popular as winter residences as those to the west of that famous city, and, indeed, their winter climate is not, on the whole, so suitable to invalids, especially to those who suffer from chest affections. The Riviera di Levante is colder and wetter than the Riviera di Ponente. It is not so well protected from the north ; the sheltering mountains are not so high, they are usually further off, and gaps occur in the chain which admit cold currents from the north and north-east.

The rainfall is considerably greater, and the relative humidity greater.

Genoa and its immediate neighbourhood is peculiarly unsuited to pulmonary invalids, as its climate is very changeable and often cold, windy, and rainy; but between Genoa and Spezia there are many spots on the Italian Riviera well suited for winter residence to those who are simply looking for a milder climate and more sunshine than can be found within our own shores. A very few are sufficiently sheltered from the prevailing winds to be adapted to delicate invalids in winter; one of these is—

Nervi, which may be regarded as almost a suburb of Genoa, from which it is only six miles distant; it lies in 44° 22′ N. lat. It is well sheltered towards the north, and fairly so towards the east, but it is more exposed to the north-east and north-west. The south-east or Sirocco is of frequent occurrence, and renders the climate, for the time, somewhat damp and relaxing. Owing to the steepness of its mountain boundaries, and the absence of good roads, there are but few walks and possible excursions, so that it is only suited to invalids seeking repose and quiet. Its climate is less tonic and exciting than the resorts in the Western Riviera, it is less windy, more humid, and has a greater number of rainy days.

The town of Nervi has some good hotels. Gardens with orange and lemon orchards occupy the level space between the town and the sea-shore, giving to the town a very picturesque aspect. A sunny and sheltered promenade has been cut along the rocky shore, and is admirably suited for invalids, as they can enjoy there a temperature twenty or more degrees higher than in the shaded streets of the town.

There are, on an average, about fifty-four rainy days from December to April, and a rainfall during the six winter months, November to April, of 25½ inches.

It would seem to be much cooler in spring than Mentone and the other western resorts; but in winter it would appear, in some seasons at any rate, to be warmer. There can be no doubt as to the mildness of its climate, as is evidenced by the growth of standard lemon-trees and an abundant subtropical vegetation. Living is less costly at Nervi than at most of the western resorts. The place is much affected by Germans.

Santa Margherita, ten miles from Nervi, is beautifully situated in a sheltered bay a little more than a mile from Rapallo, its more popular neighbour.

Rapallo is well sheltered from the north, in the same bay as Santa Margherita. It has a very sunny aspect, facing south-east. The little bay has a very narrow entrance, so that it is much shut in by a promontory to the west and another to the east. These two promontories are connected towards the north by a semicircle of hills; this natural protection from the access of cold winds gives Rapallo a very mild climate. Olive, chestnut, and fig-trees cover the lower hills; the more distant ones to the north-east rise to between two and three thousand feet above the sea.

The accommodation is good, and the prices are moderate. There are a number of beautiful walks along the coast and inland, which give it an advantage over Nervi. It has a sandy beach, which is another advantage. Its climate is no doubt warm and rather moist. It has been said to resemble that of Pisa; but its situation and surroundings are far more attractive. Its air is not so dry as at the resorts on the French Riviera, but the temperature is more equable. Altogether Rapallo has much to recommend it as a winter resort, and is growing in popularity with English invalids.

Sestri-Levante, half-way between Genoa and Spezia, is in a very picturesque but somewhat exposed situation, and has a very sunny and equable climate.

Spezia is a town with a famous arsenal, and is built at the north-west angle of a magnificent deep bay or gulf, formed chiefly by the projection of a rocky promontory to the west, about four miles in length. There are delightfully quiet valleys and sheltered bays to the east of the town, well suited for walks and excursions.

The western coast of the gulf is rugged and hilly, but the northern and eastern part is comparatively level for about three miles, and this is utilised for walks and drives. The town and gulf are open to the south and south-east, but they are protected to the north and west by steep and high mountains, whose spurs stretch down into the sea. Its climate is a mild one, its mean winter temperature is 40·6° F., but the town and bay are not protected from the prevailing wind, which is from the south, nor from the Sirocco which not unfrequently blows from the south-south-east. The climate is moderately warm, moderately moist, calm, and tolerably equable, and the air is free from dust. There are good hotels.

Spezia may be commended to the robuster sort of invalid who is not greatly dependent on protection from wind, who prefers a somewhat moist to a very dry climate, and who desires to meet with facilities for sailing, boating, riding, and a tolerably active life. Its air is said to be soothing and comforting to those who suffer from sleeplessness in the resorts of the dryer and more exciting Western Riviera. It has a fine public garden and promenade, the Marina, a great boon to invalids.

Viareggio is the only other place on this coast which need be here mentioned, situated between Spezia and Leghorn. Having a fine sandy beach, it has hitherto been chiefly known as a summer bathing-station; but its mild climate, and the immediate adjacency of large pine woods affording both shade and shelter, tend to bring it into favour as a winter resort. It is, however, somewhat exposed to mists.

It is scarcely necessary to allude to **Pisa**, only a few miles from the coast, except to mention its former reputation as a winter resort.

There is another group of winter resorts, which, although littoral stations like those on the French and Italian Riviera, have very different climatic characteristics. They are the comparatively sedative stations of the **south-west coast of France**—Arcachon, Biarritz, St. Jean de Luz, and the adjacent Spanish town, San Sebastian; and with these littoral climates we may associate the neighbouring inland health resorts of Pau and Dax.

Arcachon, as an example of a sedative, yet not a relaxing climate, no doubt possesses advantages for the treatment of certain maladies. Ten miles from the Atlantic coast (44° 7′ N. lat.), from which it is separated by high sand dunes covered with pine forests, it is protected to a great extent from the fury of the west and south-west winds by the dense forest, which also offers a protection from the winds coming from the east and south-east. To the north of the town lies the great sea basin, a harbour many miles in extent, inclosed on all sides, only communicating with the Atlantic by a narrow channel running almost due south. The north and north-east winds must pass over this basin, and they become thus somewhat warmed in winter and their irritating dryness diminished, while it is maintained that they also bring from the surface of this unusually salt sea water, and from the vast extent of sands exposed by the retreating tides, an appreciable amount of saline and other marine emanations, to give a special efficacy to the air in certain scrofulous conditions. Arcachon shares also in the equable temperature which belongs to moist, marine littoral climates. The air contains much moisture, owing to the west and south-west winds which blow in from the

Atlantic and bring much rain and mist; but, owing to the extreme porosity of the soil, which for miles and miles is wholly sand, the water is drained off from the surface as soon as it falls, so that there can never be any stagnant water on the ground. The air of the forest is impregnated with the balsamic emanations from the pine trees, peculiarly grateful to some forms of chest affections; and, moreover, it is found to be very remarkably rich in ozone.

Arcachon contains two quite distinct parts; the Plage, a level tract on the south shore of the Bassin, which is occupied by somewhat closely packed streets and houses, and is, in summer, crowded with sea-bathers; and the Ville d'Hiver, separated from the former by a high sand-hill, and consisting of numerous villa residences actually built in the forest; each house being surrounded on all sides by pine trees. The prevailing winds, north-west, west, and south-west, being sea winds, are not cold like continental winds; but they often blow with great violence, and were it not for the protection of the lofty pine trees, over the tops of which they blow, they would form a serious drawback to the climate. There is less sudden transition from day to night temperature than in the Riviera. The mean winter temperature is 44·5° F., the mean relative humidity 85 per cent., the annual rainfall about 35 inches, and there are 103 rainy days. The climate is, in short, moderately mild and soothing, and it is especially suitable to cases of irritative bronchial or laryngeal catarrh, to cases of early phthisis with tendency to congestion or inflammatory complications, and to persons of nervous temperament. It is not suited to persons of a lymphatic and torpid habit, who do better in the tonic and stimulating air of the Western Riviera. Cases of consumption and of other chronic lung diseases have certainly been arrested at Arcachon, and dyspeptic persons, in whom the dyspepsia has been complicated with hysteria, hypochondriasis, and nervous irritability, have derived great benefit from its climate. Arcachon is reached in eight hours from Paris by express train.

Biarritz (43° 29′ N. lat.) has in some respects the same qualities as Arcachon; but as it lies completely exposed to the Atlantic winds, with no protection like the pine forests of Arcachon, it is more bracing and less mild, and by no means so suitable to cases of chest disease. It is, however, well suited to some forms of nervous exhaustion and irritability. Its mean winter temperature is 45·6° F., mean relative humidity 80 per cent., and annual rainfall 49½ inches.

Its climate is bright and exhilarating for a great part of the year; the relative humidity is rather high, but owing to the dryness of the soil, the heavy falls of rain are rapidly absorbed, and the air is rarely felt to be damp. As a winter resort it is most suitable to hypochondriacal persons and to those who suffer from depressed states of the nervous system. Old Anglo-Indians are said to find it suitable to the ailments they are prone to suffer from. In the spring it is a pleasant place for a change for those who find benefit from a sea climate with a fair amount of bright sunshine.

Some asthmatics, and invalids who require no special protection from strong winds, do well there.

The town is built in a commanding position on bold and lofty cliffs which dominate from a considerable height the Bay of Biscay, and form a part of the eastern shores of the Atlantic. The broken rocky coast there is very picturesque, and Biarritz has many attractions both as a winter and a summer resort. The winter season, during which it is chiefly occupied by English visitors, extends from November to the end of March. There are beautiful sands for bathing and these are crowded in the summer and autumn. It has also a well appointed thermal bath establishment supplied by the natural salt springs of Briscous, eighteen kilometres from Biarritz.

The climate of Biarritz is a sedative one, and is in this respect contra-distinguished from the somewhat exciting climate of the Mediterranean littoral. It is also bracing as well as sedative; it could scarcely be otherwise with the strong Atlantic winds blowing over its towering cliffs and its mighty waves dashing against their feet. It is this combination of bracing and sedative properties that makes the climate of Biarritz valuable to so many chronic invalids. It is, however, too blustering and humid a climate for many forms of chest disease, and it is on that account rarely resorted to by the consumptive. Some invalids who find the resorts on the Riviera too exciting, and who become sleepless and feverish there, are benefited by being transferred to Biarritz. By the Sud-express it is reached in ten hours from Paris.

St. Jean de Luz, a little to the north of the last westward spurs of the Pyrenees, as they stretch toward the Atlantic, is beautifully situated in a fine bay a few miles south of Biarritz, with the climate of which it has much in common. It is, however, more protected from winds, being surrounded by hills to the north-east and south-west, and better suited therefore to pulmonary invalids. Owing to its vicinity to the western Pyrenees, many interesting excursions can be made from it. St. Jean de Luz, though duller than its attractive neighbour, Biarritz, has the advantage of being cheaper and of offering greater quiet and retirement for those who seek them.

About eight miles from St. Jean de Luz is **Hendaye**, the last French village, with a fine beach and a sanatorium for feeble children.

San Sebastian, the Spanish resort, only ten miles by rail from Hendaye, certainly shares the mild sedative character of the adjacent health resorts on the south-west coast of France, while it would in all probability be found warmer and more sheltered, and therefore better suited to pulmonary visitors. It is, however, chiefly resorted to in summer for its sea bathing, and has not yet been much frequented by English health-seekers.

Pau.—The climate of Pau (43° 20′ N. lat.) has often been the subject of much controversy, and has had its admirers and its detractors; the variability of the different seasons, which is found in all European health resorts, affording ample support to both parties. It appears to be generally admitted, however, that its climate is sedative, and that an unusual stillness of atmosphere has often been observed to prevail there for long periods at a time. It is well protected from the north by a series of plateaux rising behind the town, and the Pyrenean chain, at a distance of fifteen miles, affords a barrier from the enervating south winds. It is unprotected, however, to the west and east, and it is occasionally visited by severe storms. The prevailing winds are from the north and west. Its average winter temperature, from November to April, is 43·2°, but little higher than that of London. Its relative humidity is about 82 per cent., its annual rainfall 43 inches, and there are 119 rainy days in the year. The sandy, porous soil rapidly absorbs the rain as it falls. Frost and snow and cold nights are not uncommon in winter.

Compared with the French health resorts on the Riviera, it is moister, its rainfall and number of rainy days are greater, it has less sunshine and sunheat, and periods of cold weather are more common. On the other hand its temperature is more equable, and it is much freer from winds. The climate of Pau is sedative, not bracing, and it is most suitable to irritable nervous persons having a tendency to febrile excitement. To such persons, when suffering from chronic chest affections, spasmodic asthma, emphysema, bronchial catarrh, active forms of chronic phthisis with tendency to hæmorrhage and laryngeal irritation, the sedative climate of Pau may be recommended, but it is not suited to relaxed lymphatic persons, nor to sufferers from loss of nerve tone.

A small sanatorium, the Trespoey Sanatorium for Consumptives, has been built on a hill, half an hour's drive from Pau, at an elevation of about 700 feet; it is open from the middle of October to the middle of May.

Many patients who pass their winter at Pau remove in the summer to one of the adjacent Pyrenean resorts, Bagnères-de-Bigorre or Eaux Bonnes, where they escape the summer heat of the town, and where they can avail themselves, if so disposed, of a course of treatment at the mineral springs.

The town of Pau is splendidly situated, facing the entire chain of the Pyrenees at an elevation of 650 feet above the sea. It contains some very excellent hotels, a good English club, and many other social attractions. The season is from November to May. Many charming excursions can be taken from Pau as a centre. It is only a few hours to Biarritz and the shores of the Bay of Biscay, and most beautiful and interesting tours of any length can be made into the Pyrenees in the fine days of spring.

Dax, in the Department of the Landes, about midway between Pau and Arcachon, with thermal, mud, and mineral baths, is described in Part I., page 159.

Passing to the other extremity of the Iberian peninsula, we find but a very few places in the **South of Spain** suitable for winter quarters; the chief of these are Malaga, Gibraltar, San Lucar, Huelva, and Seville.

These are all in the southern portion of Andalusia, and situated between 36° 8′ (the most southern Gibraltar) and 37° 26′ (the most northern Seville) north latitude. San Lucar and Huelva are on the Atlantic south-western coast, Gibraltar and Malaga on the Mediterranean south-eastern coast of Spain, and Seville is about forty miles inland from the former.

Malaga (36° 44′ N. lat.) is the only one of these Spanish southern stations that has ever been much frequented by English invalids.

The serious defect of Malaga as a resort for invalids, notwithstanding its admirable climate, is that it is a large, densely populated, and not very healthy town, but of late years, since the improvement in the water supply, many villas have been built in the suburbs. The city is built on a flat sandy plain, and its streets are narrow and close. Its climate is, however, one of the most equable on the Continent, and it is also very dry. The rainfall is small, and there are on an average only 40 rainy days in the year; so that in some seasons the drought is very serious, and the absence of water, no doubt, at times contributes to its defective sanitary condition. There are great variations, however, in the rainfall in different years. The water supply is good and abundant.

It is doubtful if this constant sunshine and absence of moisture would prove invigorating and health-giving to the majority of invalids, unless they could at the same time live in fresh country air, which appears to be impossible there. Winter, as we understand that word in England, is almost unknown at Malaga, or is very exceptional, the mean winter temperature being 56° F.; and a whole winter may pass without the thermometer sinking to 50° F., even at night.

It is sheltered from the north, and to some extent from the east, by mountains which rise behind the town to the height of 3,000 feet. It lies open to the south and to the sea. The winds are occasionally trying, especially the prevalence in winter of the land-winds or "Terrals," which gain access to Malaga through a defect in the protecting hills to the north, and, from passing over the snow-covered sierras, are cold and dry to a degree which proves very irritating to some invalids.

Owing to the mildness of the climate, the sugar-cane and most tropical plants flourish there, and the eucalyptus has been introduced with success, and has, to some extent, improved the sanitary condition of the portions of the town where it has been planted. The orange groves are particularly fine.

There is, then, much in the climate of Malaga and the adjacent coast to recommend it as suitable winter quarters for invalids who desire to find warmth and bright sunshine in winter; but the drawbacks to Malaga, on other grounds, are very great. These are the discomforts of the hotels, the difficulty of getting well-cooked food, the absence of objects of interest in the town, and the impossibility of invalids getting any accommodation outside the town. To these must be added the trouble of getting there and the difficulty of getting away. There is either a very long land journey, twenty-six hours from Paris to Madrid, twelve hours from Madrid to Cordova, and six and a-half hours from Cordova to Malaga; or there is the sea voyage of four or five days by P. & O. steamer to Gibraltar, and another short sea trip from Gibraltar to Malaga, which is very trying in the small Spanish boats; the large boats of the Compagnie Générale Transatlantique are, however, good.

Malaga is an important summer resort for sea bathing.

Most travelled Englishmen are acquainted with **Gibraltar** (36° 7′ N. lat.), and of late years a certain number of the robuster class of English invalids have passed some part of the winter there. It has been written of as "an uncomfortable fortress where, every way the traveller turns, he finds a hill, and a different temperature at every corner of its stuffy streets." It is, however, for those who are fairly strong, and only require a little southern warmth and sunshine, a fairly healthy and pleasant place of residence from November to May, but its attractions are limited and circumscribed, and the majority of visitors begin to get tired of it after about two months, and want to go elsewhere. Then it is to be avoided in seasons when the "rock fever" is prevalent, the fear of which shortens the stay of many visitors. Its mean winter temperature is given as 54·5° F. The annual rainfall is 32 inches. One drawback to the climate of Gibraltar is the occasional prevalence of easterly wind, the Levanter, which proves irritating and very trying to most persons. The hotel accommodation has improved of late years.

Of **San Lucar** very little need be said. It is situated at the mouth of the Guadalquivir, where this famous river pours its waters into the Atlantic. It enjoys a very hot climate, but it is a dull town, situated in a treeless, sandy, undulating country. It can be reached by river steamer from Seville.

Huelva, a few miles to the north of San Lucar, on the same coast, has much more to recommend it as a winter resort. It has a fine situation at the confluence of the Rivers Odiel and Tinto, and the famous Rio Tinto mines are about twenty miles distant. It is the seat of a small English mining colony, and is also important on account of its sardine fisheries. The water supply is excellent.

Huelva has a moist, warm, and equable winter climate, and snow has never been known there. Its mean winter day temperature is 67° F., and night temperature 56·30° F. Good hotel accommodation has been provided there.

Seville (37° 24′ N. lat.) is not exactly a health resort, and yet it affords an agreeable and suitable residence in winter for certain delicate persons who require more warmth and sunshine than they can find at home. Ice and snow are said to be unknown there; and although it has occasionally a wet winter, the climate is usually dry, bright, and sunny. Its mean temperature in the coldest month of winter (January) is 52·2° F. The mean annual rainfall is about 29 inches, with 34 rainy days. It is scarcely necessary to add that it is a city full of objects of interest, and that the hotel accommodation is fair.

The Italian cities of **Rome** and **Naples**, although winter resorts greatly frequented on account of the objects of interest they present to the visitor, can scarcely be regarded as suitable health resorts for invalids. Indeed, the excitement and fatigue of sight-seeing in Rome has often done much injury to invalids who have been unwise enough to yield to its attractions. Its winter climate is very variable, the cold "tramontana" is the prevailing wind, and the warm, moist, depressing "sirocco" occasionally blows. The relative humidity in winter is 72 per cent., and in some seasons there are many wet days. No doubt the city of Rome is in a much better sanitary condition than it used to be, and one rarely hears now of "Roman fever," but the country immediately surrounding Rome is still malarious.

The spring—March, April, and part of May—is the best season for visitors. To the mental invalid who needs distractions and pleasant occupation, Rome may be useful.

Naples, like Rome, has much improved of late years in matters of sanitation; but it cannot be said to have a very suitable climate for invalids. Its mean winter temperature is 48·1° F.; it is much exposed to the cold "tramontana," one of the most prevalent winds, and a good deal of rain falls, especially in November and December. Indeed, it is often very cold in winter. The higher part of the city, the neighbourhood of Posillipo, is *best* suited for the residence of visitors. **Castellamare di Stabia, Sorrento,** and **Amalfi** are popular resorts in the immediate vicinity of Naples.

Castellamare is about seventeen miles from Naples by rail; it is a port on the Bay of Naples, and as it faces north-west it is not well suited as a residence for invalids in winter, but it is well adapted for a spring and summer resort, as its aspect tends to keep it cool in the hot season. It is apt at times to be damp and cloudy. It has sulphur and other mineral springs.

Sorrento is seven miles south-west of Castellamare, by a fine carriage drive. It is splendidly situated, with grand views over the Bay of Naples,

Vesuvius, and the island of Capri. It is a warm and sunny resort, but is exposed to north-west winds. There is good hotel accommodation there.

Amalfi, on the Gulf of Salerno, is twenty-four miles south-east of Naples. It is a most beautifully situated and interesting town. It faces south, and it is much more sheltered from the cold north wind than the preceding resorts. It is the best and sunniest winter resort in this neighbourhood, and the accommodation is good. These resorts are useful in the spring for invalids returning to Europe from Egypt and other African resorts.

Abbazia (45° 20′ N. lat.) is an Austrian winter resort, and has been termed "the Nice of the Adriatic," and "the Austrian Mentone." It is situated on the eastern shore of the peninsula of Istria at the head of the beautiful Gulf of Fiume, and is much frequented for its mild winter climate by those who wish to escape from the cold of Vienna, Prague, Buda-Pesth, and other towns of Austro-Hungary. It is also a popular sea bathing resort in summer. It is a drive of about four miles from Mattughi station, thirteen hours by rail from Vienna, and three hours from Trieste. It can also be reached by small steamer from Fiume in eighty minutes.

It enjoys complete shelter from the west by the Monte Maggiore behind it, more than 4,000 feet high, but it is imperfectly protected from the dreaded "bora" or north-east wind, and it is often visited by the sirocco, which blows there as a hot and rainy wind. It has a sunny south or south-eastern aspect, with a fine view over the Straits of Quarnero, at the top of the Adriatic, the islands of Veglia and Cherso, and the coast line of Croatia. Its mean temperature for the coldest month (January) is 40·6° F., and for the winter 42·8° to 44·6° F. The annual rainfall is large, 66 inches, snow falls on an average about five days in the winter, and severe frosts are not uncommon. Its relative humidity in winter is also rather high, 80 per cent. It will thus be seen that it is much less warm and dry than the resorts on the Western Riviera, and cannot, therefore, be attractive to English invalids in winter, but it affords the dwellers in the Austro-Hungarian cities a comparatively pleasant climate during some of the winter months. The vegetation is rich and varied—there are good hotels, with beautiful gardens and many charming walks, including a promenade of three miles along the sea coast. It is said that there are no mosquitoes there in summer.

There are many interesting and valuable climatic resorts in some of the **islands** of the Mediterranean.

In **Corsica** the only really available winter resort is the beautifully situated town of **Ajaccio** (41° 54′ N. lat.), on a fine bay facing south-west and protected from the north and the east by high mountain ranges. It is thus greatly sheltered from cold winds, but is exposed to the south-west. It has a great number of bright sunny days, but it is undoubtedly a more humid climate than the French Riviera. Its mean humidity is 80 per cent., its average winter temperature 54° F., and spring temperature 59° F. There is a moderate but not excessive daily range of temperature.

On an average there are thirty-five rainy days during the winter and spring months. A great advantage is the absence of dust and mosquitoes. The scenery is magnificent and the country interesting. Some who have spent a winter season there speak of it with enthusiasm, especially sufferers from asthma. There are beautiful drives and walks along well-kept roads, the vegetation is luxurious, and odorous shrubs and flowers are abundant, so that the whole island is fragrant with them.

Steamers belonging to the Compagnie Transatlantique, from Marseilles, perform the journey in fifteen hours, and from Nice in ten hours. There are also steamers from Leghorn to Bastia—the least stormy part of the Mediterranean—in six hours.

There is a railway from Bastia to Ajaccio passing through very fine scenery.

The climate of this place is no doubt of great value in cases of protracted convalescence from acute disease; in some cases of chronic rheumatism and gout, requiring a mild and sunny winter climate and not too stimulating an atmosphere; in cases of chronic chest disease without any tendency to active symptoms, and where there is plenty of reserve force; while it would seem to be very beneficial to certain asthmatics. It must be remembered that it is a more equable and moister climate than that of the Riviera, and warmer, and being more sedative it is more suitable to certain cases of neuralgia and insomnia. There are comfortable villas built round the town, where good accommodation can be obtained, and there are also good hotels situated at an elevation of some hundred feet above the sea.

The well-known gaseous chalybeate springs of Orezza are about eighty miles distant among the mountains in the north-eastern part of Corsica. The village of Orezza is situated about 2,000 feet above the sea and has an hotel and bath establishment. It is a place of summer, not winter resort.

In the island of **Sicily** there are four places that have been commended as winter resorts: Palermo, Taormina, Catania, and Acireale.

Catania and Acireale do not offer any great attractions to English health-seekers, and but very little need be said of them here. As a change from Palermo, when one is tired of that place, either of these towns, or both, may be visited.

Catania is a modern, popular, and busy town. Its mean winter temperature is 53·8°, and its daily range of temperature 14·5°. There is less humidity of atmosphere and less equability of temperature than at Palermo, and there is a considerable difference between the day and night temperature. There is often a great deal of wind and dust, particularly in the months of December and April. The east winds are disagreeable, and the sirocco blows at times. Catania has only 40 rainy days in the year. The low temperature at night is doubtless due to the adjacency of the snow fields of Mount Etna, at the base of which this town lies. The environs, composed of lava, are bare and desolate, and the place, though warm and sunny, is not suited to delicate invalids.

Acireale is ten miles north of Catania and nearer Messina, from which town it is about two hours by rail. It is 560 feet above the sea, on the southern slopes of Mount Etna. It possesses warm mineral springs, which are much frequented in summer, and a fine bath establishment and hotel—"Grand Albergo dei Bagni"—which is surrounded by gardens and has fine views. It has been found "cold and desolate" in winter, and is too exposed and windy for invalids. Its climate resembles that of Catania; but owing to its elevation, its atmosphere is no doubt fresher.

Taormina, from the beauty and salubrity of its situation, is a very attractive winter resort. It lies on the eastern coast of Sicily between Messina and Acireale, and is approached from the Giardini railway station by a drive of two or three miles up a very steep hill on which it is built, at an elevation of about 400 feet above the sea. It commands magnificent views over the sea and the opposite coast of Italy, and of Mount Etna, which lies to the south-west. It is reached from Naples in about fourteen hours. As to its climate, it is reported to have great equability of temperature and much sunshine, allowing of many hours being passed daily in the open air, in protected situations, from January to April. December is a rainy month. There are some famous ruins of a Greek theatre there. Excellent hotel accommodation is provided. It is a popular resort with Germans.

Palermo (38° 6′ N. lat.) is one of the most beautiful winter stations to be found in Europe. Its situation is one of great beauty, surrounded by an amphitheatre of mountains forming at each extremity an arm of the beautiful bay which the town faces.

Between the town and the mountains a richly cultivated plain rises gradually for about four miles till it reaches their base; this, from its shell-like form, has been named the Concha d'Oro. The town itself is finely built, and beautiful public and private gardens and luxuriant vegetation surround it. There is a fine promenade by the sea, the Marina, commanding magnificent views, and there are varied excursions, and objects of much interest in and around the city. There are steamers from Naples daily in about twelve hours; by this route Palermo can be reached in three days from London.

A sanatorium for invalids (the Villa Igeia) has been built in a fine situation on the coast to the north of the city, with a southern aspect and good protection from the north. The visitors all have south rooms facing the sea.

The winter climate of Palermo is warm, but it is also damp and moist. It has a good many rainy days, although its rainfall is not great. November is usually a very wet month, and visitors for the winter should not arrive before December. It has a warmer and moister winter climate than the Western Riviera, more equable and freer from those sudden and great transitions between the day and night temperature. It is a good deal exposed to winds from the north, north-east, and north-west; these, however, blow across the Mediterranean before they reach Palermo, and thus become somewhat warmed and charged with moisture. It is also subject, with the rest of the island, to occasional visitations of the African sirocco, which, no doubt, serves to raise the average winter temperature, and is felt, while it prevails, as a most pernicious influence—dry, hot, and exhausting.

The mean temperature for the coldest winter month (January) is 51·6° F. The mean daily range is about 10·5° F. The soil is damp in parts, and the glare of the sun is often found very trying to the eyes.

Apart from the trouble of getting to Palermo for those who dread a long land journey to Naples and then twelve hours of sea, it is not well suited for invalids requiring delicate care and protection from winds, or for those whom a moist and warm climate unduly relaxes and depresses; so also, like Algiers, it seems not to be suited to persons who are predisposed to bilious disorders. Its climate is somewhat of an intermediate one between that of Madeira and that of the Riviera. It is colder and dryer than Madeira, warmer, moister, and more equable than the Riviera. We may expect to find this climate suitable to those cases of chronic or sub-febrile phthisis for which a dryer and less equable climate is too exciting, or which suffer from a tendency to hæmorrhage or to dry catarrh of the larynx and trachea; also to the gouty bronchitic with tenacious, scanty secretion; it is suitable to irritable neurasthenics and to those exhausted from over-work or worry, who are likely to derive benefit from the life of brightness and the many objects of interest to be found in a large historic city in the midst of beautiful surroundings. It is not likely to suit the bronchial or asthmatic patient with profuse secretion so well as the dry air of Egypt or the Riviera. It is too damp and windy also for the rheumatic.

It has been said to be "one of the great advantages of **Malta** (35° 53′ N. lat.) as a health resort that invalids can so easily get away from it!" But it is very doubtful if invalids in the strict sense of the word ought ever to go there. A low island, nowhere rising above 600 feet from the sea level, without protection from mountains or forests, in the centre of the Mediterranean, exposed to every wind that blows, with frequent and abundant rain in the winter—such a place can scarcely be a suitable resort for delicate invalids, whatever social attractions its official society may seem to present. The climate of Malta is a very equable one, the difference between the night and day temperature not being more than 4° or 5° F. in winter; and this quality may be serviceable to some who are very sensitive to changes of temperature, and who find they avoid catarrhal attacks in such a climate. The relaxing effects of such an equable climate are certainly counteracted, to some extent, by the bracing influences of the sea winds, but in still conditions of atmosphere it must be very enervating. It should be borne in mind that seasons vary greatly at Malta, so much exposed as it is to weather, and in fine seasons it has been found a very pleasant winter resort. The mean winter temperature is 56° F.

As all the gardens are inclosed by high stone walls, to protect the trees and shrubs from the winds, the island has an unusually barren and formal appearance.

A stay of two or three weeks at Malta, in connection with a short sea voyage by a P. & O. steamer to the Mediterranean and back, may be recommended in certain cases of over-work or over-strain, where temporary repose in a soothing and yet moderately bracing climate, with cheerful surroundings, is needed.

The Island of **Corfu**, in the Ionian Sea (39° 30′ N. lat.), a few miles from the coast of Albania, owing to its somewhat inconstant and changeable winter climate, is not exactly suited for the more serious class of invalids to winter in.

From the situation of the town—facing the coast mountains of Albania, which are eight or ten miles distant—it is very insufficiently sheltered from the continental winds which, in winter, blow over the snow-topped mountains opposite it. When the wind comes from the north-east, which it frequently does, it must be unpleasantly cold; and when from the south-east, which is also a prevailing wind, it must be disagreeably relaxing. The mean temperature in January and February is said to be about 50° F., and in April about 60° F., so that it has a decidedly southern climate so far as average temperature is concerned.

The mean relative humidity varies between 70 and 80 per cent., so that it is also rather a moist climate, and there is a considerable rainfall, chiefly in the early part of the winter, with about 72 rainy days between November and April.

The island is moreover subject to fogs which often last some time; but on the other hand it is very free from dust.

Corfu is a suitable resort for the more robust class of invalids who are able to lead a fairly active life, who require plenty of exercise and sport, if it can be got, and who would be able to avail themselves of the attractive excursions for sport and pleasure which this charming island affords. As a change for a month in spring from some other southern winter resort, as in the transition from Egypt to Europe, it is highly to be commended.

The town, together with the bay, lies open to the south and south-east. There is always some movement in the air, a breeze blowing in from the sea till three in the afternoon when the land breeze sets in. The streets of the town are lively and attractive, and filled with varied picturesque costumes showing that it is a sort of link between the east and the west. The principal hotels are good, and the roads all over the island excellent.

It can be reached by steamer either from Trieste in two days or from Brindisi in twelve hours.

The beautiful island of **Capri** (40° 32′ N. lat.) in the magificent bay of Naples, and twenty-one miles from that city, is one of the most attractive of winter resorts.

The island is, for the most part, surrounded by precipitous cliffs affording only two landing places, one on its north and the other on its south side. The town of Capri, with its white-washed, flat-topped houses, its dark covered archways, and its palm-trees, has quite an Oriental aspect. Its hilly slopes are covered with vineyards and olive groves.

It is usually approached from Naples by steamboat touching at Sorrento on the way.

Capri affords a delightful winter climate, and a most comfortable residence for invalids who are not very weak or delicate, but who retain a considerable amount of physical vigour, and are able to take a good amount of exercise out of doors up and down hill.

Its insular position gives it quite a sea climate; it has been compared to a ship in mid-ocean, and the effects of a residence there has been likened to a sea voyage without its accidents and discomforts. It has the equable temperature of sea climates, and one is not exposed there to that chill, when the sun goes down, which is encountered in the Riviera, and even at Naples only twenty miles off. But Capri has also a dry climate. Much less rain falls there than on the shores of the Bay of Naples, or on the island of Ischia at the other horn of the bay. The clouds pass over the island and break on the heights behind Naples, so that there is often a great dearth of water at Capri. Owing to the amount of clear blue sky, and the reflection from the surrounding sea, this little island is very bright and sunny. On account of its form (it is somewhat saddle-shaped), the central depression, where the town is situated, enjoys considerable protection from east and west winds by the elevated ground at each end. It is exposed to the winds from the north and south; the invalid can, however, choose either side of the island for his walks. When the north wind is blowing he can confine himself to the southern side of the island, and when the wind is from the south, to the northern.

Capri has good hotel accommodation at a moderate price.

There is much to commend Capri to the more active and robust class of invalids, who desire to escape from the northern winter and get winter sunshine in combination with beautiful scenery, pure air, and comfortable entertainment. The drawbacks are its distance from home, and the difficulty and trouble of crossing to and from Naples in bad weather, so that one may be detained several days at either place; also the very few roads and paths, and the absence of English doctors. It is not suited to cases of advanced consumption, but may be recommended in early or stationary cases with but a small amount of disease and plenty of physical strength.

We have yet to notice a few climatic winter resorts, most of them **on, or adjacent to, large lakes,** as Montreux on the Lake of Geneva, Locarno on Lago Maggiore, Lugano on the lake of that name, Riva on the Lago di Garda, the adjacent resort Arco, and the not far distant Meran and Innsbruck. None of these has what can be called a warm climate, in winter some of them are decidedly cold, and some have a fair amount of moisture; but they respond, some of them, to local needs, and are also adapted to satisfy the idiosyncrasies of certain invalids, who dislike what they term the "glare" of the Mediterranean coast—or the winds of the Atlantic—or the dust and flies of Egypt and of certain other stations. Their intermediate character often renders them useful as transition resorts in spring and autumn.

Montreux is situated on the north-eastern shore of the Lake of Geneva. The district known as Montreux really comprises several villages, stretching from Clarens to Veytaux.

The village of Montreux itself enjoys a more sheltered position than any of the others. The indentation of the lake, which is here called the Bay of Montreux, is protected by the mountains around from the north and east winds, and in some degree from the north-west winds. The "bise"—the cold north-east wind—is not nearly so much felt at Montreux as at Geneva, and the temperature is more equable.

Montreux, though open, dry, and sunny, and with a considerable number of clear days, has a large rainfall, and, as has been said, must not be regarded as a warm winter climate. Its mean winter temperature is 36·5° F.

There are about 140 rainy days in the year; and the rainfall is considerable, much greater than at adjacent stations, the mean annual quantity being 46 inches.

The atmosphere is of medium humidity (annual mean 73·2 per cent.), and in some winters fogs are not unknown. Owing to its protection from winds, the air is usually calm and still.

In an average winter a good deal of cold weather must be expected at Montreux, as its mean winter and spring temperature is some 5° F. lower than that of Ventnor; but in favourable seasons, on the other hand, a good many bright, clear, sunny days may be expected and comparatively few rainy ones. In November, however, there are often many cold, damp days. The average amount of sunshine in the winter is much lower than in many other resorts, only 56·3 hours in December, and 66·9 in January. The amount of *possible* sunshine is small in the shortest day of winter, at Veytaux only 5 hours.

In spring the weather is often very variable. There are perhaps some very fine days, and then a sudden and unexpected return of cold with rain or snow; so that invalids need to take great precautions at this season. Patients often ascend to Glion at this period of the year. Few people spend the summer at Montreux, on account of the heat, but the autumn is a fine season up to the middle of October, when storms of rain frequently set in and there is occasionally a passing snow-fall.

It is an advantage at Montreux to have such mountain stations as Glion, Les Avants and Caux readily accessible; for in some seasons there is much more sunshine to be found at the higher resorts than at the lower one.

The climate of Montreux is, on the whole, somewhat sedative, and seems to suit excitable people who find they do not sleep well on the Riviera. The influence on the climate of the adjacency of a large lake, is like that of the sea on the sea-coast—it increases its equability—moderates the cold of winter and the heat of summer. It is a well-known station for the grape cure in autumn.

Locarno (46° 16′ N. lat.) is at the north or Swiss end of Lago Maggiore, and reached by a branch line from Bellinzona on the St. Gothard Railway. Being on the western shore of the lake, it has an eastern aspect. Its elevation above the sea is about 700 feet. The little town is well protected by high mountains to the north and south, less so to the west. The winds from the east and south-east are broken by the mountains which separate this lake from the Lake of Lugano. It has a rich, sub-tropical vegetation. Its winter climate is mild and sunny, with a large proportion of clear skies. The adjacency of the lake moderates the temperature of the air by its temperature (44·24° F. in winter), and by reflection of sun-heat from its surface. The mean temperature of January — the coldest month — is 35° F. There are on an average in the winter six months, about 40 days, when rain falls. Snow is rare, but there is a heavy rainfall in the autumn. Mists occasionally appear, but are of brief duration. There is but little wind in winter, and the atmosphere is very still. The winter climate may be described as sedative, mild and equable, with little wind, no dust, and much sunshine. It is a suitable intermediate station for such cases as are sent to the South—chiefly chronic affections of the respiratory, circulatory, and renal organs—seeking a quiet, restful resort, free from excitement and gaiety.

Lugano (46° N. lat.), most picturesquely situated on the lake of that name, with a station on the

St. Gothard Railway, is, like Locarno, a very suitable intermediate resort for those who have wintered in the South, or are about to do so. Its protection from prevailing cold winds is not very complete, its rainfall is considerable, and it is rather humid. Its mean temperature for the coldest winter month (January) is 34·5° F., rather colder than Locarno, and its relative humidity for the same month is 81 per cent. There is, however, a large daily average of sunshine, viz. 4.15 hours in January. Rain is rare in winter, but heavy falls usually occur in autumn and late spring.

The climate is sedative, rather humid, with much sunshine. It is suitable to some forms of bronchial catarrh, cardiac affections, rheumatism and nervous dyspepsia, and to convalescents—to those who find the Riviera district too exciting.

Riva (45° 54′ N. lat.), in Austria, is in a fine situation at the north end of the Lago di Garda, with beautiful country for excursions around. It is too little protected from the cold north and south-east winds to afford a suitable winter residence for delicate invalids. The period of sunshine in winter days is short, and the atmosphere is often damp and misty. The mean temperature for the three winter months is 38·8° F. It is better suited for a stay in autumn than in winter. On the western shore of the Garda lake, in a more protected and sunny situation, there are some resorts frequented chiefly by Germans in the winter: the best known of these is Gardone-Riviera, which has a mild, equable climate, with but little wind and dust, and is frequented by convalescents from acute disease, chronic pulmonary invalids, and neurasthenic cases.

Arco, another Austrian winter resort much frequented by Germans, is situated only three miles from Riva to the north-east, in the Sarca Valley. It has much the same winter temperature as Riva, but it is better protected from cold winds by surrounding mountains. As a winter climate it enjoys much protection from prevailing winds, has a moderate degree of humidity and much sunshine. Arco has been developed by the Austrians as a winter resort, and is provided with institutions for applications of hydrotherapy and inhalation treatment. It is visited as an alternative to the warmer southern resorts by patients who, for various reasons, may not desire or be able to visit the latter.

Meran (46° 41′ N. lat.), once the capital of Tirol, is situated about eighteen miles by rail from Botzen on the line of rail connecting Innsbruck and Verona. The situation of Meran is exceedingly picturesque, placed as it is on the southern slopes of the Alps of the Austrian Tyrol, at an elevation of from 920 to 1,180 feet above the sea, on the banks of the Passer, about half-a-mile above its confluence with the Adige. Its position is a very sheltered one, as it is surrounded on all sides by mountains, except towards the south, towards the wide and extensive valley of the Adige, where it lies fully exposed to the southern sun as well as to the full fury of the south wind, which occasionally blows with considerable violence ; but it is protected to a great extent by lofty mountains, some rising as high as 10,000 feet, to the north, the east, and the west.

It is to this exceptionally protected situation that it owes its peculiar climatic advantages.

In the first place it is an exceptionally dry climate. It has an average of only 52 rainy days in the whole year, and only 13 during the winter. On an average it has seven days of snow in the winter, so that it is not a warm climate, its mean temperature for the coldest month (January) being 32·6° F. Meran has a dry and cold winter climate ; but the cold is much better borne, is more tonic and far less depressing than in a place which is damp as well as cold. The cold is also better borne because of the absence of wind, the protecting girdle of mountains keeping off all winds except that from the south. The sun heat, owing to its exposure to the south, is very considerable, especially at mid-day, and there are an unusual number of bright sunny days in winter.

Owing to the dryness of the air, the intensity of solar radiation, and the absence of winds, invalids are able to remain in the open air at lower temperatures than would otherwise be possible. For the same reasons the difference between sun and shade temperature at mid-day is often considerable, as much as 27° F., so that while it is freezing in the shade, you may have a pleasant temperature of about 60° F. in the sun. The mean annual relative humidity is 67·8 per cent.

A medical correspondent, writing in January, remarks: "Skating has been in full swing here since early in December; and invalids and ladies are daily seen sitting on the bank looking on, and shielding themselves from the sun with shades and fans! Most people wear during the mid-day only a light overcoat; and some, none at all. The morning and the evening, after sunset, are cold, and then feeble invalids keep within the houses, which are comfortable and well warmed." There is an excellent Kurhaus with a resident physician, a staff of nurses, baths of various kinds, "pneumatic" chambers, reading rooms, restaurants, theatre, etc., etc. There are numerous good hotels and *pensions* there, as well as at the villages of Untermais and Obermais on the opposite bank of the Passer.

Patients often move further south about the end of February, when troublesome unsettled spring weather is apt to set in and to continue through March, with occasional dust storms. Its summer climate is oppressively hot, but in the autumn it is, like Montreux, a favourite locality for the grape cure.

The class of invalids to whom the climate of Meran seems best suited are those suffering from pulmonary disease, who find by experience that a dry and bracing climate suits them better than a warmer moist one, and who can bear a certain amount of cold in winter without being made uncomfortable by it, *e.g.* certain cases of chronic bronchial catarrh, of asthma and of emphysema, especially when treatment in the pneumatic chambers is desired; certain forms of chronic phthisis before the lung has broken down and where there is no tendency to hæmorrhage; and many other forms of chronic derangement of health, neurotic, anæmic, rheumatic, or scrofulous.

Innsbruck (47° 18′ N. lat.), the capital of the Tirol, possesses many attractions as a winter resort for those who are not exactly invalids but who are lacking in tone and vigour, or who need to take preventive measures against morbid tendencies by seeking in winter a dryer, clearer, and sunnier climate than our own. It is an advantage also to many to be able to get these benefits in a bright, cheerful university town surrounded by beautiful mountain and river scenery, and with those social, educational, and artistic resources which such a capital affords; and it is not too large, as it has only about 30,000 inhabitants, while it is only thirty hours from London. There is excellent accommodation for visitors in winter, when the hotels are much less crowded than in summer. Its elevation is about 1,900 feet; owing to its protection from cold north winds, and its clear, sunny atmosphere, it has a warmer winter climate than might be expected from its situation and elevation, its mean temperature in the coldest month (January) being 24·9° F. Its mean humidity in winter is 76·2 per cent. The weather is often changeable and unpleasant in October, when the winter snowfall takes place, but from November to February the sky is usually clear, the atmosphere still, and the insolation considerable. In short Innsbruck has most of the advantages of the high mountain resorts without their drawbacks.

The Grape Cure.—Montreux, Meran, Arco, as well as other resorts, are on account of the suitable quality and abundance of the grapes grown there, associated with what is known as the "grape cure."

The nutritive value of grapes is not very great, but they contain much sugar and salts of potash, and are, to many, an agreeable food, while they also possess some medicinal qualities. Although attended with aperient effects, usually it is essentially a dietetic cure, but should be taken with moderation, as the excessive quantities at one time consumed were not beneficial. It is best to begin with small quantities, which may be gradually increased. About three pounds a day is a moderate dose; two pounds is enough for pulmonary patients. As to the cases suitable for this cure, constipation is often advantageously modified by three or four pounds of grapes taken in the twenty-four hours. But, according to Prof. Lebert, cases of obstinate and aggravated constipation of long standing often resist the cure, and in such exceptional cases he has given up to five or six pounds, according to the efiect and tolerance of the cure.

Lebert found a thoroughly laxative dose of grapes (five or six pounds a day), to be very salutary in hæmorrhoidal affections without much loss of blood, also in cardiac diseases when not much advanced, and when the venous circulation began to be troubled, giving rise to pulmonary, renal, hepatic, and intestinal congestions; and further that the calculous diathesis, renal and hepatic, was sometimes modified very advantageously by grapes. He thought the cure useful also, combined with the open air life, for those who are neither ill nor well, who are fatigued by a too exciting and somewhat intemperate life, or who lead habitually a too sedentary and too laborious existence.

This cure should not be attempted except under competent and experienced medical supervision.

CHAPTER VIII.

THE WESTERN RIVIERA.

A Study of its Climate and a Survey of its Principal Resorts.

THE many picturesque towns that lie scattered along the beautiful Mediterranean coast of France and Italy have long been the favourite winter resorts of the inhabitants of Northern Europe. Some of these have enjoyed a reputation as winter health resorts for a very long period, while others have quite recently grown into popularity and renown.

Passing from west to east, the health resorts of the Western Riviera may be said to begin at Hyères, a few miles from the important arsenal of Toulon, and to end at Pegli, a few miles west of Genoa. Between these, its western and eastern limits, we have the well-known French stations, St. Raphael, Cannes, Antibes, Nice, Beaulieu, and Mentone, the principality of Monaco, with Monte Carlo; and the Italian resorts, Bordighera, Ospedaletti, San Remo, and Alassio, besides certain smaller and less known places on the coast between these.

In geographical strictness, Hyères is not included in the Western Riviera, the Riviera di Ponente, since the mountains of the Esterels, to the west of Cannes and many miles east of Hyères, form its western boundary; but as a health resort this town naturally falls into the group just indicated, with which it has much in common.

Before considering the distinguishing characteristics of each of the principal health resorts of this region, it will be convenient to discuss briefly the general characters of the climate of the whole district of the Western Riviera. The Riviera is a land of sunshine and a land of winds. It is a land of intense brilliant sunshine, and of cold chilling shade. The very intensity of its sun-heat is to some extent the cause of its manifold local currents of air. The air is scarcely ever still, although, of course, some localities are much more protected from prevailing winds than others. The climate of the Riviera, then, has conspicuous merits and conspicuous defects. But a perfect climate in winter is to be found nowhere, neither on the Riviera nor elsewhere.

We have pointed out in previous chapters that in examining the climate of any district the chief points to be considered are—1. Its temperature, with its variations. 2. The relative proportion of sunshine and cloud; of clear skies and of skies that are overcast. 3. The amount of rainfall and the number of rainy days. 4. The average humidity of the air. 5. The prevailing winds, and the amount of exposure to or protection from them afforded by local conditions.

And first as to the *temperature* of the Riviera.

The several health resorts of the Western Riviera lie between 43° and 45° N. lat., while London lies at 51° 30′; therefore from latitude alone the temperature would be higher, and the intensity of the sun's rays greater; hence the difference between sun and shade temperatures is considerable. In a room looking south and exposed to the brilliant sunshine it is summer; in a room in the same house, facing north and in the shade, it is winter. And similarly, out of doors, there is a great risk of chill in passing from sun to shade. It behoves all visitors to the Riviera constantly to bear in mind that if they would benefit by the great heat of the sun, they must take care to protect themselves against the corresponding chill of the shade.

The Riviera in winter is not a hot climate, as some persons seem to expect it should be; and, indeed, if it were altogether a hot climate it would be a far less valuable climate than it is. Still it is a climate in which the inhabitants of Northern Europe may in the winter find, on an average, much more warmth than at home. The *mean* winter and spring temperature of the Riviera (between October and May) is from 8° to 10° F. higher than that of England.

But it is not to its latitude alone that the Western Riviera owes the relative mildness of its winters, for both Genoa and Florence are within the same latitude, and they do not possess by any means the same mild winter climate. It is also to the protection from northerly winds afforded by the chain of Maritime Alps, which extends along nearly the whole of this coast, and at a sufficient elevation to prevent the cold winds that blow from Northern Europe, and over the snowy Alps of Switzerland and Savoy, from reaching the resorts lying along this part of the northern coast of the Mediterranean. Some of these resorts are better and more completely protected than others, from northerly blasts, by reason of the relative nearness to them of this mountain wall, and by the unbroken nature of the barrier it forms; while at other parts the existence of gaps in the chain, or its distance from the coast, diminishes the protection it affords, and renders some of these localities unsuited for winter resort. Thus many of the places along that part of the coast which extends from San Remo to Genoa, owing to the greater remoteness from them of the higher chain of Maritime Alps, and the comparatively low elevation of the mountains behind, are much more accessible to northerly winds than the more western towns, and much less suited for the reception of invalid winter visitors.

Another cause of the mild winter temperature of the Riviera is its southern exposure along the shores of a sea the water of which is unusually warm. It has been calculated that the temperature of the Mediterranean off this coast is 20° higher than that of the Atlantic at the same depth and in the same latitude; and that the temperature of the surface of the sea (off the coast of Cannes) has a mean excess of about 12° F. over the minimum temperature of the air, and a mean excess of 9° F. over that of the sea on our own southern coast (Falmouth). Hence it follows that the atmosphere on this coast of the Mediterranean must obtain a considerable addition of heat during winter from that which has been stored up in the sea during summer, and which is slowly diffused through the air during the colder season.

It is generally known that there is a great fall of temperature on the Riviera at sunset, and that owing to this fact the time of sunset and the hour or two which follow it are particularly dangerous to invalids and other sensitive persons. This fall of temperature at sunset is easily accounted for, and is always encountered whenever, owing to the absence of aqueous vapour in the air and the presence of clear cloudless skies, solar radiation is very powerful; for when the sun is withdrawn the whole surface of the country is plunged in shade, the air no longer derives any heat from the direct solar rays, and the temperature of the whole air is a shade temperature. But this is not the only cooling agency that comes into operation at sunset. When the sky is free from cloud and the atmosphere clear, as soon as the sun sets, the heat, which has been absorbed by the surface of the earth during sunshine, is rapidly lost by radiation into space, the air in contact with or near the ground is rapidly cooled, and the moisture it contains becomes precipitated in the form of dew, and thus the lower strata of the air become damp as well as cold at and after sunset. When the sky is overspread with clouds, these prevent the radiation of heat from the earth's surface into space and reflect it back to the earth, so that the chilling of the surface at sunset is not nearly so great when the sky is cloudy as when it is clear; it is therefore especially during clear cloudless weather that invalids must be cautious of exposing themselves to the fall of temperature and deposit of dew which occur at sunset.

The temperature rises again two or three hours after sunset, and again falls to the minimum of the twenty-four hours towards sunrise, so that it is less dangerous to be out of doors three or four hours after sunset than at the time of sunset itself

In the second place, as to *the relative proportion of sunshine and cloud;* the excess of sunny days during the winter in the Riviera over that of our winter is remarkable. If we compare Nice with London we find that during the six winter and spring months, *i.e.* between October and May, there are on the average ninety-seven clear cloudless days at Nice, and only twelve in London! We are justified, then, in saying that the Riviera is a land of sunshine.

Next, with regard to *rain*. It may be said, speaking generally, that it is a land of heavy rainfalls and few rainy days. But much more rain falls at the eastern end of the Riviera di Ponente, *i.e.* about Genoa, than at the western end, *i.e.* around Nice; *e.g.* the mean annual rainfall of Genoa being 1317 millimetres, that at Nice is 811, and that at Hyères only 746; while the rainy days from November to April, both months inclusive, number 67 at Genoa, 43·5 at Mentone, 36·2 at Nice, 45·8 at Cannes, and 37·5 at Hyères.

Compared with England, the climate of the Riviera is undoubtedly a very dry one; for a few days in autumn and spring there are torrents of rain, so that the total average rainfall may nearly equal that of the west coast of England; but the number of fine days is immensely greater, both in summer and winter, than in almost any other part of Europe.

If we compare the rainfall at Nice during the five winter months, between October and April, with that of London and that of Torquay during the same months, we find that Nice has 16·92 ins., London 9·51 ins., and Torquay 12·28 ins., so that nearly twice as much rain falls at Nice during the winter as in London. But if we compare the number of rainy days during the same period, then we have at Nice only 30·5 rainy days, while in London there are 76·5, and at Torquay 98.

It is rare to encounter continuous broken weather on the Riviera, still it does occur occasionally.

As a rule the winter rainfall is distributed in the following manner: it is common to have a heavy fall of rain in October; as many as 13 inches will often fall in that month. The next greatest rainfall is in November, then December. Next comes March; and January and February have the lowest rainfall. In April there are heavy falls of rain again, as in October.

But the Riviera, like every other locality, is subject to great variations in different seasons, and in the same months in different seasons, *e.g.* the rainfall in Mentone has been known to be as little as 0·27 inches in the November of one year, and as much as 10·12 inches in the same month in another winter.

Taking the average of a succession of winters, the Riviera is a very dry climate, the number of rainy and cloudy days being very few compared with the number of dry and clear days; but it has exceptional seasons, and some are very wet and disagreeable.

In the next place, if we compare the records of the *humidity of the air* during winter, as observed in certain stations on the Riviera, with those obtained from similar observations at certain stations at home, we get decided evidence of the superior dryness of the atmosphere of the former. Saturation being represented by 100, we get the relative humidity of the Riviera (Cannes and Mentone), as compared with London and Falmouth, represented by the following figures:

Cannes and Mentone	London	Falmouth
72·4	88	84·4

It is not an easy task to describe the *winds* of the Riviera. They are legion. The mistral, the sirocco, the Greco, the tramontana, the sea wind, the land wind, etc. Indeed, certain exposed localities on the Riviera are rendered wholly uninhabitable on account of these tormenting winds; and the relative merits of its various health resorts chiefly depend on the greater or less protection afforded them against the prevailing winds by the surrounding mountains.

The mistral is a wind which blows from the west and north-west. It is a very dry wind, and a wind which generally brings fine clear weather, although it is always attended with a falling barometer. It is a wind which blows with great fury, and owing to its dryness, raises clouds of dust. The air loses its humidity and becomes dry, cold, penetrating, and irritating. The dryness of this wind is accounted for by its losing all its moisture as it sweeps over Central France. It is especially the torment of the more westerly stations, such as Hyères and Nice, but it is also felt at times, usually with diminished violence, as far east as San Remo.

It blows more frequently in March than in any other of the winter and spring months.

The sirocco is a south-east wind, a hot African wind, which only reaches the northern shores of the Mediterranean after having crossed this sea and so become laden with moisture; hence it is a wet wind—warm, wet, and enervating. It brings to this coast the heaviest and most prolonged rains. But these rains do not usually appear until after it has blown violently for a day or two. The spring and summer are its favourite seasons, but it may occur for two or three days in any of the winter months.

The east wind, which frequently blows in spring and summer, is not very often encountered in winter, and in this region it is not the formidable and dreaded wind that it is with us. It is frequently followed by rain, and is most common from March to May, when it occasionally blows with great force.

A very disagreeable wind is the north-east wind, or Greco. It is bitingly cold, and not unfrequently brings with it sleet, hail, and even snow. Fortunately it does not blow often. It is more felt and is more frequent and severe along the eastern portions of the Riviera di Ponente than along its western parts, and Genoa owes much of the bitterness of its climate to its exposure to this wind.

The Tramontana is the name given to the north wind. Most of the health resorts along this coast are sheltered from it by the chain of mountains which rises behind them, and forms a more or less complete protection from winds coming from this quarter. The northerly winds are either completely arrested by this mountain barrier, or they blow over the tops of the mountains, and are only felt at some distance from the coast. But the barrier is in some localities not so perfect and effective against these winds as at others. Where long valleys run down in a direction due north and south, as at Ventimiglia, the north wind may have free access, and, owing to the lower elevation of the near hills, the district east of San Remo is less protected from northerly winds than the western portion of the same coast. Nice, also, as we shall see, is but imperfectly protected from these northerly winds.

Occasionally a strong wind is felt from the south-west. A wind also often blows with considerable violence from the west; this and the south-west wind are regarded by some as really "deflected mistrals."

It is well known that on sea coasts generally, in sunny weather, there is a breeze which blows from the sea on to the land during the day, while at night the reverse takes place, and a breeze is found blowing off the land on to the sea. We have explained this fully in former chapters. This wind from the sea is very much felt all along the Riviera, even as far as a mile from the sea, especially on sunny days. It begins to blow about 11 a.m., and continues till 3 or 3.30 p.m.

The foregoing is a brief account of the principal

winds which the visitor to the Riviera must expect to encounter from time to time. The greatest number of calm days occur in January and December, and the windiest months are March, April, May, and October. The strongest, as well as most frequent, winds are from the east and the south-west.

Having thus briefly considered, from a general point of view, some of the chief characters of the climate of the Western Riviera, we now propose to pass in brief review the principal resorts on this coast.

Hyères is one of the oldest health resorts on the French Riviera. It is not actually on the coast as are the other health resorts of this region, but it is about three miles distant from the sea, a plain of this extent stretching between the town and the coast. So that the exciting influence of the sea is not experienced at Hyères, and this is considered to be one of its advantages. It feels the sea breeze less than other resorts on the coast, not only because of its distance from the sea, but also because of the protection from the sea winds afforded by the islands off the coast—the Iles d'Hyères.

The town itself is built along the base of a steep rocky hill, having a southern or south-eastern aspect. This hill forms part of a small and picturesque chain of mountains which bounds the valley of Hyères to the north; mountains to the east and north-east close in the plain of Hyères in that direction, and project as a promontory into the sea, protecting it quite sufficiently from the north-east, but less completely from the east winds. On the opposite side of the valley, that is to the west and south-west, a series of hills rises and forms a kind of screen between Hyères and the roadstead of Toulon. The situation of the town is admirably chosen for gaining all the advantages possible from the heat of the sun.

Owing especially to its protection from sea breezes, and also from the north and north-east winds, and to the infrequency or mildness of the east wind, at this distance from the coast, the atmosphere at Hyères is sometimes exceedingly still and calm, unlike the other health resorts on this coast, where perfect stillness of atmosphere is rare. And the air of Hyères is neither so dry nor so keen as at Cannes or at Nice, and its climate is therefore less exciting and more soothing. It has one serious drawback. The valley is completely exposed, in its whole length, to the mistral, which from February onwards blows with great force and frequency.

The temperature records show that the climate, apart from the winds, is a very mild one. The temperature is about ten degrees warmer than in England. It seems also to be more equable than at some of the other stations. In the depth of winter the thermometer rarely falls below 44° or 45° F. The mean winter temperature is 50·6° F. There would seem to be a great difference between the valley and the town. "The town is warm, but the valley, at four hundred yards from the town, is cold." The relative humidity of the air in winter is 73 per cent.

As to the rainfall at Hyéres, it would seem to be from 28 to 30 inches in the year, and the mean for the winter six months is 16·9 inches, with an average of 41 rainy days. The winter and spring months are probably somewhat dryer than at other health resorts on the Riviera. The average amount of sunshine in winter is large—136 days of bright sunshine in the winter six months. The water supply is good, the sanitary conditions of the town are satisfactory. Invalids and visitors live for the most part in hotels, of which there are several good ones, the cost of living at them being somewhat less than at the best hotels at Cannes or Nice. There are many charming and picturesque promenades, as well as longer excursions, and in this respect Hyères is much better off than most other resorts on the Riviera. It is suited to persons of nervous temperament who dislike the seaside, and who find resorts like Mentone and Cannes too exciting. It is good for nervous, feeble children, and for some forms of gout and rheumatism. It is not bracing and stimulating enough for scrofulous cases. Scrofulous children do better on the sea-shore, and there is a sanatorium for such children (150 beds) on the peninsula of Giens, a few miles to the south of Hyères.

Other cases that do well in the winter at Hyères are convalescents from acute disease—anæmic, debilitated, and neurasthenic cases—the early stages of gouty, renal, and arterial changes; cases of cardiac weakness, of chronic catarrh of the respiratory passages, and cases of early or of chronic torpid phthisis. The climate is said to be too irritating for laryngeal phthisis, and for the highly neurotic.

Costebelle, two miles south of Hyères and only a mile from the sea, is by many much preferred to Hyères, especially by English visitors. It is built on the southern slope of a pine-covered hill (Mont des Oiseaux), and is more protected than Hyères from the mistral; it is also more wooded, less dusty, being away from high roads, but not quite so dry. It is thought to be more tonic and bracing than Hyères, being more open to the sea. Two sanatoria are in course of construction in this district for patients of the middle class—one, the Sanatorium du Mont des Oiseaux for adults (150 beds), and another, de San Salvador (150 beds), for children. Costebelle consists mainly of three excellent hotels, all under the management of M. Peyron. There are golf links at Hyères. The branch line from Toulon to Hyères leaves the main line at La Pauline.

Saint Raphael and **Valescure** are at the eastern end of the Bay of Fréjus, separated from Cannes and the Bay of Napoule by the chain of the Esterels. It is in rather a windy situation, and the ground between the coast and Valescure is low lying and damp in parts. Valescure itself is but little raised above the sea level, and its horizon is very limited; it has also the drawback of being greatly exposed to the mistral. There are no doubt charming excursions to be made into the valleys of the Esterels, and many prefer the quiet, almost rustic life of this retreat to residence in a more fashionable resort; but it cannot be said to offer any great attraction to sensitive invalids.

Cannes.—From Napoule, which is situated at the eastern base of the Esterels, and gives its name to the bay, we get a magnificent view of Cannes as it lies facing south, bathed in sunshine, stretching along the eastern end of the bay, its countless villas spreading far and wide on the undulating rising ground which lies between the sea and the lower hills, with the range of snowy Alps for the distant background. Cannes is rather the name of an extensive district than of a small coast town. Unlike any of the other health resorts on the Riviera, it is scattered over a wide tract of land, so that its eastern and western limits are some miles apart; and its attractions and beauties are not limited to and concentrated on one particular spot, but are varied and widespread. There is no sense of restraint and imprisonment in a place like Cannes, where the landscape is wide, open, and free. Corresponding with this great range and variety of territory there is a corresponding range of climate.

With regard to the climate of Cannes, in the first place, if we consider the whole district, there can be no doubt that it is less protected from winds than some of the other resorts on the Western Riviera, and that Cannes, on the whole, must be considered a rather windy place.

The protecting chain of high mountains to the north is removed to some considerable distance from the coast, and scarcely offers so complete a screen from northerly currents as it does when close to the town, as at Mentone. The Esterels present a considerable barrier to the approach of the mistral; but the protection from this wind is not complete; there is more or less of a gap between the hills to the west and those to the north-west, through which this wind is able at times to reach Cannes. The mountains to the east and to the north-east are not sufficiently high to afford a complete protection from winds coming from those quarters. The prevailing winds at Cannes come from the east, varying from north-east to south-east. A wind from the north is rare, and always feeble. Still more rare in winter is a wind blowing directly from the south.

The neighbourhood of Cannet, a village about two miles from the sea, presents many most favourable and protected sites for dwellings and for promenades; and delicate persons, especially those who suffer from chest affections, or those of sensitive, nervous temperament, who find the neighbourhood of the sea too exciting, are strongly recommended to settle in the valley of Cannet.

On an average the mean winter temperature at Cannes is about 8° higher than that of London; and, compared with other stations on this coast, Cannes is not so warm as Mentone or San Remo, while it is somewhat warmer than Nice.

There is a considerable rainfall at Cannes, about 32 inches during the winter-time (November to April), and about 58 rainy days. As elsewhere on the Riviera, there are heavy falls of rain, lasting often several days, in November and March; in the former month the rains have been known to last for three weeks! The winds which bring these rains are usually warm winds, coming from the south-east and the south-west. Between these periods rain is rare, and lasts but a few hours. Snow appears about once every two or three years, and never lies on the ground more than a few hours. A fog is a still greater rarity.

Occasionally a very wet or a very cold season is encountered.

The following reference to one of the worst

winters at Cannes may afford some idea of what a bad season there is like :—

> "We have had dreadful weather. On the 8th we woke up to find the place in deep snow, from a foot and a-half to two feet, down to the water's edge. Before this had time to melt, more fell, with a hard frost, the thermometer sometimes at 23° F. The evergreens were broken down by weight of the snow. Lemon and orange trees are killed by the frost ; even the olive trees have been frozen. The snow lay on the ground till the 17th, when a heavy rain, following a hail-storm, made it disappear."

The country around Cannes is exceedingly beautiful, and in the number, variety, and attractiveness of the possible drives and excursions into the surrounding neighbourhood, it possesses eminent advantages.

One great drawback to the pedestrian, especially in the central part of Cannes, is the dustiness of the roads, and the absence of cross-roads by which to pass from one district to another.

Cannes is provided with many excellent but expensive hotels, and numerous elegant villas. There are plenty of good shops where all the necessaries and even the luxuries of life may be procured.

In considering what cases are best suited for this climate, it must be remembered that Cannes is a bracing place, that its air is tonic and stimulating, and to some nervous and sensitive organisations exciting and irritating. But many who need a calmer and softer climate during the winter months are benefited by the change to the more tonic air of Cannes in the spring—the end of March and the beginning of April. It must be borne in mind also that at Cannes you can avail yourself of two somewhat different climates, according as you choose a residence in the neighbourhood of the sea-shore, or inland—in the valley of Cannet for example.

All invalids, except those who suffer from scrofulous or lymphatic conditions, are advised to keep away from the shore. The extreme heat of the

Boulevard de la Croisette, the fierce sunshine, the sea air, the wind, excite but do not fortify, and induce a feverish condition in a certain class of invalids.

Speaking very generally, it may be said that all scrofulous affections, especially in children, as well as all the milder forms of glandular affection and cases of retarded development, derive very great benefit from the climate of Cannes. These are cases in which the forces of growth, repair, and nutrition require flogging into activity, and the stimulating climate of the sea-shore, the air, the brilliant sunshine, the restless winds, are all needed to rouse the sluggish temperament into the vigour of health.

Nearly all cases of anæmia improve greatly at Cannes, especially if they lead a prudent and careful life, and take as much out-of-door exercise as possible; even cases of cerebral anæmia in the aged mend rapidly; these persons, however, must reside inland, away from the sea, and avoid too much exposure to direct sunshine. The same remark applies to cases of slow convalescence from acute disease. Of cases of chest disease, those of simple chronic bronchial catarrh do well by the sea-shore. Asthmatics, on the contrary, should avoid the sea, and live as far inland as possible. Cases of emphysema, of chronic pleurisies, and of chronic laryngitis also improve there. Cases of chronic consumption, under certain conditions, do exceedingly well at Cannes; and even in very advanced stages its climate will often help to prolong life for many years. But a number of minute details have to be carefully attended to in these cases, which it would be out of place to enumerate here; it is only necessary to say they must avoid the sea-shore. Certain forms of chronic gout and rheumatism, and of Bright's disease, are benefited by wintering at Cannes.

Hysterical and nervous maladies, and neuralgias, associated with general nervous irritability, should avoid Cannes, where their sufferings are often aggravated by the too exciting and irritating effects of the climate.

Grasse, which it will be convenient to notice in this place, is situated about nine miles from Cannes, nearer the mountains, on the southern slope of one of which it is built, at an elevation of about 1,000 feet above the sea. It possesses a large and well-appointed hotel, the Grand. The climate of Grasse differs somewhat from that of the towns on the coast. Its mean temperature is less than that of Cannes, owing to its elevation, and to its comparative nearness to the snow-covered Alps; but it has greater protection from cold winds, and its southern aspect ensures it abundance of sunshine, so that many winter visitors are attracted to it. Its temperature is said also to be more equable than that of Cannes. The richness of its vegetation testifies sufficiently to the mildness of the climate. The town is surrounded by immense gardens of odorous plants, the jasmine, rose, violet, orange-flower, jonquil, etc. etc.; the fabrication of perfumery being its chief industry. Its mountain air, and its distance from the sea, render it popular with those invalids who find the sea-shore unsuited to them, especially those who suffer from neuralgia, asthma, or rheumatism when on the coast. It also serves as a good transition station in the spring when the resorts on the coast become too hot. It is reached from Cannes by rail in three-quarters of an hour. It is connected also by rail with Nice.

The railway going east from Cannes first skirts the Golfe Jouan, the fine bay which is bounded on the west by the Cap de la Croisette and the Iles des Lérins, and on the east by the peninsula formed by the Cap d'Antibes, which stretches far out into the sea, and forms the western limit of the wide bay at the eastern end of which lies the town of Nice.

Antibes has a growing popularity amongst winter visitors to this coast, and many who have passed a winter season there regard it with great partiality.

Living there is somewhat cheaper than at Nice or Cannes, but its climate, though an agreeable one, is not well suited to delicate invalids, as it has very little protection from winds.

After passing Antibes, the line running nearly due north along the western shore of the Baie des Anges, the traveller finds opened out to him a very grand and extensive view of the Mediterranean, and of the Riviera coast as far east as Bordighera, while to the north he obtains a fine view of the snowy Alps behind Nice. After crossing the river Var the train soon reaches Nice, which is twenty miles east of Cannes.

Nice is resorted to as much for pleasure as for health; it is a bright and lively town of 100,000 inhabitants, and there is much gaiety there during the winter months. Its winter climate partakes of the defects as well as of the advantages of the climate of the Riviera generally; it has an abundance of sunshine in winter, consistently clear, blue, cloudless skies, and remarkably dry, bracing air, often a little too exciting for many invalids. There are fewer rainy days than at some of the other resorts on this coast, but there are occasional heavy downpours, more especially in the autumn and spring, which are the rainy seasons. The not infrequent keenness of the winds at Nice is well known, and in some seasons the wind and dust are very trying, more particularly along the sea front. As a set-off against the disadvantages of its incomplete protection from prevailing winds we must place the advantages, social and educational, of a large city and the undoubted beauty of its position and its surroundings, and especially the accessibility of its fashionable suburb Cimiez, which enjoys much greater shelter and protection from the mountains to the north of the town. This suburb is now largely resorted to, and it has some of the best and most attractive hotels in Nice, besides many beautiful villa residences. Nice itself is very imperfectly screened by surrounding mountains from the north and north-easterly winds, nor has it any shelter or protection to the west.

The meteorology of Nice has been carefully studied. Its mean annual temperature is 60·3° F., nearly the same as that of Pisa and Rome. The sea temperature at Nice varies between 53° and 61° F. The mean winter temperature is 48° F., that of January, the coldest month, 47·1°. Falls of the barometer are almost always caused by the dry north-west wind, and rains "only cause the mercury to sink gradually and almost imperceptibly." The relative humidity at Nice is small, the annual mean at 2 p.m. being 59·6. The mean proportion of sunny, cloudy, and rainy days in winter (181 days) is 88 days of sunshine, 60 days of partial sunshine, 33 days of cloud all day, and 36 rainy days. The mean annual rainfall is 32·43 inches, and 19·45 for the six winter months (November to April). Most rain falls, as elsewhere on the Riviera, in October and April; and the winds that bring rain are, according to some observers, the east, the south-west, and the north-east, while others maintain that the heaviest and longest rains come from the south-east. It has been calculated that for the whole year there are 83·4 days of strong wind, 258·8 of gentle wind, 22·8 of complete calm. March, April, and May are the windiest months. The east wind is the most common of the stormy winds, and blows 45 days in the year. The south-west wind is also a violent wind, especially at the time of the autumn equinoctial rains. The north-east wind sometimes brings hailstorms and snow. The mistral blows (from north-west or west) chiefly in February and March, and is accompanied with clouds of dust. The magnificent Promenade des Anglais, one of the finest promenades in Europe, running along the sea-shore, is especially exposed to the mistral, as is also the adjacent quarter of the town; more protected from this and other winds is the Carabacel quarter, situated about a mile inland from the shore, and therefore more under the protection of the northern hills. Still further north, about two miles from the sea, is the suburb of Cimiez, which has a much better and less exciting climate than Nice itself, and many invalids with chest complaints do well there, especially those with chronic bronchitis and asthma. Cimiez is much more sheltered from the north and other winds owing to its getting under the shelter of the high mountains to the north. It of course escapes the exciting sea winds and the stimulating saline emanations on the shore, and with its complete southern exposure gets all the advantage possible from the sunshine, without the reflection and glare from the sea.

The reflection of the sun's rays from the white soil contributes also to raise the temperature of the air. Cimiez is connected with all parts of Nice by an excellent service of electric trams, and has grown of late years immensely in popularity. It is undoubtedly a very attractive resort.

The environs of Nice are very beautiful, especially the drive eastward, to the Observatory and the Corniche road, and on to Beaulieu. The climate of Nice is useful in many cases—it is beneficial to feeble, anæmic, or scrofulous children, whose growth and nutrition require stimulating. It is a good resort for cases of senile debility with a tendency to catarrhal attacks; for cases of over-work, or chronic dyspepsia, or those with torpid livers, and tendency to mental depression; but it is too exciting for irritably nervous, sleepless cases. Cases of anæmia in young people requiring abundance of air and sunshine, in bright and stimulating surroundings, do well there. Cases of chronic catarrh of the respiratory passages, and cases of asthma often gain very great benefit by residing at Cimiez. It is suitable also to some forms of cardiac and renal disease, and to cases of chronic muscular rheumatism.

Beaulieu, only four miles from Nice and connected with it by electric tram as well as by railway, is one of the best protected and warmest resorts on the Riviera, and has undergone rapid development of late years in the provision of hotel and villa accommodation. Being so near Nice and within six miles of Monte Carlo, and on the high road between them, it has become popular for its beauty and accessibility, as well as a resort for invalids on account of its climatic advantages. These latter advantages have gained for it the title of "La Petite Afrique," for owing to its protection by high mountains on the north, north-east, and to some extent on the north-west, and to the reflection of the powerful rays of the sun by the gray rocks around the small area on which it stands, between the sea and the high rocks, it is so warm and sheltered that lemon, orange, and olive trees and many flowers flourish in great luxuriance. Many villas (including that of the Marquis of Salisbury) have been built on the surrounding heights, and some on the peninsula of St. Jean and Cap Ferrat, which, stretching out into the sea between Villefranche and Beaulieu, affords most delightful promenades on nearly level ground.

The *mean* winter temperature at Beaulieu is stated to be 51·8° F., the *minima* are relatively high, and the difference between night and day temperature is comparatively small. The air is fairly dry, the relative humidity varying between 60 and 70. Fog is practically unknown. The mistral is rarely felt, and then its severity is much modified. The prevailing wind is from the south-east. Beaulieu is a suitable resort for all those who require rest in a pure, dry, tonic air, with abundance of sunshine, and a fairly constant and mild temperature—for aged persons and delicate children; for those subject to chronic catarrhal affections of the respiratory passages; as a prophylactic in cases predisposed to pulmonary tuberculosis, or in the pyretic forms of that disease in the early stage (patients in more or less advanced stages are objected to).

Some cases of bronchial asthma (not the nervous

forms), cases of neurasthenia from over-work, with nervous and vascular depression, *not* excitable cases; certain forms of gout, and early stages of Bright's disease, chronic rheumatism, anæmia, and neuralgia do well there; but excitable neurotic cases should not be sent there. The electric tramway is now continued to Mentone.

Eze, the next station to Beaulieu, is in a well sheltered situation, and the Eden Hotel, at Cap d'Ail, only three miles from Monte Carlo, is an attractive and convenient residence.

Monaco and **Monte Carlo**, although enjoying an admirably protected situation, are less resorted to by invalids than other less favoured resorts, and for obvious reasons. It is stated that the mean annual temperature of Monaco is 2° higher than that of Mentone, and 3° higher than that of Nice, and as a proof of the greater mildness and equability of its climate it is also stated that during the exceptional winter of 1870-71, when at Cannes and at Nice the frost destroyed a number of plants recently acclimatised, the same plants at Monaco did not suffer at all, although in the open air and without shelter, and that the lemon-trees, which were severely injured at Mentone, were not at all affected at Monaco.

Mentone is but five miles east of Monaco. The bay, on the shores of which the town of Mentone is built, is bounded on the west by the low-lying Cap St. Martin, covered by forests of olive-trees, and on the east by the Cap de la Mortola. From cape to cape this bay is about four miles across, and has a south-easterly aspect. As at Cannes, the old town is built on a ridge which projects into the sea and divides off a portion of this bay to the east, this forming the smaller and eastern bay, the western division being much wider. The division of Mentone into an east bay and a west bay represents a very essential difference in climate; for the Mentone district is bounded, behind and on each side, by a sort of semicircle of high limestone mountains, some of them reaching an elevation of over 4,000 feet, and the lowest depression or gap in them being not less than 2,500 feet above the sea. The chief part of this mountain wall opposite the *western* bay is at a distance of about three miles from the town, but hills and ridges of lower elevation, from 400 to 700 feet, run down from it at right angles to the shore. Between these ridges, three principal valleys, with their torrents, stretch down from the higher mountains and open behind the western bay. Through these valleys currents of air descend from the north, and so produce a certain ventilation and movement of the atmosphere in this part of Mentone.

It is quite different with regard to the eastern bay. In the first place it is a much deeper indentation of the coast than the western bay, so that its curve is almost a semicircle. Then the hills come so close to the shore that there is scarcely any room for the town, which consists here of little more than a road and a row of houses and hotels squeezed in between the base of the mountains and the sea-shore; the mountains, however, recede a little, farther east, towards where the road ascends to the Italian frontier. Nor are there any considerable valleys opening into the eastern bay to bring cool currents of air down from the mountains. It follows that the temperature of this bay is from 2° to 3° F. higher than that of the western bay, owing to the reflection of the sun's rays by day from the surface of the bare limestone rocks which rise directly behind it, and to the gradual giving up at night of the heat absorbed during the day. There is also less movement in the air. There is said to be more humidity in the air of the east bay than in that of the west. The east bay, then, is very sheltered and very picturesque, but it is found to have a relaxing effect on some people, who also complain of a sense of being "shut in" there, and that on bright sunny days, which often succeed one another with an almost unvarying monotony, the heat and glare of the sun become really distressing.* Then there is only one level walk, and that is along the dusty high road. But for invalids whose chief care is to lounge through the winter in a warm and comparatively still atmosphere, the east bay of Mentone is well suited; while the villas and houses built in the wider eastern part of the east bay no doubt enjoy the warmest and most protected situation in Mentone. In the western bay it is quite different; here the higher mountains fall back, as has already been said, to some distance behind the town, and the houses not only stretch along the bay, but extend, in a more or less scattered way, over the gradually sloping territory which reaches from the bay to the foot of the lower ridges and the sides of their intervening valleys which come down to the north of the town. So that the west bay is not so much protected from winds as the east bay; it is more open to the south-west and to the west, and consequently gets more wind and is somewhat cooler and more bracing. The mistral is occasionally felt at Mentone, especially in the west bay. Of other winds, the east is felt chiefly along the shore, and shelter from this wind can always be obtained in the walks and drives along the valleys behind the west bay. South-south-west and south-east winds, all coming across the sea, have free access to Mentone, but these are not, as a rule, cold winds, although they may blow at times with considerable violence. From the north wind it is completely protected.

By comparing the means of the temperature records of different observers at Mentone, the following figures are obtained. Mean temperature for the months from October to May:—

	Oct.	Nov.	Dec.	Jan.	Feb.	March.	April.	May.
East Bay	65·3	55·3	50·55	49·9	50·6	53·9	58·7	65·76
West Bay	62·2	55·6	50·69	49·12	49·46	51·1	57·64	63·1

* "The eastern bay is simply a sun trap, almost intolerable all the noontide hours. Often have I sought the old town and plunged into its dark street, as into a bath, from the glare of that faint mile of great hotels and villas."—Dean Alford's "Riviera."

It will be noticed that during the months in which there is least wind, December and January, there is scarcely any difference in the temperature of the two bays, but in the windy spring months the greater protection enjoyed by the east bay is shown by its higher temperature. The lowest temperature recorded during ten consecutive winters was 25·5° F. in March, and the highest 77° F. in November. The mean daily range of temperature was found to be least in December, 9·2°, and greatest in April, 12·5°. The average rainfall from October to May inclusive is 25·61 inches, but if we omit October and May, for the remaining six months it is only 17·87 inches. The corresponding number of rainy days is 63·8 if we include October and May, 45·15 excluding them. January and February are the finest months, and have the smallest rainfall and the fewest rainy days. October is the wettest month. The average number of very fine days for the six winter months, from November to April inclusive, seems to be about 94·5, rather more than fifteen in each month. Considered generally, the climate of Mentone may be taken as a favourable example of the Riviera climate, and it has the great advantage of possessing, as it were, two climates, suited to different classes of invalids. For those who especially desire warmth and shelter and a quiet indolent life, with plenty of sunshine and sun-heat, and who like to live close to the sea, there is the mild and sedative climate of the east bay, with its southern exposure and its almost complete protection from strong winds.* For those, on the other hand, who find advantage from a more bracing air, who like to have the sun-heat tempered by cooling winds, who cannot feel at ease without "ample space and room enough" to wander free over hill and valley, or who are irritated by the

* "There is hardly a fairer scene of languid repose to be found in all this resty land. . . . There is no edge in the breeze, no sea-air breathing from the waves."—Alford's "Riviera."

monotonous beat of the tideless sea against the shore, or to whom the saline emanations from the sea prove exciting and discomforting—for such there is the west bay with hotels and villas, some on the sea-shore, some a little removed from it, some, and those the newest and best, far removed from the sea and high up on the hillside. The value of a climate of this kind in many forms of pulmonary affections, in certain chronic gouty and rheumatic conditions, in states of anæmia, in convalescence from many acute diseases, and in the many infirmities to which old age is exposed, is incontestible.

There are some very beautiful walks and drives around Mentone, but, unfortunately for the delicate, the walks are nearly all of them steep and fatiguing, so that, unless he is able to climb, the invalid's walks will probably be restricted to the somewhat windy "Promenade du Midi." This is not the case, however, at the excellent hotel at *Cap Martin*, where many level and shady walks may be had. In the adjacent valley of Gorbio, forty minutes' drive from Mentone station, a French sanatorium has been erected for the treatment of cases of tuberculosis. It is in a protected situation, facing south, at an elevation of over 800 feet, and distant two miles from the sea. The buildings and the accommodation are well arranged, and offer all the needed facilities for a satisfactory open-air cure in a beautiful situation with a sunny and tonic climate. It is known as the "Sanatorium de Gorbio."

Bordighera is the next health resort eastward from Mentone, from which it is distant about ten miles, being three miles from the Italian frontier town of Ventimiglia. Bordighera is a conspicuous object nearly all along the Western Riviera as it lies glittering in the sunshine, its houses clustered together on a promontory that projects far out into the sea. It is the only health resort on this coast that occupies a position on a promontory; all the others being built round bays or depressions in the coast. It is naturally, therefore, much exposed to winds, that is to say, to all those winds that can reach it in blowing across the sea; the east, the south-east, the south-west, and the west winds can all blow freely upon this promontory. But it is well protected by mountains to the north, north-east, and north-west, whence the coldest winds come. Moreover, it is to be remembered that all the winds that reach it must, on account of its position, come to it from the sea, and impregnated with saline emanations. And this is the sole distinguishing characteristic of the climate of Bordighera as compared with that of neighbouring stations; the predominating influence of sea air rendering it essentially bracing and tonic. For this reason, also, its temperature is probably rather more equable—warmer in the winter and cooler in the summer—than at other places on this coast.

The old town of Bordighera is built partly on the promontory itself, and this commands a fine view westward of the Riviera coast, Cap Mortola, the mountains round Mentone, the Tête de Chien above Monaco, and even, on a clear day, the Esterels, west of Cannes; eastward the view is not very remarkable, the chief objects being the two capes which form the eastern and western boundary of the Bay of San Remo (Capo Nero and Capo Verde), and the little bay and village of Ospedaletti. The *new* town has been built on level ground to the west of the promontory, on each side of the main carriage-road. This plain, thickly covered with dense olive groves, stretches for a distance of three miles in the direction of Ventimiglia, and for about a quarter of a mile inland from the shore, till it reaches the base of the hills forming its eastern and north-eastern boundary. Here some of the principal hotels and villas are built. The possession of this level tract of land near the shore, thickly covered with vegetation, gives quite a peculiar and attractive aspect to the western side of Bordighera.

"Nowhere else can you get such delightful strolls under the dense shade of the old olives without a fatiguing climb."—(*Dean Alford.*)

Bordighera is also celebrated for its palm groves. These give a remarkably Oriental aspect to the place. The largest groves are to the east of the promontory, but they abound on all sides.

Bordighera is one of the most equable of the health resorts of the Western Riviera. The new town, by its position under the cape, is greatly protected from the east and south-east. It is well protected also from the north, and fairly so from the north-west, though the mountains in this direction are distant. But it is completely exposed to the west and to the south-west. At Bordighera the mistral is a west wind, being turned completely in that direction by the mass of mountains behind Monaco, and from being forced to blow over the sea it loses somewhat of its dry and cold character. Bordighera naturally feels the local sea-breezes, which are not strong winds, more than its neighbouring resorts, and it would seem to suffer from the stronger winds in about the same proportion as these.

Its mean temperature differs very little from that of the other resorts on this coast. For the whole winter it is the same as that of Nice, a little lower than at Cannes, still lower than at Mentone. Its position on a promontory jutting out into the sea would certainly tend to make it cooler than its neighbours in the hot spring months, and would seem to point to it as a good locality for invalids to move to in order to escape the heat of this season before returning northward. As to the rainfall and number of rainy days at Bordighera, it would seem to be neither better nor worse off than its neighbours in this respect. It is especially suited to invalids who want *sea* air; to cases of torpid phthisis in its early stages, without any tendency to hæmorrhage; to cases of throat and bronchial catarrh; to cases of chronic pleurisy; those of convalescence from acute diseases, cases of anæmia, and many other conditions of constitutional feebleness. Its climate is too exciting for the very nervous and sensitive. The special facility it affords for a variety of level, shady walks cannot fail to make it attractive to a large class of invalids.

Ospedaletti.—As we continue eastward from Bordighera the interest and beauty of the coast begin to diminish. A drive of three or four miles along the coast brings us to the pretty little bay and village of Ospedaletti, shut in and protected on almost all sides by its olive-clad hills. Ospedaletti is in an advantageous situation, and is much resorted to by Germans.

San Remo.—Just beyond Ospedaletti we arrive at one of the most thriving of winter stations, the old Italian coast town of San Remo. The special recommendation of the climate of San Remo seems to be that it is less exciting than some of the resorts further west, and on that account better suited to nervous and sensitive organisations. Invalids who cannot sleep at Nice and Cannes can often sleep at San Remo. Its temperature records, compared with those of the other health resorts on this coast, show it to be as warm in winter as the warmest of them, somewhat more equable, with less difference between day and night temperature, and less difference between summer and winter temperature. Owing to the greater equability of its temperature, visitors can remain later at San Remo without feeling the weather unpleasantly hot and relaxing as in some other of the towns on the Riviera. The Italians use it in the summer as a sea bathing station. It is exceedingly well protected by a triple barrier of mountains from northerly winds, which blow over the town and are only felt far out at sea. The east wind is the strongest and most felt there, owing to the low elevation of Capo Verde and the absence of any other protection in this quarter. This and the south-east are the prevailing winds. The north-east wind blows occasionally in winter, and is a biting cold wind. The mistral, too, is felt there, more so, according to some observers, than at Mentone. San Remo has a clay soil, and on that account it is somewhat damp after heavy rains, but this is looked upon as not altogether a disadvantage, as it tends to render the air less dry and irritating. The rainfall at San Remo and the number of rainy days during the winter season appear to be less than at almost any other resort on this coast.

The accommodation provided for visitors at San Remo is good. As to the class of invalids likely to be benefited by San Remo, it is unnecessary to recapitulate what has already been said with respect to other health resorts on the Riviera. San Remo is adapted to the same class of cases, with this distinction, that the climate is rather less bracing and more soothing than that of some of the other stations, and therefore better adapted to nervous and sensitive constitutions. It is a favourite resort with Germans.

There remain but two other towns on the Western Riviera that can be spoken of as in any sense winter health resorts. They are Alassio and Pegli.

Alassio is about twenty-eight miles east of San Remo, and is best reached from the north by the line from Turin to Savona, the latter town being about twenty miles east of Alassio. Alassio is situated in a lovely bay, having a south-eastern aspect and being well protected by two headlands, Capo delle Male on the west, and Capo di Santa Croce on the east. It is also well protected by encircling hills to the north, at no great distance from the shore. It possesses an excellent beach of fine sand, and is popular with the Italians on that account as a summer bathing-place. The Riviera scenery again becomes very beautiful at Alassio. The fine hills behind the town are covered with olive trees, and there are many sheltered nooks for villas as well as admirable picturesque walks and drives in the neighbourhood.

Some of the views are remarkably beautiful and interesting.

Alassio is not so warm as San Remo, as it is rather more open to the north-east winds, and the northern hills not being so high the north wind (the tramontana) reaches a portion of the district close to the shore. The wooded hills behind the town are better suited for the residence of invalids than the sea-shore.

Pegli is really a suburb of Genoa, from which it is distant only half-an-hour by rail. But it is very much warmer than at Genoa, as it enjoys a purely local protection from cold winds by means of hills to the north as well as to the east and west. It is a little fishing and ship-building town, situated along the sea-shore looking south. It differs, no doubt, considerably in its climate from the resorts at the western extremity of the Riviera di Ponente. The humidity of the air, for one thing, is much greater, and those who have found the air of Mentone unpleasantly dry and irritating have improved much at Pegli. It has acquired a reputation for benefiting asthmatic cases.

In the foregoing brief sketch of the principal health resorts on the Western Riviera, the object has been to point out, in as concise a manner as possible, the chief characteristics of climate and situation of those several stations. It will be seen that the climate of the Riviera is by no means a perfect one. But if it has cold winds and at times blinding dust, and if the air in places is exceedingly dry and irritating, it has also an immense proportion of fine days, clear skies, and bright sunshine, when from ten in the morning until three in the afternoon an invalid can live in the open air. "The warm southern sun and the azure sky of the Mediterranean, far more than elevated temperature, constitute the advantages of this climate; fine weather rather than heat is what is here sought for." But if the Western Riviera has its drawbacks—and what climate has not?—it must be admitted that the number of localities which we there have to choose from gives us an opportunity of selection impossible to find elsewhere. And then it is a region of almost unrivalled beauty.

NOTES.

There are but few places in the **Maritime Alps** suitable, either by their elevation above the sea or by the accommodation they afford, for invalids who may wish to avoid coming north to pass the hot months of summer.

One of the most accessible is the valley of **Thorenc**, with a good hotel, kept by Mr. F. Rost, of the Grand Hotel, Grasse. It is specially arranged for the mountain air cure, and is in a beautiful situation near pine woods, at an elevation of 3,850 feet. It can accommodate 150 people, and is surrounded by a park of 1,250 acres. It is open from May 15th to October 15th. It is connected by carriage road with Grasse (omnibus twice daily in five hours) and Nice.

The climate has been spoken of very highly by physicians who have visited this valley. It is very sunny, dry, and equable, free from damp and fog, and permitting invalids to be continually in the open air. It is protected by high mountains to the north and east. Another resort is **St. Martin Lantosque** (3,120 feet above the sea, and seven hours from Nice by carriage-road); it affords fair accommodation in several hotels and *pensions*, and is becoming more and more resorted to during the summer, especially by the inhabitants of Nice. It is surrounded by beautiful scenery; the air is pure, fresh, and moderately bracing. There is, at times, a good deal of humidity of atmosphere; but the temperature is equable, and rarely fluctuates many degrees in the twenty-four hours.

The Baths of Valdiéri (about 4,300 feet above the sea), on the Italian side of the Maritime Alps, can be reached from St. Martin in five and a-half hours, either on foot or, in fine weather, by mule track. The climate is mild and equable, and the place is completely protected from winds from the north; but it is refreshed by local currents of air which are rarely very strong. The surrounding scenery is grand and picturesque; the only drawback is the difficulty of access. On the Italian side it is approached from Coni.

The Baths of **Vinadio** and those of **Certosa di Pesio** are also reached by mountain passes from St. Martin.

All the preceding resorts are approached from Nice by the Vésubie Valley. The adjacent valley of the Raya has the advantage of being traversed in its upper part by a carriage-road which connects Turin and the plains of Piedmont with the Riviera at Nice. A conveyance runs daily from Nice to Coni in eighteen hours.

In this valley is **St. Dalmas di Tendi** (3,500 feet above the sea), about fifty-three miles from Nice on the high road between Nice and Coni. It has an Etablissement for hydrotherapy, with a fine garden, which was formerly a Carthusian monastery, and it has also a fairly good hotel. It is in the midst of wild and beautiful scenery.

CHAPTER IX.

SEA VOYAGES AND SOME DISTANT CLIMATIC RESORTS.

Sea Voyages.

TRAVELLING by sea presents such great attractions to some persons, and is associated with so many discomforts to others, that it is not to be wondered at that sea voyages for invalids have both their opponents and their advocates. As a common prescription for consumptive patients it is not nearly so popular as it once was, more especially since the open-air treatment of these cases in suitably-placed sanatoria has been attended with such satisfactory results; for one of the great recommendations of a sea voyage, for such patients, was that it provided them with an out-of-door life which they now get in these sanatoria.

But before we refer to the disadvantages and drawbacks of a sea voyage, it will be advisable to mention its advantages as they are generally stated.

These are—1st, *perfect rest and quiet;* complete removal from and change of ordinary occupation and way of life; a very thorough change of scene, and perfect and enforced rest from both mental and physical labour.

2nd—The *open-air* life it provides and the *great amount of sunshine* to be enjoyed (it is quite possible, under the most favourable circumstances, to spend fifteen hours daily in the open air), and, whenever it is possible, the traveller by sea is certain to endeavour to escape from the close and not rarely unpleasant atmosphere of a small cabin into the pure air to be found on deck.

3rd—The *great purity of the air* at sea, and its entire freedom from organic dust and other impurities. In this respect it has an advantage over the air of the open country, for the latter is apt to contain the pollen of grasses and other plants which, in some persons, excite "hay fever" and "asthma." The air of the cabins may, of course, be contaminated, but the air of the open sea "is probably the purest that can be found on the surface of the globe."

4th—The *presence in sea-air of a large amount of "ozone,"* or an active form of oxygen, as well as of *particles of saline matters*, especially in stormy weather, from the sea-spray, which may exercise a beneficial influence on the respiratory mucous membrane.

5th—The great *equability of the temperature* at sea. Even in the tropics the mid-day temperature is rarely over 85° F. This refers chiefly to the *daily* variations, which rarely exceed 4° or 5° F. It must be borne in mind, as we shall see directly, that in a *long* sea voyage very considerable variations of temperature are encountered, and in a swift steamer the transitions are somewhat sudden.

6th—The *humidity of the atmosphere* (the mean relative humidity is about 73·5 per cent.) and the *high barometric pressure*, which are considered to exercise a useful *sedative* influence on certain constitutions. It is said that the body temperature averages 1° F. lower at sea on account of this sedative effect.

7th—The exhilarating and tonic effect of rapid motion through the air; for, by the continuous progress of the ship, the sea-breezes are constantly blowing over it, and the passengers are borne along without any exertion of their own. The influence of these currents of air on the body surface is no doubt important as a stimulant and a tonic, increasing evaporation from the skin, and imparting tone to the superficial blood-vessels. To these influences must be added, in *long* sea voyages, the invigorating effect of the *changes of climates experienced in passing through the different regions of the ocean.* It must, however, be admitted that although this may have a bracing effect on many, it is often injurious to the more serious and sensitive class of invalids.

The sea voyage, for persons whom it suits, may be regarded as a combination of sedative and tonic influences, increasing the appetite, stimulating the nutritive processes, and favouring repose of mind and calm sleep.

We may next notice the various kinds of sea voyages that are practicable for invalids.

There are, in the first place, the *short* voyages or trips to Madeira, or the Canaries, and back, in large ocean-going steamers; to Gibraltar, Malta, Genoa, Naples, and the various ports of the Mediterranean; then there are the short "pleasure trips," with frequent stoppages and landings, now organised at different periods of the year by the several steamship companies and by private enterprise.

2nd—There are voyages of *medium* length, such as to the West Indies and back, to Brazil and the River Plate, to the Cape and back, to India and back, and

3rd—There is the *long sea voyage*, which usually means round the Cape to New Zealand or Australia and back; or the Suez Canal route may be taken; or the voyage to India may be extended to China and Japan. For the voyage round the Cape to Australia or New Zealand the patient should leave in October and return in June; the outward voyage takes in a steamer about six weeks, and in a sailing vessel ten to fourteen weeks; there should be an interval of four to eight weeks on land; the return journey is generally made by the Suez Canal. In this trip the full effect of the ocean climate is obtained. The drawbacks are the absence of fresh vegetables and fruit, the monotony of the life and diet, especially in a sailing vessel, and the long calms with great heat in the tropics. In returning by the Canal the transition from the heat of the Red Sea to the cold winds of the Mediterranean may prove injurious, while to *sail* back round the Cape would be long and tedious.

The heat in the Red Sea is the great drawback to the eastern voyage to Ceylon, India, China, Japan, etc., which is otherwise an interesting and attractive one, and luxurious accommodation can be obtained in the fine vessels of the P. & O. fleet.

The voyage to the Cape and back, with short trips into the interior of Cape Colony, or to Natal, occupying from six to eight weeks or more, is long enough for many cases.

The trip to the West Indies may be recommended to those patients who are benefited by moist heat, but it is unsuited to those who are depressed by these conditions. It is also important to ascertain that the islands visited are free from endemic diseases. Barbados is said to be generally healthy.

The voyage to the coast towns of Brazil and to the River Plate at a suitable season is attractive from its moderate length, the number of places called at, and the fine winter climate and beautiful scenery of most of the places visited. An interesting but more adventurous trip is that from New York to San Francisco by Panama, taking twenty-eight days. From San Francisco trips can be made of varied length, in a warm climate, to other Pacific ports.

Next, as to the cases best suited to a sea voyage.

All authorities are agreed that the best results obtained from sea voyages are seen in those cases of anomalous nervous affections, unconnected with organic disease, that are induced by over-work or worry and anxiety, and often associated with disorder of the digestive organs—cases that have been termed "irritable weakness" of the nervous system. The perfect rest, the constant exposure to the invigorating sea breezes, the open-air life, the entire change of scene, all these influences combined tend to bring back the power of sleeping soundly and of digesting well, and to restore a healthy organic activity both physical and mental.

As these nervous conditions vary greatly, so the

kind of voyage suitable to their several needs varies also. For some a mere pleasure trip of a few weeks' duration is all that is necessary; for others a somewhat longer voyage may be better, as that to the Cape and back, or one in which the interest is kept alive by frequent stoppages at interesting spots, as in the voyages to the different Mediterranean ports, or to Ceylon or India and back, or to the Brazils, or the still longer voyage to China and Japan; while in some more chronic and troublesome cases, requiring a prolonged period of perfect rest, the long sea voyage to Australia or New Zealand may be most appropriate. The natural temperament and disposition of the patient must be considered, as some bear the inevitable monotony of a long sea voyage badly, and are more benefited by two or three shorter voyages with longer or shorter intervals. Perhaps the next most suitable cases for a sea voyage, and especially for a long one, are cases of chronic scrofulous disease of the joints, glands, and skin; or wounds in scrofulous persons that are slow to heal; such patients may be incapacitated by their maladies from taking much exercise in the open air, and the advantage of being carried through the open air in a ship, and constantly exposed to the tonic influences of the sea breezes, is very great Some cases of protracted and tedious convalescence from severe attacks of chest and other disease are occasionally greatly benefited by a sea voyage, especially if the patients have a fondness for the life at sea, and do not look upon it with dread or distaste.

The sea voyage in warm latitudes is also useful in some cases of hepatic and renal functional disorders; in the latter the warmth and moisture of the tropics or the sub-tropical regions, by exciting great activity of the skin, often prove especially favourable; and in the former, the alterative influence of sea air may prove very beneficial. Cases of chronic dysentery acquired during residence in hot countries, and the chronic intestinal catarrh occurring as a consequence of such attacks, are often completely cured by a voyage at sea. We often find that men invalided home suffering from the effects of tropical and malarial affections arrive in England already partly restored to health by the sea voyage. Cases of chronic catarrh of the larynx and bronchi, and some cases, but by no means all, of chronic muscular and articular rheumatism, are benefited by winter voyages to warm climates; also cases of hay fever are cured at sea.

In certain forms of debility in young people, associated with over-growth or educational strain, or dependent on other depressing influences, and which threaten to induce serious disease, a long sea voyage is often of essential service.

Such cases, especially if, perchance, accompanied by a slight cough from a relaxed or catarrhal condition of the mucous membranes of the throat or upper air passages, are not unfrequently suspected to be cases of so-called "*incipient phthisis*," and it is probably mainly owing to the exceedingly good results that are obtained in these cases from a long sea voyage, that we owe the great reputation which sea voyages formerly enjoyed in the treatment of consumption.

If we were to subtract from the so-called *cures* of consumption, attributed to sea voyages, all those that may not have been cases of consumption at all, the residue, we suspect, would be surprisingly small. But as a *preventive*, in young men with a constitutional tendency to phthisis, a long sea voyage is of great value.

The propriety of sending persons, who are undoubtedly the subjects of tubercular disease of the lungs, on a sea voyage, is a point of some doubt and difficulty. The late Sir Andrew Clark, who had himself been a naval surgeon and had had an altogether exceptional experience in connection with this subject, said:—"For my own part, when I now review the experience of the effects of sea voyages upon young invalids, I am more strongly impressed than ever I was before with the necessity of extreme caution in prescribing them."* Our own experience is certainly in accord with this view. No one can control the accidents of weather at sea, and a long voyage made in bad weather may suffice to destroy all hope of recovery in such cases. The cases in which a sea voyage may possibly be expected to be attended with benefit are those in which either the disease is limited and progressing slowly, and without fever, in young persons with constitutions otherwise healthy and vigorous, or others in which the disease, after a stage of active progress, and perhaps the formation of a limited cavity, has become stationary and quiescent, and the general health is fairly good.

In either of these conditions, if the patient has a taste for a sea-faring life, a sea voyage is calculated to be of service. But even in these cases, if there is any distaste for the sea, it is unwise to urge it.

On the impropriety and unwisdom of sending cases of advanced consumption, or cases of actively progressive disease, or cases in which the general health and strength are seriously compromised, on a long sea voyage, many have animadverted.

The late Professor Sir W. H. Flower made some pertinent observations on this point. "The principal objection," he said, "to persons in delicate health undertaking a long sea voyage is the uncertainty about the influences to which he or she may be exposed; while on land the traveller is, to a great extent, his own master, and has power to control the surrounding conditions. He may regulate the day's journey, according to strength or inclination, he may linger in such places as have agreeable associations and environments, he may hasten over those of an opposite character; but when once embarked upon a voyage, whether he finds himself crowded in a dark, close, cabin, with two or three uncongenial companions, lying on a narrow, hard shelf, port-holes rigidly closed, and the atmosphere he breathes poisoned by

* *Brit. Med. Jour.*, Dec. 20, 1890.

noisome odours, of which the sickening smell of the oil of the engines is one of the least objectionable; the rain pouring on deck making escape from his prison, even for a few minutes, impossible; when he feels he would give all his wordly possessions for a breath of pure air, or a few hours' cessation from the perpetual din of the engines within and the waves without; he is perfectly helpless, he must go through it, day after day, and night after night, until the weather changes or the voyage is ended."

Dr. Coupland Taylor, himself an invalid, commented—("The Ocean as a Health Resort in Phthisis")—on the "real hardships" of a long sea voyage in a sailing vessel to Australia, and he contends that the purity, etc., of the sea-air is, for invalids, more than outweighed by the obvious disadvantages of close, hot cabins, the weakness caused by sea-sickness, damp sea-fogs, draughty saloons, etc. In the first part of the voyage to Australia, if undertaken, as it usually is, about the month of September or October, you encounter, he says, "sea-sickness and cold winds;" and in the second part, when the hot regions are reached, the "decks are running with water from heavy dews," so that the invalid cannot sleep in the open air, and the cabins are intolerably close, shared, as they usually are, with one or two companions.

In a gale the invalid is necessarily shut up below, probably sea-sick, and may for days be confined in a close, unwholesome atmosphere, with no possibility of leaving it.

There is a pleasant time after the first fortnight, when the N.E. trade winds are reached, and until the ship enters the tropics. A fortnight passed in the humid heat of the tropics is very depressing. To the tropics succeeds the most pleasant part of the voyage, *i.e.* the S.E. trade winds between 15° and 40° S. lat., with very fine weather. After passing the Cape, further trials await the invalid, in the shape of heavy seas and great cold from the nearness of ice, and as there are no fires he can only find warmth in his bed. This lasts until he nears the west coast of Australia, and then (December) he gets into pleasant summer weather for the rest of the voyage. Of ten consumptives on board the same sailing vessel with Dr. C. Taylor, he stated that six died soon after their arrival in the colony. His conclusion was that it needs considerable bodily strength to withstand the bad weather and the great transitions incidental to the long sea voyage in a sailing vessel.

Dr. L. E. Shaw also testified from personal observation to the same effect. He say: "No one who has acted as surgeon to an invalid ship, who has seen patients with advanced phthisis suddenly transferred from their comfortable invalid homes, on land, to the small accommodation and scanty luxuries which, with the best intentions, the authorities are able to provide for them at sea; no one who has watched the fearful anxiety of these patients to get back to their homes when they find their disease progressing, and who, finally, as their best and perhaps only friend, has received their last messages for their relatives, could possibly recommend a long sea voyage as a justifiable treatment in such cases. What I would contend is that, while for the large majority of cases of phthisis, in which the patient is willing to submit to such treatment, a long sea voyage is unsuitable, whether in a sailing vessel or a steamer, for the minority, who can be safely recommended to try it, a sailing vessel is much to be preferred."

Of the voyage to New Zealand, a gentleman who sailed early in December, to avoid an English winter, gave the following account:—"The weather was very pleasant for some days after we left Teneriffe; but, as we had a following wind, the north-east trade, it got gradually warmer until the thermometer touched 83° in the cabins at 10 degrees north. Then began a process which astonished us very much. So far, we had not been any great distance from land; but as soon as we passed the Gulf of

Guinea, and while still north of the equator, the temperature began to fall, 82, 80, 79, 77, 75, 71, 71, 69, 69, 68. This, with a strong south-east trade wind in our teeth, made the ship very cool, if not cold ; and, when under the vertical sun, great-coats and rugs were required on deck after dinner. As we approached land again, towards the Cape, the thermometer rose a few degrees, touching 74° ; but, as soon as the land was left behind, it went to 71, 63, 57, 55, 52, 50, 45. These are cabin readings, and on deck 37° and 36° were the mid-day temperatures. The regular steamer-route goes to 51 degrees south, and travels on that parallel for 65 degrees ; and one soon begins to wonder whether doctors know what they are about when they recommend a voyage round the Cape. The weather, we are told, is quite normal, and a shower of sleet is just what may be looked for at midsummer here. The ship's officers consider it a very good voyage, and the captain, when he turns out of his cabin, after a week of congestion of the lungs, says the weather is beautiful. So it is, according to the log ; for there is generally plenty of fair wind, and the runs are long ; but it is not invalids' weather. I wear both summer and winter flannels, a chamois waistcoat, and, with a great-coat turned up at the neck, and lined gloves on, I manage to walk for an hour once, or it may be twice a day ; but one day this week I did not get out at all, and I had to pay for one of my walks with a mustard blister. I am not prepared to say that the cold weather has been bad for me ; for I had a troublesome cough when the weather was warmer, which I have not got now ; but it is risky, and, for a weaker man, would be dangerous."

Attention has often been drawn to the absence, on board the great ocean-going steamers, of any special arrangements for the comfort and welfare of the sick, and the absence also of single-berth cabins so necessary for invalids, especially when suffering from a disease like phthisis, which is certainly communicable under certain conditions, or from other diseases which may render them obnoxious to their fellow-travellers. If consumptive patients are sent on a sea voyage they should certainly have cabins to themselves.

Many steamers now provide a certain number of *single* cabins, and persons who are in a position to pay for superior accommodation can usually obtain it, but a sea voyage then becomes a costly affair.

There are some differences of opinion as to whether it is better to take a long sea voyage in a steamer or a sailing vessel. In favour of the steamer, it is said there is less monotony of diet, less preserved and more fresh food, less tediousness and more variety of scene, and no liability to be becalmed many days in a trying tropical atmosphere. In favour of a well-appointed sailing vessel it is urged that the cabins are more spacious, there is plenty of deck-room, no over-crowding, no unpleasant smell of oil from the engines, no jarring and unpleasant vibration from the screw disturbing rest at night. There is more leisure to enjoy and realise a sea life, the changes of temperature are more gradual, and there is a greater gain to health provided the voyage is not too long and wearisome. A steamer, it is said, hurries invalids too quickly from fog and cold to tropical heat, and from tropical heat to the icebergs of the Southern Ocean. A sailing vessel provided with means of "steaming" would be best.

Patients who should avoid long sea voyages are gouty, bilious, neuralgic, and headachy persons; persons suffering from hæmorrhoids; most forms of chronic dyspepsia, on account of the food; and all cases of grave disease, and great general debility, requiring detailed attention and care, on account of the uncertainties inseparable from sea travel.

This remark does not apply to persons who are rich enough to have a large steam yacht of their own with travelling physician and nurses.

Epileptics and the melancholy and suicidal are obviously unsuitable.

Cases of asthma should not be sent to sea without first ascertaining if they bear well sea air and ship life. Some physicians advise a sea voyage in the milder forms of diabetes, but we see no particular reason for this, and there must be a certain difficulty about the diet in long voyages.

It should also be remembered that it may prove injurious and cruel to urge a sea voyage on persons who are not good sailors, and that women do not bear sea voyages as well as men.

Distant Resorts.

Recourse to a resort far distant from England necessarily involves a sea voyage of some duration, and this may prove an insuperable objection to the large class of invalids who have a dread of the sea, and there are others whom we may be unwilling to submit to the hazards and uncertainties of a sea voyage. Distant resorts are reserved mainly for those who are termed "hardy invalids," who are not the subjects of serious attacks, but who desire entire change of scene and relief from habitual surroundings, so as to efface painful impressions or modify depressing mental states.

They may also be attractive to young persons who, having broken down in health at home, may find it expedient to seek occupation and a livelihood in other climes. There is also a certain limited class of chronic maladies that are benefited by a greater and more complete change of climatic conditions than can be obtained except at a considerable distance, such, for instance, as the climate of the West Indies.

South Africa was, before the outbreak of the Transvaal War, largely resorted to by the class of young persons we have referred to, who, together with altered climatic conditions, needed to find occupation and a livelihood. We have pointed out, in a former chapter, that under existing circumstances South

Africa is hardly a suitable country for young invalids, and it would be difficult at present to point to any particular stations where they might go with advantage. We shall only refer to a few of the better-known resorts.

The general characteristics of the climate of the South African veldt are well known, viz. low atmospheric pressure, great dryness and clearness of the atmosphere, abundant and intense sunshine, small rainfall, and a wide daily range of temperature; also great purity of the air and freedom from organic dust; but the dust and the winds are often very trying, and so are the heat and absence of shade in summer. The South African winter, which corresponds with our summer, is the best season for the phthisical, the class of invalids chiefly interested in these climates, and those of the more vigorous sort mend greatly if they are at first received into suitable sanatoria and well looked after.

Cape Town is not a suitable resort for these patients. In the winter season (May, June and July) it is humid, rainy, and windy; in summer it is dusty. Its suburbs are preferable, such as Claremont (with a sanatorium), Rondebosch, and Wynberg. Two hours from Cape Town is **Caledon** (850 feet), with thermal gaseous iron springs and a sanatorium, and **Ceres** (1,493 feet) is also easily accessible—this and **Grahamstown** (1,772 feet), in the eastern part of Cape Colony, are good transition stations between the coast and the high veldt. **Beaufort West** is higher (2,729 feet), and is midway between Cape Town and Kimberley, and, like **Cradock** (2,856 feet), is regarded as a suitable resort for consumptive patients on first arriving in South Africa. **Turkastad** (4,300 feet), **Burghersdorf** (4,554 feet), **Aliwal North** (4,330 feet), on the Orange River, have all been recommended as eligibly situated resorts. **Kimberley** (4,042 feet) has a well-appointed sanatorium; so has **Barkley West** (4,000 feet); **Bloemfontein** (4,518 feet) has been referred to in a former chapter. **Harrismith**

(5,250 feet), in the Orange River Colony, has been highly praised as a resort for the phthisical; **Maritzburg** (2,200 feet), the capital of Natal, forty-one miles from the coast, has a warm, moist climate suitable for cases of chronic laryngeal and bronchial catarrh. As we have already said, very careful inquiries should be made before invalids set out for any South African resort.

Australia. There are very few invalids to whom a resort to Australia can be recommended. Young men with some chest delicacy, but capable of pursuing an agricultural life, may find healthy occupation in some of the more favoured localities, such as Eden, in New South Wales, and Twofold Bay, in Victoria; in some parts of Gippsland, as Mount Macedon, with a good sanatorium adjacent; some resorts in the Blue Mountains, as Mount Victoria, Katoomba, Boaroolong, the Riverina plain; the Darling Downs, in Queensland. But local information should be sought and local aid secured before venturing upon such a change.

Tasmania, with a cooler, moister, and more equable climate than Australia, is resorted to by Australians for an agreeable and wholesome change. Hobart Town is a favourite and popular summer resort.

New Zealand has a climate very similar to our own, and has practically little or no interest as a climatic resort for the ordinary run of invalids.

The **West India Islands**, most of them situated within the tropics, have a characteristic warm, humid, and equable climate, which has been reported to be very beneficial to certain forms of chronic Bright's disease, as the action of the skin is greatly promoted by the moist warmth of the atmosphere, while its equability provides against chills. Cases of dry and chronic irritative catarrh of the larynx and bronchi are also soothed and relieved by the sedative climate. It has, however, the drawback of proving very relaxing to many, causing loss of appetite, and not rarely producing chronic diarrhœa; while the frequent presence of endemic disease, in some of these islands, naturally makes physicians hesitate to recommend them as winter resorts. Moreover, furious hurricanes occasionally occur, and in some of the islands volcanic activity, at times, becomes alarming.

The English island of **Jamaica**, with Kingston for its capital, affords an attractive residence, especially at a distance from the sea, at an elevation of 1,000 feet (Gordontours) or 2,000 feet (Mandeville) above the sea; and higher and cooler resorts can be found (Newcastle, 4,000 feet). The rainfall is large, 55 inches being the annual average. The dryest and best season to visit the island is from the middle of December to May.

Barbados is perhaps the most attractive and suitable resort for the English invalid. It resembles Jamaica in climate, but, unlike it, it has no high mountains. The mean annual rainfall is large, 57 inches, but from December to May is a fairly dry season, and is the best for visitors from the north. Barbados is usually free from endemic disease, and is well looked after from a sanitary point of view. Many of the other islands are very picturesque and beautiful, but they have no interest for us as health resorts for invalids.

Nassau, the capital of the Bahamas, is frequented as a winter resort chiefly by Americans. It lies to the east of Florida, and is easily reached by steamer from the mainland, from which it is distant about 200 miles. Nassau has a warm, moist, equable climate, resembling somewhat the climate of Madeira. It has a good reputation for healthfulness, and possesses good hotel accommodation. In winter the relative humidity is 83 per cent., and the mean annual rainfall is 56 inches. Its warm, moist, sedative climate suits some convalescents from acute disease, and cases of irritative laryngeal and bronchial catarrh; but it is too relaxing for the tuberculous and too damp for the rheumatic.

Bermuda (Great Bermuda) has very much the same climatic characters as Nassau; but, being a British naval station, it has also social attractions. It is rather cooler and less humid than Nassau. Its climate has been thought suitable to excitable, nervous convalescents, to irritable neurasthenics, to cases of chronic nephritis, of dry bronchitis, and to cases of pneumonia.

The last of these distant resorts which we shall now refer to, and which are of interest to European invalids, is that favoured portion of the Pacific coast of the United States which belongs to **Southern California.** This coast, with the portion of the "Pacific slope" lying directly behind it, possesses one of the most genial and *equable* climates in the world. It is under the influence of a warm ocean current from Japan, and ranges of high mountains form its northern boundary, the land sloping gradually down from these to the ocean. It has mild winters and relatively cool summers, without extremes either of heat or cold. In the northern regions of this coast the atmosphere is humid and the rainfall is considerable, but this diminishes as we pass southwards, and there is a great difference between the climate of the towns on the northern part of the coast and that of the resorts to the south. The following are the chief of these:—

San Diego and **Coronado Beach** is situated at the extreme south-western corner of California. It has an attractive winter climate, warm and relatively dry. In January, the coldest month, the mean maximum temperature is 66° F., and the mean minimum is 35° F. There are a great number of clear days, but fogs are apt to appear in April and May. The rainfall is small, only 12 inches in the year. Summer is the dry season, but the temperature is rarely very high, the mean maximum in July being 84° F. Good hotel accommodation is to be had at Coronado, where there is also a good sanatorium.

Sea bathing is pleasant during nearly the whole year. There are suitable mountain resorts for camping out close at hand.

Avalon, the chief place in Santa Catalina Island, twenty-three miles from the mainland of California, is a popular and attractive winter resort suited for an out-of-door life, and well adapted to chronic bronchial and renal cases, and to those of general debility.

Los Angeles, 300 feet above the sea, and fourteen miles from the Pacific coast, is a large town 123 miles from San Diego. It has a wet winter and a dry summer climate, but there are a great number of fine days between November and May. There are fogs in spring and autumn; some doubts have been expressed as to the sanitary state of the city, and the influence of the climate in cases of advanced phthisis has not been favourable. **Pasadena**, nine miles from Los Angeles, at an elevation of 800 to 1,000 feet, is said to be a much better winter resort for invalids. **Santa Monica** and **Long Beach** are suitable sea-bathing resorts on the adjacent coast.

Santa Barbara is resorted to in both winter and summer on account of its mild and remarkably *equable* climate. Roses bloom and strawberries ripen, out of doors, all the year round. A fair idea of the great equability of its climate may be gained by comparing its mean temperature in January (63° F. at 2 p.m., 52° F. at 9 p.m.), and in July (78° F. at 2 p.m., 65° F. at 9 p.m.). Fogs in the early morning in the summer are not unusual. Its relative humidity is 69 to 71 per cent. Open to the south, it is well protected to the north. It enjoys light breezes from the sea by day, and breezes from the mountains by night. The mean annual rainfall is 18 inches, but it is very variable, ranging from 4½ to 35 inches. As a rule there is no rain between April and November. Santa Barbara has good accommodation for visitors, with great social advantages. There are hot sulphur springs. It has been described as "a safe and delightful refuge for old and young."* Its climate is especially favourable to chronic pulmonary and bronchitic cases, and to cases of chronic nephritis.

At **Idyll-wild**, at an elevation of 5,200 feet above the sea, in the mountains, about sixty miles from the Pacific coast, a sanatorium for consumptives has been established "in an ideal situation." Its elevation is the same as that of Davos Platz, but it "has a great advantage in the fact that out-of-door occupation is available 340 days in the year." The air is dry and pure, and not unpleasantly hot in summer. The temperature only occasionally falls below freezing point in winter. It is reached by the Santa Fé railroad.†

The only other South Californian resort that need be mentioned here is **Monterey**, beautifully situated on the bay of that name, 125 miles south of San Francisco. It has a sedative, equable climate, and outdoor life is agreeable all the year round. Accommodation for invalids is good. It is a resort especially recommended in cases of nervous debility and exhaustion, neurasthenia and insomnia. It is not, however, well suited to consumptive invalids.

The advantage of these South Californian resorts to European invalids of a certain type—young persons requiring occupation in a genial and suitable climate—is that they afford a means of obtaining a livelihood to those who are industrious, and who can devote a certain amount of capital to fruit growing and other agricultural pursuits.

* Cohen's System of Physiologic Therapeutics.

† *Ibid.*

CHAPTER X.

THE APPLICATION AND SELECTION OF CLIMATES. TREATMENT IN SANATORIA.

In our account of particular climatic resorts we have pointed out, especially in the more important, the kind of cases for the treatment of which they are appropriate; we must now indicate very briefly, in a general sense, the kind of climatic resorts suited to particular maladies.

As in treatment by mineral springs, treatment by climate is only applicable to cases of chronic disease, and to a certain number only of these; and in *incurable* forms of chronic disease we must be on our guard how we yield to the pressure of patients and their friends to send cases on long journeys in search of a doubtful remedy; such journeys can only be attended with disappointment and distress.

We should also keep in view the fact that the usefulness of particular climates is liable to be seriously modified and disturbed by the uncertainties of weather, and that in our statements and recommendations with regard to particular places, we can only rely on *averages*, and cannot be responsible for particular seasons, any more than the captain of a ship can be accountable for storms at sea! There is almost always, therefore, an element of risk in change of climate. But in some cases more than others, very much of that risk can be eliminated by proper care and caution; and we may repeat here what we have said elsewhere that "it is possible to make good use of a bad climate and bad use of a good one," and, in the case of consumptive invalids, that "care without climate is more important than climate without care."

Diseases of the respiratory organs, and especially *pulmonary consumption*, have always been regarded as especially benefited by climatic treatment, but of late years it has become more and more evident that climatic influences afford an important auxiliary factor in the restoration or maintenance of health in many other maladies; still the climatic treatment of so widely spread a disease as phthisis will always be of predominant interest and claim our first consideration.

The following is extracted from the address we had the honour of giving at the British Congress on Tuberculosis (July, 1901), on the Climatic Treatment of Consumption.*

The objects of treatment by climate in cases of pulmonary tuberculosis are the following:

(*a*) To arrest catarrhal conditions of the air passages.

(*b*) To improve nervous and circulatory tone.

(*c*) To increase the activity of the digestive functions, and thus stimulate nutrition by promoting the desire and increasing the power to take exercise.

(*d*) To raise the moral tone—by no means an unimportant matter—by affording a clear, bright, and cheerful environment.

(*e*) To diminish by its asepticity bacterial activity.

It must be a question for consideration whether so-called "open-air treatment," without regard to suitable climatic conditions, will do all this. It should be our object when practicable to place the consumptive patient under conditions and in circumstances where, without risk or injury, he may obtain the most complete and perfect aëration of the lungs possible.

If you place a feeble catarrhal patient in the open air in a damp and cold climate, you will risk an increase of the catarrh, and this will diminish pulmonary aëration by blocking up the air passages. The modern "open-air" treatment is only "new" in its manner of carrying out this idea of hyperaëration

* *Transactions* of the British Congress on Tuberculosis.

of the diseased lungs, and we must be especially careful, in applying it, to avoid the risk of aggravating catarrhal conditions. This has now been fully admitted by some of the most strenuous advocates of open-air treatment *per se.*

The recommendation of a long sea voyage as a cure for phthisis doubtless had its origin in the idea of pulmonary hyperaëration. It was an early form of "open-air" treatment, but with grave drawbacks and risks to which we have already referred.*

It may be interesting to mention that, between two and three centuries ago, Sydenham seems to have had in his mind also this same idea of hyperaëration of the lungs in the treatment of consumption. He says, in "A Short Treatise of Consumption":

> "The best remedy hitherto discovered . . . is riding sufficiently long journeys on horseback, provided this exercise be long enough continued. . . . For, in reality, the Peruvian bark is not more certainly curative of an intermittent fever than riding is of consumption."

And again :

> "But the principal assistant in the cure of this disease is riding on horseback every day, insomuch that whoever has recourse to this exercise in order to his cure, need not be tied down to observe any rules in point of diet, nor be debarred of any kind of solid or liquid aliment, as the cure depends wholly upon exercise."

Sydenham, in recognising, in the treatment of phthisis, the value of increasing pulmonary aëration, by long-continued horse exercise, clearly anticipated the modern idea of open-air treatment of this disease.

Now climatic treatment is essentially "open-air" treatment ; and the appropriate selection of a climate must depend on the suitability of that climate to open-air life in the particular cases we have to deal with.

* *See* chapter on Sea Voyages, p. 697.

It is difficult to establish any precise and rigid classification of the cases best suited to particular places, because in many cases, and especially in very early cases, and in quiescent chronic cases, with a limited area of local disease, the patients will do well and obtain arrest of the disease in a variety of places with somewhat different climatic conditions.

One of the most remarkable arrests of phthisis we have ever seen in an advanced stage—that is, with a considerable area of consolidation and excavation in the upper lobe of the left lung—occurred in London.

In another of the best results we have ever seen, in a case in a fairly advanced stage, the patient never went further from home than Hastings. The disease in the lungs has been arrested for some years.

Another advanced case that we have watched for many years has done well in a variety of places; she has wintered on the Riviera, in Algiers, in South Africa, at Orotava, at Montreux, at Cairo; but she will not go where she cannot get social entertainment, and for that reason she prefers Egypt.

These instances show how difficult it sometimes is to draw minute and precise conclusions as to the suitability of different places, from the results observed in individual cases. Many chronic stationary cases, with fair general health, travel about to different winter resorts in successive seasons and appear to benefit more or less in all.

All are agreed that early cases with a very limited area of local disease, with little or no fever, with integrity of the digestive functions, and in young and otherwise healthy adults, do well, and are frequently cured, in a variety of climates, provided they live a perfectly hygienic, open-air life. They recover probably more speedily in altitude climates than elsewhere.

There is also a general agreement that decidedly advanced dyspnœic cases should not, as a rule, be sent far from home, more especially if there is any pyrexia. It will, however, occasionally happen that such patients amongst the upper classes insist on change and get very restless at home, and they often rally a little on removal to some bright resort.

Of climates in which we have known distinct benefit follow, in such advanced chronic cases, we would especially cite Madeira and Malaga. These advanced cases are generally associated with bronchial catarrh, and the warm, equable, and moist climate of these places soothe the cough, favour expectoration, and allow of the patient being much in the open air.

The idea that formerly prevailed that a warm, moist, and equable climate was the best for consumptives had a certain foundation in the suitability of such climates to the advanced catarrhal cases. There was little idea of *cure* associated with these climates, because consumption was then regarded as incurable, but it was thought that they prolonged life, and made the slow process of dying less painful.

The quality of equability in a climate was at one time greatly over-rated. Indeed, we nowadays avoid an equable climate when seeking a cure for early cases of pulmonary tuberculosis. We rather choose a climate with a very wide diurnal range of temperature, if it is a dry climate, as the Engadine or the desert climate in Egypt.

Wide diurnal variations of temperature exert a bracing, invigorating, tonic effect, especially when they follow a certain regularity. What renders our own climate so very trying at times is that, although very variable, the variations of temperature follow no regularity. We get a week or ten days of very cold, fine, dry weather, and then, just as the organism is adapting itself to the dry external cold, it changes, and we get a spell of moist, wet, south-westerly winds, to be followed, after a few days, by a return of severely cold weather; and so on. It is on this account that our climate can never be well suited to the out-of-door treatment of cases of catarrhal phthisis.

There is no great difficulty in deciding what to do with cases at the very onset; we must be greatly influenced by questions of age, sex, temperament, occupation, social conditions, and constitutional tendency. Such cases will get well in a variety of places with careful management.

Nor is there much room for hesitation as to what course is best to follow in decidedly advanced cases. The progressive febrile cases are best in bed with an abundant supply of fresh air. It is the moderately advanced case that calls for careful discrimination, and is the most difficult to decide about.

It is now that the question of constitutional tendency comes into the foreground. Tuberculosis being an infective disease attended with greater or less dissemination of toxic substances throughout the organism, we find, as we do with the attacks of other infective microbes, varying degrees of reaction, of susceptibility, or infectibility, in different types of constitution.

It has been thought that the gouty constitution is antagonistic to tuberculous infection. Our impression is that the rheumatic constitution is so also, and that the latter is especially prone to develop the slow, fibroid, pleurogenic form of phthisis.

This form is not, in our opinion, well suited to altitude climates. These cases do best in a warm and dry climate, such as the more protected resorts of the Riviera and the desert climate, as in Upper Egypt or Biskra. Setting aside this group, the high mountain resorts have doubtless the widest range of applicability to moderately advanced cases. There are, however, certain other cases that do not improve in these resorts. Early or moderately advanced cases, with manifest cachexia, gastric disturbance, and more or less fever, do not do well in these or, as far as we are aware, in other resorts. A mild marine climate perhaps suits these cachectic cases best.

Cases with laryngeal or intestinal complications should not be sent to the mountains.

Cases of much emphysema complicating tuberculous infiltration, or tubercle invading emphysematous lungs will perhaps express better what we mean, are unsuited to altitude resorts. Cases of this latter group are prone to attacks of almost continuous and peculiarly uncontrollable hæmorrhage, and are most unpromising. As might be expected, cases with renal complication do not do well in the mountains, and if in such resorts albuminuria makes its appearance the patient should be removed to a warmer climate.

A peculiar sensitiveness to cold is a very decided drawback to wintering in the mountains; for although the patient may be mending, so far as the local disease is concerned, he or she is always depressed and unhappy.

In our own country, in which sanatorium treatment is becoming justly popular, we must seek for localities in which the worst characteristics of our changeable, insular climate are least felt, and where we can profit by what is best in it.

We have to consider the prevalence of fog and mist in many low-lying localities, the exposure to north-east and easterly winds in some, and to wet south-westerly gales in others.

What the consumptive patient most needs, for his cure, is a combination of climate and sanatorium treatment.

The gains to be obtained from a suitable climate in cases of consumption are these:—

(*a*) It relieves or removes catarrhal conditions accompanying the disease in a number of cases.

(*b*) It raises nervous and vascular tone.

(*c*) It increases muscular energy and the ability as well as the desire for exercise.

(*d*) By rendering an open-air life possible, it increases the aëration of the lungs and diminishes the activity of bacterial agencies, one of the most essential conditions of arrest and cure of the disease.

(*e*) It improves the tone and promotes the activity

of the digestive functions, and so enables the patient to take the large amount of food which is needed to heighten his state of nutrition.

(*f*) And, finally, it improves the moral and mental state by surrounding the patient with a bright, cheerful, and hopeful environment.

Next as to the selection of climates for different cases:

1. Cases seen at the very commencement of the disease, and who are otherwise in good health, may be permitted a certain amount of choice in the selection of a climate, provided it allows of many hours being spent daily in the open air, and that they are placed under admittedly hygienic conditions. A choice may be made from climates of altitude, the desert climate, the inland plateaux of South Africa, the sea voyage for those with a decided liking for the sea, and suitably placed sanatoria.

2. For progressive febrile cases, repose in bed or on a couch at home, in the best conditions practicable for the free access of air and sunshine to their apartments.

3. For advanced cases home is best, if the conditions of home life are favourable, or the warm marine climates, with cheerful surroundings, if home life is unfavourable or change is urgently desired.

4. For catarrhal cases warm, soothing climates like Madeira or Teneriffe are best.

5. For rheumatic or gouty cases of the fibroid or pleurogenic type, dry, marine climates or the desert climate are most suitable.

6. For the so-called "scrofulous cases," if free from catarrh, fairly bracing marine climates; if with catarrh, mild marine climates should be prescribed.

7. For most other moderately advanced cases, with the limitations already mentioned, the climate of the high mountains, above the cloud belt, is the most curative.

Chronic Bronchial and Laryngeal Catarrh; Pulmonary Emphysema.—Chronic catarrhs of the respiratory mucous membrane are greatly under the influence of climatic conditions.

We do not share the view that the cold dry air of high mountain valleys is useful, even in young subjects, who are *actually* the subjects of these catarrhal conditions; but we think them of great value in the *intervals* between the attacks, or, when an attack has passed away, as a preventive of the tendency to them. In such cases the influence of the mountain climate should be sought in the summer, and, if things go well, the residence might be prolonged into the winter. We have known cases in which a period of five or six weeks, in summer and autumn, spent in the Engadine, for several years in succession, has, by its bracing and tonic influence, quite removed this tendency to catarrhal attacks. But in elderly and feeble subjects the mountain climate should never be prescribed for these affections, for they are then very frequently accompanied by pulmonary emphysema and dilated right heart, and sometimes by much dyspnœa on exertion, which the rarefied air of these elevations greatly aggravates. Such patients also want *level* walks if they are to take any walking exercise. The slightest ascent will often cause them much uneasiness.

If the case is one of "dry" catarrh and in a gouty subject, a warm, rather moist, equable, sedative climate, of which Madeira may be taken as a type, is the best. But Madeira or the Canaries are too far off for most patients, and we have to be content with something less perfect. Algiers, Palermo, Malaga, Ajaccio, are also far off, but suitable. Pau is a rather uncertain climate, and Biarritz is often very windy. Arcachon suits some, but a warmer climate is more advantageous. In this country the moist climate of Penzance, Falmouth, or Torquay is the best.

For those cases with much expectoration it is better to choose a warm, dry winter climate, such as Egypt and the resorts of the Riviera (the Austrians use also Meran and Arco in such cases). The Riviera resorts are very useful when proper precautions are taken to avoid the chill of the late afternoon. The bronchitic patient, in the short days of winter on the Riviera, should be within doors by three in the afternoon. There is also a certain range of climate to choose from in that region—the climate of Bordighera and San Remo is more sedative and less exciting than that of Cannes and Nice. Cimiez and Cannet are more tonic than Beaulieu or Mentone, where much warmth may be found, especially in the eastern bay of Mentone. Hyères and Costebelle are more sedative than some of the resorts further east. At Nice cases of chronic bronchitis and emphysema can also obtain treatment at a well-arranged inhalatorium, under the skilful direction of Mons. Vos, and many patients find the combination of inhalation treatment with the climatic influences in this resort of great service. Our best home resorts for these cases are Hastings, Ventnor, Bournemouth, and Sidmouth. Cases complicated with albuminuria, however slight, should never be sent to the mountains; they do best in Egypt or on the Riviera. In cases in which *emphysema* is the predominating condition, Meran often proves a useful winter resort, where pneumatic treatment can be applied. Its climate is a dry, bright, but cold one. The same kind of treatment can be obtained at Reichenhall in the summer and autumn.

The foregoing remarks are applicable also, to a great extent, to those troublesome cases of *naso-pharyngeal catarrh* so common in some families. In young subjects we should place rather more stress on the great advantage of bracing treatment in high altitude stations, as a preventive measure; and in scrofulous cases the advantage of a long sea voyage carried out under favourable circumstances, or, still better, a series of sea trips, of comparatively brief duration, in sunny seas, may prove of great value.

We are not sanguine as to the value of change of climate in cases of *bronchiectasis;* but if it is thought desirable to try its effect, the same climates as are suitable for chronic bronchial catarrh, with abundant expectoration, should be chosen.

Chronic pleurisy, adhesions in the apical regions, and the remains of pleuritic effusions, require the same climatic treatment in cases of early phthisis.

Asthma.—The purely nervous or *spasmodic* form of asthma is extremely capricious in its behaviour at different places, so that it is scarcely possible to predict, without previous trial, what place will or will not suit the individual patient. It is not quite the same with the catarrhal form—the cases that have followed and been caused by, and are associated with, attacks of bronchial catarrh. In such cases a primary condition of successful treatment is to select a climate in which the catarrh will be relieved.

With regard to the first group of cases, if the asthmatic attacks occur in young people, especially in young children, the climate of the high Alps may afford prospects of a cure—Davos and St. Moritz are the best localities, as in either educational advantages can be obtained. It is advisable for the patient to begin residence in the summer or autumn, and continue through the winter. More than one season will usually be necessary.

Adult patients and patients advanced in years, with a dry, irritating cough, and very sensitive respiratory mucous membrane, will sometimes be greatly benefited by the sedative, warm and moist climate of Madeira, especially at the higher resorts in the island, or by the somewhat more tonic resorts of Algiers, Ajaccio, Palermo, or even Pau and Arcachon; in England, Torquay or Falmouth or Penzance may be tried. Cases with profuse expectoration do better in the dryer climate of Egypt or the Riviera. We have seen some excellent results from a winter or two at Cannet or Cimiez—going on to Grasse in the late spring. We have also seen remarkable relief of the spasmodic attacks follow a change from London to Folkestone. Attempts have been made to treat asthmatic patients advanced in life, at high altitudes; but inasmuch as in all these cases a certain amount of pulmonary emphysema is sure to exist, the attempts have not only failed, but, in some instances, have been disastrous.

Hay asthma and hay fever require a marine climate; such cases need to be actually on the sea, or surrounded by sea, on a small rocky island without vegetation; or if this is not practicable, to be on the sea coast away from vegetation.

Diseases of the Circulatory System.—The climatic treatment of cardiac affections must be determined to some extent by individual considerations; especially as to age and condition, the extent and nature of the cardiac lesions, and the presence or absence of complications.

The cardiac patient requires a climate free from extremes—where the air is pure and invigorating without being either cold, dry and exciting, or hot, moist, and relaxing. Shelter from cold winds is desirable; plenty of sunshine, and as dry an atmosphere as is compatible with a certain degree of equability. If gastro-hepatic troubles complicate the case it is usually best to avoid the seaside and choose a mildly bracing inland resort at a moderate elevation. Near London we have such resorts in Tunbridge Wells, Sevenoaks, Crowborough, Haslemere, and, at a greater distance, Malvern. The possibility of a variety of level walks is most important for the cardiac patient.

As a rule it is not advisable to send cardiac patients far from home—but if in the summer, or autumn, a trip to Switzerland or the Black Forest seems desirable, places of quite moderate elevation should be chosen, between 1,000 and 3,000 feet, where level walks can be had, as Interlaken, Glion, Meiringen, Triberg, Baden-Baden; and younger subjects with well compensated mitral lesions may go higher—to St. Beatenberg, Les Avants, Engelberg and the like. High elevations should be avoided unless in quite exceptional cases. If the case is complicated with bronchial catarrh and a tendency to emphysema, great caution must be observed in the selection of a winter climate. Some cases of this kind do best in a mild, equable marine climate, or in the more protected resorts on the Riviera, as Beaulieu, Costebelle, Mentone, or Bordighera. In our own southern coasts Hastings, the sheltered part of Eastbourne away from the sea, West Worthing, Bournemouth, Sidmouth, and Torquay present suitable winter resorts ; the object being to exercise a soothing influence on the irritable bronchial mucous membrane and to promote, by sun-warmth, the circulation in the skin, and so relieve the labour of the heart.

It is an error to send cardiac cases to a dry, exciting climate like Egypt, with a wide diurnal range of temperature, bringing risk of chill.

The sedative winter climate of Pau suits some cases.

The cardiac invalid requires in summer a clear, fresh atmosphere, mildly tonic but not exciting, and in winter, warmth, sunshine, and protection from chill. In all advanced cases a restful and peaceful *entourage* is needful—for these rest is the best tonic.

Dyspepsia.—The dyspeptic can scarcely expect to be cured by climate, but there are certain climates which tend to aggravate his malady, and others which help to remove it.

Change *per se* and the distractions of travel often prove of much service to the nervous dyspeptic and to the dyspeptic whose malady has been aggravated, if not induced, by too close application to business or study. Climates which by their bracing air and attractive scenery provoke to active exercise often prove most valuable and remedial resources to this class of invalid ; we therefore find removal from lowlands to mountain regions most useful.

Most dyspeptics complain that they are apt to get worse at the seaside—to become "bilious," constipated, and to lose appetite and become depressed. This is more particularly the case with coast towns which are on a level with the sea and have what is known as "strong" sea air. If the visitors can live on a cliff, high above the sea, as at Folkestone, or on high ground at a little distance from the sea, as at Eastbourne, we hear less of these complaints. Such patients, however, are better at bracing inland resorts, as at Hindhead or Crowborough or Malvern.

If there is a tendency to hepatic congestion and hæmorrhoids these patients do not bear well the higher mountain stations, and should not go beyond 3,000 or 4,000 feet—Engelberg, Grindelwald, Chamounix are suitable.

The pleasant sunny resorts of the French Riviera often agree well in winter with many dyspeptics if they choose a residence removed some distance from the sea.

Chronic Nephritis.—Cases of chronic Bright's disease, that are well enough to leave home, should seek a winter climate which favours a free circulation in the skin and increased cutaneous activity, for there is a close relation between the functions of the kidneys and those of the skin. Any check to the action of the skin throws additional work on the kidneys. It is usual to recommend a warm and dry climate for such cases in winter, such as the Egyptian resorts—Mena, Helouan, Luxor, Assouan—but the drawbacks to this kind of climate, apart from its distance from home, is the wide daily range of temperature and the risk of chill to the surface from the great differences between day and night and sun and shade temperatures, so that constant care and caution to avoid such chill are needful; and although in such a dry and warm climate the loss of water from the skin is promoted, it is questionable whether the solids which should be got rid of by the skin are excreted in the same proportion. It will be found that climates which are more equable, if not quite so dry, suit some cases better—as the warmest of the Riviera resorts: Mentone, Beaulieu, Bordighera. The climate of Algiers, although moister, is more equable, and cases of Bright's disease do fairly well there. The same may be said of Ajaccio and Palermo.

In America the extremely equable coast resorts of Southern California—especially Passadena and Monterey—have been found to provide a very suitable winter climate for cases of chronic nephritis.

We have known such cases do extremely well at Madeira, and their lives have appeared to be greatly prolonged by passing the winter in that island, although, as is well known, its climate is not a dry one. The dryer climate of the Canary Islands should answer still better. We have been assured, on good authority, that the warm, equable, though moist climate of the West Indies has been found to suit some forms of Bright's disease particularly well. At Barbados, between December and May, there is very little rain, and the mean relative humidity is only 72 per cent. The skin appears to act very freely in those warm and rather moist climates. The prevalence of cold winds is one of the most prejudicial conditions for sufferers from renal disease, and patients who cannot leave England should choose a residence protected as much as possible from them—Bournemouth, Sidmouth, Torquay, Salcombe, Falmouth—a sheltered spot in either of these localities would be suitable. It is desirable, in these cases, to consider the patient's experience as to the effect of different climates upon him, as some find a warm, sedative climate suits them, but others a dry, stimulating one.

In cases of *Chronic Pyelitis* and cases of *Chronic Vesical Catarrh* the climatic indications are identical with the foregoing, but much must not be expected from climate alone in these cases; the avoidance, however, of a cold, windy, and damp atmosphere in winter is an undoubted advantage. The usefulness of a diet consisting greatly of milk, in those maladies, must not be overlooked, and, in the summer, resort may be had to one of the numerous subalpine stations in Switzerland, the Tyrol, or the Black Forest, where the milk cure is carried out.

Nervous Affections, Nervous Exhaustion or Neurasthenia, Nervous Irritability and Depression, Hysteria, Neuritis, and Neuralgia from Nervous Exhaustion, Tabes Dorsalis, Graves' Disease.— We have here grouped together a number of diseases of the nervous system which admit, in varying degrees, of beneficial treatment by change of climate. In some of these conditions, in which morbid mental states are prominent, as unhealthy habits of introspection and self-regard, undue anxiety and unfounded apprehensions, often leading to insomnia, also tendencies to hysterical manifestations —all these states are often favourably affected by removal from home influences and the habitual environment, and their replacement by the occupations and interests which travel affords in bright, sunny, and tonic climates, with cheerful social surroundings and objects of artistic, historic, and general interest. In summer and autumn we may suggest recourse to picturesque mountain and lake regions in Switzerland, Italy, or the Tyrol, or a yachting cruise in the Mediterranean ; in the winter a tour in Egypt or Algiers, or visits to the historic cities of Southern Italy and Sicily. When expense is not a consideration, a variety of interesting and health-giving tours can be devised. A less costly, but a very useful expedient, when the patients are active and vigorous, is a walking tour in the Swiss mountains or through Normandy and Brittany, with congenial companionship. Inattention to social considerations will often lead to the failure of these measures, for the class of patients we are thinking of are particularly sensitive to social influences, and an uncongenial or unsuitable environment or association will undo any good that climatic change might otherwise bring about.

Some instances and examples of the nervous maladies we have enumerated above will be found to present so great an amount of nervous and muscular exhaustion that absolute rest—a "rest cure" in short —is needed at starting, and a climate must be chosen, dry, sunny, tonic, and cheerful, where the patient may recline for many hours daily in the open air. This is possible in sheltered inland, wooded resorts in England, or in mountain resorts of medium elevation in the Black Forest, Switzerland, and the Tyrol. In winter the warmer and more sheltered resorts of the Riviera, or for some cases the more sedative climate of the south-west of France, as Biarritz, Pau, or Arcachon, may be selected.

When there is "irritable weakness" of the nervous system, a course of simple thermal baths in a cheerful mountain or forest region often proves very serviceable—we may name Gastein, Bagnères-de-Bigorre, Wildbad, and Schlangenbad. Neuralgic cases require dry warmth in winter, and tonic, dry, mountain air in summer, but not too cold.

Neurasthenic states, especially those that have been induced by overwork or much worry and anxiety, obtain very great benefit from mountain resorts where they can get "glacier air" in summer (Pontresina, Mürren, Adelboden, Grindelwald), and from the Nile voyage in a dahabeeah in winter; other patients who are fond of the sea may take a sea voyage to India or to the Cape, or the West Indies, or Brazil, etc., according to the season of the year, but the patient's tastes and wishes should be consulted, as it is most undesirable to launch such a patient upon a voyage which is distasteful to him.

Tabetic cases are often benefited in summer by thermal baths in the stations we have mentioned above; and in winter yachting in sunny seas, or the Nile voyage, may prove of service. In some a prolonged sojourn at mountain resorts of moderate elevation, where pleasant level walks can be obtained, is attended with improvement. When *Insomnia* accompanies any of these conditions we shall usually have to avoid all exciting climates, all resorts close to the sea coast, and choose quiet, sedative resorts, sheltered from high winds. The air of high mountain valleys proves soothing and refreshing to some cases; the more moderate elevations are preferred by others. Each case must be dealt with according to individual peculiarities.

Cases of *Graves' Disease* are usually more benefited by change of climate than by any other kind of treatment, as we have pointed out elsewhere.* We have seen excellent results attend removal to, and a long stay in, such sedative and tonic seaside resorts as Westgate, Folkestone, Hastings, Brighton, or other similar stations. But it must be a long stay, usually not less than six months. Biarritz is a very suitable winter resort. Many German authorities prescribe high mountain climates, such as Davos and the Engadine. Professor Erb says he has "seen excellent results" from a residence in these resorts.† Nothnagel, Eulenberg, and H. Weber have expressed similar opinions.

Gout, Rheumatism, Rheumatoid Arthritis.—Sufferers from these affections require similar climatic treatment. They are all influenced unfavourably by cold, windy and damp localities, and they are all benefited by residence in warm and dry situations. Indeed the mere removal from a dwelling on a damp clay soil, to an abode on a dry gravelly one, will make a great difference to the comfort of sufferers from chronic rheumatism. These cases rarely obtain any benefit from our sea-coast resorts—unless from the dryer and warmer ones in summer, with residence somewhat removed from the sea, and on a dry soil above the sea level. Gouty subjects are apt to become dyspeptic and bilious in what is known as "strong" sea air, and for rheumatic subjects most of our seaside resorts are too humid or too windy.

* "Manual of Medical Treatment," New Edition, vol. i., p. 489.

† "Winter Cures in the High Mountains."

Dry inland resorts with southern aspect, and protected from cold winds, are most suitable. Gouty patients are usually also unsuited to high altitudes, especially if they are subject to hepatic torpor and hæmorrhoids; and rheumatic patients not unfrequently find their symptoms aggravated by the cold and variable temperatures of these regions. Many of those patients, however, find, in the summer and autumn, treatment with simple thermal baths at quite moderate elevations useful—as at Gastein, Ragatz, and Wildbad. The most suitable winter resorts are either the warm, dry Riviera stations, with residence removed a little from the sea-shore, as Hyères, Cannes, Nice, Mentone, Bordighera, San Remo, etc., and where pleasant level walks can be obtained, as regular exercise in the open air is most important for the gouty, favouring as it does oxidation and the removal of waste, and tending to counteract constipation; or in the case of patients who are fairly vigorous and enjoy travelling, the desert resorts in Egypt or Algiers are suitable—Helouan, Luxor, Assouan, or Hammam R'Irha and Biskra. The warmer and dryer resorts are especially appropriate to the cases with tendency to arterial and renal changes.

With regard to convalescents from attacks of acute rheumatism, it is important, as we have elsewhere pointed out, that they should not be hurried away from home, as they require, above all things, a prolonged period of repose, to save the cardiac valves as much as possible from all strain and excitement. Dry and sunny inland resorts are best suited to those cases, the nearer home the better.

The prohibition of sea climates does not apply to young subjects of rheumatoid arthritis—for some of these cases appear to have affinities with scrofula, and may do well at the seaside or even on the sea. The foregoing remarks apply also to *neuralgic* cases in the gouty and rheumatic.

Diabetes.—There is not much to be expected

from climatic treatment in cases of diabetes, and as so much depends on diet and supervision, in all the serious forms of this disease, removal from the care of home (unless to a suitable sanatorium) is rarely advisable, and we should always bear in mind that the more serious forms bear the fatigue and excitement of travel *very badly*. Many such cases have been brought to a premature end by the fatigue of indiscreet travelling. When the symptom of glycosuria is only an incident of the gouty constitution, and is associated with obesity, the same resorts as we have recommended for the gouty should be prescribed, and note should especially be taken of the need of facilities for walking exercise, which is most useful in these cases.

In the cases of medium severity it is not unusual to encounter much restlessness, and a great desire to try the effect of change to a warmer and sunnier climate in winter. The accessibility and cheerfulness of the Riviera resorts may, in such cases, be recommended, with many cautions as to the avoidance of excitement and over-exertion. Cases that have benefited by treatment at one or other of the spas which are usually recommended in this disease in the summer, may advantageously take an after-cure at a medium mountain elevation.

Anæmia and Chlorosis.—In selecting a climate for cases of chronic anæmia and chlorosis we have, in the first place, to consider the need of *absolute rest* in some cases where there is much cardiac weakness and nervous exhaustion, and the desirability, in other less advanced cases that retain a certain amount of muscular strength, of promoting moderate daily exercise. In all cases we desire a bright, tonic air, plenty of sunshine, agreeable surroundings, and cheerful social conditions. We must avoid damp, relaxing situations, and all localities which are too cold for sitting or reclining in the open air. The anæmic patient should not be sent to a climate where there is any risk of feeling chilled.

In summer our own sea-coast resorts offer a great choice of sunny localities, where many hours each day may be spent in the open air. There are the more bracing resorts on the north and east coasts—Scarborough, Whitby, Cromer, Lowestoft—for those who are able to bear a tonic, stimulating, dry marine climate; while we can find climates bracing in various degrees at the south coast resorts, between Westgate and Southsea, and milder and more sedative climates in the resorts further west.

If the sea-coast fails to agree with certain cases, as is not uncommon, especially the dyspeptic and bilious cases, we must select such tonic inland resorts as are accessible, and are in dry, healthy situations. Tunbridge Wells, Crowborough, Haslemere, and Hindhead and Malvern are suitable places; or, in Scotland, Pitlochry, Braemar, and many other highland retreats, are very suitable for the less severe cases which are able to enjoy gentle out-of-door exercise. Ilkley and Ben Rhydding, in Yorkshire, are adapted to the same class of cases.

For young and fairly active anæmics the Swiss mountain resorts, at moderate elevations, often prove most beneficial, and if great improvement occurs at the lower elevations the patient can pass on to the higher and more bracing ones. By moving from place to place, at short distances, and within moderate limits, which it is quite easy to do in Switzerland or the Tyrol, the moral and mental advantage of frequent change of scene and surroundings is notable, particularly in those cases with a tendency to nervous irritability. In winter we should select for these cases a climate which is dry and sunny and which permits of being much in the open air. The resorts of the Riviera are very appropriate, especially those where patients can live at some little distance from the coast, as Hyères, Cannet, Cimiez, and Bordighera. Montreux and the surrounding resorts on the Lake of Geneva, Lugano, Locarno on the Italian lakes, or

Arco, near the Lago di Guarda, are more sedative than the Riviera resorts.

In short, the suitable resorts are those which enable the patient to be much in the open air, either for complete repose, in the severe cases requiring a *rest* cure, or for graduated exercise in those who are more vigorous. We should see that the food arrangements are satisfactory; and a good test of the suitability of the climate is an improvement in appetite. Yachting in smooth waters and sunny seas may suit some patients who like the sea.

Malarial Cachexia.—The subjects of malarial cachexia require much the same climatic conditions as the foregoing. They especially require protection from cold, damp winds, exposure to which is apt to bring back attacks of fever.

In summer, dry and sunny situations in the Alps are suitable, at quite moderate elevations at first, which may be followed by resort to the more bracing high altitude stations. Places like Engelberg, St. Beatenberg, or Grindelwald may be succeeded by Mürren, Davos, or the Engadine. Glion, Caux, Les Avants are suitable resorts, and convenient for passing readily from a lower to a higher elevation. Appropriate resorts at home are Tunbridge Wells, Crowborough, Hindhead, Malvern, Ilkley, Braemar. In winter the warmer and more protected Riviera resorts are most useful.

Paroxysmal Hæmoglobinuria.—Cases of this disease especially need removal to a warm climate in winter, as exposure to cold and damp is apt to induce an attack in the predisposed. A decidedly *warm* climate should be chosen, such as India, Ceylon, the West Indies, or the warmer Egyptian resorts, Teneriffe and the like. Such patients should depart for their destination before the cold winter weather sets in, and should be cautioned to avoid all exposure to chill.

Scrofula.—The climates most suitable to the treatment of the various forms of scrofula are maritime climates. Sea air, combined with sea bathing, when the season permits, has a remarkable influence in promoting and quickening the nutritive changes necessary to recovery in these cases. Our own coasts supply almost everything that can be needed in this direction, and delicate scrofulous children, or the children of families in which such tendencies are known to exist, should be educated and brought up at the seaside. The results obtained at the Margate sanatorium are most striking, and many other of our seaside resorts can show equally good results. A sea voyage is also useful for young boys if suitable opportunities occur.

There are, however, a certain few delicate children with whom sea air disagrees, and for these the mountain resorts often give excellent results. And there are delicate scrofulous children, with retarded development and catarrhal tendencies, who are very sensitive to cold, and who seem to need more of the stimulating effect of sunshine than can be obtained on our shores; for these the warmer winter climate of the Riviera resorts, or those on the south-west coast of France, or in Algiers, or the frequented resorts in the Mediterranean islands, are of great help in furthering normal development.

The *Climacteric* period in women is often associated with troublesome nervous and circulatory symptoms, vague apprehensions, insomnia, palpitations, flatulent dyspepsia, etc., which may need recourse to change of climate. In these cases moral, social and mental influences play an important *rôle*, and in prescribing change we must be guided in our selection by what is likely to be agreeable to the patient. As a rule, exciting climates are best avoided, and a combination of tonic and sedative influences is the desideratum. Biarritz and Pau in winter are suitable, and so are Montreux and the surrounding resorts, or Lugano and Locarno. On the Riviera the less exciting situations are best, as Hyères, Cannet, Mentone, Bordighera, San Remo,

Rapallo. Ajaccio and the Sicilian resorts are also suitable. In summer, well wooded and shady places at moderate elevations in the Black Forest, or in Switzerland, are suitable, and in some cases it will be found that the higher elevations prove more calming to the nervous symptoms than lower resorts. A combination of simple thermal baths with mountain or forest air, as at Gastein, Ragatz, or Schlangenbad, often has a very soothing effect. A well-arranged tour to interesting places in healthy localities, with congenial companionship, will sometimes be the best resource.

Senility.—Change of climate often proves useful in warding off, or retarding, the loss of power and debility which accompany advancing years.

Aged persons are also more liable to suffer from serious chill from exposure in winter to great cold, or sudden and frequent changes of temperature, and they need protection from such injurious conditions. Prosper Merimée spoke of the sun as "le grand arbitre des santés humaines, Monseigneur le Soleil ;" and winter sunshine, clear skies, and a certain amount of warmth are the climatic conditions favourable to the prolongation of the life of aged people.

The search after winter sunshine is not, therefore, an unwise pursuit in old age. It may be obtained in many places—Cannes, Nice, San Remo, and other Riviera resorts, Egypt, Castellamare, the Sicilian resorts, Biarritz, Algiers, short sea voyages in sunny seas, etc., according to individual tastes and wishes. It is usually desirable to select places which present some intellectual interests, and where good food and cooking (of much importance at this age) can be obtained. In the summer and autumn a combination of mild mountain or forest air, with simple thermal baths, as at Gastein or Wildbad, is also most serviceable.

Convalescence from acute disease. We should not be in a hurry to remove from their homes patients who are recovering from attacks of acute disease; it is much better that they should remain, for some time, under the same watchful care that has attended them through the acute attack. It is only when the convalescence is retarded, and the patient appears to be making little or no progress, that a change should be advised—in the summer a change from residence in town to a well-wooded country district, at a good elevation, and offering some protected spots for reclining out of doors, or for gentle exercise; or if the patient is fond of the seaside, to a quiet resort on the coast, with agreeable surroundings. If this is not sufficient, a Black Forest resort or a Swiss resort, at a moderate elevation, may be chosen—not going higher than 2,500 or 3,000 feet at first.

In winter a warmer and sunnier climate may be needed, and then we must consult the patient's tastes and feelings, if they are reasonable; there is a great choice of resorts on the Riviera, or at the upper part of the Lake of Geneva, or on the south-west coast of France (Biarritz, St. Jean de Luz); or a visit to Egypt may be practicable; or a sea voyage may be best suited to those hardier convalescents who love the sea.

Treatment in Sanatoria.

Of late years the system of treating consumptive patients in "open-air" sanatoria has grown rapidly. No one can doubt the great advantage to the consumptive patient that he should be constantly under the observation, care, and direction of competent and experienced physicians, and that his daily life should be subject to personal medical supervision.

In a suitable, well-organised sanatorium he is kept in pure open air, so as to secure constant *hyper-aëration* of the lungs; his diet is physiologically adapted to his powers of digestion (not so excessive as to induce dyspepsia); the hours of meals, of sleep, of exercise are wisely adapted to individual needs and aptitudes; and the tonic influences, when requisite, of hydrotherapeutic measures are obtainable. The many cases that need entire or relative rest for a long period are ensured it, and when the capacity and fitness for exercise are acquired it is duly graduated to the physical strength of each patient. In short, in a well ordered sanatorium, everything that can conduce to the patient's cure is effectively enjoined and enforced, and everything that can hinder recovery is removed and forbidden.

That the application of such a system should have been attended by excellent results can occasion no surprise. But in addition to its beneficial curative influence on the patients submitted to this treatment, it has another strong recommendation in that it removes the consumptive patient from a position of danger to others—the danger of communicating the disease to those with whom he would be, in his own home, in close association. Sanatorium treatment must therefore be estimated, not only for its curative influence, but also for its efficacy as a preventive of the spread of this disease. Its best effects are seen in young adults who present signs of the earliest stage of the disease; but this is the case with all other methods of treatment of phthisis, and, like all forms of climatic treatment, its idea and aims are to augment the resisting power of the patient so that he may be able to overcome the activities of the agents of infection.

The mode of carrying out this treatment varies somewhat according to the views of "open-air" treatment that may be entertained by the various medical directors of these institutions. Some are extremists, and advocate keeping patients in the open air night and day, in all weathers, and exposed to all the winds that blow. Others are more cautious, and consider it of some importance to have the sanatorium placed where the climatic conditions are favourable, with a sunny, southern aspect, on a dry soil, with pine woods near at hand, and where the atmosphere is comparatively still, and there is protection from chilling winds. Dr. Gordon, of Exeter, has shown, we think conclusively, that exposure to strong winds is injurious to the phthisical, and Dr. Howard Sinclair observes: "The aphorism that strong winds are poison to the consumptive cannot be too strongly insisted on."

It seems to be generally admitted that, where it is possible, the sanatoria should be placed in high altitude resorts, as they give the best results; but where this is not practicable, as must be the case in providing such institutions for the working classes, it is desirable to build them in the country, in healthy districts, in well sheltered situations, with pure, dry air, and as near as possible to the usual habitations of the patients.

In the opinion of some physicians it is not possible to afford the patient, in his own home, under any circumstances, the advantages and protection from imprudences that he will get in a sanatorium. We can hardly share so extreme an opinion. We believe an intelligent patient, anxious to be cured, and convinced of the curative power of the conditions prevailing in sanatoria, and with the means needed to secure constant medical supervision, can be provided with "open-air" treatment at home as well as in such institutions, although, no doubt, a temporary residence in a well directed sanatorium would serve as a useful introduction and education for home treatment.

The shortest time limit that can safely be estimated for efficient treatment in a sanatorium is six months—some estimate it at a much longer period; but six months is a long time for a working man to be away from his work, and it has been shown that unless, after his discharge, he can be kept employed in some healthful open-air pursuit, there is great danger of an early return of disease.

Those who do not bear well the extreme open-air treatment are persons advanced in years, catarrhal subjects, persons abnormally sensitive to cold, persons with habitually delicate appetites, and young children.

Men are said to bear it better than women. The most recent statistics seem to show that the results of sanatorium treatment are not quite so satisfactory as was at one time stated. That it distinctly has its limitations is clear, and it cannot be regarded as doing away with the need for climatic treatment, but rather as an alternative, when climatic change cannot be obtained, or as an adjunct to it.

What is most urgently needed is the provision of asylums for advanced and hopeless cases, so as to prevent the spread of the disease in the overcrowded dwellings of the poor.

LIST OF SANATORIA.

England and Wales.

The London Sanatorium (64 beds). Pinewood, Wokingham, Berks. Address: Secretary, London Open Air Sanatorium, 20, Hanover Square, W.

Bournemouth, Alderney Manor Sanatorium, Parkstone (25 beds). Medical director: Dr. Denton Johns.

Bournemouth, Overton Hall Sanatorium (16 beds). Medical directors: Drs. Pott and Stein.

Bournemouth, Stourfield Park Sanatorium (45 beds). Medical officer: Dr. F. Fowler.

Bournemouth, Brinklea Sanatorium (10 beds). Medical director: Dr. Kinsey Morgan.

Bourne Castle Sanatorium, Belroughton, Worcestershire. Elevation, 750 feet. Resident physician: Dr. Phillpot.

Belle-Vue Sanatorium, Shotley Bridge, near Durham (10 beds). Resident physician: Dr. E. W. Diver.

Cotswold Sanatorium (37 beds). Elevation, 800 feet. Medical officer: Dr. Pruen.

Chiltern Hills Sanatorium, near Reading. Elevation, 375 feet. Physician: Dr. Esther Colebrook.

Crooksbury Sanatorium, near Farnham, Surrey (20 beds). Medical director: Dr. Walters.

Dartmoor Sanatorium, near Chagford, Devon. Elevation, 750 feet. Resident physician: Dr. A. Scott-Smith.

Dunston Park Sanatorium, Paignton, S. Devon (16 beds). Medical officer: Dr. T. Carson Fisher.

East Anglian Sanatorium, Nayland, near Bures, Suffolk (35 beds). Medical director: Dr. Jane Walker.

Harbourne Sanatorium, High Haldon, Ashford, Kent (20 beds). Medical officer: Dr. P. Paget.

Hailey Sanatorium, Ipsden (Chiltern Hills), Goring, near Reading (12 beds). Medical director: Dr. Reinhardt.

Linford Sanatorium, Ringwood, New Forest, Hants (15 beds). Physician: Dr. Mander-Smith.

Moorcote Sanatorium, Eversley, Winchfield, Hants (12 beds). Resident physician: Dr. W. L. Baker.

Mundesley Sanatorium, near Cromer (15 beds). Medical officer: Dr. Fanning.

Mendip Hills Sanatorium, Hill Grove, Over Wells, Somerset (20 beds). Elevation, 850 feet. Medical officer: Dr. Muthu.

Nordrach-upon-Mendip, near Wells, Somerset (37 beds). Elevation, 862 feet. Medical directors: Drs. Thurnam and Gwynne.

Nordrach-in-Wales, Pendyffryn Hall, Penmaenmawr, N. Wales (20 beds). Elevation, 1,000 feet. Physician: Dr. Morton Wilson.

Painswick Sanatorium, Cotswold Hills, Gloucestershire. Elevation, 600 feet. Physician: Dr. W. McCall.

Rudgwick Sanatorium, near Horsham, Sussex (12 beds). Medical director: Dr. Annie McCall.

Timbercombe, Spaxton, near Bridgewater, Somerset (10 beds). Medical officer: Dr. Brown.

Vale of Clwyd Sanatorium, Llanbedr Hall, Ruthin, N. Wales. Elevation, 450 feet. Physicians: Drs. Grace-Calvert and C. E. Fish.

Whitmead Hill Sanatorium, Tilford, near Farnham, Surrey (19 beds). Medical director: Dr. Hurd-Wood.

Scotland.

Grampian Sanatorium, Kingussie. Elevation, 860 feet (20 beds). Medical director: Dr. de Watteville.

Nordrach-on-Dee Sanatorium, Banebury, Aberdeen (36 beds). Physician: Dr. Lawson.

Woodburn Sanatorium, Morning Side, Edinburgh (20 beds). Resident physician: Dr. Galbraith.

Ireland.

Altadore Sanatorium, Kilpedder, Co. Wicklow (18 beds). Medical officer: Dr. J. C. Smyth.

Rossclare Sanatorium, Irvinestown, Fermanagh (17 beds). Medical officer: Dr. P. S. Hichens.

Rostrevor Sanatorium, Co. Down (20 beds). Resident physician: Dr. Howard Sinclair.

France.

The **Canigou** Sanatorium, near Vernet les Bains (hot sulphur springs), in the Pyrénees Orientales (100 beds). Elevation. 2,300 feet. Medical director: Dr. Giresse. Open all the year.

The Sanatorium **d'Aubrac**, in the Monts **d'Aubrac**, in the Dept. Aveyron (60 beds in a chalet and adjoining courts). Elevation, 4,600 feet. Only for patients in the earlier stage, or the *prétuberculeux*. Open all the year. Physicians: Drs. de Moneau and Fauvel.

Sanatorium **de Durtol**, Puy de Dôme (32 beds). Receives patients with advanced lesions of the *torpid* form, with only a moderate amount of fever, and general condition good. Proprietor: Dr. Sabourin.

Sanatorium **de Gelos**, near Pau, is associated with one at **Eaux Bonnes, Basses-Pyrenées**. The first, with 15 beds, is open from October to May; the second, with 10 beds, from May to October. At Eaux Bonnes patients can combine the sulphur water treatment with sanatorium treatment. Elevation, 2,625 feet. For torpid cases with much catarrh. Medical director: Dr. Portes.

The **Trespœy** Sanatorium, also near Pau (14 beds). Proprietor: Dr. Crouzet.

Sanatorium **de Gorbio**, in the Vallée de Gorbio, **Mentone**. Elevation, 820 feet. Distance from the sea, two miles (58 beds). It is open from Oct. 21 to June 15. (*See* also p. 689.) Physician: Dr. Malibran.

Sanatorium **de Meung-sur-Loire**, Dept. Loiret (17 beds). Elevation, 413 feet. Open all the year. Receives all curable forms of tuberculosis. 84 miles from Paris, 10 miles from Orleans. Physicians: Drs. Leriche and Sarrot.

Sanatorium **des Puis à Lamotte-Beuvron**, Dept. Loir-et-Cher (22 beds). Elevation, 426 feet. 61 miles from Paris, 14 miles from Orleans. Physician: Dr. Heroe.

Sanatoria in course of construction, in the vicinity of **Hyères**, for middle class patients: **Sanatorium Philanthropique du Mont des Oiseaux** (150 beds). For adults. **Sanatorium d'Enfants de San Salvador** (150 beds).

Algiers.

Sanatorium **d'Alger** (100 beds, 60 of which are devoted to *assisted* patients in a separate section). Elevation, 656 feet. Receives cases needing a warm winter climate, such as torpid, subacute forms, with extensive lesions, and cases with laryngeal, intestinal or renal complications.

Italy.

Palermo, Villa Igeia (200 beds). Appears to be more of an hotel than a sanatorium.

Germany.

Brehmer Sanatorium (the parent of such institutions), Görbersdorf, Silesia, near Friedland (156 beds of the first class, 179 beds of the second class). Medical director: Dr. Rudolf Kobert.

Falkenstein Sanatorium (one of the earliest instituted), Cronberg, near Frankfort (112 beds). Medical officers: Drs. Hess and Besold.

Hohenhonnef Sanatorium, on the Rhine, station Honnef (109 beds). Medical director: Dr. Meissen.

Laubbach Sanatorium, near Coblenz-on-the-Rhine (113 beds). Medical director: Dr. Achtermann.

Nordrach Sanatorium, near Biberachzell, Black Forest (45 beds). Medical director: Dr. Walther.

Schomberg Sanatorium, near Liebenzell, Pforzheim, Black Forest (50 beds). Medical director: Dr. Adolf Koch.

St. Blasien Sanatorium, railway station Albbrück, near Basel, Black Forest (62 beds). Medical director: Dr. A. Sander.

Wherawald Sanatorium, near Todtmoos, Black Forest (98 beds). Medical director: Dr. Lips.

Reiboldsgrun Sanatorium, near Auerbach, Saxony (108 beds). Medical director: Dr. Wolff-Immermann.

Fréland Sanatorium, near Aubure, Haute Alsace.

Rehburg Sanatorium, Bad-Rehburg, Hanover (20 beds). Medical director: Dr. Michaelis.

Switzerland.

Davos and Davos-Dorf.

The Schatz-Alp Sanatorium, 1,000 feet above Davos (120 beds). Chief physician: Dr. L. Spengler.

Dr. Turban's Sanatorium (80 beds).

Dr. Dannegger's Sanatorium (40 beds).

Sanatorium Schweizerhof. Physician: Dr. Peters.

Sanatorium du Midi. Physician: Dr. Michel.

Sanatorium Davos-Dorf. Physician: Dr. C. Dönz.

Neues Sanatorium, Davos-Dorf. Physician: Dr. Philippi.

International Sanatorium. Physician: Dr. P. Humbert.

Sanatorium Clavadel. Physician: Dr. Frey.

Arosa Sanatorium. Physician: Dr. Herwig.

Leysin Sanatoria, elevation 4,783 feet, in the Vaudois Alps, near Aigle. (See p. 583.)

Teneriffe. Guimar Sanatorium. Physician: Dr. J. L. Salmund.

INDEX.

I.—MINERAL WATERS AND BATHS AND THE DISEASES IN WHICH THEY ARE USED.

A

Aachen, 52
Abano, 75
Acne, Treatment for, 450
Acquarossa, 75
Acqui, 76
Æsculap water, 76
After-cures, 50
Aibling, 76
Aigle les Bains, 76
Aix en Provence, 76
Aix la Chapelle, 52—55
Aix les Bains, 55—64
Albuminuria, Treatment for, 442
Alet, 76
Alexandersbad, 77
Alexisbad, 77
Alkaline baths, Preparation of, 44
Alkaline earthy springs, 15
Alkaline waters, 10; Action of, in baths, 30; Action of, taken internally, 35—38
Allevard, 65—67
Alvaneu-bad, 77
Amélie les Bains, 67—69
Amenorrhœa, Treatment for, 452
Amphion, 181
Anæmia and chlorosis, Treatment for, 385—389
Andabre, 77
Andeer Pignieu, 78
Antogast, 78
Apenta water, 69
Apollinaris water, 70—72
Archena, 78
Argelès-Gazost, 78
Arnstadt, 79
Aromatic baths, Preparation of, 43
Arsenical waters, 20; Action of, taken internally, 42
Arterio-sclerosis, Treatment for, 439
Articular rheumatism, Treatment for, 411
Ashby-de-la-Zouch, 72
Askern Spa, 73
Assmannshausen, 79
Asthma, Treatment for, 431
Astringent baths, Preparation of, 44
Audinac, 79
Auerbach, 79
Augustusbad, 79
Aulus, 79
Aussee, 80
Austria (*see* Germany)
"Austrian selters water," 340
Auteuil, 80
Ax les Thermes, 74

B

Baassen, 127
Bad-Boll, 130
Baden (in Austria), 83
Baden (in Switzerland), 83—85
Baden-Baden, 80—83
Badenweiler, 85
Bad-Hall, 212
Bad Linda, 252
Bad-Salzbrunn, 281
Bagnères-de-Bigorre, 86—88
Bagnères de Luchon, 244—249
Bagni Caldi, 243
Bagni di Lucca, 243
Bagnoles de l'Orne, 88—90
Bagnoli, 127
Bagnols les Bains, 127
Bains (Vosges), 127
Bakewell, 128
Balaruc, 90
Ballynahinch, 128
Ballyspellan, 128
Barbotan, 128
Barèges, 91—93
Bartfeld, 128
Barzun, 128, 317
Bath, 94—98
Baths, Preparation of, 22—24; Action of indifferent thermal, 26; Action of common salt, 28; Action of gaseous thermal salt, 29; Action of alkaline, 30; Action of bitter water, 30; Action of chalybeate, 30; Action of earthy springs, 31; Action of sulphur, 32; Preparation of aromatic and medicated, 43; Pine-needle, 43; Alkaline, 44; Astringent, 44; Peat, 44; Mud, 44; Gas, 45; Sun and light, 47; Electric light, 47; Electric, 47;

Application of, for alleviation and cure of disease, 382—456
Battaglia, 98
Bauche, La, 128
Belgium, Simple thermal waters in, 7; Chalybeate waters in, 14
Bentheim, 129
Berchtesgaden, 99
Berg, 129
Berg and Canstatt, 132
Berka, 129
Bertrich, 100
Bex, 101
Bibra, 129
Bile ducts, Treatment for diseases of, 424—426
Bilin, 129
Birmenstorf, 129
Birresborn, 129
Bitter waters, 12; Action of, in baths, 30; Action of, taken internally, 38; Apenta, 69; Æsculap, 76; Franz Joseph, 191; Friedrichshall, 192; Grau, 198; Hunyadi Janos, 214; Kissingen, 219; Pullna, 292; Reichenhall, 295
Bocklet, 130
Boll, 130
Borjom, 130
Bormio, 103
Borszek, 130
Bosnia, Sulphur spring in, 19
Boulou, Le, 104
Bourbon Lancy, 105—107
Bourbon l'Archambaut, 107—110
Bourbonne les Bains, 110—112
Bourboule, La, 113—116
Bramstedt, 130
Bremerbad, 131
Brides les Bains, 116—119
Bridge of Allan, 131
Bridge of Earn, 131
Brine baths, Action of, 28
Briscous, 131
Bromides and iodides, Waters containing, 20, 42
Bronchial catarrh, Treatment for, 429—431
Brückenau, 120—122
Builth Wells, 122
Bukowine, 131
Burtscheid, 52, 53, 131
Bussang (Vosges), 122—124
Buxton, 124—127
Buzias, 131

C

Cadeac, 157
Calcareous springs, 15; Action of, in baths, 31; Action of, taken internally, 40
Calculi, Treatment for, 441
Cambo, 131
Canstatt and Berg, 132
Capvern, 157
Carabana, 157
Cardiac diseases, Treatment for, 432—440
Carlsbad, 133—141
Carratraca, 157
Casamicciola, 157
Casséra-Verduzan, 157
Castellamare di Stabia, 157
Castiglione, 157
Castleconnell, 157
Castro-Caro, 157
Catarrh, bronchial, Treatment for, 429—431
Cauterets, 141—144
Cerebral hyperæmia, Treatment for, 445
Ceresole-Reale, 157
Challes, 144—146
Chalybeate waters, 13; Action of, in baths, 30; Action of, taken internally, 39
Charlottenbrunn, 158
Châteauneuf, 158
Chatelguyon, 146—148
Chaudes Aigues, 158
Chaudfontaine, 158
Cheltenham, 148
Chianciano, 158
Chloride waters, 8
Chlorosis, Treatment for, 385—389
Chorea, Treatment for, 448
Circulatory system, Treatment for diseases of, 432—440
Cirrhosis, Treatment for, 424
Civillina, 158
Civita Vecchia, 158
Classification of mineral springs, 5—21
Colitis, muco-membranous, Treatment for, 422—424
Composition of mineral springs, 3—5
Condillac, 158
Congestion of liver, Treatment for, 424
Constipation, habitual, Treatment for, 421
Contrexéville, 149—156
Counter indications of treatment by mineral waters, 382—384
Cours-les-Bains, 159
Court Saint Etienne, 159
Couzan table water, 159, 338
Cransac, 159
Croft Spa, 159
Csiz, 159
Cudown, 159
Cusset, 159, 367
Cutaneous diseases, Treatment for, 448—451

D

Dax, 159—162
Diabetes, Treatment for, 394—399
Diarrhœa, chronic, Treatment for, 422—424
Diet, Importance of, 49

Digestive organs, Treatment for diseases of, 417–421
Digne, 165
Dinkholder-Brunnen, 165
Dinsdale-on-Tees, 165
Dirsdorp, 165
Ditzenbach, 165
Doberan, 165
Douches, Various forms of, 24
Driburg-Bad, 162
Droitwich, 163—165
Dürkheim, 165
Dürrenberg, 165
Dürrheim, 166
Dysmenorrhœa, Treatment for, 453
Dyspepsia, Treatment for, 417—421

E

Earthy springs, 15; Action of, in baths, 31; Action of, taken internally, 40
Eaux Bonnes, 166—170
Eaux Chaudes, 170
Eberswalde, 182
Eczema, Treatment for, 449
Eilsen, 182
Electric bath, 47
Electric light bath, 47
Elmen, 182
Elöpatak, 183
Elster, 171
Emphysema, chronic, Treatment for, 431
Ems, 173—175
Encausse, 183
Enghien, 175—177
Erdöbenye, 183
Escaldas, Les, 183
Essentuke, 183
Euzet, 183
Evaux, 183
Evian, 177—181
Exercises, Mechanical, at different spas, 48

F

Fachingen, 190
Farnbuhl, 190
Fatty liver, Treatment for, 424
Faulenseebad, 190
Female genital organs, Treatment for diseases of, 451–456
Fideris, 190
Finneck, 303
Fitero, 191
Flinsberg, 191
Flitwick, 191
Forges-les-Eaux, 184
France, Simple thermal waters in, 7; Common salt waters in, 9; Simple alkaline waters in, 11; Alkaline and common salt springs in, 11; Bitter waters in, 13; Chalybeate waters in, 14; Earthy springs in, 16; Sulphur springs in, 17. (Each mineral spring is entered under its own name)
Frankenhausen, 191
Franzensbad, 185—190
Franz Joseph, 191
Freiersbach, 191
Friedrichshall, 192
Frienwalde, 191
Fuered, 192
Furunculosis, chronic, Treatment for, 451
Fuscherbad, 192

G

Gallstones, Treatment for, 424
Gandersheim, 197
Gas baths, 45
Gaseous thermal salt baths, 29
Gastein, 192—195
Genital organs, female, Treatment for diseases of, 451–456
Germany and Austria, Simple thermal waters in, 7; Common salt waters in, 9; Simple alkaline waters in, 11; Alkaline and common salt springs in, 12; Alkaline and sodium sulphate waters in, 12; Bitter waters in, 13; Chalybeate waters in, 14; Earthy springs in, 16; Sulphur springs in, 18. (Each mineral spring is entered under its own name)
Giesshuebl-Puchstein, 197
Gilsland Spa, 197
Gleichenberg, 195
Glycosuria and diabetes, Treatment for, 394—399
Gmunden, 197
Goczal Kowitz, 197
Godesberg, 197
Gonten, 197
Göppingen, 197
Gottleuba, 198
Gout, and uric acid diathesis, Treatment for, 399—405
Grau, 198
Gravel, Treatment for, 441
Great Britain, Simple thermal waters in, 6; Common salt waters in, 9; Bitter waters in, 12; Chalybeate waters in, 14; Sulphate of iron springs in, 15; Earthy spring in, 15; Sulphur springs in, 17. (Each mineral spring is entered under its own name)
Greece, Sulphur spring in, 19
Greifswald, 198
Grenzach, 198
Gréoulx, 198
Griesbach, 198
Gurnigelbad, 198
Gymnastics at spas, 48

H

Haarlem, 212
Habsburger-Bad, 327
Hæmorrhoids, Treatment for, 422
Hall (Bad-Hall), 212
Hall (in Austrian Tyrol), 212
Hall (Swäbisch Hall), 212
Hallein, 212
Hamm, 212
Hammam R'Irha, 198—200
Hapsal, 212
Harkany, 213
Harrogate, 200—203
Harzburg, 213
Heart diseases (*see* Cardiac diseases)
Heilbrunn, 213
Heilbrunnen, 351
Heiligen Kreuzbad, 213
Helouan les Bains, 203
Hercules-Bad, 213
Hermannsbad (in Saxony), 213
Hermannsbad (in Silesia), 213
Heustrich, 204—207
Homburg, 207—212
Honnef, 213
Hot sand baths, 45
Hunyadi Janos, 214
Hyperæmia, cerebral, Treatment for, 445
Hysteria, Treatment for, 448
Hythe, 498

I

Ilidze, 216
Imnau, 216
Impaludism, Treatment for, 415
Indifferent thermal waters, 6; their action applied externally, 26—28; their action taken internally, 34
Infantile paralysis, Treatment for, 447
Inhalation of mineral waters, 24
Innichen, 216
Inowrazlaw, 216
Inselbad, 216
Insomnia, Treatment for, 448
Iodides and bromides, Waters containing, 20, 42
Ireland, Sulphur springs in, 17
Iron waters, 13; Action of, in baths, 30; Action of, taken internally, 39
Ischia, 214
Ischl, 214
Italy, Simple thermal waters in, 7; Common salt waters in, 10; Simple alkaline waters in, 11; Alkaline and common salt springs in, 12; chalybeate waters in, 14; Earthy springs in, 16; Sulphur springs in, 18. (Each mineral spring is entered under its own name)
Ivonicz, 216
Ivonitch, 216

J

Jagstfeld, 216
Jalcznovodsk, 217
Jaundice, chronic, Treatment for, 425
Johannis table water, 217
Johannisbad, 217
Juliushall, 217

K

Kainzenbad, 224
Karlsbad, 224
Kellberg, 224
Kidney, gouty, Treatment for, 442
Kiedrich, 224
Kissingen, 217—221
Kissingen Well (Harrogate), 200, 2.2
Koenigsdorf-Jastrzemb, 224
Koenigswart, 224
Koesen, 225
Kohlgrub, 225
Kolberg, 225
Krankenheil Tölz, 351
Krapina Töplitz, 225
Kreuth, 225
Kreuznach, 221—224
Krynica, 225

L

Ladis, 250
La Lenk, 233
La Malou, 225—228
La Motte les Bains, 228—230
La Mouillère, 230
Landeck, 250
Langenau, 251
Langenbrücken, 251
Längenfeld, 250
Langensalza, 251
Langen-Schwalbach, 330—332
La Preste, 292
Laryngitis, chronic, Treatment for, 427
Lauchstädt, 251
Laurvik, 251
Lausigk, 251
Lavey, 231
Leamington, 232
Ledesma, 251
Leixlip Spa, 251
Lenk, 233
Le Prese, 292
Leucorrhœa, Treatment for, 454
Leukerbad, 284—286
Levico, 236
Lichen, Treatment for, 451
Liebenstein, 252
Liebenzell, 252
Liebwerda, 252
Light baths, 47

Linda-Pausa, 252
Lipetsk, 252
Lipik, 252
Lippspringe, 237
Lisdoonvarna, 237
Lithiasis, Treatment for, 405
Liver and bile ducts, Treatment for diseases of, 424—426
Llandrindod Wells, 238—240
Llangammarch, 240
Llanwrtyd Wells, 241
Lobenstein, 252
Locomotor ataxy, Treatment for, 445
Loèche les Bains, 284—286
Lons le Saunier, 252
Lostorf, 253
Louisen baths (Franzensbad), 187
Lucan, 242
Lucca, 243
Luchon, 244—249
Luhatschowitz, 253
Lumbago, Treatment for, 412
Luxemburg, Common salt waters in, 10
Luxeuil les Bains, 249
Luz, 316
Lye or alkaline baths, Preparation of, 44

M

Malarial affections, chronic, Treatment for, 415
Mallow, 266
Malou, La, 225—228
Marcols, 266
Marienbad, 253—256
Marlioz, 64
Martigny les Bains, 266
Massage, 48
Matlock Bath, 257
Medicated baths, Preparation of, 43
Meinberg, 266
Melksham, 267
Mendorf, 267
Menorrhagia, Treatment for, 453
Metallic poisoning, chronic, Treatment for, 394
Middlesbrough, 339
Middlewich, 267
Mineral peat baths, Preparation of, 44
Mineral springs, Description of principal, 52—381
Mineral waters, Nature of, 1; Definition of, 3; Composition of, 3; Varying temperature of, 4; classification of, 5—21; modes of application, 22; their action when applied externally, 24—33; their action when taken internally, 33—42; Counter indications of treatment by, 382—384; for anæmia and chlorosis, 385—389; for scrofula and tubercle, 389; for pulmonary tuberculosis, 390—392; for syphilis, 392—394; for chronic metallic poisoning, 394; for glycosuria and diabetes, 394—399; for gout and the uric acid diathesis, 399—405; for lithiasis, 405; for oxaluria, 406; for phosphaturia, 407; for obesity, 407—409; for rheumatism, 409—413; for sciatica, 413; for rheumatoid arthritis, 413; for chronic malarial affections, 415; for diseases of the digestive organs, 417—421; for constipation, 421; for hæmorrhoids, 422; for chronic diarrhœa and muco-membranous colitis, 422—424; for diseases of liver and bile ducts, 424—426; for diseases of the respiratory organs, 426—429; for bronchial catarrh, 429—431; for chronic emphysema, 431; for asthma, 431; for diseases of circulatory system, 432—440; for renal and urinary disorders, 440—443; for diseases of nervous system, 443—448; for cutaneous diseases, 448—451; for diseases of the female genital organs, 451—456
Miscarriages, tendency to, Treatment for, 455
Mitterbad, 267
Moffat, 267
Molitg, 267
Monsumano, 267
Mont Dore, 257—265
Monte Catini, 265
Montegrotto, 268
Montemayor, 268
Monte Ortone, 268
Montmirail, 268
Montrond, 268
Moor baths, Preparation and action of, 44
Morgins, 268
Mouillère, La, 230
Muco-membranous colitis, Treatment for, 422—424
Mud baths, Preparation and action of, 44
Munster-am-Stein, 268
Muriated waters, 8
Muscular rheumatism, Treatment for, 411

N

Nantwich, 268
Nauheim, 269—274
Nenndorf, 279
Nephritis, interstitial, Treatment for, 442
Néris, 274—276
Nervous system, Treatment for diseases of, 443—448
Neuenahr, 277—279
Neuenhain, 279
Neuhaus (Bavaria), 279

Neuhaus (Styria), 279
Neu-Ragoczi, 279
Neuralgia, chronic, Treatment for, 447
Neuralgia of large nerves, Treatment for, 413
Neurasthenia, Treatment for, 448
Neuritis, Treatment for, 446
Neuroses, Treatment for, 448
Neustadt-Eberswalde, 280
Niederbronn, 280
Niederlangenau, 251
Niedernau, 280
Niederselters, 341
Norway, Sulphur springs in, 19

O

Oberlahnstein-am-Rhein, 281
Obersalzbrunn, 281
Obesity, Treatment for, 407—409
Obladis, 250
Oeynhausen, 280
Offenbach-am-Main, 281
Oldesloe, 281
Olette, 281
Ontaneda, 282
Orb, 282
Orezza, 282
Oriol, 282
Osteo-arthritis, Treatment for, 413
Oxaluria, Treatment for, 406

P

Panticosa, 289
Parad, 290
Paralysis, infantile, Treatment for, 447
Paralysis, Treatment for, 444
Pardoux table water, 106
Passugg, 290
Peat baths, Preparation of, 44
Peiden, 290
Pejo, 290
Pestrin, 290
Petersthal, 290
Pfaeffers, 293
Pfriem's method of heating water for baths, 23
Pharyngitis, Treatment for, 427
Phlebitis, Treatment for, 439
Phosphaturia, Treatment for, 407
Piatigorsk, 290
Pierrefonds, 282
Pietrapola, 290
Pine-needle bath, Preparation and action of, 43
Pit-Keathly water, 131
Pityriasis, Treatment for, 451
Plombières, 283—286
Ponte Seraglio, 243
Poretta, 290
Portugal, Simple alkaline waters in, 11; Sulphur springs in, 19
Pöstyen, 292
Pougues les Eaux, 286
Pouillon, 291
Pozzuoli, 291
Preblau, 291
Préchacq-les-Bains, 291
Pré-Saint-Didier, 292
Prese, Le, 292
Preste, La, 292
Prurigo, Treatment for, 451
Pruritus, Treatment for, 451
Psoriasis, Treatment for, 450
Pulina, 292
Pulmonary tuberculosis, Treatment for, 380—382
Purton Spa, 292
Puzzichello, 292
Pyrmont, 287—289
Pystjan, 292

R

Rabbi, 303
Radein, 303
Ragatz-Pfaeffers, 293
Rajeczfürdö, 303
Rappoltsweiler, 303
Rastenburg and Finneck, 303
Ratzes, 304
Recoaro, 304
Rehburg, 304
Rehme-Oeynhausen, 280
Reiboldsgrün, 304
Reichenhall, 294
Reinerz, 304
Rietbad, 304
Remoncourt, 304
Renal disorders, Treatment for, 440—443
Renlaigue, 304
Rennes les Bains, 304
Respiratory organs, Treatment for diseases of, 426—429
Reutlingen, 304
Rheinfelden, 295—297
Rheumatic neuralgia, Treatment for, 413
Rheumatism, chronic, articular, and muscular, Treatment for, 409—415
Rheumatoid arthritis, Treatment for, 409, 413
Rhino-pharyngitis, Treatment for, 427
Rio, 305
Rippoldsau, 297
Rohitsch, 305
Römerbad and Tüffer, 305
Roncas-Blanc, 305
Roncegno, 298
Ronneberg, 305
Ronneby, 305
Rosenheim, 305
Rothenbrunnen, 305
Rothenfelde, 305
Rouzat, 305
Royat les Bains, 299—303
Rubinat-Llorach, 305

Russia, Simple alkaline waters in, 11; Alkaline and common salt springs in, 12; Sulphur springs in, 19

S

Sacedon, 338
Sail les Bains, 338
Sail sous Couzan, 338
St. Alban, 338
St. Amand, 306
St. Antoine de Guagno, 338
St. Boès, 338
St. Christan, 307—309
St. Galmier, 338
St. Gervais, 309
St. Honoré, 310
St. Laurent les Bains, 338
St. Maurice, 370
St. Moritz-Bad, 311—314
St. Nectaire, 314—316
St. Olafs, 338
St. Sauveur, 316
St. Vallier, 338
St. Yorre, 338
Salies-de-Béarn, 317—319
Salies du Salut, 338
Salins-du-Jura, 319
Salins Moutiers, 116, 119
Salso Maggiore, 320—326
Salt (common) waters, 8; their action when applied externally, 28
Saltburn by the Sea, 338
Salvator, 339
Salzbrunn, 339
Salzburg, 339
Salzdetfurth, 339
Salzerbad, 339
Salzhausen, 339
Salzschlirf, 326
Salzuflen, 339
Salzungen, 339
Sanatorium du Canigou, 359
San Bernardino, 339
Sanct Lorenz, 340
Sand baths, Hot, 45
Sandefjord, 340
Sandrock, 340
San Marco, 340
San Pedro do Sul, 340
San Pietro Montagone, 340
Santa Agueda, 340
Santa Catarina, 340
Santenay, 340
Saxon, 340
Schandau, 341
Schimberg, 341
Schinznach, 327
Schlangenbad, 328—330
Schmalkalden, 341
Schmiedeberg, 341
Schwäbisch Hall, 212
Schwalbach, 330—332
Schwalheim table water, 270, 341
Schwarz method of heating water for baths, 23
Schwarzbach, 341
Schwefelberg, 341
Schweizerhalle, 341
Sciacca, 341
Sciatica, Treatment for, 413, 447
Scotch Douche, 24
Scrofula, Treatment for, 389
Sea-mud baths, 45
Segeberg, 341
Selters, 341
Serneus, 341
Shanklin, 341
Shap Wells, 342
Simple alkaline waters, 10
Simple thermal waters, 6
Siradan, Sainte Marie, 342
Skin diseases, Treatment for, 448—451
Soden, 332
Soden a Werra, 342
Soden-Salzmunster, 342
Sodenthal, 342
Sodium chloride waters, 8
Sodium sulphide waters, 19
Sodium waters, 19; their action taken internally, 35
Solis, 342
Sotsass table water, 345
Soulzmatt, 342
Spa, 333—336
Spain and Portugal, Simple thermal waters in, 7; Common salt waters in, 10; Bitter waters in, 13; Sulphur springs in, 18. (Each mineral spring is entered under its own name)
Spring water, Chemical composition of, 2
Springs, Mineral (*see* Mineral waters)
Srebernik, 342
Stachelberg, 342
Stafford, 342
Steben, 342
Sterility, Treatment for, 456
Stoney Middleton, 342
Strathpeffer, 336
Submarine douche, 24
Suderode, 342
Sulis water, 97
Sulphur and sodium chloride waters, 19
Sulphur waters, 16; Subdivision of, 19; Action of, in baths, 32; inhalation of, 33; Action of, taken internally, 41
Sulphuretted hydrogen gas bath, 46
Sulphuretted hydrogen springs, 19
Sulphurous peat baths, 45
Sulza, 342
Sulzbach, 343
Sulzbrunn, 343
Sun baths, 47
Swanlinbar, 343
Switzerland, Simple thermal waters in, 7; Common salt waters in, 10; Simple alkaline waters in, 11; Alkaline and

sodium sulphate waters in, 12; Bitter waters in, 13; Chalybeate waters in, 14; Earthy springs in, 16. (Each mineral spring is entered under its own name)
Sylvanès, 343
Syphilis, Treatment for, 382—394
Szczawnica, 343
Szkleno, 343

T

Tabes, Treatment for, 445
Tabiano, 350
Table Waters: Aix la Chapelle, 55, 57; Apollinaris, 70—72; Sulis, 97; Pardoux, 108; Condillac, 158; Couzan, 159; Giesshuebl-Puchstein, 197; Johannis, 217; La Vernière, 226; Lenk, 233; Levico, 236; Schwalheimerbrunnen, 270; Couzan, 338; St. Alban, 338; St. Galmier, 338; Selters, 341; Soulzmatt, 342; Sotsass, 345; Törmisstein, 351; Impératrice, 358; St. Jean, 358; Vichy, 359—368
Tarasp-Schuls, 343—347
Teinach, 350
Tennstedt, 351
Teplitz, 347—349
Termini-Imersee, 351
Thale, 351
Thonon, 351
Tiefenkasten, 351
Tobelbad, 351
Tölz, 351
Topusco, 352
Törmisstein, 351
Tracheitis, Treatment for, 427
Traunstein, 352
Trefriw, 352
Trenczin Töplitz, 352
Trillo, 352
Tuberculosis, pulmonary, Treatment for, 390—392
Tuberculosis, Treatment for, 389
Tüffer, 305
Tunbridge Wells, 349
Tusnad, 352

U

Ueberlingen, 354
Urberoaga de Alzola, 354
Uriage, 352—354
Uric acid diathesis, Treatment for, 399—405
Urinary disorders, Treatment for, 440—443
Urticaria, Treatment for, 451
Ussat, 355
Uterine fibroids, Treatment for, 455

V

Valdieri, 369
Vallacabras, 369
Vals, 355—358, 369
Val Sinestra, 369
Vegri di Valdagno, 370
Veldes, 370
Vernet les Bains, 358
Vicarello, 370
Vichy, 359—368
Vic le Comte, 370
Vic sur Cère, 370
Vidago, 370
Villa, 243
Villach, 370
Vinadio, 370
Viterbo, 370
Vittel, 368
Voeslau, 370

W

Warasdin-Teplitz, 380
Warmbad, 380
Warmbrunn, 381
Waters, Mineral (*see* Mineral waters)
Weilbach, 370
Weissenburg, 371
Werl, 381
Werne, 381
Wiesbaden, 372—375
Wildbad, 375—377
Wildbad-Gastein, 192—195
Wildegg, 381
Wildungen, 377—379
Wimpfen, 381
Wipfeld, 381
Wittekind, 381
Woodhall Spa, 379
Writer's Cramp, Treatment for, 448

Y

Yverdon, 381

Z

Zalzon, 381

II.—CLIMATES AND CLIMATIC RESORTS, AND DISEASES TREATED IN THEM.

A

Abbazia, 648
Aberdeen, 536
Aberdovey, 520
Aberystwith, 520
Achensee, 602
Achill, 532
Acireale, 651
Adamello, 594
Adelboden, 589, 597
Airolo, 592
Ajaccio, 649
Alagna, 599
Alassio, 693
Aldeburgh, 528
Algiers, 628—631; Sanatoria in, 744
Aliwal North, 709
Alps, maritime, Resorts in the, 695
Alt-Prags, 595
Alum Bay, 509
Amalfi, 647, 648
Anæmia and chlorosis, Climatic treatment of, 734—736
Andermatt, 587, 596
Andes, Resorts in the, 605
Antibes, 680
Appenzell, 603
Arcachon, 551, 638—640
Arco, 660
Ardrossan, 535
Arolla, 592
Arosa, 581—583
Arran, Isle of, 535
Assouan, 614
Asthma, Climatic treatment of, 725
Audierne, 551
Australia, 710
Avalon, 713
Avants, Les, 585, 601
Avranches, 545
Azores, 622

B

Bad Fideris, 601
Bad Gurnigel, 599
Ballybunnion, 532
Baltic resorts (*see* Continental seaside resorts)
Bangor, 521
Barbados, 711
Barfleur, 545
Barkley West, 709
Barmouth, 520
Baths of Leuk, 596
Beaufort West, 709
Beaulieu, 683—685
Beaumaris, 521
Bell-Alp, 590
Berck-sur-Mer, 538
Berg-Dievenon, 550
Bermuda, 711
Berwick, North, 535
Beuzeval, 543
Bevers, 563
Bexhill-on-Sea, 499
Beyrout, 618
Biarritz, 551, 640
Birchington-on-Sea, 492
Biskra, 633
Blackpool, 522
Blankenburghe, 548
Bloemendaal, 549
Bloemfontein, 608, 709
Bognor, 504
Bordighera, 689—692
Boscastle, 517
Boscombe, 509
Boulder, 606
Boulogne-sur-Mer, 538
Bournemouth, 509
Bray, 534
Brennerbad, 595
Bridlington Quay, 525
Brighton, 501—503
Brittany seaside resorts (*see* Continental seaside resorts)
Broadstairs, 494
Bronchial catarrh, Climatic treatment of, 722—725
Bronchiectasis, Climatic treatment of, 724
Broughty Ferry, 536
Bude, 517
Budleigh Salterton, 512
Buncrana, 532
Bundoran, 532
Burgenstock, 602
Burghersdorf, 709

C

Cabourg, 544
Cairo, 613
Calais, 538
Caledon, 709
California, Southern, 712—714
Campfer, 561
Canary Islands, 622—627
Cancale, 545
Cannes, 676—680
Cañon City, 607
Cap de la Hague, 545
Cape Town, 709
Capri, 655—657
Cardiac affections, Climatic treatment of, 726
Castellamare di Stabia, 647
Catania, 650
Catarrh, chronic, Climatic treatment of, 722—725, 729
Caux, 585
Celerina, 562

Ceres, 709
Ceresole-Reale, 594
Certosa di Pesio, Baths of, 695
Chamounix, 600
Champéry, 596
Chandolin, 592
Channel Islands, 546
Charnex, 603
Châteaux d'Oex, 600
Chaumont, 600
Cheimsee Hotel, 604
Cherbourg, 545
Chesière, 596
Chlorosis, Climatic treatment of, 734—736
Circulatory system, Climatic treatment of diseases of, 726
Clacton-on-Sea, 528
Classification, of Climates, 475—477; of English and Welsh seaside resorts, 529—531
Clavadel, 581
Climacteric period in women, Climatic treatment of, 737
Climates, 457—475; Classification of, 475—477; Characters and restorative action of sea and mountain, 478—491; Application and selection of, 715—739
Clovelly, 517
Colorado Springs, 606
Colwyn Bay, 522
Comballaz, 597
Concarneau, 551
Consumption, Mountain-air cure for, 566—580; Climatic treatment of, 716—722
Continental seaside resorts, 538—554
Convalescence, Climatic treatment of, 738
Conway, 521
Cordilleras, Resorts in the, 605
Corfu, 654
Coronado Beach, 712
Corsica, 649
Cortina, 595
Costebelle, 675
Courmayeur, 598
Courseulles, 544
Cowes, 505
Cradock, 709
Cresta, 562
Croisic, Le, 552
Cromer, 525—527
Crotoy, Le, 539
Cruden Bay, 537
Cuzco, 605

D

Davos Dorfli, 567
Davos Platz, 566—569, 579
Dawlish, 512
Dax, 643
Deauville, 542
Denver, 605
Diabetes, Climatic treatment of, 733
Dieppe, 539
Dinard, 546
Dingle, 532
Dissentis, 599
Divonne, 604
Donaghadee, 533
Dornoch, 537
Douarnenez, 551
Dover, 496
Dovercourt, 528
Duin-en-Dal, 549
Dunkirk, 538
Dyspepsia, Climatic treatment of, 727

E

Eastbourne, 499—501
Eggischhorn, 590
Egypt as a winter resort, 610—618
Engadine, Climatic resorts in the, 555
Engelberg, 601
England, Seaside resorts in, 492—519, 522—529; Classification of seaside resorts in, 529—531; Sanatoria in, 742
Engstlen Alp, 591
Estes Park, 607
Etretat, 541
Evolena, 597
Exmouth, 512
Eze, 685

F

Falmouth, 516
Fécamp, 540
Felixstowe, 528
Felsenegg, 602
Filey, 525
Flushing, 516
Folkestone, 495
France, Sanatoria in, 744. (Each resort is under its own name)
Freshwater Bay, 509
Frohburg, 603
Funchal, 620—622

G

Gais, 601
Gastein, 596
Geissbach Hotel, 604
Genoa, 635
Gerardmer, 603
Germany, Sanatoria in, 745. (Each resort is under its own name)
Gibraltar, 645
Glengariff, 532
Glenwood, 607
Glion, 575, 586
Gorbio, 689
Gorleston-on-Sea, 527

Gornergrat, 590
Gossensass, 588
Gout, Climatic treatment of, 732
Grahamstown, 709
Grange, 523
Granville, 545
Grape Cure, 663
Grasse, 680
Graves' disease, Climatic treatment of, 730—732
Great Yarmouth, 527
Gressonay-la-Trinité, 594
Gressonay St. Jean, 594
Greystones, 534
Gries, 595
Grindelwald, 600
Gryon, 600
Guimar, 626

H

Hæmoglobinuria, paroxysmal, Climatic treatment of, 736
Haifa, 618
Hammam Meskoutine, 632
Hammam R'Irha, 631
Harrismith, 709
Harwich, 528
Hastings, 498
Havre, Le, 542
Hay asthma, Climatic treatment of, 726
Hayling Island, 504
Heart affections, Climatic treatment of, 726
Heiden, 575, 603
Heiligenblut, 595
Heiligen Damm, 550
Heligoland, 549
Helouan les Bains, 613
Hendaye, 641
Heringsdorf, 550
Herne Bay, 492
Heyst, 548
Höchenschwand, 601
Höhlenstein, 595
Hohwald, 604
Hollywood, 533
Home-Varaville, 544
Honfleur, 542
Hospenthal, 596
Houle, La, 546
Houlgate, 543
Howth, 534
Huancayo, 604
Huelva, 646
Hunstanton, 525
Hyères, 673—675
Hysteria, Climatic treatment of, 730—732
Hythe, 496

I

Idyll-wild, 714
Ilfracombe, 518
Innsbruck, 663
Insomnia, Climatic treatment of, 731
Ireland, Seaside resorts in, 531—534; Sanatoria in, 743
Isle of Arran, 535
Isle of Wight, 505—509
Italy, Sanatoria in, 744. (Each resort is under its own name)

J

Jamaica, 710
Jauja, 604

K

Karrersee, The, 594
Kilkee, 532
Kilrush, 532
Kimberley, 709
Klosters, 601
Knocke, 548
Kochel, 604
Kolberg, 551
Kranz, 551
Kurhaus Axenstein, 579

L

Ladis, 595
Lago Mesurina, 595
Laguna, 626
La Houle, 546
Langrune-sur-Mer, 544
La Paz, 605
Largo, 536
Laryngeal catarrh, chronic, Climatic treatment of, 722—725
Las Palmas, 623
La Tremblade, 552
Le Croisic, 552
Le Crotoy, 539
Le Havre, 542
Lengenfeld, 596
Lenk, 600
Les Avants, 585, 601
Les Petites Dalles, 541
Les Sables d'Olonne, 552
Le Tréport, 539
Leysin, 583
Lima, 604
Lion-sur-Mer, 544
Littlehampton, 503
Littlestone-on-Sea, 498
Llandudno, 521
Locarno, 659
Long Beach, 713
Los Angeles, 713
Lower Engadine, Climatic resorts in the, 565
Lowestoft, 527
Luc-sur-Mer, 544
Lugano, 659
Luxor, 614

Lyme Regis, 511
Lynmouth, 518
Lynton, 518

M

Macugnaga, 594
Madeira, 619—622
Maderaner-Thal, 596
Magglingen, 602
Malaga, 643—645
Malahide, 534
Malarial cachexia, Climatic treatment of, 736
Mallirany, 532
Malta, 653
Manitou Park, 607
Margate, 493
Maritzburg, 710
Mena House, 613
Mentone, 685—689
Meran, 661—663
Mexico, 605
Milford-on-Sea, 509
Milltown-Malbay, 532
Misdroy, 550
Mistral wind, 671
Mogador, 627
Monaco, 685
Monnetier, 603
Montana, 584
Mont de Caux, 585
Monte Carlo, 685
Monte Generoso, 599
Monterey, 714
Montreux, 657—659
Morecambe, 523
Morgins, 596
Morocco, 627
Mountain air, Characters and restorative action of, 478—491
Mountain climatic resorts, 555—608
Mountain sickness, Symptoms of, 487
Mount Pilatus, 591
Mumbles, 519
Mundesley, 527
Mürren, 593

N

Nairn, 537
Naples, 646, 647
Nassau, 710
Nephritis, chronic, Climatic treatment of, 728
Nervi, 635
Nervous affections, Climatic treatment of, 730—732
Neuralgia, Climatic treatment of, 730—732
Neurasthenia, Climatic treatment of, 730—732
Neuritis, Climatic treatment of, 730—732
New Brighton, 522
Newcastle, 534
Newport (Ireland), 532
New Prags, 595
Newquay, 517
New Zealand, 710
Nice, 681—683
Niederdorf, 595
Nieuport Bains, 548
Norderney, 550
North Berwick, 535
North Sea resorts (*see* Continental *and* English seaside resorts)

O

Oban, 535
Obermais, 662
Obertsdorf, 603
Obladis, 595
Orezza, 650
Ormond Dessus, 597
Orotava, 624—626
Orriccleth, 520
Ospedaletti, 692
Ostend, 548

P

Paimpol, 547
Palermo, 651—653
Parknasilla, 532
Paroxysmal hæmoglobinuria, Climatic treatment of, 736
Pasadena, 713
Pau, 642
Pax, La, 605
Pegli, 694
Penarth, 519
Penmaenmawr, 521
Penzance, 516
Peruvian Andes, Resorts in, 604
Pharyngeal catarrh, chronic, Climatic treatment of, 724
Phthisis (*see* Consumption)
Pleurisy, chronic, Climatic treatment of, 725
Pontresina, 563
Pornic, 551
Portrush, 533
Port Stewart, 533
Pragser-Wildsee, 595
Pralognan, 596
Promontogno, 600
Pueblo, 605
Pulmonary emphysema, Climatic treatment of, 722—724
Pwllheli, 520
Pyelitis, chronic, Climatic treatment of, 729

Q

Queenstown, 531
Quito, 605

R

Ragenwalde, 551
Ramsgate, 495
Rapallo, 636
Redcar, 523
Rheumatism, Climatic treatment of, 732
Rheumatoid arthritis, Climatic treatment of, 732
Rhone Glacier Hotel, 593
Rhyl, 522
Rieder-Alp, 591
Rieder Furka, 591
Riffel-Alp, 589
Riffel-berg, 589
Rigi, The, 592
Riva, 660
Riviera di Levante, 634
Riviera, Western, 665—696
Rocky Mountains, Resorts in, 605—608
Rome, 646
Roscoff, 547
Rostrevor, 533
Rothesay, 534
Royan, 551
Ryde, 505

S

S. Vaast la Hogue, 544
Saanen, 600
St. Andrews, 536
St. Aubin-sur-Mer, 544
St. Beatenberg, 587, 599
St. Bees, 523
St. Blasien, 603
St. Cergnes, 600
St. Dalmas di Tendi, 695
St. Helens, 506
St. Ives, 517
St. Jean de Luz, 641
St. Leonards, 498
St. Malo, 546
St. Margaret's Bay, 495
St. Martin Lantosque, 695
St. Moritz, 555—559; as a winter resort, 569
St. Pair, 545
St. Raphael, 675
St. Valéry en Caux, 540
St. Valéry-sur-Somme, 539
Salcombe, 516
Saltburn-on-the-Sea, 523
Samaden, 562
Sanatoria, Treatment in, 739—742; List of, 742—745
San Barnardino, 593
Sandgate, 497
San Diego, 712
Sandown, 506
San Lucar, 646
San Lui Park, 607
San Remo, 692
San Sebastian, 641
Santa Barbara, 713
Santa Catarina, 593
Santa Cruz, 624
Santa Fé de Bogota, 605
Santa Margherita, 636
Santa Monica, 713
Sassnitz, 550
Scarborough, 524
Scheideck, Great, 591
Scheveningen, 548
Schliersee, 603
Schluchsee, 602
Schlucht, 599
Schluderbach, 595
Schönbrunn, 603
Schönfels, 602
Schröcken, 598
Schwarzsee, 590
Scilly Islands, 516
Scotland, Seaside resorts in, 534—537; Sanatoria in, 743
Scrofula, Climatic treatment of, 736
Sea air, Characters and restorative action of, 478—491
Seaford, 501
Seaside resorts: English, 492—519, 522—531; Welsh, 519—522; Irish, 531—534; Scottish, 534—537; Continental, 538—554
Sea voyages, Advantages and disadvantages of, 697—708
Seelisberg, 603
Seewis, 574, 601
Semmering, 596
Senility, Climatic treatment of, 738
Sestri Levante, 636
Seville, 646
Shanklin, 507
Sheringham, 527
Sicily, 650
Sidmouth, 512
Silloth, 523
Sils, 560
Silva Plana, 561
Sirocco wind, 671
Soglio, 600
Sorrento, 647
South Africa, Resorts in, 608, 708—710
Southbourne-on-Sea, 510
Southend, 529
Southport, 522
Southsea, 504
Southwold, 528
Spanish seaside resorts, 553
Spezia, 637
Starnberg, 604
Steinach, 595
Stonehaven, 536
Stoos Hotel and Kurhaus, 597
Sulden, 592
Summer mountain resorts, 589—608
Swanage, 510
Swinemünde, 550
Switzerland, Sanatoria in, 745. (Each resort is under its own name)
Syria, Winter resorts in, 618

T

Tabes dorsalis, Climatic treatment of, 730—732

Tacaronte, 626
Tangier, 627
Taormina, 651
Tarasp-Bad, 565
Tasmania, 710
Teignmouth, 513
Tenby, 519
Thorencs, Valley of, 695
Thusis, 574, 603
Tintagel, 517
Toblach, 595
Torquay, 514
Totland Bay, 509
Towyn, 520
Trafoi, 594
Tralee, 532
Tramontana wind, 672
Tramore, 531
Travemünde, 550
Tréguier, 547
Tremblade, La, 551
Tréport, Le, 539
Triberg, 603
Trieste, 553
Trouville, 542
Turkastad, 709
Turma, 604

U

Uetliberg Hotel, 602
Untermais, 662
Upper Engadine, Climatic resorts in the, 555—565

V

Valdieri, Baths of, 695
Valescure, 675
Ventnor, 507—509
Vesical catarrh, Climatic treatment of, 729
Veules, 540
Viareggio, 553, 637
Vilaflor, 626
Villars-sur-Allon, 598
Villers-sur-Mer, 543
Villerville, 542
Vinadio, 695
Vorauen, 603
Vorder-Todtmoos, 603
Vulpera, 565

W

Waidring, 603
Walchensee, 603
Waldhaus-Flims, 599
Wales, Seaside resorts in, 519—522; Classification of seaside resorts in, 529—530; Sanatoria in, 742
Walton-on-the-Naze, 528
Warnemünde, 550
Waterville, 532
Weissbad, 603
Weissenstein (in Carinthia), 595
Weissenstein (in Swiss Jura), 597
Wengern Alp, 591
Westerplatte, 551
Westgate-on-Sea, 493
West Indian Islands, 710
Weston-super-Mare, 519
Westport, 532
Westward Ho, 517
Weymouth, 511
Whitby, 523
Wiesen, 581
Wildbad Innichen, 595
Winter and summer mountain resorts, 555—589
Winter health resorts, 609—696
Worthing, 503

Y

Yarmouth, Great, 527
Yarmouth (Isle of Wight), 509
Yport, 541

Z

Zandvoort, 549
Zell-am-See, 603
Zermatt, 594
Zinal, 594
Zoppot, 551
Zug, 565

PRINTED BY CASSELL & COMPANY, LIMITED, LA BELLE SAUVAGE, LONDON, E.C.

MANUALS FOR
Students and Practitioners of Medicine

Published by CASSELL & COMPANY.

A Manual of Operative Surgery.

By Sir Frederick Treves, Bart., K.C.V.O., C.B., F.R.C.S., LL.D. Revised by the Author and **Jonathan Hutchinson, Jun., F.R.C.S.**, Surgeon to the London Hospital, Examiner in Surgery Royal Army Medical Department. With 450 Illustrations. In Two Volumes, ***42s.*** Supplied in sets only.

A Manual of Medical Treatment or Clinical Therapeutics.

By I. Burney Yeo, M.D., F.R.C.P. With Illustrations. *New and Revised Edition.* Two Vols. ***21s.*** net.

"It is a book rom which the most skilled therapeutist has something to learn, a book which the more ordinary physician, no matter how frequently he appeals to it, will surely find a true guide, philosopher and friend. One thought at the time that improvement on the first edition would be next to impossible. Success, however, is a wonderful stimulant to an author, hence we have a thoroughly revised, extended, and modernised Edition of the *Manual of Medical Therapeutics* which is likely to remain for some time to come the standard work on the subject in the English language. We feel at liberty to give the book unqualified praise, and almost constrained, not only to recommend it, but also to urge it upon all who do not possess it, yet are ambitiousof becoming polished practical surgeons."—*The Medical Press and Circular.*

Surgical Diseases of the Kidney and Ureter.

By Henry Morris, M.A., M.B. Lond., F.R.C.S. Chairman of the Court of Examiners and recently a Vice-President of the Royal College of Surgeons, Senior Surgeon to the Middlesex Hospital, &c. With 2 Chromo Plates and numerous Engravings. Two Vols. ***42s.*** net.

"The soundest and most authoritative teaching, expressed in the clearest and brightest phrasing. British surgery may justly pride itself on having produced so admirable and worthy a treatise."—*British Medical Journal.*

Tumours, Innocent and Malignant: Their Clinical Characters and Appropriate Treatment.

By J. Bland-Sutton, F.R.C.S., Surgeon to the Chelsea Hospital for Women, etc. With 312 Engravings. *New and Revised Edition.* ***21s.***

"A work which must have entailed on its author the expenditure of infinite labour and patience, and which there can be little question will rank high among works of class."—*The Lancet.*

The Therapeutics of Mineral Springs and Climates.

By I. Burney Yeo, M.D., F.R.C.P. ***12s. 6d.*** net. (In preparation.)

This is a new and revised edition of Dr. Yeo's "Climate and Health Resorts."

Tropical Diseases.

A Manual of the Diseases of Warm Climates. By **Sir Patrick Manson, K.C.M.G., M.D., LL.D. Aberd., F.R.C.P., C.M.G., F.R.S.** With Two Coloured Plates and 130 Illustrations. *New Edition.* ***10s. 6d.*** net.

"It is a good book, conceived and written in a scientific spirit and well up to date and—not to admit in these utilitarian days a practical view of its merits—it strikes us as sound and judicious in regard to the general dietetic and therapeutical treatment of the maladies which it describes. The volume is of a handy size and admirably illustrated."—*The Lancet.*

Diseases of the Skin.

An Outline of the Principles and Practice of Dermatology. By **Malcolm Morris,** Surgeon to the Skin Department, St. Mary's Hospital, London. With Two Coloured Plates, 36 Plain Plates, and Numerous Illustrations. *New Edition.* ***10s. 6d.*** net.

Surgical Applied Anatomy.

By **Sir Frederick Treves, Bart., K.C.V.O., C.B., F.R.C.S., LL.D.,** assisted by **Arthur Keith, M.D., F.R.C.S.** With 80 Illustrations. New and Enlarged Edition. ***9s.***

Oral Sepsis as a Cause of Disease.

By **W. Hunter, M.D., F.R.C.P.** ***3s. 6d.***

Intestinal Obstruction.

Its Varieties, with their Pathology, Diagnosis, and Treatment. By **Sir Frederick Treves, Bart., K.C.V.O., C.B., F.R.C.S., LL.D.** *Illustrated.* ***21s.***

Orthopædic Surgery.

A Text-book of the Pathology and Treatment of Deformities. By **J. Jackson Clarke, M.B. Lond., F.R.C.S.** With 309 Illustrations. ***21s.***

"Based upon a sound knowledge of pathology, Mr. Clarke's descriptions are illustrated by numerous cases drawn from his extensive hospital experience, whilst their value is enhanced by the frequent reference which he makes to the work of others, and by numerous photographs, drawings, and diagrams."—*Medical Chronicle.*

Medical Diseases of Infancy and Childhood.

By **Dawson Williams, M.D. Lond.,** Fellow of the Royal College of Physicians of London, and of University College, London; Consulting Physician to the East London Hospital for Children, Shadwell. With 18 Full-page Plates and numerous Illustrations. ***10s. 6d.***

Diseases of Women.

A Clinical Guide to their Diagnosis and Treatment. By **George Ernest Herman, M.B. Lond., F.R.C.P.,** Senior Obstetric Physician to, and Lecturer on Midwifery at, the London Hospital; Examiner in Midwifery to the University of Cambridge and the Royal College of Physicians, &c. &c. With upwards of 250 Illustrations. New and Revised Edition. Price ***25s.***

Ringworm. In the Light of Recent Research. Pathology—Treatment—Prophylaxis. By **Malcolm Morris**, Surgeon to the Skin Department, St. Mary's Hospital, London. With 22 Microphotographs and a Coloured Plate. ***7s. 6d.***

"Mr. Malcolm Morris has now given the profession a most excellent, concise, and readable account of Ringworm, viewed from the modern standpoint; and we heartily commend his book to the attention of every practitioner."—*Dublin Medical Journal.*

A System of Surgery. Edited by **Sir Frederick Treves, Bart., K.C.V.O., C.B., F.R.C.S., LL.D.** *Seventh Thousand.* Each Vol. contains Two Coloured Plates and Several Hundred Original Woodcut Illustrations by CHARLES BERJEAU, F.L.S., and others. Complete in two volumes, price ***48s.***

A List of Contributors, with Contents, will be forwarded on application.

Diseases of the Joints and Spine. By **Howard Marsh, F.R.C.S.**, Professor of Surgery in the University of Cambridge, &c. *New and Revised Edition.* With 79 Illustrations. ***12s. 6d.***

"This volume is excellently planned. Mr. Marsh brings to bear upon it keen critical acumen."—*Liverpool Medico-Chirurgical Journal.*

Surgical Diseases of the Ovaries and Fallopian Tubes, including Tubal Pregnancy. By **J. Bland-Sutton, F.R.C.S.**, Surgeon to the Chelsea Hospital for Women, Assistant Surgeon to the Middlesex Hospital. With 146 Illustrations. ***21s.***

"We have nothing but praise for the contents of the book."—*Edinburgh Medical Journal.*

Difficult Labour. A Guide to its Management. For Students and Practitioners. By **G. Ernest Herman, M.B. Lond., F.R.C.P.**, Senior Obstetric Physician to the London Hospital, &c. With 165 Illustrations. *New and Revised Edition.* ***12s. 6d.***

"The book is well arranged and profusely illustrated with excellent diagrams. It is a decided acquisition to the literature of midwifery, and we have pleasure in recommending it to all interested in the subject."—*Glasgow Medical Journal.*

On the Origin and Progress of Renal Surgery, with Special Reference to Stone in the Kidney and Ureter; and to the Surgical Treatment of Calculous Anuria. Being the Hunterian Lectures for 1898. Together with a Critical Examination of Subparietal Injuries of the Ureter. By **Henry Morris, M.A., M.B. Lond., F.R.C.S.**, Chairman of the Court of Examiners of the Royal College of Surgeons, &c. &c. With 28 Illustrations. ***6s.***

Surgical Diseases of Children. By **Edmund Owen, M.B., F.R.C.S.,** Consulting Surgeon to the Hospital for Sick Children, Great Ormond Street; Surgeon to St. Mary's Hospital, &c. &c. With 5 Chromo Plates and 120 Engravings. ***21s.***

"Mr. Owen's volume will rank as an invaluable *résumé* of the subject on which it treats."—*Medical Press and Circular.*

Diseases of the Tongue. By **H. T. Butlin, F.R.C.S., D.C.L.,** Consulting Surgeon and Lecturer on Clinical Surgery to St. Bartholomew's Hospital, and **Walter G. Spencer, M.S., M.B. Lond., F.R.C.S.,** Surgeon to Westminster Hospital, &c. With Chromo Plates and Engravings. *New and Revised Edition.* ***21s.***

The Rectum and Anus, Their Diseases and Treatment. By **Sir Charles B. Ball, Hon. M.Ch. Dublin, F.R.C.S.I.,** &c., Surgeon and Clinical Teacher at Sir P. Dun's Hospital, and Regius Professor of Surgery, University of Dublin. With Chromo Plates and 61 Engravings. ***9s.***

"As a full, clear, and trustworthy description of the diseases which it deals with, it is certainly second to none in the language. The author is evidently well read in the literature of the subject, and has nowhere failed to describe what is best up to date. The model of what such a work should be."—*Bristol Medico-Chirurgical Journal.*

Diseases of the Breast. By **Thomas Bryant, F.R.C.S.,** &c., Surgeon to, and Lecturer on Surgery at, Guy's Hospital. With 8 Chromo Plates and numerous Engravings. ***9s.***

"Mr. Bryant is so well known, both as an author and a surgeon, that we are absolved from the necessity of speaking fully or critically of his work."—*The Lancet.*

Syphilis. By **Jonathan Hutchinson, F.R.S., F.R.C.S.,** Consulting Surgeon to the London Hospital and to the Royal London Ophthalmic Hospital. With 8 Chromo Plates. *Seventh Thousand.* ***9s.***

The student, no matter what may be his age, will find in this compact treatise a valuable presentation of a vastly important subject. We know of no better or more comprehensive treatise on syphilis."—*Medical News, Philadelphia.*

Insanity and Allied Neuroses. By **George H. Savage, M.D.,** Lecturer on Mental Diseases at Guy's Hospital, &c. With 19 Illustrations. *Eighth Thousand.* ***9s.***

"Dr. Savage's grouping of insanity is practical and convenient, and the observations on each group are acute, extensive, and well arranged."—*The Lancet.*

Clinical Methods: A Guide to the Practical Study of Medicine. By **Robert Hutchison, M.D., F.R.C.P.,** Assistant Physician to the London Hospital, &c., and **Harry Rainy, M.A., F.R.C.P. Ed., F.R.S.E.,** formerly University Tutor in Clinical Medicine, Royal Infirmary, Edinburgh. With 8 Coloured Plates and upwards of 150 Illustrations. *New and Enlarged Edition.* ***10s. 6d.***

The Tale of a Field Hospital. By

Sir Frederick Treves, Bart., K.C.V.O., C.B., F.R.C.S., LL.D. With 14 Illustrations. Cloth, *5s.*; leather, *6s.*

Cookery for Common Ailments. By

A Fellow of the Royal College of Physicians, and **Phyllis Browne.** Limp cloth. *1s.*

"Cram-full of information, overflowing with helpful detail and invaluable advice."—*Pall Mall Gazette.*

Handbook of Nursing for the Home and for the

Hospital. By **Catherine J. Wood,** Lady Superintendent of the Hospital for Sick Children, Great Ormond Street. *Twenty-first Thousand. 1s. 6d.*; cloth, *2s.*

"A book which every mother of a family ought to have, as well as every nurse under training."—*Guardian.*

The Practical Nursing of Infants and Children.

By **Frank Cole Madden, M.B., B.S. Melb., F.R.C.S.** 288 pp., crown 8vo. *3s. 6d.*

Advice to Women on the Care of their Health, Before, During, and After Confinement.

By **Florence Stacpoole,** Diplomée of the London Obstetrical Society, etc. etc. *New and Enlarged Edition, 2s.*

"Is written very sensibly, and with no affectation of superior knowledge, but simply and directly to meet obvious wants in private home nursing."—*Glasgow Herald.*

Our Sick and How to Take Care of Them;

or, Plain Teaching on Sick Nursing at Home. By **Florence Stacpoole.** *Fourth Edition.* Paper covers, *1s.*; or cloth, *1s. 6d.*

"Well written and very much to the point. The book will be valuable to anyone called upon to perform the responsible and arduous duty of nursing the sick."—*British Medical Journal.*

CASSELL & COMPANY'S COMPLETE CATALOGUE, *containing particulars of upwards of One Thousand Volumes, including Bibles and Religious Works, Illustrated and Fine Art Volumes, Children's Books, Dictionaries, Educational Works, History, Natural History, Household and Domestic Treatises, Science, Travels, &c., together with a Synopsis of their numerous Illustrated Serial Publications, sent post free on application.*

CASSELL & COMPANY, LIMITED, *Ludgate Hill, London: Paris, New York & Melbourne.*

Lightning Source UK Ltd.
Milton Keynes UK
15 May 2010

154178UK00001B/28/P